Handbook of Medical and Healthcare Technologies

Borko Furht · Ankur Agarwal
Editors

Handbook of Medical and Healthcare Technologies

Springer

Editors
Borko Furht
Ankur Agarwal
Department of Computer Science and Engineering
Florida Atlantic University
Boca Raton
FL, USA

ISBN 978-1-4614-8494-3 ISBN 978-1-4614-8495-0 (eBook)
DOI 10.1007/978-1-4614-8495-0
Springer New York Heidelberg Dordrecht London

Library of Congress Control Number: 2013953231

Printed on acid-free paper

Springer is part of Springer Science+Business Media (www.springer.com)

Preface

This Handbook is carefully edited book—contributors are worldwide experts in the field of medical and healthcare technologies. The scope of the book includes leading edge technologies including breakthroughs in tissue engineering, nanotechnology in medicine, innovative medical image techniques, knowledge mining techniques in medicine, cloud computing applications in medicine, personalized medicine, mobile medical and healthcare applications, health informatics, and other innovative technologies.

Medical and Healthcare Technology refers to a wide range of healthcare products that are used to diagnose, monitor, and threat diseases or medical conditions affecting humans. Recent advances in mobile and wireless technologies, medical imaging, nano- and telemedicine, knowledge and data mining, information technology, and other interdisciplinary areas, provided a framework for a significant growth of the field and introduction of innovative products and systems. The Handbook will present the current state-of-the-art in this explosive field, and introduce innovative systems, applications, and techniques developed by experts in the field worldwide.

The Handbook comprises of two parts, which consist of 22 chapters. The first part on *Medical Technologies* includes chapters dealing with medical information retrieval, tissue engineering techniques, 3D medical imaging, nanotechnology innovations in medicine, medical wireless sensor networks, and knowledge mining techniques in medicine. The second part on *Healthcare Technologies* covers topics such as prediction hospital readmission risk, modeling e-health framework, personal Web in healthcare, security issues for medical records, and personalized services in healthcare.

With the dramatic growth of data intensive computing and systems and their applications, this Handbook can be the definitive resource for persons working in this field as researchers, scientists, medical and healthcare, and users. This book is intended for a wide variety of people including academicians, designers, developers, educators, engineers, practitioners, and researchers and graduate students. This book can also be beneficial for business managers, entrepreneurs, and investors. The book can have a great potential to be adopted as a textbook in current and new courses on Medical and Healthcare Technologies.

The main features of this Handbook can be summarized as:

1. The Handbook describes and evaluates the current state-of-the-art in the field of medical and healthcare technologies.
2. It presents current latest achievements in the hot areas of medical technology including medical imaging, advanced personalized diagnostics and therapeutics, personalized medical systems, knowledge mining and bioinformatics techniques, and mobile medical and healthcare systems.
3. Contributors to the Handbook are the leading researchers from academia and practitioners from industry.

We would like to thank the authors for their contributions. Without their expertise and effort this Handbook would never come to fruition. Springer editors and staff also deserve our sincere recognition for their support throughout the project.

Borko Furht
Ankur Agarwal

Contents

Part I
Medical Technologies

Chapter 1
Mobile Medical and Healthcare Applications

Ankur Agarwal, Borko Furht and Mamata Yenagi

The invention of high data connectivity on mobile devices has opened the doors of innovative applications in healthcare and medical technologies. The current generations of smart phones are considered as handheld computers rather than as phones. Smart phones have advantages like continuous uninterrupted data stream, powerful computing power, portability, large memories, wide screens, capability to support multimedia application software compared to other wireless communication technology. This technology is being widely used in health care industry known as m-health. Mobile applications can lower costs and improve the quality of healthcare as well as help in prevention, all of which can improve health outcomes over the long term. This chapter provides a brief overview of various mobile applications in healthcare domain. We will discuss what is mobile health, how can we achieve it. We will discuss different smart phone applications in the market today and how are they affecting the global world. This paper covers applications targeting patients and healthcare providers.

Introduction

Mobile devices and applications have gained more popularity than other newer technologies. Mobile devices have reached more people around the globe than any other systems like road systems, water works, power grids, transportation. 3G and 4G connectivity have a large impact on all aspects of life. Mobile services provide a way for private and public sectors to reach different communities of the society one of which is health.

A. Agarwal (✉) · B. Furht · M. Yenagi
Florida Atlantic University, Boca Raton, Florida, USA
e-mail: ankur@cse.fau.edu

B. Furht
e-mail: bfurht@fau.edu

B. Furht and A. Agarwal (eds.), *Handbook of Medical and Healthcare Technologies*,
DOI: 10.1007/978-1-4614-8495-0_1, © Springer Science+Business Media New York 2013

The medical field is changing dramatically with mobile systems and devices. Mobile technology used in providing healthcare is referred as mobile health or m-health. Different mobile devices are used for m-health apps such as tablets, push to talk devices, cell phones, PDAs, Smart phones. Among these devices Smart phones are gaining more popularity in the usage of m-health apps. m-health apps offer fast and new way of accumulating health information without the use of full fledge work station or computer. With a smart phone or mobile device such as tablet information can be quickly exchanged between patient and health care provider and even connect the patient monitoring device to healthcare provider. Doctors are incorporating them into their practices to be more effective and efficient. Patients are using them to monitor specific aspects of their health, fill in gaps in their medical care, and take more responsibility for their well-being. Therefore m-health is a phenomenon that is here to stay and is expected to rapidly progress in its evolution in the years to come. There is therefore great scope to harness the potential of mobile applications to improve the health care. We will discuss the different mobile devices used for health care applications in the chapter. We will also discuss what are different kinds of mobile applications are there for healthcare.

Methodology

What is m-health

The rapid expansion of mobile information and communication technologies in healthcare sector has created a variety of new opportunities to deliver healthcare services to patients, and healthcare providers. m-health is the way of providing healthcare services through mobile technology platforms on wireless and cellular networks. m-health brings revolutionary change by allowing the medical providers to reach out to their patients and continuously monitor them anytime and anywhere. During the months of September, October and November of 2011 approximately 16.9 million people used mobile phones to access health information. The number of users using smart phones is increasing exponentially. As the number of smart phones increase the opportunities and penetration of m-health is expected to increase.

Why m-health

Mobile phones have several sensors integrated in the system. These sensors are the hardware sensors such as gyroscope, compass, accelerometer, temperature sensor among others and software sensors which allow us to monitor our likes, dislikes location and other socially important attributes through the help of various social networks. Such capability can be exploited to provide meaningful applications for simplifying the daily lives. Further, the average interaction of a human with the mobile device has increased while the interaction with the person computer has reduced at the same time. This trend has opened the opportunities for the developer community to capture the consumer attention with new innovative application. Since phone is a personal device, and is expected to stay with the same person almost all time therefore is it much easier to provide the access to the information or monitoring related services through the same device. Further, the cellphone is integrated with multicore processor, fast memory, high definition camera, WiFi, Bluetooth, NFC (Near Field Communication), high data connective rate among others, and therefore it serves as an integration platform for deploying technology through software and hardware integration. Healthcare on the other hand is always expensive and provides good market opportunities for the business community. Therefore this became a natural opportunity market for business community to provide healthcare services in a cost effective manner. Today there are wode range of m-health applications through which patients can interact with health care providers with features like mobile scheduling, wait time check in offices and emergency rooms, mobile prescription refills. Therefore m-health saves a lot of time for both patients and health care organizations which providing efficiency to the overall system.

m-health Approach

m-health is has evolved in forms of innovative mobile applications in the area of healthcare technologies on a smart device. There are 3 main issues in m-health: Access, Quality and Value. "Access" means accessing data from anywhere and anytime, "Quality" includes providing high level health care by establishing integrated information system and "Value" includes provision for effective and efficient health care delivery. All these issues are solved by the use of present generation mobile devices such as smart phones, tablets, push to talk devices, PDAs. 3G and 4G connectivity provides wide variety of services to all the mobile users such as voice services, interactive video services, quality images, mobile payments, m-commerce, and location based services. With such type of services a wide variety of m-health applications are being developed which will facilitate remote monitoring, assisted living, personal wellness, prevention, diagnostics, m-prescriptions, follow ups and access to patient records (Fig. 1.1).

The m-health industry is at gained an extraordinary momentum with the total revenue rising at a very fast pace. To realize m-health's potential, it needs strong leadership and long term support in terms of strategically policies from government, technology, health and finance sectors of the society. This alliance between these different sectors will provide great inputs to m-health industry such as new technology handsets, finance and market regulations and rules for using bandwidth. It also ensures that output will be as per the requirements of health sector. Recently Food and Drug Administration (FDA) has embraced the m-health technology and issued policies and procedures for accepting m-health applications. Health and well-being/wellness

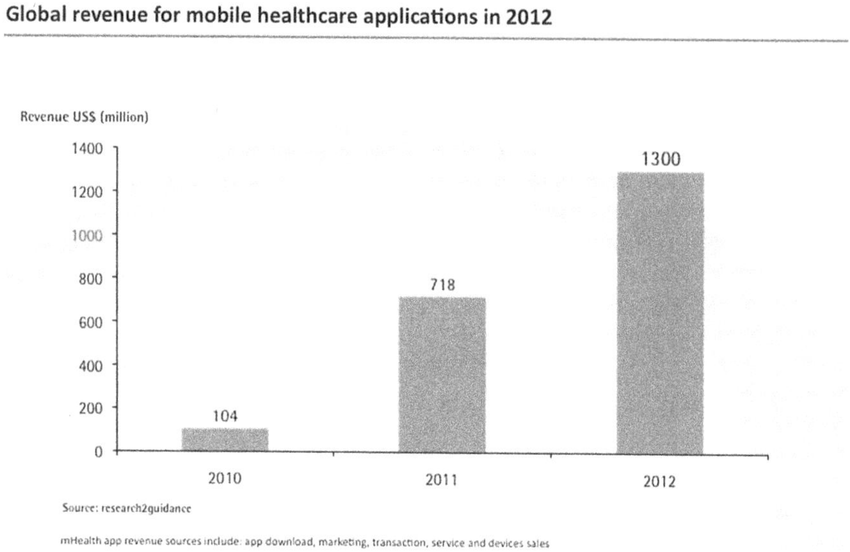

Fig. 1.1 Global Revenue for m-health Applications [Taken from [2]]

applications are estimated to make up about 40 % of smart phone applications being developed currently. This is one of the fasted growing segments in mobile application domain and is set to benefit both, patients and healthcare providers. According to research2guidance [2] m-health app market has seen a sevenfold increase in total revenues in 2011 as compared to year 2010. research2guidance [2] has also made the prediction that m-health app will reach US $ 1.3 billion in the year 2012. It also makes clear that the growth is exponential in mobile health industry. The total growth of USD 1.3Billion is very small compared to $7 trillion global health industry. This clearly demonstrates the future opportunities and potential growth for m-health.

Role of Smart Devices in Healthcare

The current generation of smart mobile device includes the smartphone, tablets, push-to-talk devices. Smartphones specifically are taking the prominent place to reach the internet. Two or Three among five persons who own mobile phone has a Smartphone. According to forecast made by Frost and Sullivan [1], the Smartphone penetration in North America is to surge from 23.9 % from 2009 to 67.1 % by the year 2015. Doctors are said to be the highest adopters. The graphical representation of the forecast is shown below in Fig. 1.2.

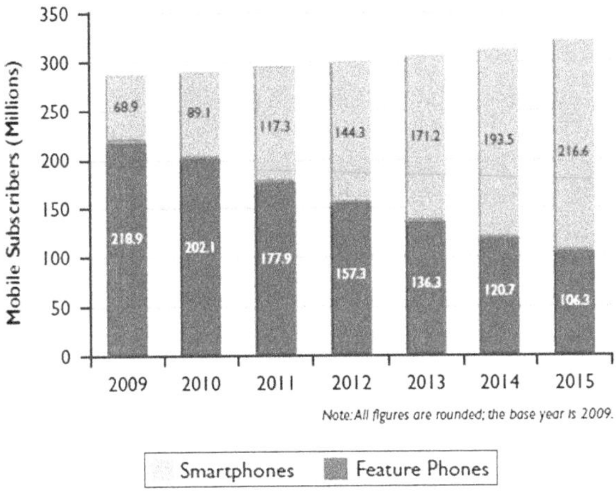

Fig. 1.2 Smartphone Market: Mobile Device Connections Forecast (2009 to 2015) [Source : [1]]

Smart mobile technology has emerged as significant communication technology in the current society. Such a rapid progress in mobile technology has transformed many aspects of our life. One of these aspects is health care. Some of the platforms available today are Apple ios, Android, Rim blackberry, Symbian and Windows. The potential for the creation of simple and easy to download apps for smart phones has created a new trend in health care. GPS and location enabled smart phones offer advanced applications like assisting independent living of persons with disabilities and long tern chronic diseases. According to research2guidance [2], a long awaited revolution in mobile healthcare is set to happen. Both healthcare provider and consumer are embracing smartphones as a way to improving healthcare. research2guidance [2] says Smartphone applications become killer applications for mobile health solutions. Out of 1.4 billion Smartphone users, Smartphone applications will help healthcare to successfully reach 500 million people by 2015.

Healthcare Mobile Applications

It is clear that the potential for mobile communication has tremendously increased newer and advanced technology in all the aspects of life and health care is one of them. These mobile applications provide easy and cost effective healthcare anywhere anytime. According to research2guidance [2] currently there are 17,000 m-health application in major app stores. Approximately 74 % of these applications are adhering to paid business model. The basic features of these applications include ability to record vital signs, track health progress, access health notes and send secured info to healthcare provider among other features. Some of these mobile applications [3–10] are categorized in this section:

Chronic Disease Management Applications

For patients who are suffering from chronic health conditions such as diabetes, asthma, or heart disease among others, good health management requires making adequate decisions on daily basis. Smart phone applications assist this process by where and when decisions are made. Such monitoring helps to prevent situations when a more expensive and time consuming treatment is required such as hospitalization. For example if blood glucose of a diabetic patient falres up, application will inform the patient about its status without the hospital visit. Below is the list of areas in which mobile applications have been developed and deployed:

a) Glucose monitoring
b) Reminders for testing breathing for Asthma patients
c) Symptom Checkers
d) Heart rate monitoring
e) Food consumption logging tool

Remote Monitoring Applications

To promote safety and injury preventions these applications play an important role. These applications assist mainly elderly and disabled patients. Fall detection and location tracking technologies monitor patients in terms of location, balance and gait. There is an tremendous incrase in remote monitoring devices and apps. Below is the category for such applications:

a) Remote heart monitoring
b) ECG viewer
c) Lifescan for patients with diabetes
d) Oxygen level remote check
e) Telemedicine

Diagnostic Tool Applications

These are the applications which require integration with diagnostic tools. Such applications allow the patients to connect the one or more monitoring devices for making the measurements and further get the results instantaneously. Further the applications upload the results to the healthcare providers. These applications in general diagnostic category mainly are developed in the following domains:

a) Digital imaging
b) MRI/X-Ray viewing apps
c) Electronic chart review
d) Lab results review

Personal Wellness and Healthy Living

These are the applications which provide health news and information along with other functionalities. Applications for wellness can be categorized into several groups like fitness, nutrition, diet and overall quality of life. The category applications are classified into following sub-domain:

a) Pregnancy and baby development
b) Healthy eating
c) Diet assistance
d) Exercise and fitness

Access to Health Information Applications

These applications include Personal Health Record (PHR) technologies. Such applications allow patients to track their health care services, view their health records and manage their health. This category includes:

a) Capzule PHR
b) Cloud PHR
c) Family and health PHR

Medication Adherence Applications

These applications provide proper education to both health care providers and patients. Further such applications are used for scheduling and reminder of events, such as reminder for taking the pills. Other applications such as prescription refill requests and patient educational resources would also fall under this category. This category includes

a) Virtual pill box apps
b) Medication reminder apps
c) Dosecast apps
d) Family medication apps

Miscellaneous Applications

These applications include appointment scheduling and reminders, remote dictation, surgery scheduling, interoffice communication. Such applications help both patient and health care organization to work effectively by managing time.

Overview of Mobile Applications

DrawMD

Visible Health's DrawMD is a free iPad app that lets physicians show patients exactly what a surgical or other procedure will entail. Conceived by surgical oncologists, it provides interactive diagrams in nine specialties, giving doctors visual tools to help explain complex medical and surgical procedures. Users can select a pre-populated anatomical image or upload their own. They can sketch, stamp, and type directly on the image. The images and notes can be shared with patients during consultations and emailed to them. Figure 1.3 illustrates a screen from DrawMD showing the coronal view of nose.

DrawMD diagrams are not just for doctors to show patients what is going on with their bodies. Patients can also use the diagrams to get their doctors to answer their questions and illustrate where stents have been placed, for example, or where other procedures were done. DrawMD's specialties include anesthesiology, critical

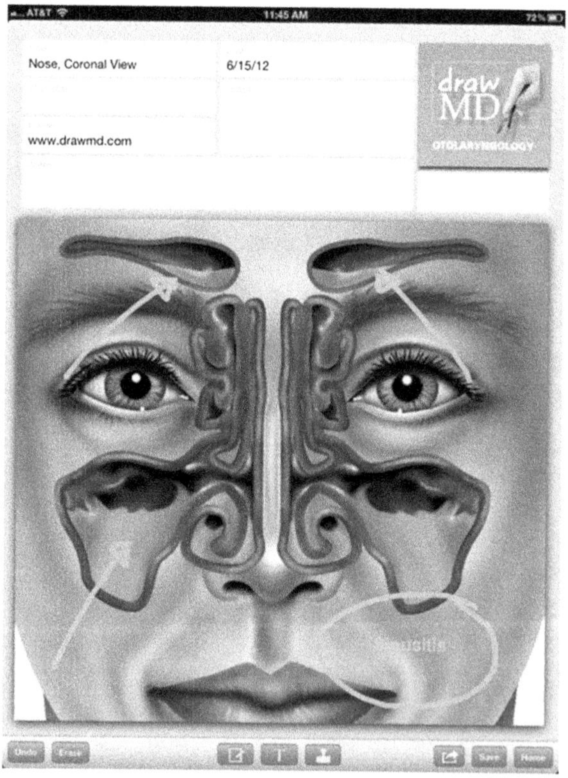

Fig. 1.3 DrawMD screen—Coronal view of nose

care, cardiology, otolaryngology, female pelvic surgery, general and vascular surgery, ob/gyn, orthopedics, and urology.

Visible Body

Visible Body's 3D Human Anatomy Atlas gives medical students, doctors, and patients an up-close look at all the systems of the human body. Available for Apple iPad, iPhone, and Google Android, the app provides detailed, anatomically accurate 3-D models of more than 2,500 individual structures and hundreds of definitions body systems, organs, vasculature, and nerves. A panel of physicians and anatomists reviews the anatomical content in the atlas for accuracy, says Visible Body. The current release includes content covered in undergraduate-level anatomy and physiology courses, according to the company. Figure 1.4 illustrates an example screen from Visible Body.

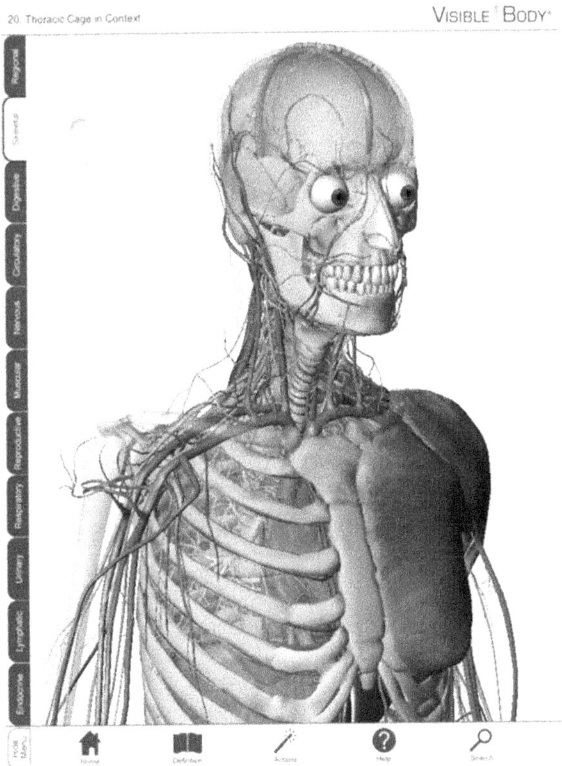

Fig. 1.4 Human Anatomy Atlas is included in the app Visible Body

VaxNation

Students at Baylor College of Medicine, Rice University, and the University of Texas School of Public Health have developed VaxNation, an online vaccination tracker. The patent enters information such as birth date, vaccinations that he/she had, and the dates of those immunizations, and VaxNation provides age-appropriate recommendations based on the Centers for Disease Control and Prevention's guidelines.

Families can set up joint accounts, and accounts can be linked to Facebook and Twitter so that information about immunizations can be shared. The app helps locate clinics, provides email reminders when immunizations are needed, and offers educational information. VaxNation won first prize in the Institute of Medicine and the National Academy of Engineering's Go Viral to Improve Health collegiate challenge. Figure 1.5 illustrates a screen shot from VaxNation showing vaccine chart.

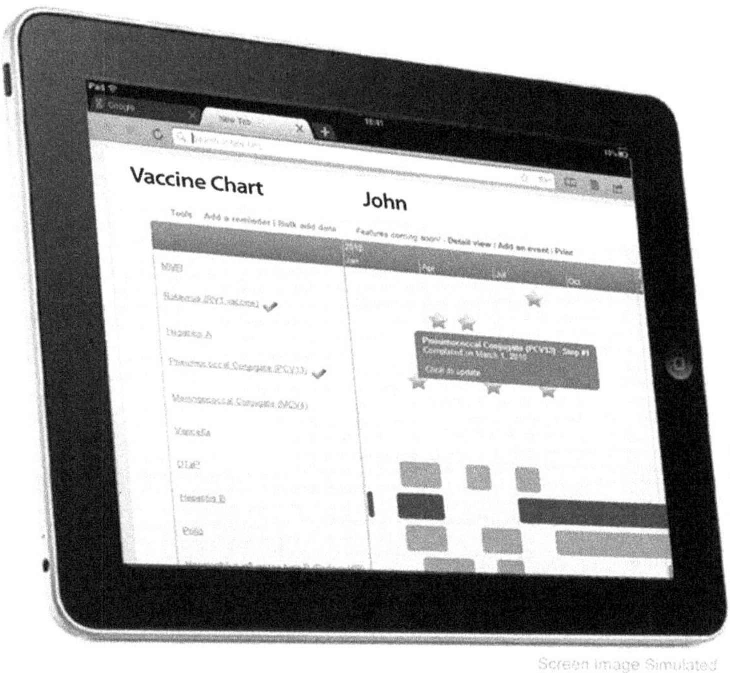

Fig. 1.5 VaxNation example: Vaccine Chart for a patient John

EZ Derm EHR

EZ Derm's iPad-based electronic health record system lets dermatologists do what they need to do just by talking. Specifically designed for dermatology, the app incorporates Nuance Communications' cloud-based medical speech recognition technology so clinicians can dictate notes and other clinical information into the system and navigate within the app. EZ Derm also provides physicians with anatomically accurate 3-D body maps on which they can make notes using touch technology. And it has integrated clinical decision-support that includes diagnosis information, workup algorithms, and suggested treatments. Doctors can use the app's telephony, videoconferencing, and texting capabilities to communicate with colleagues, staff, and patients. Figure 1.6 shows a screen from EZ Derm EHR application.

Mayo Clinic Patient Application

The Mayo Clinic Patient App provides patients with a range of tools to help them navigate the healthcare provider's medical campuses and processes. This free iPhone and iPad app provides patients with secure access to their medical records, appointment schedules, and lab results. It provides maps of the medical facilities and directions to patients' appointment venues and other facilities. The app also lets patients stay in touch with Mayo staff to make appointments and provides health management tips from Mayo's online resources, as well as a list of clinical trials that patients might be interested in (Fig. 1.7).

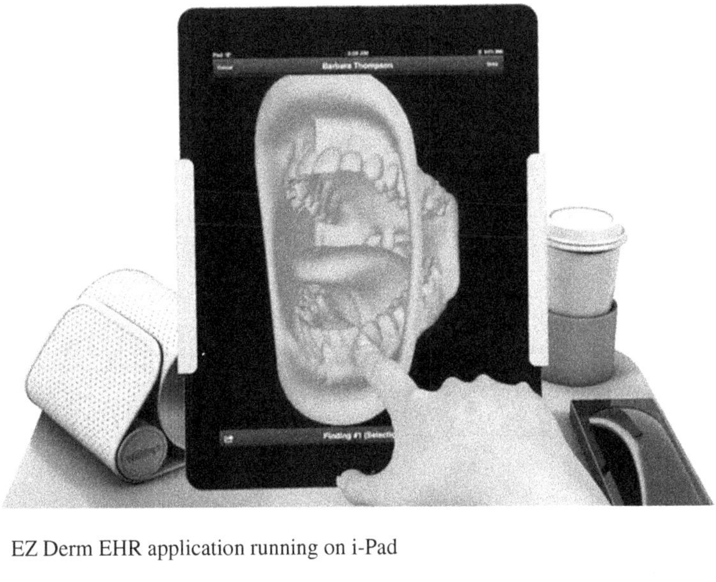

Fig. 1.6 EZ Derm EHR application running on i-Pad

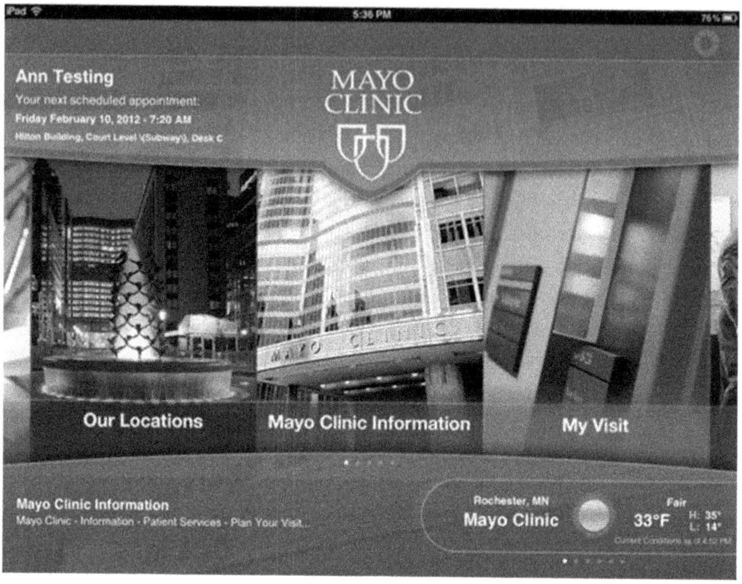

Fig. 1.7 Mayo Clinic Patient Application

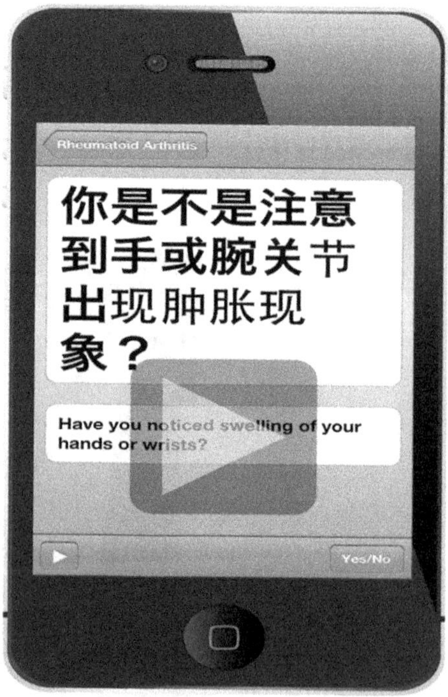

Fig. 1.8 MedSpeak application provides the doctor's communication with Chinese patients

MedSpeak

For physicians who need to communicate with Mandarin- or Cantonese-speaking patients, QxMD Software's MedSpeak Mandarin and Cantonese Translators could be lifesavers. The apps provides more than 3,300 medical phrases, with English text and Mandarin or Cantonese translations in both written and audio formats. Nursing, rehabilitation, pharmacy, and medical topics are covered, and content can be sorted by category, topic, and symptom. Figure 1.8 shows an example screen.

Conclusion

Healthcare applications on mobile platforms have tremendoud potential to impove the healthcare needs in a cost effective manner. The diversity and quality of medical apps shows the iPad and other mobile systems have become more than just tablets for consuming everyday content. Rather, it shows the iPad now possesses the ability to improve the physician workflow, and as we demonstrated in our videos, offers the ability to improve the patient physician relationship.

References

1. Frost and Sullivan, white paper, "Mobile Devices and Healthcare: What's New, What Fits and How to Decide", 2012.
2. Research2guidance, "Global Health Market Report 2010–2015", 2010.
3. Colin Konschak and Ram Devaloor, whiet paper " Mobile Applications in Health Care", 2011.
4. Darrel West, "How Mobile Devices are changing the Health Care", in Issues in Technology innovation, May 2012.
5. Center for technology and aging, draft postion paper, "mhealth technologies: applications to benefit older adults", March 2011.
6. Raj Gururajan, San Murugesan and Jeffrey Soar, "Bringing Mobile Technologies in Support of Healthcare", Cutter IT Journal Article, August 2005.
7. Jane Sarasohn - Kahn, "How Smart Phones are Changing Healthcare for Consumers and Providers", April 2010.
8. RedaChouffani, "The Different Types of Mobile Healthcare Apps", January 2011.
9. Maged N Kamel Boulos, Steve Wheeler, Carlos Tavares and Ray Jones," How Smart Phones are Changing the Face of Mobile and Participatory Healthcare: an Overview with an example from eCAALYX", April 2011.
10. Doctors and Patients go Mobile, Information Week, Health Care, February/March 2013.

Chapter 2
Medical Information Retrieval Enhanced with User's Query Expanded with Tag-Neighbors

Frederico Durao, Karunakar Bayyapu, Guandong Xu, Peter Dolog and Ricardo Lage

Abstract Under-specified queries often lead to undesirable search results that do not contain the information needed. This problem gets worse when it comes to medical information, a natural human demand everywhere. Existing search engines on the Web often are unable to handle medical search well because they do not consider its special requirements. Often a medical information searcher is uncertain about his exact questions and unfamiliar with medical terminology. To overcome the limitations of under-specified queries, we utilize tags to enhance information retrieval capabilities by expanding users' original queries with context-relevant information. We compute a set of significant tag neighbor candidates based on the neighbor frequency and weight, and utilize the qualified tag neighbors to expand an entry query. The proposed approach is evaluated by using MedWorm medical article collection and results show considerable precision improvements over state-of-the-art approaches.

F. Durao (✉) · P. Dolog · R. Lage
IWIS- Intelligent Web and Information Systems, Aalborg University, Computer Science Department, Room 2.2.05, Selma Lagerlöfs Vej 300, DK-9220 Aalborg-East, Denmark
e-mail: fred@cs.aau.dk

P. Dolog
e-mail: dolog@cs.aau.dk

R. Lage e-mail: ricardol@cs.aau.dk · K. Bayyapu
CBS - Center for Biological Sequence Analysis, Technical University of Denmark, Department of Systems Biology, Building 208, Room 020, DK-2800 Kongens Lyngby, Denmark
e-mail: karun@cbs.dtu.dk

G. Xu
Center for Applied Informatics, Victoria University, PO Box 14428, MelbourneVIC 8001, Australia
e-mail: guandong.xu@vu.edu.au

B. Furht and A. Agarwal (eds.), *Handbook of Medical and Healthcare Technologies*,
DOI: 10.1007/978-1-4614-8495-0_2,

Introduction

Inadequate domain knowledge in the medical field can be considered on of the reasons why users under-specified queries often lead to undesired search results in the context of medical information retrieval. Either the results do not contain the information they seek or there is no existence of semantically related resources in the repository. For instance, web search over recent outbreaks of highly pathogenic avian *influenza* virus with the query *influenza* would return a list of documents containing the query term that do not necessarily address the needed information about the specific avian virus. In this scenario, at least three issues affecting the quality of the web-based search result are evident. One, a query with single term based information retrieval may not yield a satisfactory performance [18]. Second, in the document repository of the search engine, there might exist hundreds of thousands articles matching the requested query. With such an amount of information, it is impossible to locate the desired information by simply browsing through all contents [8] of returned results. The third reason is related to domain knowledge requirements. Because conventional search engines focus on generic information search, domain specific results are usually not taken into consideration. Thus, a simple word-based search does not produce relevant search results in specific domains such as the medical field [20]. As a consequence of such issues relating to query-based searches, only 25–50 % of the relevant articles on a given topic are retrieved in searches performed in specific domains [18]. In other words, sparse and incomplete query terms may result in information overload, thereby increasing the noise presented in search results. Hence, the importance of enriching a query increases in such scenarios.

To face and attenuate the drawbacks of under-specified queries, we utilize tag neighbors to enhance information retrieval capabilities by expanding the user's original query. Tags are free-style terms used for annotations indicating the user's own perceptions or conceptual judgments about the tagged resources. We focus on tags that are assigned to medical document collection in web repositories such as PubMed [36] and MedWorm [31]. We believe that by expanding the user's query with tags assigned to this web resources, we can attenuate the problem of user-specified queries and improve the retrieval of relevant results. The purpose of query expansion is therefore to make up for the gap between the user query and its result containing the desired and relevant documents. In a nutshell, we compute a set of significant tag neighbor candidates based on the tag neighbor frequency and weight, and utilize the most frequent and weighted tag neighbors to expand an entry query that has terms matching the tags. For instance, the query *influenza* will automatically map with the higher frequency tag neighbor term *contagious* by our method when looking for query *influenza* on a domain-specific web search engine. Thus, the search will be refined by retrieving documents with the words *influenza* and *contagious* in their contents. Furthermore, related terms are also searchable. Take the previous query, for example. Documents indexed with medical terms that include the word *influenza* (e.g., influenza contagious viral) will also be returned depending on the neighbor frequency and weight.

We implemented our method as a web-based search system with contents extracted and indexed from the medical article repository MedWorm that is available to the public on the Web. We carry out experiments with MeSH (Medical Subject Headings) [33] vocabulary search queries to evaluate the performance of our method in the developed system. The experimental results show that retrieval effectiveness can be improved with the Mean Average Precision (MAP) by +39 % over and above the traditional information retrieval method.

[1] The main contributions of this paper are summarized as follows:

- An algorithm for tag neighborhood generation, that searches for the neighboring words of all tags occurring in the document corpus and computes the neighbor's frequency and weight;
- Tag neighborhood selection for the expansion of a given query based on the neighbor frequency and weight. The expanded query seeks to obtain documents that not only refer to the given query but also to related concepts based on their neighbors;
- A comparative experimental evaluation that assesses the quality of search results over a baseline and state-of-the-art approaches;
- A specialized analysis of which medical categories this approach is most recommended to be applied.

The rest of the paper is structured as follows. Section "Motivation Scenario" shows the motivation scenario. Section "Related Work" reviews the related research undertaken in this area. Section "Tag Neighbor-based Query Expansion" presents our approach of expanding query for document search with tag neighbors. Section "Experimental Evaluation" describes the experimental setup, evaluation methodology, metrics and results. Section "Discussion" discusses the results of the query expansions carried out into the evaluation. Section "Limitations and Points of Improvements" outlines the limitations of the work and points of improvements. Section "Conclusion and Future Work" concludes the paper and outlines future works.

Motivation Scenario

The primary goal of expanding a user's query is to provide the user with results that match his real intention when formulating a query. In the context of this work, our application is aimed at helping the layman users in querying a medical database. Due to the lack of expertise or knowledge of specialized vocabulary, one might be confronted with such vocabulary when searching for articles that address scientific medical terms.

---

[1] This journal version was previously published at the *International Conference on Information Science and Applications (ICISA 2011)* [12] and the main differences from previous work to this are: (i) enhancement of related work by including new comparative studies and (ii) extension of evaluation by comparing our results against state-of-the-art approaches.

In order to motivate our approach, we show a scenario where a user is searching for articles addressing the topic diabetes. Intuitively, he puts in the query "diabetes" and receives as result hundreds of articles containing the term "diabetes" in the text content. If the search results do not look promising, the user will reformulate the query, either by putting in a completely different one or expanding the current query with new terms. Our approach will step in exactly at that point by anticipating this step of query reformulation.

Assuming the user has decided to look into the retrieved articles, if he browses the first 10 documents, the user will likely notice that his query *diabetes* is usually followed by other related terms such as *insulin*, *glucose*, *blood*, *pancreas*, etc. Due to this connection between the terms, we believe that they are strong candidates for composing the user's new query in case of reformulation. Motivated by this premise, we utilize related terms to expand the user's query in order to better meet user's need. The question is: how do we know which terms will be included in the user's query? In fact, we do not know this in advance but we can rely on the tags assigned to the medical articles. In brief, tags are keywords assigned to documents (or video, audio, etc.) with the usual purpose of conceptualization [34, 40]. Tags are then valuable pieces of information to describe or categorize the topic addressed in the article. We believe that tags are propitious to the user's query, thereby allowing us to calculate the expanded terms.

In this sense, we consider all tags and generate a list of related terms for each tag, i.e., what we call *tag neighbors*. This list is pre-computed and allows us to quickly expand the user's query once a user issues a query that matches an existing tag(s) in the system. As a result, the search engine retrieves those articles containing the user entry query with the expanded terms. Back to the example, if the user issues the query *diabetes* to the search engine, such a query will be expanded with the qualified tags such as *insulin*, *hormone*, *glucose*, *blood*, *pancreas*. The search results will contain documents that address diabetes but also articles of related terms. On the one hand, the results will be closer to the user's expectations while on the other hand they will be enriched by articles addressing related information. In summary, this study tries to combine the utility of tags with a technique for query expansion, aimed at helping users with improved quality search results.

Related Work

Keyword-based search is a widely used approach in information retrieval for retrieving needed information from the content database. However, ordinary users often lack sufficient domain knowledge to properly choose query keywords, which greatly affects the information retrieval performance. In addition, search queries are usually short in length [22] and ambiguous in meaning expression [37]. Due to these difficulties, it is widely recognized that query formulation is a challenging obstacle in improving search quality. Query expansion is considered as an effective strategy in enhancing keyword based queries [25] that are widely used in search engines and database systems. A commonly used query expansion method is to add related queries from a set of candidate queries which are explicitly or implicitly related to the semantics of input query from the co-occurrence of queries of previous users. Query expansion has been studied for many years from the perspectives of keyword or knowledge based approaches. The research efforts on related query suggestion could be categorized into the three types of strategies according to the feature space source used by them: (1) Keyword based suggestion is a simplest approach, which intuitively considers the candidate queries having common words with a current input query to be related. However, the very small word overlap between short Web queries makes it hard to accurately determinate the similar terms. One reason is probably that a term may be meant for different meanings by different users (i.e. polysemy), e.g., apple is related to fruit or computer. The other reason is that different terms may have a similar meaning (i.e. synonymy), e.g., car and automobile. (2) Pseudo relevance based approach does not involve the user feedback, instead assumes the retrieved results by search engines are relevant. It induces the similarity between the two queries by enriching query expressions with additional features (e.g., terms and URLs) from the top results returned by search engines [46]. The pseudo relevance reflects the viewpoints of general search engines, but contains no evidence of individual users' judgments. (3) Implicit relevance based suggestion captures the relatedness of queries from the clicked search results of Web logs, i.e., user navigational behaviors [29, 32]. It demonstrates advantages over the pseudo relevance because the click choices made by a large number of users do suggest a certain level of relevance from the viewing point of actual users. Among these studies, all efforts are focused on measuring the relatedness of queries from explicit or implicit semantics, but engage a large volume of external resources [2] such as keyword indexing, ontologies, search engines or web log files, therefore resulting in additional overheads. Different from these, in this paper, we aim to utilize user tagging information, which is equivalent to a semantic representation of perception or judgment by users on resources, to especially address the document retrieval in medical domain via neighboring tag expansion approach. Below we first review the existing works related to our approach from two-folds.

Query Expansion in the Medical Domain

Query expansion requires a term selection stage where the system presents the query expansion terms to the users in a reasonable order [13]. The order should preferably be one in which the terms that are most likely to be useful are close to the top of the list. In addition, heuristic decisions can also be applied during this stage, for example, poor terms are excluded from the term list instead of being given low weights. [6] proposed an information-theoretic approach to automatic query expansion, which is based on Information Theory, assigning scores to various candidate expansion terms. These scores are used to select and weight expansion terms within Rocchio's framework for query re-weighting. This approach was compared with other query expansion techniques via empirical studies. They claimed that their approach was able to achieve a better retrieval effectiveness on several performance measures. Similar to our model, [6] weight candidate terms for query expansion with the goal of achieving better retrieval effectiveness. On the other hand they do not explore tags as means of providing additional semantics to the query expansion.

[27] investigated the effectiveness of using MeSH in PubMed through its automatic query expansion process: Automatic Term Mapping (ATM) and concluded that the retrieval performance was improved but the improvement may not affect end PubMed users in realistic situations. Although our approach has applied a different technique, our evaluation shows that we also achieved improvements on the performance with the query expansion. Likewise [27], we outline some drawbacks of our approach. Specifically, we identify which medical categories our information retrieval does not perform properly and achieve low precision rates.

[3] explored two strategies for query expansion utilizing medical subject headings (MeSH) ontology to improve the effectiveness of medical image retrieval systems. In order to achieve greater effectiveness in the expansion, the search text was analyzed to identify which terms were most amenable to being expanded. To perform the expansions, the authors utilized the hierarchical structure by which the MeSH descriptors are organized. Two strategies for selecting the terms to be expanded in each query were studied. The first consisted of identifying the medical concepts using the unified medical language system meta thesaurus. In the second strategy the text of the query was divided into n-grams, resulting in sequences corresponding to MeSH descriptors. In our work, the textual content was the target item to be retrieve rather than image. In addition to that, we did not utilize any ontology for finding out relations between documents. In our approach, free will tags were utilized to infer correlation between related documents and then improve precision of medical information retrieval.

A knowledge-based query expansion method [26] exploits UMLS (Unified Medical Language System), a large thesaurus in the biomedical domain constructed by Library National of Medicine knowledge source. The goal is to append the original query with additional terms that are specifically relevant to the query's scenario. The exploration of UMLS knowledge is done by mapping a large text of collection ImageCLEFMed(CLEF-Cross Language Evaluation Forum) to UMLS concepts, and expanding queries and documents automatically based on semantic relations in the UMLS hierarchy [9]. The exploitation of semantic relations from a knowledge base is what most differ their work from ours. In our work we do not maintain any knowledge base such as a domain ontology to perform the query expansion. Instead, we harvest the implicit semantic relations inherit within the nearest candidate terms (see details in Sect. "Tag Neighbor-based Query Expansion".

[8] presented a method to expand queries with a medical ontology in order to improve an IR system. The aim is to improve a multi modal retrieval system by expanding the user's query with MeSH descriptors. They have combined two independent subsystems to retrieve textual and visual information. The evaluation of this system is carried out using the collection queries, and relevance judgments are provided by the ImageCLEF medical task organization. Moreover, they compared the

use of a traditional Information Retrieval (IR) system, an IR system with medical knowledge, a Content-Based Information Retrieval(CBIR) system and a mixed system with information from these systems. Finally, the results showed that the use of medical ontology to expand the queries greatly improves the system. Similar to [26], [8] also relies on an ontology to perform the query expansion. Unlike our approach they benefit from a second resource, which is the visual information. This information enriches the semantics of the search queries with taxonomic concepts.

Concept-based query expansion for retrieving gene related publications from MEDLINE was investigated by [30]. The approach is based on exploiting the direct links between genes and other biological concepts obtained from public biological databases. These networks of associations are implemented through direct relations in the integration database. Images are also more important and varied in the medical domain, as they become available in a digital form. Despite the fact that images are language-independent, they are often accompanied by textual features such as associated captions, titles and articles that strongly improve the retrieval quality. Link relations are not considered in our approach. However we see a potential study of tagging activity between documents. This analysis could bias the weighing of the search score.

In [27] authors used approximately the same data source for query expansion on different knowledge domains. However, to the best of our knowledge, this is the first attempt to use *tags* for query expansion to enhance information retrieval performance in the medical domain.

Tagging and Folksonomy

A *tag* is a one-unit word or label that describes a piece of information. In social tagging, in contrast to taxonomies developed by subject specialists using authorized terms determined by professionals, people use their own keywords to describe websites for future discovery and retrieval [5]. The resulting list of tags of information and objects is often termed a "folksonomy", a classification done by untrained individuals, i.e folks [44]. The term "folksonomy" is a combination of folk and taxonomy to describe the social classification phenomenon. Folksonomy provides user-created metadata rather than the professional created an author created metadata [24]. The tags are the core of folksonomy that can be seen as good keywords for describing the respective web pages from various aspects of domain ontology [15].

Tags in Medical bookmarking systems are usually assigned to organize and share resources on the Web. By tagging, users label resources freely and subjectively, based on their sense of values [34]. [10] method showed that an effective tagger for medical terms related to diseases, injuries, drugs, medical devices, and medical procedures can be built using words from a robust medical term list along with a probabilistic term classifier that uses local context to disambiguate terms being used in a medical sense from terms being used in a non-medical sense. [21] proposed a semantic tagger that provides high level concept information for phrases in clinical documents, which enriches the medical information tracking system that supports decision making or quality assurance of medical treatment. Tagging systems in the medical field have focused on the lexical level of syntactic and semantic tagging. [38] and [39] performed semantic tagging on terms lexically using the Unified Medical Language System (UMLS). [41] explores the use of "purpose tagging" to better capture the intent of the user when using tags to improve search results. The authors evaluate their work in a case study but do not provide a quantitative analysis of improvements in the search results. Also, their prototype, although designed to ease the task, expects the users to explicitly attribute purpose tags to the tagged resources. The disadvantage of this approach is to make the tagging activity a little more complex, reducing the simplicity of straightforward labeling. [14] highlights the importance tags as semantic representations and interpretations of information in search engines and social information systems. This work in particular converges to our objective of exploring the representativeness of tags to find information. Aligned with this work, [28] presents MedSearch, a search engine specialized in retrieving medical documents to people in general. The goal of the search engine, similar to our approach, is to address the challenges of providing the user with meaningful medical search results given under specified queries. The authors specifically address the problem of queries with longer sentences that describe their intent (e.g., description of symptoms) without the proper use of the related and shorter technical terms. The new features they add to the search engine include the ability to write longer sentences in plain English. It also rewrites longer sentences into smaller versions with more appropriated terms. Finally, it diversifies the search results with pages from various medical aspects of the searched medical conditions and presents the user with alternative queries. To evaluate both the relevance and diversity of the search results, the authors propose a single metric, usefulness. According to them, a search result is considered useful if it is relevant to the query and if most of its relevant content does not appear in other search results ranked higher in the list. They compare their approach with Google Health and Healthline, showing better results on their approach. In the case of our approach, the comparison was not possible because the metric used was different. Moreover, our work is focused on the use of tags to capture user interest and improve personalized search results in the medical domain and not on proposing new features to a search engine.

Tag Neighbor-based Query Expansion

In this section, we discuss the query expansion approach. First, we provide an overview of the query search system and then explain the generation of tag neighbors and the query expansion procedure. In order to test our approach, we develop a keyword-based search system which supports search by user-entry queries. The framework of the proposed approach is depicted in Fig. 2.1. Steps (1) and (2) are a preprocessing phase concerned with data extraction, database storage and neighborhood

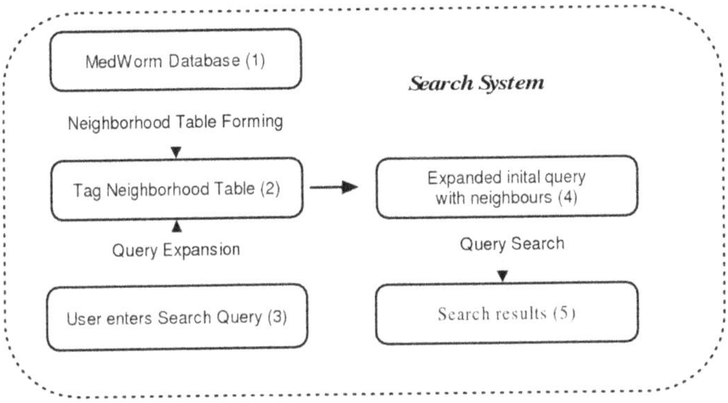

Fig. 2.1 The framework of expanded query search system with tag neighbor expansion

forming. In Step (3), the user query is entered, and then expanded in Step (4). The last one, Step (5), presents the results to the user..

Generating Tag Neighbors

The basic idea proposed in this paper is to expand the user query with related tag neighbors in order to retrieve more closely related documents. Thus, we utilize the (term) neighbors, appearing before or after the query terms that match one or more tags assigned to the document concerned. The neighbors are selected terms extracted and analyzed from the document's textual content. The rationale behind this approach is the observation that such kinds of tags, i.e., the tag neighbors, appear in specific blocks or in pairs within the content of a document. In the context of medical documents, this phenomenon is sometimes predominantly observed. For instance, the words "pandemic, H1N1, influenza, contagious, viral?" are often used concurrently.

To realize the task of expanding the initial query terms provided by a user during a search, we first define and retrieve tag neighbors from the document corpus. This is a pre-processing algorithm as described below.

1. Let T be the set of all tags assigned to the whole corpus. For each tag $t \in T$, we search for documents using t as an entry query.
2. For each retrieved document, we fetch the n terms before and after each occurrence of the tag t in the document. There are two main intuitions that justify why we did not utilize all terms but n before and after t: (i) terms relatively distant (e.g., $n \geq 6$) from t are usually semantically unrelated to t because they appear in other sentences of the text thus possibly discussing other aspects/subjects. The terms tend to receive extremely low values and thus becoming strong candidate of being outliers, (ii) The limitation of n terms also increases the efficiency for computing the tag neighbors since a subset of whole terms will be considered.

3. To assure minimal quality of the neighbor candidates, we analyze the fetched terms, remove possible invalid characters using the constraint those present in the list of stop words. The qualified terms are now represented by C, i.e. the set of candidate neighbors for the tag $t \in T$.
4. For each term $c \in C$, we calculate its weight based on its distance from the tag $t \in T$. We assume 1 unit the distance from t to the immediate term c after or before it. The distance to the second term is 2 units and so forth until the $|n|th$ unit. We assume that the further away the term c is from tag t, the less relevant it is. The function $w(t, c)$ that weighs the distance between a tag $t \in T$ and a candidate neighbor c is defined as:

$$w(t, c) = \sum_{i=1}^{|c|} \frac{1}{d(t, c_i)}, \forall c \in C \tag{2.1}$$

   where $d(t, c_i)$ is the distance between the occurrence i of candidate neighbor c and the tag $t \in T$, and $|c|$ is the total number of occurrences of candidate neighbor c near tag t.
5. For each candidate neighbor $c \in C$, we calculate the neighborhood frequency for its respective tag $t \in T$. i.e.

$$f(c) = \frac{|c|}{|C|} \tag{2.2}$$

   where $|C|$ is the total number of candidate neighbors for the particular tag t.
6. The neighborhood frequency function $nf(t, c)$, that takes into account the weights and frequency is defined as follows:

$$nf(t, c) = w(t, c).f(c) \tag{2.3}$$

The calculus of the tag neighbors runs on the dataset as a data pre-processing procedure. After computing the most frequent and highest weight tag neighbors, we select those whose final scores are above a threshold α to ensure minimal quality during the expansion. The threshold α is defined by at least nf(t,c) within the highest standard deviation from the best ranked neighbor. This avoids the need for defining an absolute number of neighbors to be retrieved, and guarantees that low frequent neighbors are selected. The set of tag neighbors will finally be saved in a (hash) tag neighborhood table. In this table, each tag points to its respective set of neighbors.

Working Example on Generating Tag Neighbors

In Sect. "Generating Tag Neighbors", we described the method for computing tag neighbor frequency and weight. Based on this, we select neighbors with the higher frequency and weight for the original query. Based on this, we select which neighbors have higher frequency and weight for the original query. Formally, let t be the tag and

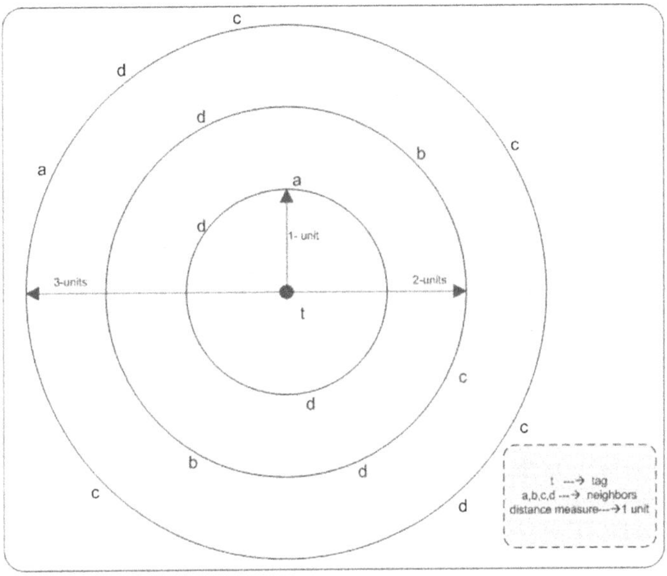

Fig. 2.2 Example of a concept view of a tag and neighbors distance relationship graph

Table 2.1 Tag neighbors weight and frequency from Fig. 2.2

T, C	w(t,c)	f(c)	nf(t,c)
t, a	0.665	0.13	0.086
t, b	0.5	0.13	0.065
t, c	1.83	0.3	0.549
t, d	3.66	0.4	1.464

$C = \{c_0, c_1, \ldots, c_{|C|}\}$ be the candidate neighbors set. Then, every $c_i(1 \leq i \leq |C|)$ can be instituted as a potential expansion for tag t. According to Fig. 2.2, t is the tag and $\{a, b, c, d\} \in C$ are the candidate neighbors. The total occurrence with the number of candidate neighbors is 15 (i.e. $|C| = 15$). The tag a occurs twice, b occurs twice, c occurs five times, and d occurs six times. According to these occurrences, we compute the weight function $w(t, c)$ by considering the distance of each candidate neighbor from the original tag. Particularly, in the case of the candidate neighbor a, two distances are evidenced, the first 1 unit and the second 3 units. Thus $w(t, c) = 0.665$ according to Eq. 2.1. The frequency of each candidate neighbor is each candidate neighbor divided by the total number of candidate neighbor with respect to tag t, i.e. $\frac{|c|_{each_a}}{|C|} = 2/15 = 0.13$. Finally the neighborhood function that multiplies the frequencies by the weights is $nf(t, a) = w(t, a) \cdot f(a) = 0.086$. This procedure is repeated throughout the remaining candidate tag neighbors. Table 2.1 shows the results of all candidates for each function as explained in the previous section.

The selection of most qualified neighbors is based on the $nf(t, c)$ value analysis. For instance, (see Fig. 2.2), candidate neighbor d is more likely to be selected instead of candidate a, since $nf(t, d) > nf(t, a)$. The selection ordering of tag neighbors is the following: $\{d,\ c,\ a\ and\ b\}$.

Expanding Query with Tag Neighbors

In theory, every query has neighbors in the content with the chance to get an expansion. Once the tag neighbors are processed, queries provided by the user for searching documents can benefit from the query expansion, which denote the relevant degree between the expansion query and the original query. We consider only certain sets of neighbors to expand queries, and we select top k neighbors to generate a new expanded query by adding all the terms (see in Fig. 2.3).

The important structure of the query expansion is thus: given T as a set of all tags occurring in the document corpus and a query consisting of terms $Q = \{q_i\,|q_i \in Q, i = 1, 2, \ldots z\}$, where z is the number of terms that occur in Q. For each term $q_i \in Q \cap T$ we define $Q' \subset Q$ as $Q' = \{q'_i\,|q'_i \in T \cap Q, i = 1, 2, \ldots m\}$, where m is the number of tags that occur in Q'.

For each one $q'_i \in Q'$, we retrieve all previously processed neighbors C and select all neighbors $C' \subset C$ ranked above the threshold α (see Sect. "Generating Tag Neighbors"). Finally, we add all retrieved neighbors C' to Q' expanding it to $Q_{expanded} = Q' \cup C'$. Once this process is repeated for all tag queries q'_i, we perform the search using the newly expanded $Q_{expanded}$ expressed in the form of a query vector with a traditional information retrieval algorithm, such as in [4].

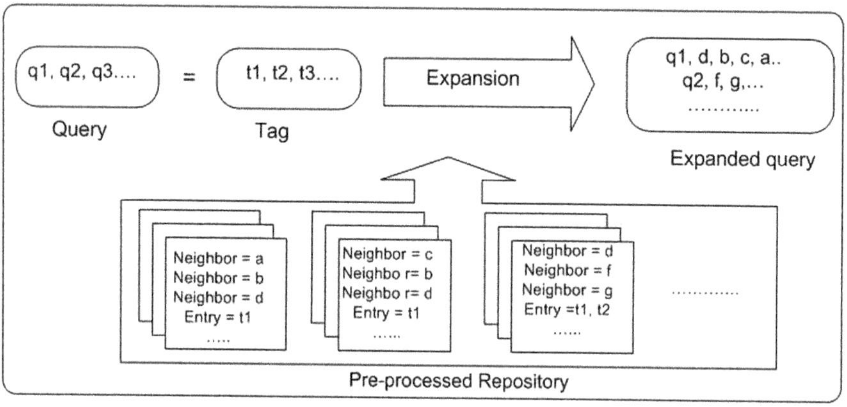

Fig. 2.3 Query expansion process with tag neighbors

Working Example on Expanding Query with Tag Neighbors

In order to illustrate the query expansion, we continue working on the previous example from Fig. 2.2 where t is the tag and a, b, c, d are the candidate neighbors. Assuming that a given query q matches the tag t, the query expansion procedure begins.

According to Eq. (2.3), the tag neighbors (whose neighborhood function values $nf(t, c) > \alpha$) of tag t are selected from the pre-processed neighborhood table. The selection order will depend on the neighborhood function values. In Table 2.1, the candidate neighbors selection order follows d, c, b, a since their $nf(t, c)$ values are $1.464, 0.549, 0.065, 0.086$, respectively, i.e. the given query q expands with d first and then follows c, b, a. Therefore, the expanded query q' formation is equal to $\{t \wedge d, t \wedge c, t \wedge b, t \wedge a\}$. Finally, the search system performs the search with the expanded query q'.

Experimental Evaluation

In this section, we describe the experimental design that supports the evaluation of our proposal and the evaluation results achieved from the experiment. The goal of this evaluation is to show that document search, enhanced by the tag neighbor expansion, results in an improvement of document retrieval effectiveness in comparison with baseline and state-of-the-art approaches. In the following sections, we detail the data collection, methodology, and metrics used in the experiment.

Dataset and Experimental Setup

Data

In order to test our approach, we crawled the article repository in MedWorm system during April 2010. MedWorm is a medical RSS(Really Simple Syndication) feed provider as well as a search engine built on data collected from RSS feeds. We downloaded the contents into our local database. After stemming out the entity attributes from the data, four data files, namely user, resource, tags and quads, were obtained for our experiments. The fourth file represents the links between users, resources and tags. Using these data files, we generated SQL scripts to insert all data into the database. The resulting dataset comprises 949 users, 13,509 tags and 26,1501 documents. Currently, this data is available at [19].

Queries

The proposed approach is evaluated with MeSH (Medical Subject Headings) vocabulary(i.e., queries), which are in MedWorm dataset. Selected queries are related to the MeSH tree structure-2011 [2]C-diseases. The MeSH thesaurus is a National Library of Medicine's (NLM) controlled vocabulary for subject indexing and searching for journal articles in MEDLINE, books, journal titles, and non-print materials in NLM's catalog [8]. These headings, also known as descriptors, are organized into 16 categories: category A for anatomic terms, category B for organisms, C for diseases, D for drugs and chemical, etc. However, we only consider C-diseases category due to the specific purpose of our project. This category is further divided into 26 subcategories as C01, C02,..., C26. Table 2.2 shows sample sub category *MeSH queries* and their candidate neighbors with frequencies.

Experimental Setup

After data storage, we indexed the stemmed words in order to build up the search space. We utilize the processed indexing and content database to compute the tag neighborhood and calculate the neighbor frequency and weight as described in sect. "Generating Tag Neighbors". As a result, we ended up with 15,175,334 tag neighbors with an average of approximately 9 highly ranked candidate neighbors per tag when selecting a higher value of neighborhood function threshold $\alpha = 0.6$ ("Generating Tag Neighbors").

The Web-Based Search Tool

To evaluate the approach we developed a keyword-based search tool based on the Lucene search engine. The Lucene search engine is utilized for searching documents as well as for indexing them. Lucene is a high performance, fully featured text search engine library written in Java [17]. In brief, our tool operates by maintaining a

Table 2.2 Sample MeSH queries and their TOP 4 Neighbors followed by their frequencies

Query	1	2	3	4
Influenza	Contagious {0.41}	Viral{0.35}	Infection{0.31}	Cold{0.28}
Cancer	Metastasize {0.34}	Malignant{0.33}	Infection{0.31}	Tumor{0.19}
Diabetes	Insulin {0.45}	Hormone{0.42}	Glucose{0.38}	Blood{0.30}
Overdose	Drug {0.31}	Blood{0.27}	Hemoglobin{0.19}	Injection{0.11}
Diarrhoea	Intestinal{0.32}	Bacteria{0.28}	Fluid{0.25}	Digestion{0.18}
Chemotherapy	Blood{0.40}	Cancer{0.36}	Treatment{0.24}	Tumor {0.12}

[2] http://www.nlm.nih.gov/mesh/trees.html

comprehensive index of Medworm documents that are crawled from the MedWorm website. The index structure is composed by a field "content" that comprises the document terms and a field "docID" referencing the document meta-information in the database. When a user submits a query to the tool, the query expansion takes place and the reformulated query terms are compared against index terms for relevant items in the search engine index. An overall relevancy score for each document is computed according to how many terms occur in the index, and how important these terms are for that item. The search score is given by the federated Lucene model.

The index is utilized exclusively for searching however the all meta information about the document and other entities such as user and tags are stored in a relational database. To make the search tool available for online usage, we created a web application where users can issue queries, retrieve results and download them. The web application was developed based on JBoss seam framework, an open source development platform for building rich Internet applications in Java. Seam integrates technologies such as Asynchronous JavaScript and XML (AJAX), JavaServer Faces (JSF), Java Persistence (JPA), Enterprise Java Beans (EJB 3.0) [45].

Evaluation Methodology and Metrics

The methodology for inferring relevance assessments is based on the ranked lists of documents submitted in response to a given query and the number of documents relevant to the query. For the human relevance assessment, we chose 106 MeSH queries according to [26] from 26 sub categories of selected C category of MeSH-2011 vocabulary. However, 6 queries did not have any information in our database. So, we compute the relevant assessment for 100 queries. Each query is evaluated by the top-10 and top-20 retrieved documents. For the relevance assessment, we invited in total twenty experts who are familiar with medical domains to browse through the whole content of documents and assess whether they were relevant. The experts invited were ten biological and medical PhD students and ten employees of the FP7 ICT project M-Eco (Medical Ecosystem Personalized Event-Based Surveillance). Each participant evaluated five queries, i.e. at least 20 documents per query were assessed. In particular, six of them evaluated six queries. To make the evaluation less exhaustive, since the results of four methods were analyzed, we designed the interface of the Web-based system to display the search results of two methods in parallel and simultaneously. At last, we averaged the precision rate from the experts' evaluations.

Analysis of Precision

Our analysis was based on observation over the precision of our search engine. We compared our precision results against results obtained from a baseline query search that relies on the simple user entry query without expansion and two other state-of-the-art approaches, [26] and [8]. In a nutshell, [8] expands the user's query with MeSH descriptors, while [26] exploits UMLS (Unified Medical Language System), a large thesaurus in the biomedical domain, to append the original query with additional terms where explicit semantic relations are found. In order to compare our approach against [26] and [8], we discarded our own tag neighborhood table and expanded the user's query with terms found at the MeSH descriptors and at the semantic network UMLS [43]. For instance, at UMLS there is a semantic statement "*Body Substance—causes—Acquired Abnormality*". If the user's query matches "Body Substance", then the term "Acquired Abnormality" will be considered. Needless to say, all semantic relations are investigated in the UMLS corpus.

Because the evaluation took place specifically in the top-10 and top-20 retrieved documents, we are unable to perform a realistic recall analysis. As pointed out by [7], the recall should determine the ability of search engines to obtain all or most of the relevant documents in the corpus. Thus, it requires knowledge not just of the relevant and retrieved ones but also those not retrieved. Since we do not have the precise knowledge of all relevant items within the entire corpus, it is very likely that we might perform an inaccurate and non-realistic recall analysis. On the other hand, we understand that this demanding analysis must be conducted in a future experiment.

Aiming at fully reflecting the performance comparisons across related works, we adopted MAP (Mean Average Precision), nDCG (Normalized Discounted Cumulative Gain) and P@n, i.e. precision of the first n retrieved documents as in the Text Retrieval Conference (TREC) [42]. The Text Retrieval Conference is an on-going series of workshops focusing on a list of different information retrieval (IR) research areas, or tracks. In particular, MAP, P@10, P@20 and nDCG at positions 10 and 20 are utilized in our assessment. While the nDCG indicates how good the search results were to an optimal ranking, $P@n$ reflects the percentage of documents in the top n of the ranked list that are relevant to the query. $P@n$ is defined as follows.

$$P@n = \frac{\textit{number of relevant documents in top n results}}{n} \tag{2.4}$$

MAP stands for the mean of the average precision scores for a set of queries. The average precision (AP) for a single query is the mean of the precision after each relevant document is retrieved.

$$AP = \frac{\sum_{n=1}^{N} P@n \times rel(n)}{\textit{number of relevant documents}} AP = \frac{\sum_{n=1}^{N} P@n}{\textit{number of relevant documents}} \tag{2.5}$$

where n is the rank, and N is the number of retrieved documents. Finally, MAP is obtained by averaging the AP values over the set of queries.

$$MAP = \frac{\sum_{q=1}^{Q} AP(q)}{|Q|} \tag{2.6}$$

where Q is the number of queries and $|Q|$ is the amount of queries.

The nDCG is a commonly used standard evaluation metric indicating that highly relevant documents are more useful when appearing earlier in a search engine result list. However since we are considering a limited (top 10 and top 20) subset of search results, the DCG at position p should be normalized. Therefore, we calculate the nDCG at position p, which is defined as:

$$nDCG_p = \frac{DCG_p}{IDCG_p} \tag{2.7}$$

where the discounted CG (Cumulative Gain) accumulated at a particular rank position p is defined as:

$$DCG_p = \sum_{i=1}^{n} \frac{2^{rel_i} - 1}{\log_2(1+i)} \tag{2.8}$$

where the relevance values of documents (rel_i) range between 0 and 1 [23]. For calculating the nCGG at positions $p = 10$ and $p = 20$, for each query, we had to create an ideal ordering as pointed out in [23].

Empirical Evaluation of Tag Neighbors Quality

Besides the search performance assessment, we also performed an empirical analysis of tag neighbors quality on the given dataset since the performance of our approach is highly dependent on the quality of the tag neighbors utilized in the query expansion. In order to empirically assess such quality, first we set up the threshold ($\alpha > 0.6$) to cut off the unwanted tag neighbors and then, we sorted the tag neighbors by their neighborhood function values in descending order. Last, we invited the experts to assess the degree of relevance between the tag neighbors and parent tags.

Evaluation Results

Performance Results

Table 2.3 summarizes the overall performance measures (MAP, P@10, P@20, nDCG@10 and nDCG@20) achieved by our approach plus the baseline, MeSH, and UMLS-based approaches. As seen in the results on Table 2.3, the baseline achieved the worst precision rates among all the methods. Our approach outperformed all compared approaches but our precision results were nearly equal to the MeSH results. The reason is simple. Since our queries were random selection of MeSH database, all queries achieved reasonable query expansion and subsequent relevant retrievals. On the other hand, the expansion on the UMLS-based approach were never guaranteed,

Table 2.3 Comparison of the performance over 100 queries

Metrics	Baseline	Our approach	MeSH	UMLS
MAP	0.353	0.491	0.477	0.452
P@10	0.399	0.523	0.501	0.510
P@20	0.367	0.509	0.491	0.496
nDCG@10	0.512	0.649	0.627	0.503
nDCG@20	0.432	0.623	0.620	0.499

Table 2.4 Statistics about a sample MeSH sub categories, queries and performance measures

MeSH subcategory (Diseases)	Query (Expansion size)	Baseline (P@10)	Approach (P@10)	Baseline (P@20)	Approach (P@20)
Bacterial infections [C01]	Infection (16)	0.689	**0.798**	0.673	**0.789**
Virus diseases[C02]	Arbovirus (11)	0.646	**0.783**	0.641	**0.769**
Parasitic diseases[C03]	Helminthiasis (7)	0.459	0.632	0.435	0.612
Neoplasms[C04]	Hamartoma (1)	0.145	0.145	0.112	0.112
Musculoskeletal [C05]	Dysostoses (9)	0.654	0.711	0.632	0.697
Digestive system diseases[C06]	Cholangitis (8)	0.599	0.688	0.572	0.671
Stomatognathic [C07]	Mouth (13)	0.701	**0.796**	0.699	**0.785**
Respiratory tract [C08]	Lung disease (17)	0.764	**0.802**	0.732	**0.798**
Otorhinolaryngologic [C09]	Nose disease (5)	0.356	0.422	0.325	0.413
Nervous system [C10]	Brain injuries (12)	0.712	**0.794**	0.705	**0.786**

thus performing at a level that is at least equal to the baseline approach. Both MESH and UMLS-based approaches outperformed the baseline. We also applied the *t-test* method to assesses whether the precision average of the compared approaches to our approach was statistically significant. In all cases (MAP, P@10, P@20, nDCG@10 and nDCG@20) we observed $p - value \geq 0.05$, meaning that our method achieved higher value precision rates but was also statistically significant.

Table 2.4 shows the sample statistics at different precision levels. The first column depicts sub-categories of the MeSH headings, and the second column gives the query information which we used for search. The third column gives the amount of the best (for threshold $\alpha > 0.6$) available tag neighbors to expand the original query. The last four columns give the retrieval precision by P@10 and P@20. The MeSH and UMLS-based approaches were not considered in this demonstration.

Tag Neighborhood Results for Query Expansion

As already pointed out in Sect. "Empirical Evaluation of Tag Neighbors Quality", the quality of the search retrieval depends on the tag neighbors' quality. Tags semantically related or capable of describing a fact/epidemy can be considered high quality. For instance, the tags "2009", "flu", "Mexico" and "pandemic" can quickly remind one about the outbreak of a new strain of influenza that infected many people in Mexico in March and April of 2009. Similarly, the tags "influenza", "flu", "gripe" are terms that refer to an infectious disease caused by RNA viruses that affects birds and mammals. On the other hand, tags such as "data mining", "H1N1", and "market shares", if taken as neighbors, should probably be considered low quality since: (i) they are loosely related at the semantic level; and (ii) they do not lead to any special case in recent years. Yes, they can be related but for particular reasons and in a context that will not be of interest to many. For this reason, this group of tags should be rated as low quality.

In order to validate the tag neighbors' quality, we consulted 10 health surveillance experts of M-Eco project ("Evaluation Methodology and Metrics") to analyze the 20 most frequent tag neighbors derived from 575 tags as eventual queries, albeit randomly chosen, from our database. Also worth mentioning is that the 575 tags were generated from the same document corpus (261,501) utilized for measuring the recommendation performance. The assessment members have extensive knowledge in the medical surveillance area given that some have conducted research for many years while others have actually worked for federal institutions responsible for disease control and prevention. The evaluation criteria of the subjective assessment were based on the degree of relatedness between the tag and the tag neighbors. Based on his own experience, each evaluator had to indicate whether a single neighbor was related (or not) to the original tag.

The sample size was calculated according to [1] with the confidence level set to 95 % and confidence interval set to 4 %. Each neighbor was asked to be evaluated individually, regardless of whether it was related or not to the parent tag. As a result, according to the expert assessment, 83 % of the tag neighbors were correctly related to the parent tag while only 17 % were loosely semantically related or inadequate. This assessment was crucial to the give credibility of results expressed in Table 2.3. We observed that many terms within the set of items corresponding to the 17 % are mostly non-medical terms, generally verbs and nouns. As part of our future works, we aim at validating such terms by consulting a medical dictionary or domain ontology vocabularies when generating the tag neighborhood table.

Discussion

In this work, we present the application of tags neighbors as an auxiliary resource toward effective information retrieval in the medical domain. The satisfactory precision results obtained with the evaluation demonstrate the potential of the approach and allow us to discuss and compare our results with other approaches.

Related Work Comparison

In order to judge the relative effectiveness of our approach, we compare our results with related studies that also address the query expansion as an instrument for effective information retrieval in the medical domain.

Focused on the mean average precision (MAP) values, [27], which applied MeSH descriptors to expand the queries by adding medical information, obtained 0.3095 on the ImageCLEPmed 2006 dataset. [26], an approach based on a knowledge-based query expansion, achieved 0.474, whereas [30] achieved 0.425. In comparison with such a related work [27], we obtained MAP improvements at 58, 3.5 and 15 % respectively. Although we observe better results over compared approaches, this analysis should be moderately judged due to the fact that might exist differences in the evaluation methodology or dataset. On the other hand, this comparison gives an overview of the MAP performance among related approaches.

Obtained Results and MeSH Sub Categories

As explained previously, the queries issued during the experimental evaluation belongs to specific medical(MeSH) categories. By having this information available, we were able to analyze in which categories our approach performs better. Table 2.4 shows a MeSH sub category followed by sample queries with their performance outcomes at P@10 and P@20. As shown there, the query *lung disease* generates 17 expansions and achieves P@10 at 0.802 and P@20 at 0.798. *Hamartoma* has only one expansion term and P@10 at 0.145 and P@20 is 0.112, which is almost equal to baseline search performance.

We also observe that our approach achieves better performance for the categories Bacterial Infections and mycoses [C01], Respiratory Tract Diseases[C08], Nervous System Diseases [C10], Stomatognathic Diseases[C07], Virus Diseases[C02] MeSH categories. On the other hand, our approach gives very poor results for Neoplasms[C04] MeSH sub category since the query expansion is limited to one tag neighbor. This indicates that queries with more expandable terms have the higher retrieval performance, while the low amount of expandable terms has much less performance, close to the baseline. Bold numbers in the table indicate the top performances.

From this analysis, we obtained satisfactory results however its effectiveness for particular categories does not perform as expected. This input opens a request for further improvements on categories such as Neoplasm [C04]. This will likely require a deeper analysis of the dataset that were utilized for the evaluation.

Limitations and Points of Improvements

Although the approach has achieved more satisfactory performance results compared to the baseline approach, it still has certain limitations and hence points for improvement. These issues occur because dealing with tags is no trivial task. Since users can assign tags that are free of grammatical norms and merely based on what they have in mind, inconveniences such as sparsity, misspelling or lack of semantics can sometimes occur [34].

When tagging data that are either insufficiently available or do not equally cover all resources, this tag sparsity might degrade considerably the performance of the approach. If only a few tags are available, the tag neighborhood table will reduce the probability of matching any user's query considerably. As a result, in only very few specific cases, there will be a query expansion. Another issue concerns the tag syntax, especially since no syntax control may be guaranteed and users can assign them to the documents based on their sense of value. In the case where tags are commonly misspelled, the tag neighborhood table will not increase because misspelled tags will not match terms in the documents. As a consequence, the term neighbors will not be retrieved, thus lowering the level of recall performance.

The meaning of the tagging data does not pose a problem because it is not specified along with the tag itself; instead, it resides in the tagger's head. For this reason, it is difficult to understand and/or agree on some tag assignments because the explanation given by the tagger is not available. It is practically impossible to judge which case there is a hidden reason for such a tagging or did he mean something else [16]. In addition, *polysemy* can take place, in which the same tag can have different meanings, or *synonymy*, wherein the same concept can be represented by different tags. For example, the tag "orange" might refer to the fruit, the color or the French telephony company [35], i.e. the polysemy case. The lack of semantic distinction may lead to the generation of inaccurate retrieval. For improvement, this needs to be tackled in our future works given that users may be provided with results unrelated to the intended meaning of their queries.

The quality of the tag expansions depends on the tag neighbor terms of documents. In our model, we aim at quantifying this by addressing the frequency and distance of neighbors to the target tag. From a semantic perspective, the statistical relatedness raised by our model does not guarantee a taxonomic or semantic relation. As a point of improvement, we look forward to combining our model with an analysis of specialized medical dictionaries or domain ontology vocabularies that explicitly establish such relations. A reference work addressing the semantic evaluation in ontologies of tags can be seen in the work of [11].

Conclusion and Future Work

In this paper, we proposed an approach of using tag neighbors for query expansion. Such approach supports users with complementary information provided by the most frequent and weighted tag neighbors occurring in the document corpus. We implemented our approach in a search system with contents extracted and indexed from the *MedWorm* medical article database. The evaluation results have shown that our proposed approach achieved substantial improvement on mean average precision and different stages of precisions compared with the same metrics of the traditional information retrieval algorithm.

As a future work, we aim at improving the quality of tag neighbors by comparing then against medical specialized dictionaries or domain ontology vocabularies. Further, we plan to realize more experimental studies necessary to validate the scalability and feasibility of the proposed approach in a broader scope. Finally, we aim at combining the current approach with other techniques previously explored such as collaborative filtering.

Acknowledgments This work has been partially supported by FP7 ICT project M-Eco: Medical Ecosystem Personalized Event-Based Surveillance under grant number 247829. This journal is a extended version of previously published paper at the International Conference on Information Science and Applications (ICISA 2011).

References

1. Anderson TW, Anderson TW (1984) An Introduction to Multivariate Statistical Analysis, 2nd Edition, 2nd edn. Wiley-Interscience
2. Andreou A (2005) Agissilaos andreou. Master thesis, Agissilaos Andreou
3. Azcárate M, Vázquez J, López M (2012) Improving image retrieval effectiveness via query expansion using mesh hierarchical structure. Journal of the American Medical Informatics Association
4. Baeza-Yates RA, Ribeiro-Neto B (1999) Modern Information Retrieval. Addison-Wesley
5. Bianco CE (2009) Medical librarians' uses and perceptions of social tagging. Journal of the Medical Library Association : JMLA 97(2):136–139
6. Carpineto C, de Mori R, Romano G, Bigi B (2001) An information-theoretic approach to automatic query expansion. ACM Trans Inf Syst 19(1):1–27
7. Clarke SJ, Willett P (1997) Estimating the recall performance of web search engines. Aslib Proceedings 49(7):184–189
8. Daz-Galiano M, Martn-Valdivia M, Urea-Lpez L (2009) Query expansion with a medical ontology to improve a multimodal information retrieval system. Computers in Biology and Medicine 39(4):396–403
9. Diem LTH, Chevallet JP, Thuy DTB (2007) Thesaurus-based query and document expansion in conceptual indexing with umls pp 242–246
10. Dozier C, Kondadadi R, Al-Kofahi K, Chaudhary M, Guo X (2007) Fast tagging of medical terms in legal text. In: Proceedings of the 11th international conference on Artificial intelligence and law, ACM, New York, NY, USA, ICAIL '07, pp 253–260
11. Durao F, Dolog P (2010) Extending a hybrid tag-based recommender system with personalization. In: SAC '10: Proceedings of the 2010 ACM Symposium on Applied Computing, ACM, New York, NY, USA, pp 1723–1727

12. Durao F, Bayyapu K, Xu G, Dolog P, Lage R (2011) Using tag-neighbors for query expansion in medical information retrieval. International Conference on Information Science and Applications 0:1–9
13. Efthimiadis EN (1993) A user-centred evaluation of ranking algorithms for interactive query expansion. In: SIGIR '93: Proceedings of the 16th annual international ACM SIGIR conference on Research and development in information retrieval, ACM, New York, NY, USA, pp 146–159
14. Fu WT, Kannampallil T, Kang R, He J (2010) Semantic imitation in social tagging. ACM Trans Comput-Hum Interact 17:12:1–12:37
15. Gordon-Murnane L (2006) Social bookmarking, folksonomies, and web 2.0 tools. Searcher Mag Database Prof (6):26–28
16. Gruber T (2008) Collective knowledge systems: Where the social web meets the semantic web. Web Semant 6:4–13
17. Hatcher E, Gospodnetic O (2004) Lucene in Action (In Action series). Manning Publications Co., Greenwich, CT, USA
18. Hersh WR, David M, Hickam H (1998) How well do physicians use electronic information retrieval systems? a framework for investigation and systematic review
19. IWISPlatform (2012)https://sourceforge.net/projects/iwis/files/
20. Jain H, Thao C, Zhao H (2010) Enhancing electronic medical record retrieval through semantic query expansion. Information Systems and E-Business Management pp 1–17
21. Jang H, Song SK, Myaeng SH (2006) Semantic tagging for medical knowledge tracking. In: Engineering in Medicine and Biology Society, 2006. EMBS '06.28th Annual International Conference of the IEEE
22. Jansen BJ, Spink A, Bateman J, Saracevic T (1998) Real life information retrieval: a study of user queries on the web. SIGIR Forum 32(1):5–17
23. Järvelin K, Kekäläinen J (2002) Cumulated gain-based evaluation of ir techniques. ACM Trans Inf Syst 20(4):422–446
24. Jin S, Lin H, Su S (2009) Query expansion based on folksonomy tag co-occurrence analysis. Granular Computing, 2009, GRC '09 IEEE International Conference on pp 300–305
25. Kelly D, Cushing A, Dostert M, Niu X, Gyllstrom K (2010) Effects of popularity and quality on the usage of query suggestions during information search. In:Proceedings of the 28th international conference on Human factors in computing systems, ACM, New York, NY, USA, CHI '10, pp 45–54
26. Liu Z, Chu WW (2005) Knowledge-based query expansion to support scenario-specific retrieval of medical free text. In: SAC '05: Proceedings of the 2005 ACM symposium on Applied computing, ACM, New York, NY, USA, pp 1076–1083
27. Lu Z, Kim W, Wilbur W (2009) Evaluation of query expansion using mesh in pubmed. Information Retrieval 12:69–80
28. Luo G, Tang C, Yang H, Wei X (2008) Medsearch: a specialized search engine for medical information retrieval. In: Proceeding of the 17th ACM conference on Information and knowledge management, ACM, New York, NY, USA, CIKM '08, pp 143–152
29. Ma H, Yang H, King I, Lyu MR (2008) Learning latent semantic relations from clickthrough data for query suggestion. In: Proceedings of the 17th ACM conference on Information and knowledge management, ACM, New York, NY, USA, CIKM '08, pp 709–718
30. Matos S, Arrais J, Maia-Rodrigues J, Oliveira J (2010) Concept-based query expansion for retrieving gene related publications from medline. BMC Bioinformatics 11(1):212
31. MedWorm (2012) http://www.medworm.com
32. Mei Q, Zhou D, Church K (2008) Query suggestion using hitting time. In: Proceedings of the 17th ACM conference on Information and knowledge management, ACM, New York, NY, USA, CIKM '08, pp 469–478
33. MeSH (2012) http://www.nlm.nih.gov/mesh
34. Milicevic A, Nanopoulos A, Ivanovic M (2010) Social tagging in recommender systems: a survey of the state-of-the-art and possible extensions. Artificial Intelligence Review 33(3): 187–209
35. Orange (2012) http://www.orange.com

36. PubMed (2012) http://www.medworm.com
37. Ravid G, Bar-Ilan J, Baruchson-Arbib S, Rafaeli S (2007) Popularityand findability through log analysis of search terms and queries: the case of a multilingual public service website. J Inf Sci 33(5):567–583
38. Ruch P, Wagner J, Bouillon P, Baud RH, Rassinoux AM, Scherrer JR (1999) Medtag:tag-like semantics for medical document indexing
39. SB J (1999) A semantic lexicon for medical language processing pp 205–218
40. Smith G (2007) Tagging: People-powered Metadata for the Social Web (Voices That Matter). New Riders Press
41. Strohmaier M (2008) Purpose tagging: capturing user intent to assist goal-oriented social search. In: Proceeding of the 2008 ACM workshop on Search in social media, ACM, New York, NY, USA, SSM '08, pp 35–42
42. TREC (2012) http://trec.nist.gov
43. UMLS (2012) http://semanticnetwork.nlm.nih.gov/Download/RelationalFiles/SRSTRE2
44. West J (2007) Subject headings 2.0: Folksonomies and tags. Library Media Connection 25(7):58–59
45. Yuan MJ, Orshalick J, Heute T (2009) Seam Framework: Experience the Evolution of Java EE, 2nd edn. Prentice Hall PTR, Upper Saddle River, NJ, USA
46. Yue W, Chen Z, Lu X, Lin F, Liu J (2005) Using query expansion and classification for information retrieval. In: Semantics, Knowledge and Grid, 2005. SKG '05. First International Conference on, p 31

Chapter 3
Medical Technology Breakthroughs in Tissue Engineering

Mirjana Pavlovic , John Mayfield and Bela Balint

Mankind is searching for a key to longevity and there is no doubt that stem cells could be an important answer to this problem.
Ratajczak M.

Introduction

Powerful developments in Tissue Engineering multidisciplinary field have yielded a novel set of tissue replacement parts and implementation strategies. This chapter would bring the newest information on the medical breakthroughs in tissue engineering (TE) on all three levels that specify TE as particular entity: cells, scaffolds (biomaterials) and reactive molecules, discovered and invented to orchestrate the reparative and curative aspects of TE. It will involve technologies for detection and distinction of different types of stem cells (embryonic and adult): hematopoietic stem cells (HS), very small embryonic stem cells (VSEL) cells, mesenchymal stem cells (MSC) from different sources, and scaffolds as a platform for 3-D growth of tissue, computer aided TE (CATE), inject-printing of cells, transplantation without a donor, and other "state of the art" entities and issues along with this exciting and expansively evolving research field that is definitely changing the future of medical approaches. Among the major challenges now facing TE is the need for more complex functionality, as well as both functional and biomechanical stability in laboratory-grown tissues destined for transplantation. The continued success of TE and eventual development

M. Pavlovic (✉) J. Mayfield
Department of Computer and Electrical Engineering and Computer Science,
Florida Atlantic University, Boca Raton, FL, USA
e-mail: mpavlovi@fau.edu

B. Balint
Military Medical Academy, Belgrade, Serbia

B. Furht and A. Agarwal (eds.), *Handbook of Medical and Healthcare Technologies*,
DOI: 10.1007/978-1-4614-8495-0_3,

of true human replacement parts will grow from the convergence of engineering and basic research advances in stem cell, tissue, matrix, growth factors, and developmental biology, as well as materials science and bioinformatics.

Background and Significance

It is a matter of common sense that tissue engineering development is based upon stem cell research as a fundamental approach. An integral overview on fundamental and clinical research in the stem-cell field, with emphasis on history, controversies, new concepts, their meaning and applicability is an evolving matter. Stem cells (SCs) are now known to have unlimited self-renewal and large proliferative capacity, as well as a high potential for differentiation into all blood cells or other somatic cell types, in natural setting in situ and after "conventional" therapeutic use. Their application in the fields of regenerative medicine and tissue engineering (TE) is emerging from those fundamental capabilities that are still the matter of intensive research studies. Thus, these toti-, pluri- and/or multipotent SCs are capable of providing complete, stable and long-term reconstitution of hematopoiesis that was the basis for the clinical use of SCs in allogeneic or autologous transplant setting [1]. A striking feature of SCs is a great plasticity and ability to give rise to differentiated cells of numerous lineages—such as osteocytes, chondrocytes, cardiomyocytes, hepatocytes, even endothelial cells [1]. This differentiating capacity emphasizes their potential role in a wide spectrum of different therapeutical scenarios. In this chapter we have particularly stressed out the possibility of implantation of these cells into humans in order to reconstruct destroyed tissues/organs (regenerative medicine and TE), which is also supported by the basic research done on the SC differentiation and replacement (TE itself). Thus, SCs open novel viewpoints and perspectives in the treatment of diseases—as it is the case with the TE and regenerative medicine. It is difficult to make a sharp distinction between these disciplines since they depend on each other. Stem cells are nowadays being called a "panacea" or a "cure-all" in many diseases—although their functional role is not yet well known—and it is clear now that they are being involved in numerous areas of cell-mediated therapeutic approaches. The chapter is also dealing with advantages and disadvantages of regenerative stem cell therapy, as well as the results of different (routs of) applications and discussion of possibilities for their improvement, where appropriate. Although both: TE and regenerative medicine are strongly based upon the fundamental stem cell research development, it is clear that stem cell replacement so far, does not answer all questions about potential curative aspects of any particular disease. We have discussed both: invasive (bone marrow transplanted-BMT) and non-invasive (mobilization) approaches to stem cell therapy in TE of acute myocardial infarction (AMI) and underlined some of the results of their application in experimental and clinical settings. Altogether, the data strongly suggest the inevitable necessity for further development of this field of research and its clinical applicability, which belongs to the near future, and will require generations of enthusiastic researchers and clinicians to completely develop, distinctively categorize, and apply the concepts of regenerative stem cell therapy and tissue engineering into clinical arena.

Tissue Engineering: Definition and Technology

According to very global NIH definition, Tissue engineering (TE) is an emerging multidisciplinary field involving biology, medicine, and engineering that is likely to revolutionize the ways we improve the health and quality of life for millions of people worldwide by restoring, maintaining, or enhancing tissue and organ function. It involves integral thinking and collaboration of multidisciplinary approaches that have evolved thanks to breakthroughs in medical technology through history and especially during last decade [2–8]. Some of them are so essential and critical for the development of the filed that have to be thoroughly comprehended and elaborated. It is impossible to integrate all of them into one chapter, but is of great importance to emphasize those which present the basis for TE emergence and evolution. These breakthroughs are of course different research and clinical medical approaches in stem cell treatment, scaffolds microfabrication, 3-D growth of tissue, Computer-Aided Tissue Engineering concept (CATE), ink-jet printing of the cells and liquid scaffolds, transplantation without a donor, and other techniques/technologies of great relevance for advance of TE. Let us see what each of them means in TE development.

Medical Technology Breakthroughs

- *"Development of Cell patterns for possible TE use and technology of multiple staining-Flow Cytometry"*

The first use of stem cells in humans was done by E. Donald Thomas whose work was later recognized with a Nobel Prize and Physiology or Medicine [1]. His work showed that bone marrow cells infused intravenously could repopulate the bone marrow and produce new blood cells. His work also reduced the likelihood of developing a life-threatening complication known as graft-versus-host disease (GVHD). With the availability of the stem cell growth factors most hematopoietic stem cell transplantation procedures are now performed using stem cells collected from the peripheral blood rather than from the bone marrow. Collecting peripheral blood stem cells provides a bigger graft, does not require that the donor be subjected to general anesthesia collect the graft, results in a shorter time to engraftment, and may provide for a lower long-term relapse rate [1]. The first recorded attempt at cellular therapy occurred in 1912 when German physicians attempted to treat hypothyroid children with thyroid cells [1]. Cellular therapy, as practiced today, was developed in the early 1930s by Paul Niehans, MD (1882–1971), a Swiss physician who became known as "the father of cell therapy" [9]. It soon became popular with celebrities as a means of rejuvenation. A 1990 article in *In Health* magazine described Niehans as a "public relations genius" and stated that the Clinic La Preire, which he had founded in Clarens-Montreaux, Switzerland, had attracted 65,000 patients. Its (1999) one-week "revitalization program" costed about $8,000. However, Niehans made a great breakthrough in the last century by applying cell based therapy, which was unimaginable before him.

Generally, the Stem Cell (SC)—compartment is divided into *embryonic* and tissue specific or *adult* SCs. *Embryonic SCs* (ES or ESC) are by definition the "master cells" with the largest spectrum of differentiation potential, e.g. capable of differentiating into every type of cells either *in vitro* or in vivo [6–8, 10–13]. Thanks to the presence of embryonic body, these cells have ability to develop into three primary layers: endoderm, ectoderm and mesoderm. The discovery of SCs inside cell mass of embryos and in adult tissue has revolutionized the medical field by introducing new therapeutic dimensions into previously untreatable diseases and injuries [13]. Several experimental or preclinical studies have suggested that application of embryonic SC could be promising in the treatment of various diseases. However, recognition of appropriate ethical aspects, regulatory acts and standardization in embryonic SC mediated regenerative medicine is needed as it is still the matter of controversy. Besides, permanent, persistent and accurate updating of the facts regarding their immunologic characteristics is an essential requirement for safe clinical application of SCs. Some authors stand that the initial theory that embryonic SCs are ignored by immunocompetent hosts was overlooked. On the contrary, it is even more evident that embryonic SCs could protect themselves actively by several immunomodulatory mechanisms against T lymphocytes and natural killer cells of host, and actively participate in immune-mediated events [12].

Recent isolation of fetal SCs from several sources either at the early stages of development or during the later trimesters of gestation, sharing similar growth kinetics and expressing pluripotency markers, provides strong support to the statement that these cells may be biologically closer to embryonic SCs . In fact, they represent intermediates between embryonic and *adult mesenchymal* SCs with regards to proliferation rates and plasticity features, thus being able to confer an advantage over postnatal mesenchymal SCs derived from conventional adult sources [11].

Historically, bone marrow was the primary source of SCs for transplant. However, peripheral blood and umbilical (cord) blood are also currently used as sources. SCs derived from these sources may have therapeutic potential (without severe adverse effects) only when given to the individual from whom they were derived (autologous transplants) or from an immunologically matched donor (allogeneic transplants) [2–4].

Despite the fact that the ideal type and source of cells have not yet been defined, immature SCs are capable of colonizing different tissues due to ability of homing and trans-differentiation or lineage-plasticity, in the settings of regenerative medicine [3–7]. Furthermore, there are several facts suggesting that adult SCs and even differentiated somatic cells, under appropriate microenvironmental cues or signals, are able to be "reprogrammed" and contribute to a much wider spectrum of differentiated progeny than previously anticipated. This has been demonstrated by using tissue-specific SCs—which like embryonic SCs—do not express CD45 as an exclusive hematopoietic marker [10]. Consequently, adult mesenchymal SCs and endothelial precursors are clinically applicable for cell-mediated, regenerative therapy of patients with myocardial, brain, vascular, liver, pancreas and some other tissue damages [2, 3, 14–21].

Allogeneic transplants are still the most efficient treatment for patients with liver failure. However, there is a lack of donors and some alternative therapeutic approaches are needed. Transplantation of mature hepatocytes has been evaluated, but the long–term efficacy remains unclear and the paucity of donor cells limits this strategy. The use of SC-therapy transplantation is perhaps a more promising alternative approach.

The intensification of myeloablative radio-chemotherapy, enlarged use of SC transplants, as well as the introduction of cell-mediated therapeutic approaches in regenerative medicine resulted in increased needs for both specific blood-derived progenitor/cells and practical operating procedures inducing minimized cellular damages during their collection or processing and storage in frozen state. Therefore, successful performance of SC transplantats or cell-mediated therapy requires efficient collection, processing, and (cryo) preservation procedures for obtaining an acceptable cell yield and post-thawing recovery, as well as advantageous clinical outcome.

In South Korea, Woo Suk Hwang of Seoul National University was known as the cloning king and his lab enjoyed strong support—and funding—from the South Korean government. It helps that therapeutic cloning was (and still is) much less controversial in South Korea than in the West. And unlike most of the rest of the world, the Korean public offers almost unequivocal support. Hwang says that a poll showed that more than 70 % of South Koreans agree with therapeutic cloning, whereas a recent poll in the US suggests 75 % are opposed to it. Two factors in particular seemed to be critical to Hwang's success. First, an incredible 1200 nuclear transfers (on cow and sheep cells) would take place every day in his lab. It really has been a case of practice makes almost perfect. Second, was the supply of eggs. South Korean law allows Hwang to use fresh eggs from young women who are prepared to donate their eggs by undergoing ovarian stimulation, which can be a risky and painful procedure. Yet, the results of Hwang have been withdrawn at the certain point as false. Was it political issue? Or was it true? It seems that this drama continues and we have to wait for the final scenario.

In the UK, by contrast, scientists are only allowed to use eggs rejected or left over from IVF treatment. A group in Newcastle, UK (2005) announced that they had cloned a very early stage embryo, but this took 36 leftover eggs and the team failed to isolate any stem cells from the embryo. Hwang's team found that when the eggs used come from donors under 30, an average of only 14 eggs were needed to generate a cell line, a 16-fold improvement in efficiency from only a year ago. He has also reduced the use of animal "feeder cells" to nourish the developing embryos, making it less likely that the stem cells will become infected with viruses or prion diseases. When it comes to cloning techniques, Hwang's laboratory is now way ahead of the field, says stem cell biologist Stephen Minger of King's College London, who recently visited Korea. "There is a good chance that the US will be left behind," he says. And really, the wind came from the other side when after Dr. Hwang withdraw his discovery as not having meritory values, Dr. Stojkovic (9-)from New Castle (now in Serbia, Leskovac) has shown that analysis of arrested embryos demonstrated that these embryos express pluripotency marker genes such OCT4, NANOG, and REX1. Derived hESC lines also expressed specific pluripotency markers (TRA-1-60, TRA-1-81, SSEA4, alkaline phosphatase, OCT4, NANOG, TERT, and REX1) and differentiated under *in vitro* and in vivo conditions into derivatives of all three germ layers [7]. All of the new lines, including lines derived from late arrested embryos, have had normal karyotypes [7]. These results demonstrate that arrested embryos are additional valuable resources to surplus and donated developing embryos, and should be used to study early human development or derive pluripotent hESC [7]. The line of work of this researcher and his groups is actually the first one which has clearly and with no doubts with regards to reproducibility, demonstrated the possibility of establishing embryonic human cell line. The use of ESC in therapy of different diseases is more problematic then the story that precedes their establishment. They are actually allogeneic transplants which need immunosuppression or in vitro intervention called stem cell genetic (therapeutic) cloning, where embryonal cell is fused into hybrid with the nucleus of chosen adult cell in order to continue self-renewal and repair the desired tissue line or organ (nuclear gene transfer technique) (Fig. 3.1).

This is a critical issue from both scientific and clinical point of view, given that the concept of VSELs (very small embryonic like adult, non-hematopoietic stem cells) have been recently discovered, and proved by Dr, Ratjczak's group [6–8, 10–13]. This emerging new concept raises the questions whether these cells should be used at all, if VSELs can already replace them, successfully? Not only that, but quite a distinct CD34- population of mesenchymal stem cells (MSCs) has been isolated from adult tissues, including bone marrow, and defined phenotypically, and functionally as a distinguished category of adult stem cells with respect to hematopoietic stem cells and VSELs.

What is the best candidate for regenerative therapy in humans, then? This requires a lot of further work and methodological advances, and will make the field of stem

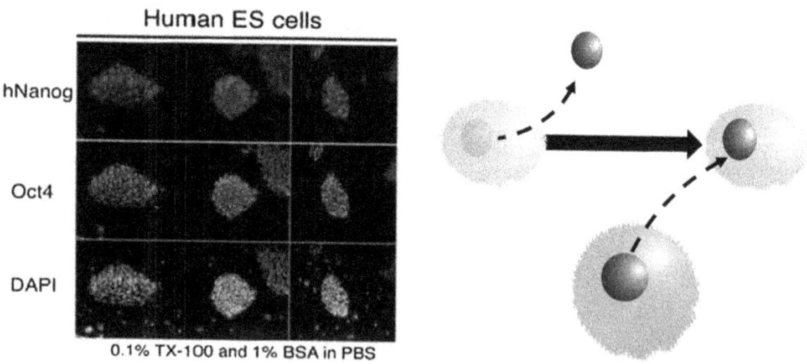

Fig. 3.1 Embryonic stem-cells: markers and therapeutic cloning

cell therapy more intriguing and closer to clearer ideas in optimizing patterns for different application (clinical) scenarios. However, the staining methods with *fluorescent labeling* of phenotypic surface molecules and *Flow Cytometry* detection of phenotypic and later on functional markers, were the significant breakthrough in identification of the stem cell sources and sole patterns: the basis for development of TE.

State of the Art

What are Stem Cells in Essence and What is Steamness?

Stem cells are the key subset of cells in the body functioning as ancestor cells to produce a variety of types of functionally specialized mature cells (differentiation) in a given tissue, while at the same time maintaining the capacity to continuously divide and reproduce themselves (self-renewal) [1]. This self-renewal process is controlled by intrinsic genetic pathways that are subject to regulation by extrinsic signals from the microenvironment in which stem cells reside [1, 9]. Stem cells play essential roles ranging from embryonic development and organogenesis (embryonic and fetal stem cells) to tissue homeostasis and regeneration (adult stem cells). Stem cell development is a complex process in which a precise balance is maintained among different cell events including self-renewal, differentiation, apoptosis (programmed cell death), and migration. Loss of this balance tends to lead to uncontrolled cell growth/death, thereby developing into a variety of diseases including tissue defects or cancer [9, 22]. Stem cell ageing involves a slow deterioration of tissue function, including an elimination of new growth, and decreased capacity for repair. Aging is also associated with increased cancer incidence in all tissues that contain stem cells [2]. These observations suggest a link between aging and stem cell function because stem cells drive growth and regeneration in most tissues, and because many cancers are thought to arise from the transformation of stem cells [2, 3]. One possibility is that much of age-related morbidity in mammals is determined by the influence of aging on stem cell function. It is found that stem cells from the hematopoietic and nervous systems undergo strikingly conserved changes in their properties as they age [2, 3]. The testing of the hypothesis that there are conserved changes in gene expression within stem cells that regulate these age-related changes in function is going on. One can hypothesize that stem cell aging is influenced by genes that regulate the proliferative activity of stem cells during development, as well as by genes that protect stem cells from the wear and tear of adult life. If we can identify these genes we might better understand the aging process. During development, stem cells divide and produce more specialized cells. Stem cells are also present in the adult in far lesser numbers, then in embryo, fetus or children. The role of adult stem cells (also called somatic stem cells) is believed to be replacement of damaged and injured tissue. Observed in continually-replenished cells such as blood cells [4–8] cells of adipose tissues [8] olfactory lining epithelial cells [8], amniotic cells [8] and skin cells, stem cells have recently been found in neural tissue, as well [6–8, 10].

Organ regeneration has long been believed to be through organ-specific and tissue-specific stem cells. Hematopoietic stem cells (HCS) were believed to replenish blood cells, stem cells of the gut to replace cells of the gut and so on. Recently, using cell lineage tracking [10], stem cells from one organ have been discovered that divide to form cells of another organ. Hematopoietic stem cells can give rise to liver, brain and kidney cells [10–16]. This plasticity of adult stem cells has been observed not only under experimental conditions, but also in people who have received bone marrow transplants [17, 18]. Tissue regeneration is achieved by two mechanisms: (1) Circulating stem cells divide and differentiate under appropriate signaling by cytokines and growth factors, e.g. blood cells; and (2) Differentiated cells which are capable of division can also self-repair (e.g. hepatocytes, endothelial cells, smooth muscle cells, keratinocytes and fibroblasts). These fully differentiated cells are limited to local repair. For more extensive repair, stem cells are maintained in the quiescent state, and can then be activated and mobilized to the required site [18, 19]. The diagram of stem-cell self-renewal and differentiation is given in Fig. 3.2.

For wound healing in the skin, epidermal stem cells and bone-marrow progenitor cells both contribute [23]. Thus, it is likely that organ-specific progenitors and hematopoietic stem cells are involved in repair, even for other organ repair. In summary, stem cells could be described as:

- Foundation cells for every organ, tissue and cell in the body
- A "blank microchip" that can ultimately be programmed to perform any number of specialized tasks
- Undifferentiated "blank" cells that do not yet have a specific function
- Self-sustaining and capable of replicating themselves for long periods of time
- Under proper conditions, begin to develop into specialized tissues and organs

These unique characteristics make stem cells very promising potential for supplying cells and tissues instead of organs in a spectrum of devastating diseases from

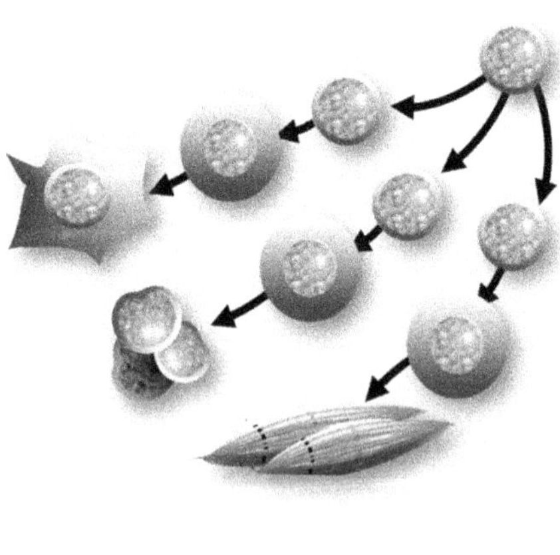

Fig. 3.2 Diagram of stem-cell self-renewal and differentiation

diabetes type1 to stroke, spinal cord injuries, and myocardial infarction. In the situation when the number of people needing organ and tissue transplants exceed the number of donated organs and tissues, this is the promise and hope, which deserves a deep and serious consideration. However, despite rapidly growing knowledge on adult stem cell sources, features and use, there are still some fundamental remaining questions regarding them that include: Does only one common type of stem cell migrate to different organs and repair tissue or are there multiple types of stem cells? Does every organ have stem cells (some of which have not yet been discovered)? Are the stem cells programmed to divide a finite number of times or do they have unlimited cell proliferation capacity?

Types of Stem Cells

A. According to their functionality, stem cells can be divided in two categories: normal and cancer stem cells.

1. *Normal stem cells* are immature cells that can replicate, or renew them, and are able to differentiate, or mature into all the cells that an organism or particular organ system needs. In other words, they possess a kind of immortality marked as self-renewal because these cells can divide indefinitely to produce more copies of them. Each stem cell is unspecialized, but it can produce progeny that mature into the various cell types of, say, the brain or the immune system. Once this maturation occurs, these adult stem cell heirs may divide rapidly but only a limited number of times [1, 9, 22]. The primary purpose of **adult stem cells** is healing. Finding out how adult stem cells store information and transform themselves into other cells with different properties is a fascinating topic for exploration. Stem cells are so named because cells are derived from a main stem or mother set of cells. This is similar to a tree trunk that provides the stem from which other cells grow and branch out into other types of cells.

2. *Cancer stem cells*. Finding cancers' stem cells is a rapidly growing area of research. These cancer-causing cells, which make up a tiny fraction of cells within tumors, have properties similar to those of stem cells. Cancer stem cells make up only a tiny number of the total cancer cells in a leukemia patient, which makes the cells next to impossible to find. Therefore, it seems that promise of this line of research can only be realized, by studying adult stem cells as well as embryonic stem cells (ES). The latter are still ethical problem and therefore substantially controversial because an early embryo is destroyed when researchers remove stem cells from it. An alternative is to take the stem cells from embryos that carry a genetic defect for specific diseases. Are cancer cells transformed normal stem cells? Researchers have traditionally thought of cancer as a collection of cells, all growing exponentially. According to the new research, conventional cancer therapies do an effective job killing the majority of cells within the tumor, but they may miss cancer stem cells. As a result, cancers often recur [2]. Even hematologic and some non-hematologic malignancies treated by autologous stem cell transplant and high dose chemotherapy,

have shown that regardless of survival rate of some cancers, the final outcome is death, due to recurrence of cancer. The reason is (among others) in the fact that clinicians are injecting also cancer cells with healthy stem cells during re-infusion after apheresis collection, which accumulate and renew with a time to the critical level causing relapse or death. Ontogeny (development of an organism) and oncology (cancer development) share many common features. From the 1870s the connection between development and cancer has been reported for various types of cancers. Existence of "cancer stem cells" with aberrant cell division has also been reported more recently. The connection between cancer and development is clearly evident in special type of tumors known as teratocarcinomas (from Greek *teratos* which means *miracle*). As early as 1862, Virchow discovered that the germ cell tumor teratocarcinoma is made up of embryonic cells [24]. In 1970, Stevens derived embryonic carcinoma cells from teratocarcinoma (a spontaneous tumor of germ cells that resembles development gone awry) [25]. This tumor may contain several types of epithelia: areas of bone, cartilage, muscle, fat, hair, yolk sac, and placenta. These specialized tissues are often adjacent to an area of rapidly dividing unspecialized cells. The teratocarcinomas are able to differentiate into normal mature cells when transplanted into another animal. This alternation between developmental and tumor cells status demonstrates how closely development and cancer are related. The present-day challenge is to decode the common molecular mechanism and genes involved in self-renewal for cancer cells and stem cells.

Common features of normal adult stem cells

B. Normal stem cells, with respect to their origin, further can be classified as: embryonic, fetal, cord blood and adult stem cells [1, 14, 15].

Self-regeneration is the ability of any kind of stem cells to divide and produce more stem cells. During early development, the cell division is symmetrical i.e. each cell divides to give rise to daughter cells each with the same potential. Later in development, the cell divides asymmetrically with one of the daughter cells produced also a stem cell and the other a more differentiated cell (Fig 3.2). Here we meet the problem with cultivation of adult stem cells since most of the media applied, induce early differentiation. Therefore, they were expanded either by cloning, transfer through NOD/SCID mice, or adoptive humanized mouse model, which all have their advantages and disadvantages, and still do not satisfy the optimal needs for expansion and later on- therapeutical use of adult stem cells [22].

For that reason, the mobilization of stem cells from intact bone marrow emerged as an idea to replace the *in vitro* manipulation and do the job *in vivo*. Unfortunately, some individuals are poor mobilizers and some of them do not respond to mobilizers at all [14]. And this is the limitation of otherwise splendidly designed clinical approach. Therefore, a lot of basic research is necessary to expand this field of stem cell application and with the better knowledge of the self-renewal control mechanism, it will largely lead to efficient improvement, since researchers will be able to control it and use the principals for better tuned expansion.

Potential Use of Stem Cells: New Concepts and Trials

What are the Potential Uses of Adult Human Stem Cells in General Tissues?

The experimental and clinical trials have shown both in animal models and humans the neovascularization and myocardial tissue repair through transdifferentiation into myocardiocites, or some other mechanism. Repair of damaged organ/tissue (myocardial, neuronal, liver, cartilage, bone, etc.) is shown mostly in animal models. Maybe the most illustrative of all is the bunch of experimental data suggesting the great potential for stem cell differentiation and homing into damaged tissues either when mobilized or injected into the tissue of interest after apheresis or BM puncture, with or without cryopreservation [26–46]. Although the adult stem cell regenerative therapy after BM aspiration and apheresis injection into coronary arteries is becoming more and more successful [27, 29, 47] the most evident success of mesenchymal stem cell (MSC) treatment at regenerative therapy level in clinical arena is seen so far in *osteogenesis imperfecta* where the results with diseased children are amazing in terms that they are dramatically visible and easily reproducible [48]. Yet, due to the obstacles already mentioned above, this is not the case with nervous system regenerative treatment, especially in humans.

Organogenesis from Adult Stem Cells and Problems with Different Tissues

How do a small number of stem cells give rise to a complex three dimensional tissue with different types of mature cells in different locations? This is the most fundamental question in organogenesis. The hematopoietic and nervous systems employ very different strategies for generating diversity from stem cells. The hematopoietic system assiduously avoids regional specialization by stem cells. Hematopoietic stem cells are distributed in different hematopoietic compartments throughout the body during fetal and adult life, and yet these spatially distinct stem cells do not exhibit intrinsic differences in the types of cells they generate [12]. This contrasts with the nervous system, where even small differences in position are associated with the acquisition of different fates by stem cells.

While local environmental differences play an important role in this generation of "neural diversity," we must accept that intrinsic differences between stem cells are also critical. Part of the reason why different types of cells are generated in different regions of the nervous system is that intrinsically different types of stem cells are present in different regions of the nervous system. To understand the molecular basis for the regional patterning of neural stem cell function, we are now studying how these differences are encoded.

Therapeutic Implications for TCSCs as a New Concept

To prove the stem-cells derived from bone marrow (BM) and peripheral blood, including hematopoietic stem cells, are indeed transformed into solid-organ specific cells, several conditions must be met:

1. The origin of the exogenous cell integrated into solid-organ time must be documented by cell marking, preferably at the single-cell level
2. Cell should be processed with a minimum of "ex vivo" manipulation (e.g. culturing) which may make them more susceptible to crossing lineages.
3. The exogenous cells must be shown to have become an integral morphologic part of the newly acquired tissue.
4. Transformed cells must be shown to have acquired the function of the particular organ into which it has been integrated both by expressing organ-specific proteins and by showing specific organ function.

Organ/Tissue specific niche (like in BM, liver, etc.)—exists as a deposit (storage) of the adult stem cells in a specific location (Fig. 3.3). These cells are circulating in a very low number in the blood. Accumulating evidence suggests that stem cells may also actively migrate/circulate in the postnatal period of life. Stem cell trafficking /circulation may be one of the crucial mechanisms that maintains the pool of stem cells dispersed in stem cell niches of the same tissue, that are spread throughout different anatomical areas of the body. This phenomenon is very well described for HSC, but other, already tissue committed stem cells (TCSC) (for example, endothelial, skeletal muscle, skeletal or neural stem cells) are probably circulating as well.

BM is the home of migrating stem cells with not only hematopoietic stem cells within their niches, but also a small number of TCSC, which might be the reason why many authors think that HSC may transdifferentiate, although we do not have a direct proof for that. They might have plasticity, but not necessarily the "transdifferentional"

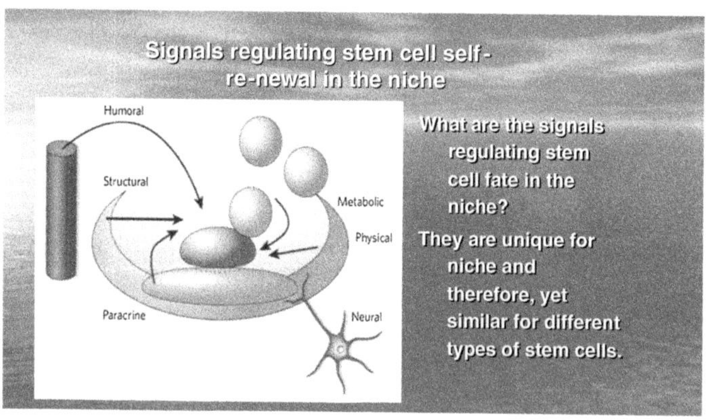

Fig. 3.3 Niche-the microenvironment of stem cells

potential [49–55]. What is differentiated in the tissue of injection might be TCSC characteristic for that tissue. It has been shown that number of these cells is decreased with ageing (long living and short living mice and humans). It would be interesting to identify genes that are responsible for tissue distribution/expansion of TCSC. These genes could be involved in controlling the life span of the mammals. Therefore, BM stem cells are a heterogeneous population of cells with HSC and TCSC, the morphological and functional characteristics of which are different from HSC. Their number among BM MNC is very low (1 cell per 1000–10000 BM MNC) within young mammals and might play a role in small injuries [49, 50].

In severe injuries however, like heart infarct or stroke they have no possibility to reveal their full therapeutic potential. The allocation of these cells to the damaged areas depends on homing signals that maybe inefficient in the presence of some other cytokines or proteolytic enzymes that are released from damaged tissue-associated leukocytes and macrophages. We can envision, for example that metallo-proteinases released from inflammatory cells may degrade SDF-1 locally, and thus perturb homing of CXCR4 + TCSC. There is possibility that these cells while "trapped" in BM are still in: "dormant" stage-not fully functional and need the appropriate activation signals by unknown factors [49–54]. These cells also, at least in some cases could be attracted to the inflammatory areas, and if not properly incorporated into the damaged tissue they may transform and initiate tumor growth. In summary, between the pool of tissue committed stem cells, there are probably those already committed to trans-differentiate into neural cells, or cells of tissues and organs other ten neural, but we still do not have the control over their tracking, homing and finally regenerative capacity in the given tissue, which is a fundamental prerequisite for successful regenerative therapy (Fig. 3.4).

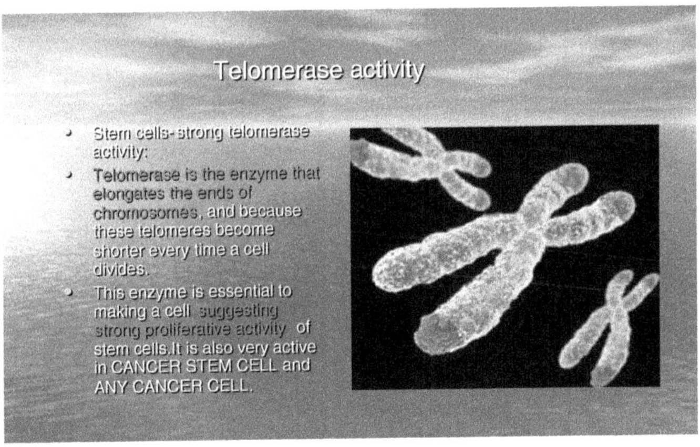

Fig. 3.4 Telomerase activity is very high in stem cells

The Concept of VSEL

In a discovery that has the potential to change the face of stem cell research, a University of Louisville scientist has identified cells in the adult body that seem to behave like embryonic stem cells [6–8]. The cells, drawn from adult bone marrow, look like embryonic stem cells and appear to mimic their ability to multiply and develop into other kinds of cells. The finding, presented the first time at the 47th Annual Meeting of the American Society of Hematology (ASH) in Atlanta, was announced December 12 at the society's news conference [6]. A study by Ratajczak's team published in 2005 year in the journal "Leukemia" was the first to identify a type of stem cell in adult bone marrow that acts differently than other marrow stem cells. The newly-identified cells, called "very small embryonic-like" (VSEL) stem cells, have the same ultrastructure and protein markers as embryonic stem cells [8]. Ratajczak and several other researchers from University of Louisville in the presentation at the ASH meeting showed that VSEL stem cells mobilize into the bloodstream to help repair damaged tissue following a stroke [56]. In further research advance, Ratajczak's team also has grown VSEL cells in a lab and has stimulated them to change into nerve, heart and pancreas cells. The difference in markers between HSC and VSELs in mouse are shown in Fig. 3.5, while the differences in ultrastructure are shown in Fig. 3.6.

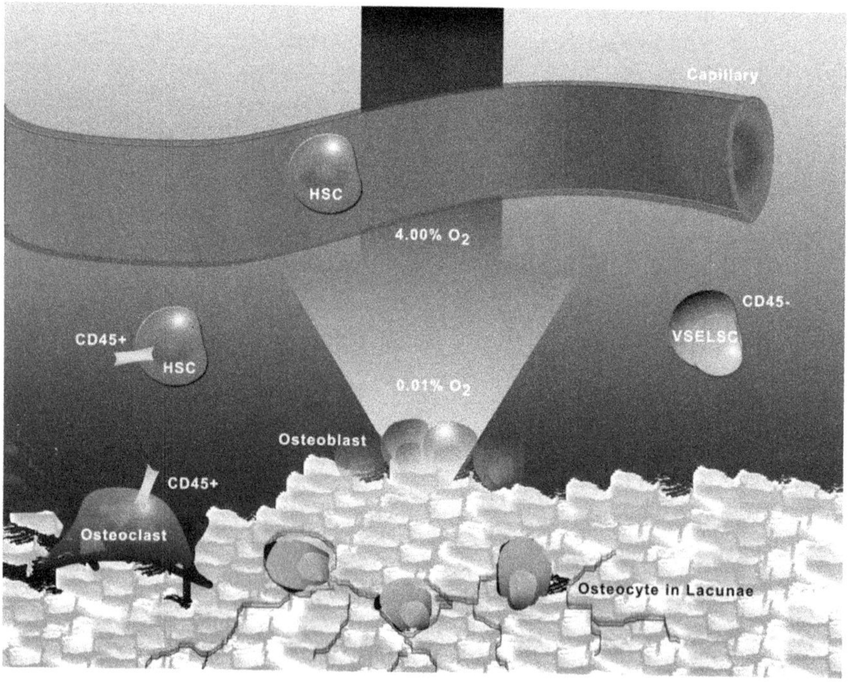

Fig. 3.5 (1 and 2) Differences in phenotypes (external and internal markers) between HSC and VSEL from mouse bone marrow

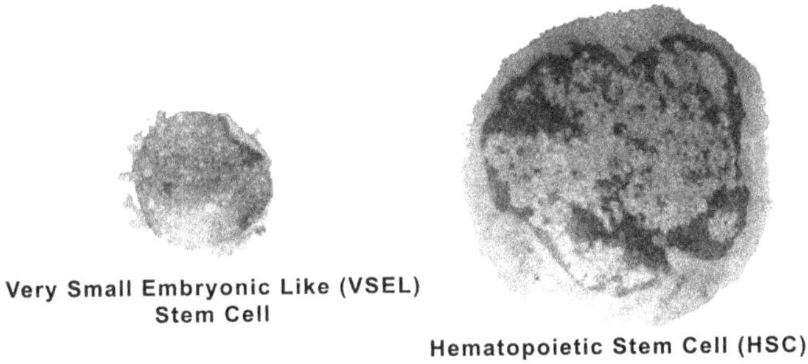

Fig. 3.6 Ultrastructural and phenotypic differences between mouse VSEL and HSC

Along with this new concept, there is a premise that in regenerative therapy done before, with hematopoietic stem cells (considered to have plasticity and multipotency) the VSELs were "contaminants" that actually contributed to positive regenerative clinical outcome, since they have those capabilities. This is an interesting concept which should be seriously considered in humans. But, since VSELs have been found in human cord blood and bone marrow [55], they seem to be of a critical importance for consideration of stem cell transplant choice based upon the phenotype and number of stem cells aimed to be transplanted within a given clinical scenario.

The concept of Mesenchymal Stem-Cell

Many human tissues are the source of stem cells responsible for tissue development and regeneration. Beside BM, (*bone marrow stromal stem cells*, BMSCs), currently it is considered that dental pulp is practically the most approachable and the most important source of adult mesenchymal stem cells [17, 18]. Within the last eight years, several populations of stem cells from dental pulp were isolated and characterized: (1) (*dental pulp stem cells*-DPSCs), (2) (*stem cells from human exfoliated decidual teeth*, SHEDs) and (3) (*immature dental pulp cells*, IDPCs) [17, 18]. These cells are of the ectomesenchymal origin, located in perivascular niche, highly proliferative, clonogenic, multipotent and similar to BMSCs (Table 3.1).

In *in vitro* conditions, they can differentiate with certain intercellular differences toward odontoblasts, hondrocytes, osteoblasts, adipocytes, neurons/glial cells, smooth and sceletal muscle cells. In *in vivo*, conditions, after implantation, they show different potential for dentine formation, as well as osteogenesis; after transplantation in mouse with compromised immune system, they make good grafts in different tissues and are capable of migrating into the brain, where they survive a certain time while reaching neurogenic phenotype. DPSCs have immunomodulatory effect , as they can be involved into immune response during infection of dental pulpe by NF-kB activation, and by inhibiting T-lymphocyte proliferation, suggesting their immunosuppressive effect [18]. The future research should give us the complex data on the molecular and functional characteristics of dental pulp stem cells, as well as differences between different populations of these cells. Such research would fundamentally contribute to the better knowledge on the dental pulp stem cells, which is necessary due to their potential clinical application in *in vivo* cell transplantation,

Table 3.1 Expression of protein or gene profiles in some dental stem cells in *in vitro* cultivation and relationship toward BMSC

Antigen	DPSC	SHED	PDLSC	BMSC
CD14	–	–	–	–
CD34	–	–	–	–
CD44	++	++	++	++
CD45	–	–	–	–
CD106	+	+/–	+/–	++
CD146	++/+/–	++/+/–	++/+/–	++/+/–
3G5	+/–	+/–	+/–	+/–
Stro-1	++/+/–	++/+/–	++/+/–	++/+/–
α-smooth muscle actin	++/–	++/–	++/–	++/+/–
Colagen type-I	++	++	++	++
Colagen type-III	++/+	++/+/–	++/+/–	++/+
Alkaline phosphatase	++/+/–	++/+/–	++/+/	++/+/
Osteocalcin	++/+	++/+/–	++/–	+/–
Osteonectin	++/+	++/+	++/+	++/+
Osteopontin	+/–	+/–	+/–	+/–
Sialoprotein of the bone	–	–	–	–
Skleraksis	+	+	++	+
Sialophosphoprotein of the dentine	–	–	–	–

DPSC Dental pulp stem cells, *SHED* stem cells from human exfoliated decidual teeth, *PDLSC* periodontal ligament stem cells, (++) strong expression, (+) weak expression, (–) negative, (/) subpopulation

tissue engineering, and gene therapy (*in vivo* and ex vivo). Actually, by the isolation of IDPCs, which are the most primitive, but also the most plastic, (similar to embryonic stem cells), they are opening the new perspectives in a potential therapeutic application of these cells not only in regeneration of dentine, but also the regeneration of periodontal tissue and bone-junctional tissue of craniofacial region, as well as in the therapy of neurotrauma, myocardial infarction and connective tissue damage (Figs. 3.7, 3.8).

Mobilization as a New Non-invasive Therapeutical Concept and New Medical Technology Approach

The classification of patients into"good" or "poor" mobilizers is based on CD34+ cell count in their peripheral blood (PB) after granulocyte-colony-stimulating factor (G-CSF) injection. CD34+ cells mobilized into peripheral blood (PB) are considered a more convenient source of hematopoietic stem and progenitor cells than their bone marrow (BM) counterparts, in autologous transplantation protocols. Beside going through a less invasive collection procedure than BM aspiration, leukapheresed CD34+ cell collections ensure a rapid hematologic recovery as a function of trans-

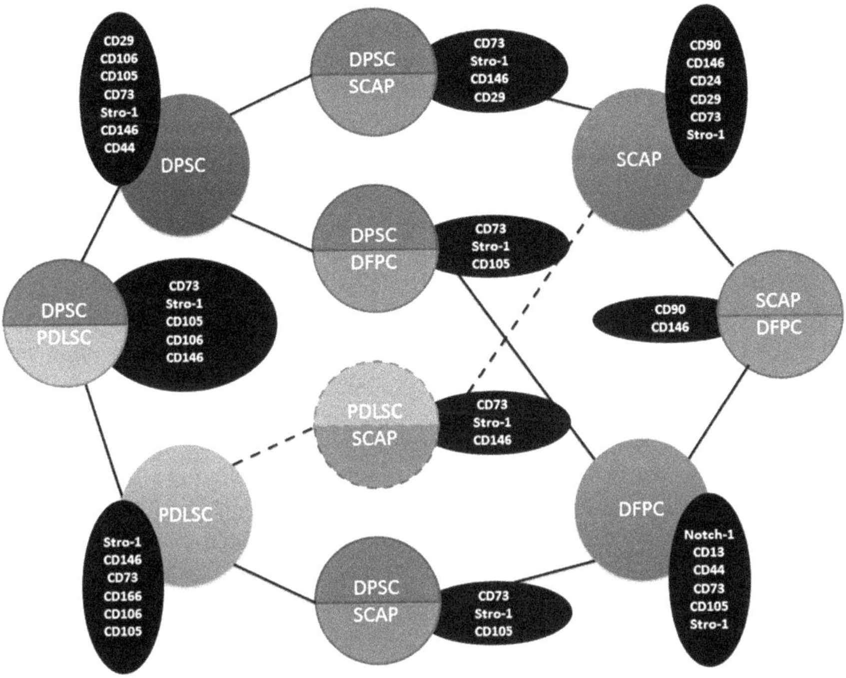

Fig. 3.7 The most important superficial cellular markers of dental pulp stem cell according to Morsczeck et al. Clin Oral Invest 2008; 12:113–118 (19). DPSC dental pulp stem cell, DFPC dental follicular precursor cell, SCAP stem cell of apical papilla, PDLSC periodontal ligament stem cell

Fig. 3.8 Mesenchymal stem cells (with courtesy of Prof. Dr. Vera Todorovic)

planted dose of these cells, and their cell cycle status. Patients unable to mobilize sufficient number of CD34+ cells for efficient transplantation procedure are designated as poor mobilizers. Whereas numerous studies were dedicated to defining predictive factors for successful mobilization, only a few characterized the phenotype of mobilized CD34+ in good versus poor mobilizers and none explored the functional and metabolic properties of mobilized cells in these two groups of patients.

Thus, Ivanovic et al. [35] hypothesized that, apart from their mobilization from marrow to the blood, the response to G-CSF of CD34+ cells also includes activation of proliferation, metabolic activity, and proliferative capacity. In this study, mobilized PB CD34+ cells purified from samples obtained by cytapheresis of multiple myeloma or non-Hodgkin's lymphoma patients of both good (>50 CD34+ cells/mL) and poor (<50 CD34+ cells/mL) mobilizers, were studied. The initial cell cycle state of CD34+ cells after selection and their kinetics of activation (exit from G0 phase) during ex vivo culture were analyzed. Their proliferative capacity was estimated on the basis of ex vivo generation of total cells, CD34+ cells, and colony-forming cells (CFCs), in a standardized expansion culture [11–19]. Indirect insight in metabolic activity was obtained on the basis of their survival (viability and apoptosis follow-up) during the 7-day-long conservation in hypothermia (4 °C) in the air or in atmosphere containing 3 % O_2/6 % CO_2. The results have shown that CD34+ cells obtained from good mobilizers were in lower proportion in the G0 phase, their activation in a cytokine-stimulated culture was accelerated, and they exhibited a lower ex vivo expansion efficiency than those from poor mobilizers (). The resistance to hypothermia of good mobilizers' CD34+ cells is impaired. The inevitable conclusion was that a good response to G-CSF mobilization treatment is associated with a higher degree of proliferative and metabolic activation of mobilized CD34+ cells with a decrease in their expansion capacity (Fig. 3.9).

Unlike other mobilizing agents requiring multi-day mobilization, AMD3100 enables mobilized donors to undergo mobilization and apheresis on the same day. The combination of excellent therapeutic benefits as well as ease of use indicates that AMD3100 could be a powerful tool to ameliorate tissue ischemia in the diabetic environment.

Factor (G-CSF) decreases expression of adhesive molecules in a population of BM CD34+ cells and intensifies the entry in the circulation of CD34+ cells in G0/G1 phases2 prepared for BM homing and reactivation. The major axis responsible for homing of PB progenitor cells seems to be CXCR4/SDF-1/HIF1 (Fig. 3.10).

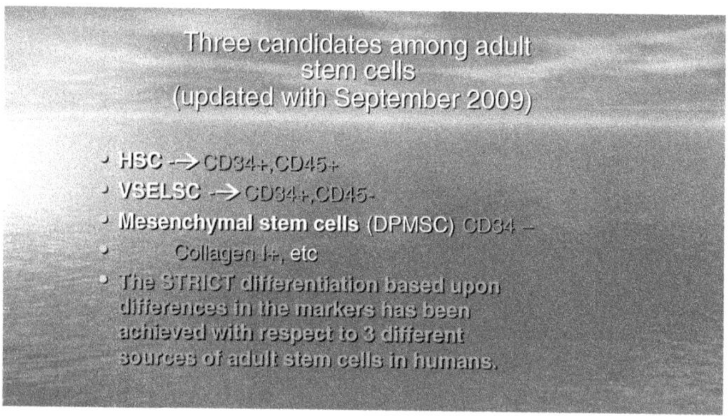

Fig. 3.9 Three distinct types of adult stem cells that can potentially be used in TE

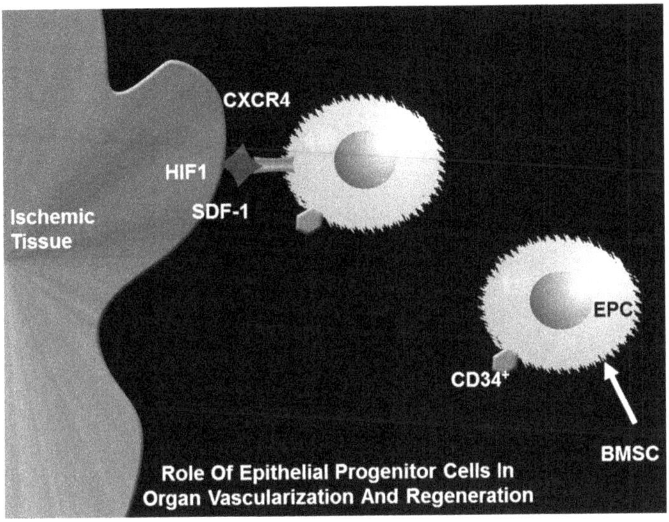

Fig. 3.10 The molecular basis of stem cell homing into hypoxic (damaged) tissues

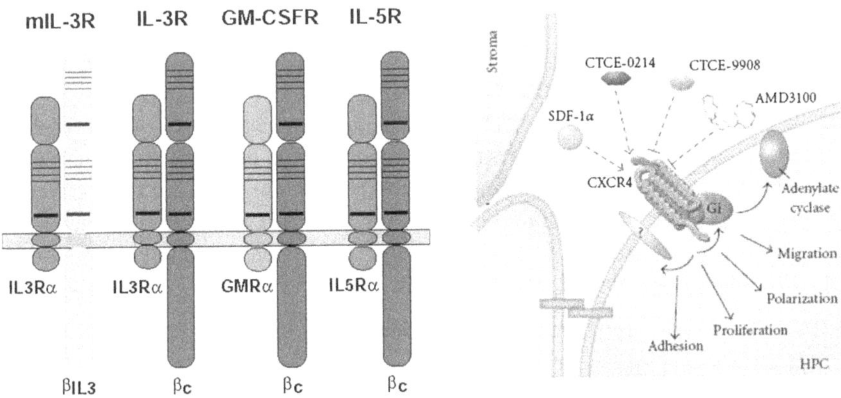

Fig. 3.11 Mobilizing agents and distinction between their mechanism of action

Very late adhesion molecule-4 (VLA-4) is another molecule identified as the receptor primarily responsible for cell trafficking expressed in all mononuclear hematopoietic cells that also acts as a co-stimulatory molecule influencing cell activation and differentiation. VLA-4 and leukocyte function-associated molecule-1 are expressed less in poor than in good mobilizers' CD34+ cells, while VLA-4 alone is expressed less in the G0 phase of cell cycle.

Altogether these data suggest that differences between poor and good mobilizers' CD34+ cells involve their trafficking capacity, but also their cell cycle status and activation. Still, one should keep in mind that the progenitors and stem cells of different classes, belonging to CD34+ population, respond *in vitro* to G-CSF stimulation by increased proliferation and/or differentiation (Figs. 3.11, 3.12).

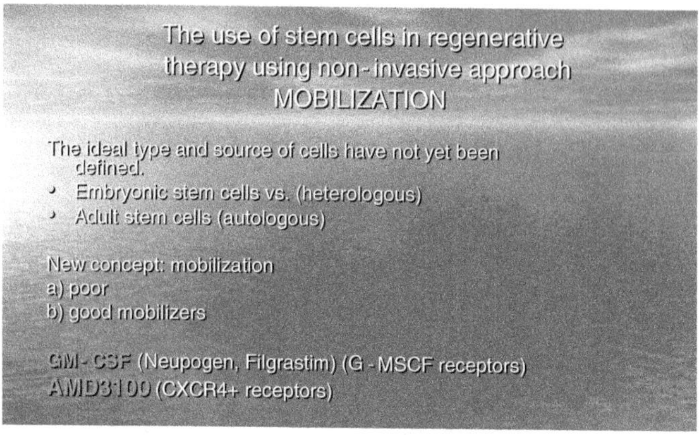

Fig. 3.12 Mechanism of action of growth factor and AMD3100

What are the Results of Stem Cell-Therapy Within Tissues or the TE Basics?

(*a*) *Neuronal*

The idea behind stem cell therapy is to isolate such cells, multiply them *in vitro* and then use them at optimal number and differentiation level to successfully replace damaged tissue. This is exactly as is done to repair skin in burns victims. Adult stem cells offer hope for cell therapy to treat diseases in the future because ethical issues do not impede their use. In addition, if the patient's own cells are used, immunological compatibility is not an issue. However, ES cells have been found to be superior for both differentiation potential and ability to divide in culture.

Two concepts are useful to describe characteristics of adult stem cells:

Plasticity is a newly recognized ability of stem cells to expand their potential beyond the tissue from which they are derived. For example, dental pulp stem cells develop into tissue of the teeth but can also develop into neural tissue [17, 18]. That is capacity of stem cells to transdifferentiate into other types of cells and it is different for distinct stem cell types.

Transdifferentiation is the direct conversion of one cell type to another [11], e.g. transdifferentiation of pancreatic cells into hepatic cells and vice versa has been reported in both animals and humans as has the transdifferentiation of blood cells into brain cells and vice versa [11]. This can be attributed to the very well documented ultrastructure of deepest adult stem cell ancestor found so far, VSEL, forming embryonic bodies, the phenomenon that is found only in embryonic cells, meaning that they contain derivatives of all the three primary cell layers—mesoderm, ectoderm and endoderm. Intercellular liaisons and addition of the substances that support differentiation (such as retinoic acid, hexametilen-disacetanide and methylsulphoxide) are inducing differentiation in all three primary cell layers. In general, brain is so complex not only in different cell types with different functions, but in integral brain cell circuits leading to a certain function, so that it requires a specially developed strategy, probably much complex then heart stem cell regenerative therapy, or some other. Therefore, we believe the results vary dependent on experimental settings, animal models used and human studies, which are proportionally rare and as yet not analyzed in details. It is extremely important to emphasize that within the spectrum of neurodegenerative diseases, a different spectrum of cell types is affected; therefore, different types of neurons are required for the replacement. Consequently, the strategy for each particular neurological disorder or injury must be elaborated according to specific criteria with respect to the location (central or peripheral), type of damaged tissues (neurons or glial cells) and degree of differentiation of the adult stem cells used for particular damage (stem cells in self-renewal stage, early or late progenitors). It is also of great importance to know and decide how to manipulate the stem cell application (administration) in order to get the best therapeutical outcome. All of these prerequisites must be fulfilled when designing the strategy for particular neural regenerative adult stem cell approach. In general, brain is so complex not only in different cell types with different functions, but in INTEGRAL BRAIN CELL CIRQUITS leading to a certain function, so that it requires a specially developed strategy, probably much complex then heart stem cell therapy. The results vary dependent on experimental settings, animal models used and human studies, which are rare and as yet not analyzed in details.

"Experimental" denotes data drawn from non-human settings, BMT bone marrow transplantation. It is important to mention that within the spectrum of neurodegenerative diseases, a different spectrum of cell types is affected; therefore, different types of neurons are required for the replacement. In stroke, occlusion of a cerebral artery leads to focal ischemia in a restricted CNS region. Many different types of neurons and glial cells degenerate in stroke. It has not yet been convincingly demonstrated that neuronal replacement induces symptomatic relief in individuals who have suffered strokes. In the only reported clinical trial, persons with stroke affected basal ganglia received implants of neurons generated from the human NT-2 teratocarcinoma cell line into the infracted area. Whether the new neurons formed after stroke are functional, is unknown. There is no substantial new neuron formation in the cerebral cortex after stroke (Table 3.2).

Recent findings in rodents suggest an alternative approach to cell therapy in stroke based upon self-repair:

Citation: *Journal of Neuroscience Research*, Feb. 2007, "Manipulation of proliferation and differentiation of human bone marrow derived neural stem cells *in vitro* and *in vivo*".

Stem cells taken from adult human bone marrow have been manipulated by scientists at the Maxine Dunitz Neurosurgical Institute at Cedars-Sinai Medical Center to generate aggregates of cells called spheres that are similar to those derived from neural stem cells of the brain. In addition, the bone marrow-derived stem cells, which could be differentiated into neurons and other cells making up the central nervous system, spread far and wide and behaved like neural stem cells when transplanted into the brain tissue of chicken embryos. Results of the experiments, described in

Table 3.2 Application of stem-cell regenerative therapy in neurological diseases: experimental and clinical data

Disease category	Model	Stem-cell source	Route of cell application	Outcome	Study
Neurodegenerative diseases	Experimental BMT	BM cells	Intraperitoneal	Generation of cells expressing neuronal markers	*Mezey et al. (2003)*
	Experimental BMT	BM cells	Intravenous	Generation of cells expressing neuronal markers	*Brazelton et al. (2003*
	Clinical BMT (allogeneic)	BM cells	Intravenous	Generation of cells expressing neuronal markers	*Mezey et al. (2003) (Y-chromosome determined by FISH on female samples)*
	Clinical BMT (allogeneic)	BM cells	Intravenous	Possible formation of Purkinje neurons	*Weimann et al. (2003)*
Middle cerebral artery occlusion (stroke)	Experimental cord blood transplantation	Stem-cells derived from umbilical cord blood	Intravenous	Improved functional recovery from neurological deficit	*Chen et al. (2005)*
	Clinical Mesenchymal BMSC autologous transplant	MSCs transplantation	Intravenous	Improved functional recovery	*Bang et al. (2005)*
	Experimental Mice B16, 129	Neural TCSCs	*In vitro* mobilization chemoattraction experiment	Chemoattraction of neural TCSCs to supernatant from damaged brain tissue	*Kucia/Ratajczak (2006)*

the February 2007 of the *Journal of Neuroscience Research*, support the concept of using bone marrow-derived stem cells to create therapies to treat brain tumors, strokes and neurodegenerative diseases. Progressing from the rat study to experiments with human cells and transplantation into mammal brain tissue, the research team continues to build a foundation for translating laboratory research into human clinical trials. The replacement of damaged brain cells with healthy cells cultured from stem cells is considered to potentially be a promising therapy for the treatment of stroke, neurodegenerative disorders and even brain tumors, but finding a reliable source for generating neural cells for transplantation has been a challenge. The use of embryonic and fetal tissue has raised ethical questions among some, and brings with it the possibility of immune rejection. And while neural stem cells can be taken from brain tissue, the removal of healthy tissue from a patient's brain introduces a new set of safety, practicality and ethical issues.

(b)Heart

In humans, the biological limitations to cardiac regenerative growth create both **a clinical imperative**—to offset cell death in acute ischemic injury and chronic heart failure—and **a clinical opportunity**; that is, for using cells, genes, and proteins to rescue cardiac muscle cell number, or in other ways promote more efficacious cardiac repair. Recent experimental studies and early-phase clinical trials lend credence to the visionary goal of enhancing cardiac repair as an achievable therapeutic target. Coronary heart disease is currently the principal cause of death in the United States. In 1997, 1.1 million Americans were diagnosed with acute myocardial infarction (MI), and 800,000 patients underwent coronary revascularization. In patients with MI, scar tissue develops in the area of infarction resulting in a decrease in cardiac contractility. This damage is irreversible and can result in heart failure since cardiac cells can not repair themselves.

During stem cell infusion due to organ damage with the goal to repair it, injury to a target organ is sensed by distant stem cells, which migrate to the site of damage and undergo alternate stem cell differentiation [10, 11]. These events promote structural and functional repair. This high degree of stem cell plasticity led researchers to investigate if dead myocardium could be restored by transplanting bone marrow cells. Investigators have demonstrated that multipotent adult bone marrow hematopoeitic stem cells and mesenchymal stem cells can repopulate infarcted rodent myocardium and differentiate into both cardiomyocytes and new blood vessels. One of the first clinical studies done on the heart reported that autologous intracoronary mononuclear bone marrow cell transplantation is safe and appears to improve cardiac function and myocardial perfusion in patients after acute MI (n = 10) [11]. However, the authors concluded that further experimental studies, controlled prospective clinical trials, and variations of cell preparations are needed to determine the role of this new procedure for the treatment of patients after acute MI [11].

Based on the hematopoietic reconstitution, the team from Belgrade Medical Military School (Balint et al.) have analyzed their results of various SC-harvesting protocols with optimized cell source, collection time-point and processed blood volume, CD34-threshold dose, immature vs. mature CD34-subset ratio in harvest, as well as cryopreservation system applied [2–4, 9, 22]. In those studies, the use of large volume vs. conventional (repetitive) apheresis resulted in improved overall CD34$^+$ yield and elevated cell viability (7-AAD flow cytometric assay). They have also confirmed that the best survival rate of very primitive hematopoietic SCs (Marrow Repopulating Ability cells—MRA) was obtained when 10 % dimethyl-sulfoxide (DMSO) was combined with microprocessor-controlled freezing by compensation of released heat of fusion [9]. Finally, higher immature vs. mature CD34-subset ratio in harvest was correlated with rapid hematopoietic reconstitution and better marrow repopulation ability (long-term engraftment), as well as organ repair (regenerative potential) [4].

Protocols for Stem-Cell Therapy in AMI (Different Authors)

Heart failure—a severe deficiency in ventricular pump function—arises through a finite number of terminal effector mechanisms, regardless of the cause. These include: defects intrinsic to cardiac muscle cells' contractility due to altered expression or operation of calcium-cycling proteins, components of the sarcomere, and enzymes for cardiac energy production; defects extrinsic to cardiac muscle cells, such as interstitial fibrosis, affecting organ-level compliance; and myocyte loss, unmatched by myocyte replacement. Cardiac regeneration is robust for certain organisms such as the newt and zebrafish, in which total replacement can transpire even for an amputated limb, fin, or tail, via production of an undifferentiated cell mass called the blastema [1]. Such a degree of restorative growth might also be dependent on the retention of proliferative potential in a subset of adult cardiomyocytes [9] and is impossible in mammals under normal, unassisted biological circumstances. Several complementary strategies can be foreseen as potentially aiding this process: overriding cell-cycle checkpoints that constrain the reactive proliferation of ventricular myocytes [22]; supplementing the cytoprotective mechanisms that occur naturally, or inhibiting pro-death pathways [2, 3]; supplementing the angiogenic mechanisms that occur naturally using defined growth factors or vessel-forming cells [4, 5]; or providing exogenous cells as a surrogate or precursor for cardiac muscle itself [6–8].

Among these conceptual possibilities, cell implantation in various forms has been the first strategy to be translated from bench to bedside. The possibility of tissue repair by autologous adult progenitor cells—suggested by the auspicious findings in experimental studies of various cell sources—immediately captured the attention of clinicians confronted with the disabling, life-threatening circumstance of patients who suffer from heart failure in acute or chronic ischemic heart disease. The promise of cellular cardiomyogenesis and neovascularization, individually or in tandem, offered altogether novel opportunities for treatment, tailored to the underlying pathobiology.

Existing trials use intracoronary delivery routes (over-the-wire balloon catheters), intramuscular delivery via catheters (e.g., the NOGA system for electromechanical mapping), or direct injection during cardiac surgery. Not represented here are the theoretical potentials for systemic delivery, suggested by the homing of some cell types to infarcted myocardium, and strategies to mobilize endogenous cells from other tissue sites to the heart.

Mechanisms of action. Progenitor cells (EPC) may improve functional recovery of infarcted or failing myocardium by various potential mechanisms, including direct or indirect improvement of neovascularization. Paracrine factors released by progenitor cells may inhibit cardiac apoptosis, affect remodeling, or enhance endogenous repair (e.g., by tissue-resident progenitor cells). Differentiation into cardiomyocytes of both stem and EP-cells, may contribute to cardiac regeneration. The extent to which these different mechanisms are active may critically depend on the cell type and setting, such as acute or chronic injury.

Summary on the Protocols Used for Stem Cell Therapy and Myocardial Tissue Regeneration in AMI in Humans

Bone marrow is, at present, the most frequent source of cells used for clinical cardiac repair [11–13, 15]. It contains a complex assortment of progenitor cells, including HSCs; so-called side population (SP) cells, defined by their ability to expel a Hoechst dye, which account for most if not all long-term self-renewal [24] and reconstitute the full panoply of hematopoietic lineages after single-cell grafting [25]; mesenchymal stem cells or stromal cells [57]; and multipotential adult progenitor cells (MAPCs), a subset of mesenchymal stem cells (MSCs) [58]. Bone marrow is aspirated under local or general anesthesia, the entire mononuclear cell fraction is obtained (a heterogeneous mix of the above-mentioned cells), or specific subpopulations are purified, and isolated cells are injected into the heart without need of further ex vivo expansion. Expansion in cell culture could be desirable or essential, though, if defined but minute subpopulations prove to be advantageous [58].

Last, **peripheral blood-derived progenitor cells** are used both for clinical cardiac repair [12] and for neovascularization in peripheral arterial occlusive disease [5]. These circulating cells (endothelial progenitor cells [EPCs]) are bone marrow derived [59], and, historically, therapeutic angiogenesis is the objective of virtually all clinical studies using bone marrow or its circulating derivatives for ischemic myocardium. For clinical use, EPCs are isolated from mononuclear blood cells and selected ex vivo by culturing in "endothelium-specific" medium for 3 days, prior to reinjection into the heart. The added hypothesis that such cells also might transdifferentiate to create new cardiomyocytes [60] is unrelated to the clinical studies' origin and dispensable to their rationale. Critiques of the clinical studies—where based on the absence or paucity of myocyte formation in mice [61–63]—raise useful questions as to the mechanisms for success (as measured to date by improvements in ventricular pump function), but overlook this most salient point, namely, the actual rationale.

On the horizon of being tested for potential clinical application are other progenitor/stem cell populations: **fat tissue-derived multipotent stem cells** [64]; **multipotential cells from bone marrow or skeletal muscle** (minuscule subpopulations, distinct from the unfractionated bone marrow and the myoblasts used in current trials) [58, 65]; **somatic stem cells from placental cord blood** [26]; and **cardiac-resident**

progenitor cells that have a heightened predisposition to adopt the cardiac muscle fate [27–31]. In each of these newer cases, techniques to isolate and purify the numerically minor population of potent cells will need to be optimized for clinical use, and enabling data from mammals larger than the mouse will surely be warranted.

Routs of application Thus far, progenitor cells for cardiac repair have been delivered in 3 ways: via an intracoronary arterial route or by injection of the ventricular wall via a percutaneous endocardial or surgical epicardial approach . The advantage of intracoronary infusion—using standard balloon catheters—is that cells can travel directly into myocardial regions in which nutrient blood flow and oxygen supply are preserved, which hence ensures a favorable environment for cells' survival, a prerequisite for stable engraftment. Conversely, homing of intra-arterially applied progenitor cells requires migration out of the vessel into the surrounding tissue, so that unperfused regions of the myocardium are targeted far less efficiently, if at all. Moreover, whereas bone marrow-derived and blood-derived progenitor cells are known to extravasate and migrate to ischemic areas [32], skeletal myoblasts do not and furthermore may even obstruct the microcirculation after intra-arterial administration, leading to embolic myocardial damage.

By contrast, **direct delivery of progenitor cells into scar tissue or areas of hibernating myocardium by catheter-based needle injection, direct injection during open-heart surgery, and minimally invasive thoracoscopic procedures** are not limited by cell uptake from the circulation or by embolic risk. An offsetting consideration is the risk of ventricular perforation, which may limit the use of direct needle injection into freshly infarcted hearts. In addition, it is hard to envisage that progenitor cells injected into uniformly necrotic tissue—lacking the syncytium of live muscle cells that may furnish instructive signals and lacking blood flow for the delivery of oxygen and nutrients—would receive the necessary cues and environment to engraft and differentiate. Most cells, if injected directly, simply die [33]. For this reason, electromechanical mapping of viable but "hibernating" myocardium may be useful to pinpoint the preferred regions for injection [13]. Finally, in diffuse diseases such as dilated nonischemic cardiomyopathy, focal deposits of directly injected cells might be poorly matched to the underlying anatomy and physiology.

Cell Mobilization as Medical Technology Breakthrough in Heart Regeneration and Revascularisation

The first hints that cytokine-induced mobilization may be a way to enhance cardiac repair came as an extrapolation of findings of results from efforts to increase EPC levels for neovascularization in another context—hind limb ischemia. Indeed, VEGF [40] and GM-CSF [41] were found to augment EPC levels and improve neovascularization, and subsequent studies documented EPC mobilization by numerous other proangiogenic growth factors—stromal cell-derived factor-1 (SDF-1), angiopoietin-1, placental growth factor, and erythropoietin [42–44]. A wide array of interventions even more accessible clinically than growth factor administration enhance the number of circulating EPCs in adults, including treatment with HMG CoA reductase inhibitors (statins) and estrogens as well as exercise [45, 46, 66]. Most studies confirmed an improvement in endothelial regeneration or neovascularization by mobilizing agents. However, such functional improvements may not rely entirely on EPC mobilization but may also—at least in part—be explained by direct proangiogenic or antiapoptotic effects. Hence, as discussed as a recurring theme in this review, the existence of known (and potential unknown) pleiotropic modes of action complicates the interpretation of regenerative therapies, even in cases where the beneficial effect is clear-cut and assured (Fig. 3.3).

A shift in emphasis from the heart's vessels to the heart itself was prompted by the report that bone marrow-derived cells can differentiate into cardiomyocytes when injected into injured myocardium and regenerate the heart effectively [60]. Based on this discovery, hematopoietic stem cell-mobilizing factors—G-CSF and SCF (Kit ligand)–were used to improve cardiac regeneration experimentally [47], which quickly led to the initiation of clinical trials studying the ability of G-CSF to mobilize stem/progenitor cells in patients with coronary artery disease. This cytokine is used routinely in the treatment of humans, e.g., to help in harvesting cells for bone marrow transplantation. Although results from these first small trials do not permit any conclusion of efficacy, the safety of G-CSF in acute myocardial infarction has already come into question [48]. The observed increase in restenosis may be partially explained by the study design (which precluded the standard clinical practice of promptly stenting the obstructed vessel), but the rise in leukocyte number to leukemic levels may be directly responsible, via plaque growth or destabilization. Adverse vascular events have also been attributed to G-CSF in patients with intractable angina who were not candidates for revascularization and even in patients without cardiac disease [49]. In the future, it may be preferable to use strategies that augment circulating progenitor cells without causing massive inflammation (Table 3.3).

A second open question regarding systemic mobilization is whether enough progenitor cells will home where needed, to the sites of cardiac injury [50]. Systemically administered human progenitor cells were predominantly trapped by the spleen when given to athymic nude rats [32], and cardiac regeneration elicited by treatment with G-CSF plus SCF was documented only for animals lacking a spleen [47]. The use of leukocyte-mobilizing cytokines might be most worthwhile combined with selective enhancements of progenitor cell homing or as a prelude to isolating cells for local delivery [50] (Table 3.4).

Numerous studies carried out in the past few years have demonstrated, that the intracoronary SC-therapy has to be considered as a safe therapeutic procedure in heart disease, when damaged myocardium must be regenerated [6, 14–18]. This kind of cell-mediated therapy with autologous BM-derived SCs is acceptable ethically and medically, except for the small numbers of patients with bone marrow disease or infiltration. A typical human infarct involves the loss of about 1×10^9 cardiomyocytes and many researchers investigated endogenous or exogenous SCs with the capacity to differentiate into cardiomyocytes and repopulate lost myocardium [17]. Clinical trials confirmed that transplantation of autologous SCs improved cardiac function

Table 3.3 Inspiration and driving force for clinical studies: animal models

Donald Orlic (NIH, Bethesda, Maryland) (mice) (2001) Nature	Hamano H (Japan)(2001)(Sheep, rabbit model of hindlimb ischemia, Lewis rats-autologous BM transplants)
A. Mouse (Orlic et al. 2001)	B. SHEEP (Hirata, Hamano, 2001, 2003, Bell, 2003)
AMI->same	AMI->ligation of circumflex arterial branches
Mobilization (non-invasive) Lin-c-kitPOS BMC from syngeneic animals SCF and G-CSF	BM biopsy (surgical, invasive method)
29 BMC in normal to 7,200 in cytokine-treated animals	4.22×10^8 cells/3 ml
$3\times10^4-2\times10^5$/5 ml PBS Injected 2.5 ml PBS containing cells	Injected in 10 sites across the Infracted area through the reopened thoracotomy

Basic postulates: the best established source for adult stem cells is the BM. It contains different cell types-HSCs posses plasticity and transdifferentiate into myocardial cells

after myocardial infarction and in chronic coronary heart disease. It is also demonstrated that the age of infarction is most likely irrelevant to regenerative potency of applied SCs [14]. In SC-therapy, the critical problem is to replace injured myocardial cells with new contractile tissue—i.e. to regenerate or create new contractile cardiac tissue. The pathways involved in cardiac differentiation, experimental and preclinical studies have suggested that stem cell pre-treatment to direct SC (trans) differentiation prior to cell application may be a more efficacious strategy for inducing cardiac regeneration [15].

(*c*) *Other tissues*

Although the most developed, excitable tissues (heart and neural tissue) are the ultimate goal of stem cell therapy, and due to that, mostly experimentally and clinically trailed, other, more simple organs and tissues are also the matter of study and therapeutical treatments. Not only that visible and known organ's and tissue's damages are treated (bone fractions, skin lesions,) but such a complex diseases like Lupus Erythemtosus Systemicus, Autism, peripheral arterial disease, Osteogenesis Imperfecta, Liver diseases) are treated with more or less success with stem cells of different sources and types . The more one is trying to widespread this approach, the more he realizes the need for further knowledge. Transplant of hepatic stem/progenitor cells or hepatocyte-like cells derived from multipotent SCs led to donor cell-mediated repopulation of the liver and improved survival rates [19, 50].Our clinical studies showed that implantation of autologous SCs into damaged/ischemic area induces their homing and subsequent trans-differentiation into the cell lineages of host organ, including collateral vessel formation [6]. To be precise, angiogenetic growth-factors (or genes encoding for these proteins) promote the development of collateral microvessels, the process known as therapeutic angio-neogenesis or neovascularization [3, 6].

Table 3.4 Clinical trials of intracoronary progenitor cells for acute myocardial infarction

Study	*N*	Days after MI	Cell type	Cell preparation (volume/purification/culture)	Mean cell no. ($\times 10^6$)	Safety	Myocardial function
Strauer et al. [11]	10	8	BMCs	40 ml/Ficoll/overnight (Teflon)	28	+	Regional Contractillity ↑ (LVA); endsystolic volume ↓ (LVA); perfusion ↑ (Scintigraphy)
TOPCARE-AMI [12, 16, 122]	59	4.9	CPCs	250 ml/blood/3 days	16	+	Global contractility ↑ (LVA/MRI); end systolic volume ↓ (LVA/MRI); viability ↑ (MRI);
			BMCs	50 ml/Ficoll/none	213		flow reserve ↑ (Doppler); similar results for both cell types
BOOST [15]	30 vs. 30 randomized controls	4.8	BMCs	150 ml/gelatin-polysuccinate sedimentation/none	2,460	+	Global Contractility ↑ (MRI)
Fernandez-Aviles et al. (123)	20	13.5	BMCs	50 ml/Ficoll/overnight(Teflon)	78	+	Global Contractillity ↑ (MRI); end Systolic Volume ↓ (MRI)

↑ indicates increase, ↓ indicates decrease, + denotes lack of adverse events. *BMC* bone marrow-derived cell, *CPC* circulating progenitor cell (EPCs), *LVA* LV cineangiography, *MI* myocardial infarction

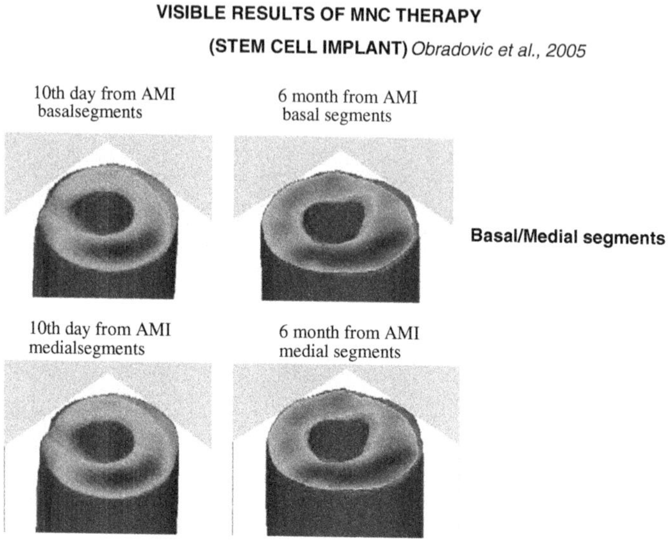

Fig. 3.13 SPEC of the 1st patient 10 days and 6 months after AMI

The overall data strongly suggest that this is not a simple mechanical-transplantational approach, but rather organized and at several levels stratified research in order to understand the conditions required for particular regenerative treatment. Once, the general mechanisms governing the process of differentiation, de-differentiation, successful homing, and optimal conditions of microenvironment for each particular damage are completely understood, the physicians will be able to apply the best possible therapeutical approach using the best possible stem-cell patterns in order to get the best possible individual therapeutic outcome (Fig. 3.13).

Stem Cells and Tissue Engineering: Comprehension

Within just the past 6 years, several early clinical studies have been published, ranging from case reports to formal trials, deploying a range of differing cell-based therapies with the shared objective of improving cardiac repair [10–15]. Clinical follow-up for as long as a couple of years is now available for some patients [16, 17]. Despite their different strategies and cells, and lack of double-blinded controls, these small initial human trials in general point to a functional improvement. Yet, key questions remain open. Understanding better just why and how grafting works will be essential, alongside needed empirical trials, to engineer the soundest future for regenerative therapy in human heart disease .Cells in current human trials include skeletal muscle myoblasts, unfractionated bone marrow, and circulating (endothelial) progenitor cells. Cells in preclinical studies include bone marrow MSCs, multipotent cells from other sources, and novel progenitor or stem cells discovered in the adult myocardium.

Ultimately, it must be proven that cellular therapy aimed at cardiac repair not only improves pump function but also reduces mortality, morbidity, or both.

Beyond safety, beyond efficacy, what else do we need to know clinically? For ischemic disease, the technical armament is in hand for treating patients' hearts with progenitor cells but still at a very early stage—rudimentary experimental knowledge is being applied in the clinical arena, yet a variety of pivotal but straightforward utilitarian questions still remain unanswered (optimal patient selection, usefulness of repeated treatments, optimal number of stem-cells, their quality, source, etc.). Nonischemic heart disease has yet to be addressed at all.

More complex and challenging is a series of pathobiological concerns, which have sent the scientific community from bedside to bench and back again. Certain patients' cells may be unsatisfactory, in their naive and unmanipulated state, which is now prompting systematic dissection of each step in progenitor cell function, from recruitment to plasticity. This task, in turn, is complicated by the fact that we do not yet understand the mechanisms underlying cell-based cardiac repair. For instance, the efficacy of skeletal muscle myoblasts [67] provided the impetus for human trials of skeletal muscle cells, but in the rabbit, diastolic functions are improved even by injected fibroblasts [38] and systolic performance improved to the same degree with bone marrow-derived cells as with skeletal muscle ones [39]. Along with the issue of skeletal muscle cells' electrical isolation from host myocardium, this prompts the question of how mechanical improvements arise even in this ostensibly straightforward instance. Another reason to consider potential indirect mechanisms is that studies have called into question the extent to which bone marrow-derived cells implanted in the heart form cardiomyocytes [61–63]. The majority of this review is, therefore, devoted to the biological horizons—namely mobilization, homing, neoangiogenesis, and cardiac differentiation , and to evolving new insights that may enable cell therapy for cardiac repair to surpass the present state of the art. Current challenges for cell-based therapy in cardiac repair include identifying the origins of the novel cardiac progenitor and stem cells found within the heart, pinpointing the biologically active cells from bone marrow and other mixed populations, optimizing cell mobilization and homing, augmenting grafted cells' survival, defining the cues for cardiac differentiation, promoting donor cell proliferation ex vivo (or, if safe, *in vivo*), and exploiting cell therapy as a platform for secretory signals. Through this diversifying and integral approach at the same time, the field of tissue engineering is arising as a new developing solid platform for optimizing arrangements of different regenerative modules within different scenarios. This largely developing field is involving basic postulates of mathematical, physical and physiological sciences integrated in the most probably optimal solutions for each particular case.

Summary and Conclusions on the Role of Stem Cells in TE

Hematopoietic stem cell transplantation remains a risky procedure with many possible complications. It has traditionally been reserved for patients with life-threatening diseases, such as malignancies. While occasionally used experimentally in nonmalignant and nonhematologic indications such as severe disabling autoimmune and cardiovascular diseases, the risk of fatal complications appears too high to gain wider acceptance [56]. Yet, this is the most-well known and the most developed stem-cell regenerative approach, given that if successfully engrafted, it repopulates and later on recruits the new, healthy bone marrow cells in circulation.

Embryonic stem-cell research is still the matter if controversies at a very stratified levels, although many researchers agree that it might be the source of stem cells with the highest differentiation potential.

Apparently, basic adult stem cell research is still evolving, and is the matter of everchanging issues. Due to our extensive studies, but yet limited knowledge on their behavior and potentials, it is not yet easy to determine how to act in clinical arena. It is obvious that each approach to any particular disease or damage has to be optimized within team work and by bridging the gap between fundamental and clinical studies. Knowing molecular level in depth, will help clinicians to orcestrate the team work and overcome critical obstacles in each particular scenario. There is no doubt that adult stem cell therapy (and probably embryonic as well) belong to the future, but we have to act as that we shall belong to the future, as well. Continuous efforts in both molecular and clinical directions will lead to the unique and optimal plan for each particular regenerative treatment. Are we too far away from that goal or not, it will be shown very soon.

- *Microfabrication of scaffolds and 3-D growth of tissues*

As the research field of particular stem cell patterns and their optimization for the cellular therapy and TE purposes is still evolving, one of the most significant/fundamental achievements in the TE filed is definitely the development of the scaffolds as the cell supporters and strong motivation for 3-D growth of tissue. So far, cell culture done on different surfaces enabled two-dimensional/ planar growth of cells which could not reproduce all of the tissue dimensions neither their complex architecture. Thus, scaffolds represent an important component in TE. What is also important it is to know the guide- lines for selecting scaffolds and the major scaffolding approaches as the part of specific TE design [53]. As the role of TE is to restore, replace or regenerate defective tissue, it is apparently multitask area providing a complex evolution of the new-growing components of defective tissue. We have seen that one of the possibilities is transplantation of stem cells, however it does function in particular occasions and is not the answer to all tissue damages that require reparation. Therefore, development of scaffolds with consecutive 3-D growth of the cells was one the most striking technological breakthroughs in this field.

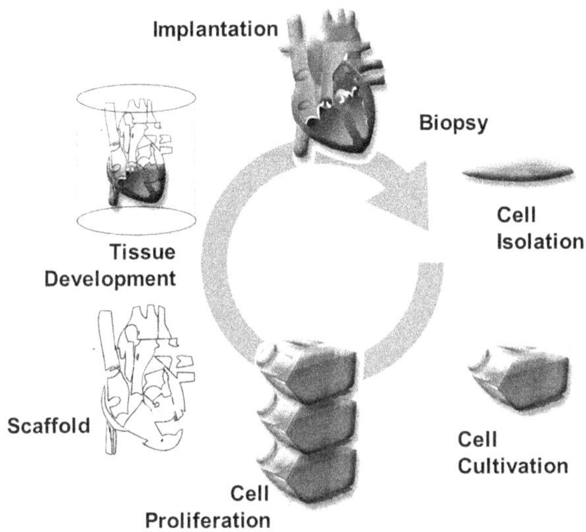

Fig. 3.14 Principles of TE

Scaffolds have the origin in biomaterials that have to be biocompatible, biodegradable and bio-resorbable in order to fully satisfy its role in supporting the 3-D growth of the cells chosen for tissue damage repair [54]. It is not easy neither to find (natural) nor to manufacture (fabricated) such material. Therefore, the technology of scaffolds is still developing as a separate scientific approach. The technologies for micro-fabrication are numerous and not the matter of this chapter. The key of the structure are holes in the architecture of the scaffolds on different levels (Fig. 3.14) that are no bigger than 50 μm and represent a physical challenge for cells to go through. This is causing three-dimensional growth and differentiation at the same time which results in a piece of tissue either in the organism or in the dish, where it will be taken from in order to be implanted into right spot. So, using the scaffolds and Growth factors from ECM (regulatory cytokines) a suitable biochemical and biomechanical microenvironment is created and cell multiplication fills the scaffold with the tissue and allows the cells to grow into the correct shape. When implanted into the body, the seeded scaffold becomes integrated concomitantly supporting and directing cell proliferation. As the cells proliferate and differentiate, the scaffolds slowly biodegrade, gradually allowing blood vessels and host cytokines to make contact with the cells [55]. Through this process, the scaffold further biodegrades while the cells proliferate and differentiate into desired tissue. Finally, the scaffold completely dissolves and the formed tissue starts functioning in its new surrounding.

- *Computer Aided Tissue Engineering (CATE) as a leading concept*

The inevitable consequence of the recent revolution in the biological sciences and bioengineering has brought about the new field of computer-aided tissue engineering (CATE). It really highlights the interdisciplinary nature of this technology breakthrough. Particular focus in this field is placed on rapid prototyping and direct digital fabrication for cell and organs, construction of tissue analogues and precursors of 3-D scaffolds (209, 210). This emerging field encompasses computer-aided design (CAD), image processing, manufacturing and solid-free-form fabrication (SFF) for modeling, designing simulation and manufacturing of biological tissue and organ substitutes (210). This involves imaging based 3D model reconstruction, computer aided-tissue informatics, with a wide array of image modalities, DNA microarrays, etc., computer-aided cell analysis (cell counting, geometry, chromosomal counting interpreting fluorescence data, etc.), computer-aided tissue identification and analysis, computer-aided tissue scaffold design and manufacturing.

- *Ink-jet printing of the cells and liquid scaffolds*

Organ printing is today possible thanks to application of brilliant idea that cells can be printed onto scaffolds as it is the ink [68, 69]. This in essence, very simple technique provides a broad spectrum of TE maneuvers including the very fast recovery from large burns, the event that is extremely useful and highly necessary in those situations. Today many cell types can be printed as bio-ink using ink-jet printers: the cells survive, maintain their phenotype, differentiate and show function. They can be printed uniformly and homogeneously into confluent layers. They can be printed into 3-D structures. However, there are considerable technical barriers in the development of this emerging inkjet printing technology, such as the ability of the modified printers to deliver viable cells and the capability of the inkjet printing to fabricate functional, viable and functionally vascularized 3-D configurations [68, 69]. This is the future problem which needs to be gradually solved.

- *Transplantation without a donor*

For more than century, medical doctors were looking for alternative solutions to help address the shortage of organs for those needing transplantation. The whole concept of this greatest probably technological breakthrough in TE is that patient can use his own tissue in order to replace damaged organ. Dr. Anthony Atala is doing that now with the bladder [70–75]. After a small biopsy, patient's own cells are shaped, grown on three-dimensional polymer mold in the shape of a bladder and eventually the temporary scaffold deteriorates inside the body, leaving behind, a healthy, functional organ. Most important is that since the cells are taken from the patient, the body will not reject the organ grown in that manner.

- *Other techniques of great relevance for advance of TE*

Tissue engineering is a very complex and multidisciplinary field. Many discoveries are in tight relationship with the development of the idea. Looking into the roots, probably the discovery of microscope was the most important for establishment of the theory of the cell. Compact light microscope is later on upgraded into microscope with phase contrast which has enabled scientists to see through the medium the cells that they were growing, including stem cells. Electron microscopy will give the ultrastructure and inspire biochemistry to develop in order to explain molecular conversions and other processes in the cells. Atomic force microscope will help understanding of chemical content of the cells. The CO_2 incubator will later on enable the growth of the cells in culture and afterwards in tissue culture .Development of fluorescent labeling and Flow Cytometer in combination with fluorescent microscope will enable molecular detection and phenotypic distinction between the cells. This had incredible impact on development of stem cell theories and concepts. The explosion and evolution of the field is infinite. The future world will due to that have more comfortable and much higher quality of life and probably the life itself will be somewhat longer although humans will never fly.

References

1. Rees ink HW, Panzer S, Deter M, Gabriel C, Lambermont M, Deneys V, Sondag D, Dickmeiss E, Fischer-Nielsen A, Korhonen M, Krusius T, Ali A, Tiberghien P, Schrezenmeier H, Tonn T, Seifried E, Klüter H, Politis C, Stavropoulou-Gioka A, Parara M, Flesland Ø, Nascimento F, Balint B, Fernández PM, Bart T, Chen FE, Pamphilon DH. International Forum: New cellular therapies: Is there a role for transfusion services? Vox Sanguinis 2009; 97: 77–90.
2. Balint B, Ljubenov M, Stamatović D, Todorović M, Pavlović M, Ostojić G, et al. Stem cell harvesting protocol research in autologous transplantation setting: large volume vs. conventional cytapheresis Vojnosanit Preg 2008; 65(7): 545–51.
3. Balint B. Stem and progenitor cell harvesting, extracorporeal "graft engineering" and clinical use - initial expansion vs. current dillemas. Clin Appl Immunol 2006; 5(1): 518–27.
4. Balint B, Stamatovic D, Todorovic M, Jevtic M, Ostojic G, Pavlovic M, et al. Stem cells in the arrangement of bone marrow repopulation and regenerative medicine. Vojnosanit Pregl 2007; 64(7): 481–4.
5. Balint B, Todorovic M, Jevtic M, Ostojic G, Ristanovic E, Vojvodic D, et al. The use of stem cells for marrow repopulation and in the field of regenerative medicine. Mak Med Pregl 2009; 63 (Suppl 75): 12–7.
6. Kucia M, Reca R, Jala Vr, Dawn B, Ratajczak J, Ratajczak MZ. Bone Maroow as home of heterogeneous populations of nonhematopoietic stem cells. Leukemia 2005, 19: 1118–1127.
7. Kucia M, Ratajczak J, and Ratajczak ZM. Bone Marrow as a source of circulating CXR4+ tissue-commited Stem Cells, Biology of the cell 2005; 97; 133–146.
8. Kucia M, Ratajczak J, Ratjczak MX. Are bone marrow cells plastic or heterogeneous-that is the question. Exp Hematol 2005; 33(6): 613–23.
9. G.T.-J. Huang, S. Gronthos and S. Shi: Mesenchymal Stem Cells Derived from Dental Tissues vs. Those from Other Sources: Their Biology and Role in Regenerative Medicine.*J DENT RES 2009* 88: 792.
10. Ratajczak J, Miekus K, Kucia M, Zhang J, Reca R, Dvorak P, and Ratajczak MZ. Embryonic stemcell-derived microvesicles reprogram hematopoietic progenitors: evidence for horizontal transfer of mRNA and protein delivery. Leukemia 2006, 20: 847–856.
11. Kucia M, Wojakowski W, Ryan R, Machalinski B, Gozdzik J, Majka M, Baran J, Ratajczak J, and Ratjczak MZ. The migration of bone marrow-derived non-hematopoietic tissue-commited stem cells is regulated in and SDF-1-, HGF-, and LIF dependent manner. Arch Immunol et Ther Exp 2006, 54, 2: 121–135.
12. Kucia M, Zhang YP, Reac R, Wysoczynski M, Machalinski B, Majka M, Ildstad ST, Ratajczak JU, Chields CB, and Ratajczak MZ. Cells enriched in markers of neural tissue-commited stem cells reside in the bone marrow and are mobilized into the peripheral blood following stroke. Leukemia 2006, 20: 18–28.

13. Kucia M, Reca R, Campbell FR, Surma-Zuba E, Majka M, Ratajczak M, and Ratajczak MZ A population of very small embryonic - like (VSEL) CXR4+SSEA-1+Oct4+ stem cells identified in adult bone marrow. Leukemia 2006, 20: 857–69.
14. Wagers AJ, Sherwood RI, Christensen JL, Weissman IL. Little evidence for developmental plasticity of adult hematopoietic stem cells. Science 2002; 297: 2256–9.
15. Alvarez A, Unda F, Cañavate ML, Hilario E. Stem cell and regenerative medicine. Curr Stem Cell Res Ther 2009 Dec 1. [Epub ahead of print].
16. Obradovic S, Balint B, GligiC B, RusoviC S, Baskot B, Ristic-Angelkov A, et al. Intracoronary non-selective implantation of high-dose mononuclear bone-marrow cells for large myocardial infarction in subacute phase improves long-term left ventricle function but causes high rate of restenosis. Clin Appl Immunol. In Press 2009.
17. Todorović V, Marković D, Milošević-Jovčić N, Petakov M, Balint B, Čolić M et al. Dental pulp stem cells - potential significance in regenerative medicine. Stom Glas S 2008; 55: 170–9.
18. Todorović V, Nikolić I, Glibetić M, Balint B. Humane embrionalne matične ćelije - dosadašnja saznanja. Anest Reanim Transfuziol 2006; 34: 109–127.
19. Kuçi S, Kuçi Z, Latifi-Pupovci H, Niethammer D, Handgretinger R, Schumm M, Bruchelt G, Bader P, Klingebiel T. Adult stem cells as an alternative source of multipotential (pluripotential) cells in regenerative medicine. Curr Stem Cell Res Ther 2009; 4(2): 107–17.
20. Pappa KI, Anagnou NP. Novel sources of fetal stem cells: where do they fit on the developmental continuum? Regen Med 2009; 4(3): 423–33.
21. Utermöhlen O, Baschuk N, Abdullah Z, Engelmann A, Siebolts U, Wickenhauser C, et al. Immunologic hurdles of therapeutic stem cell transplantation. Biol Chem 2009 Jul 30. [Epub ahead of print].
22. Balint B, Ivanović Z, Petakov M, Taseski J, Jovčić G, Stojanović N, et al. The cryopreservation protocol optimal for progenitor recovery is not optimal for preservation of marrow repopulating ability. Bone Marrow Transplant 1999; 23(6): 613–9.
23. Mayorga M, Finan A, Penn M. Pre-transplantation specification of stem cells to cardiac lineage for regeneration of cardiac tissue. Stem Cell Rev Rep 2009; 5(1): 51–60.
24. Reinecke H, Minami E, Zhu WZ, Laflamme MA. Cardiogenic differentiation and transdifferentiation of progenitor cells. Circ Res 2008; 103(10): 1058–71.
25. Biehl JK, Russell B. Introduction to stem cell therapy. J Cardiovasc Nurs 2009; 24(2): 98–103.
26. Voskoboynik A, Simon-Blecher N, Soen Y, Rinkevich B, De Tomaso AW, Ishizuka KJ, Weissman IL "Striving for normality: whole body regeneration through a series of abnormal generations." FASEB J 2007.
27. Körbling M, and Estrov, Z: Adult Stem Cells for Tissue Repair –A New Therapeutic Concept? N Engl J Med 2003;349:570–82.
28. Tsai, R.Y.L. (2004) A Molecular View of Stem Cell and Cancer Cell Self-renewal. Intl. J. Biochem. Cell Biol. 36, 684–694.
29. Cai, J., Weiss M.L., Rao, M.S. (2004) In Search of "stemness". Exp. Hematol. 32, 585–598.
30. Doyonnas, R., Blau, H.M. (2004) What is the Future of Stem Cell Research? Stem Cell Handbook ed. by Sell, S. 491–499.
31. Nosrat I.V., Smith, C. A., Mullally P., Olson L., Nosrat C.A. (2004) Dental Pulp Cells Provide Neurotrophic Support for Dopaminergic Neurons and Differentiate into Neurons in vitro; implications for Tissue Engineering and Repair in the Nervous System. Eur. J. of Neurosci. 19, 2388–2398.
32. Shen C-N, Horb ME, Slack JMW, Tosh, D. (2003) Transdifferentiation of Pancreas to Liver. Mech. Dev.120, 107–116.
33. Priller, J. (2004) From Marrow to Brain. Adult Stem Cells ed. by Turksen, K. 215–233.
34. de Wynter, E.A. (2003) What is the future of Cord blood stem cells? Cytotech. 41, 133–138.
35. Ivanovic Z, Ardilouze L, Jeanne M, Bertot A, Lafarge X, Duchez P, Vlaski M, Milpied N, Pavlovic M, Kovacevic-Filipovic M, Boiron JM, Praloran V.: CD34+ cells obtained from "good mobilizers" are more activated and exhibit lower ex vivo expansion efficiency than their counterparts from "poor mobilizers". (Accepted for publishing in Transfusion, Manuscript ID :Trans-2009-0156.R1), 2009.

36. Shi S, Gronthos S. Perivascular niche of postnatal mesenchimal stem cells in human bone marrow and dental pulp. J Bone Miner Res 2003; 18:696–704.
37. Todorovic V, Nikolic I, Glibetic M, Balint B: Human embryonic stem cells:current knowledge. Anest Rean Thransf 34, 2/3,2006:109–127.
38. Zhang W, Walboomers XF, Van Kuppevelt TH, et al. In vivo evaluation of human dental pulp stem cells differentiated towards multiple lineages. J Tissue Eng Regen Med 2008; 2:117–25.
39. TodorovicV, Markovic D, Milosevic-Jovcic N, Petakov M, Balint B, Colic M, Milenkovic A, Colak I, Jokanovic V, Nikolic N: Matične ćelije zubne pulpe i njihov potencijalni značaj u regenerativnoj medicini Stomatološki glasnik Srbije, 2008, 55, 3: 170–179.
40. Pavlovic M.: VSELs concept (Review) 2008, MNE Medica, No 1, Year I, Jul 2008, pp 16–17, ref. p. 43.
41. Pavlovic M, Balint B: The use of stem cells to repair cardiac tissue. Anest Reanim Transfuziol 2006; 34: 129–50.
42. McCulloch, E.A. (2004) Normal and Leukemic Hematopietic Stem cells and Lineages. Stem Cell Handbook ed. by Sell, S. 119–131.
43. Fraser, J.K., Schreiber, R.E., Zuk, P.A., Hedrick, M.H. (2004) Adult Stem Cell Therapy for the Heart. Intl. J. Biochem. Cell Biol. 36, 658–666.
44. Cohen, S., Leor, J. (2004) Rebuilding Broken Hearts. Scientific American Nov. 2004, 45–51.
45. Lindblad, W.J. (2004) Stem cells in Dermal Wound Healing. Stem Cell Handbook ed. by Sell, S. 101–105.
46. Draper, J.S. Moore, H., Andrews, P.W. (2003) Embryonal Carcinoma Cells. Human Embryonic Stem Cells ed. Chiu, A. Y., Rao, M.S. 63–87.
47. Stevens LC. Experimental production of testicular teratomas in mice of strains 129, A/He, and their F1hybrids. *J Natl Cancer Inst.* 1970;44:923–929.
48. Jean-Marc Muller*, Lucie Chevrier, Ste'phanie Cochaud, Annie-Claire Meunier, Corinne Chadeneau :Hedgehog, Notch and Wnt developmental pathways as targets for anti-cancer drugs.www.drygdiscoverytoday.com, 2008:285–291.
49. Beachy PA, Karhadkar SS, Berman DM. Tissue repair and stem cell renewal in carcinogenesis. Nature. 2004, 432(7015):324–331.
50. Reya T, Clevers H : Wnt signalling in stem cells and cancer. Nature. 2005 434(7035):843–50.
51. Molofsky, A V, Pardal R, Iwashita T, In-Kyung Park, Clarke M F. and Morrison SJ. Bmi-1 dependence distinguishes neural stem cell self-renewal from progenitor proliferation
52. Bracken AP, Dietrich N, Pasini D, Hansen HK, Helin K: Genes Dev. May 1, 2006 20: 1123–1136; Published in Advance April 17, 2006, doi:10.1101/gad.381706 Genome-wide mapping of Polycomb target genes unravels their roles in cell fate transitions. Metabolism and cancer August 1, 2009, 23 (15).
53. Kruger MG, Mosher TJ, Bixby S, Joseph N, Iwashita T and MorrisonSJ. Neural Crest Stem Cells Persist in the Adult Gut but Undergo Changes in Self-Renewal, Neuronal Subtype Potential, and Factor Responsiveness. Neuron, 35, I4, 657–669, 2002.
54. Kruger G, Mosher J, Tsai Y, Yeager K, Iwashita T, Gariepy C, Morrison S: Temporally Distinct Requirements for Endothelin Receptor B in the Generation and Migration of Gut Neural Crest Stem Cells.*Neuron*, Volume 40, Issue 5, Pages 917–929, 2003.
55. Morrison SJ: Neuronal potential and lineage determination by neural stem cells. Current Opinion in Cell Biology, 13, Issue 6, 1:666–672, 2001.
56. Gaiano N, Nye JS, Fishell G: Radial glial identity is promoted by Notch1 signaling in the murine forebrain.*Neuron* 2000, 26:395–404.
57. Kakinuma S, Nakauchi H, Watanabe M. Hepatic stem/progenitor cells and stem-cell transplantation for the treatment of liver disease. J Gastroenterol 2009; 44(3): 167–72.
58. Crook JM, Kobayashi NR. Human stem cells for modeling neurological disorders: accelerating the drug discovery pipeline. J Cell Biochem 2008; 105(6): 1361–6.
59. Andres RH, Choi R, Steinberg GK, Guzman R. Potential of adult neural stem cells in stroke therapy. Regen Med 2008; 3(6): 893–905.
60. Pavlovic, M.: VSELs concept (Review) 2008, MNE Medica, No 1, Year I, Jul 2008, pp 16–17, ref. p. 43.

61. Pavlovic M, Balint B. The use of stem cells to repair cardiac tissue. Anest Reanim Transfuziol 2006.
62. Sell, S. (2004) Stem cells. Stem Cell Handbook ed. by Sell, S. 1–18.
63. Forbes, S.J., Vig, P., Poulsom, R., Wright, N.A., Alison, M.R. (2002) Adult Stem Cell Plasticity: New Pathways of Tissue Regeneration become Visible. Clin. Sci. 103, 355–369.
64. Weinberg RA. Tumor suppressor genes. Science. 1991 Nov 22; 254 (5035):1138–1146.
65. Weissman I, "Stem cell research: paths to cancer therapies and regenerative medicine." JAMA 2005; 294: 11: 1359–66.
66. VIRCHOW, R., 1863 *Cellular Pathology as Based upon Physiological and Pathological Histology*. J. B. Lippincott, Philadelphia.
67. Daadi MM, Steinberg GK. Manufacturing neurons from human embryonic stem cells: biological and regulatory aspects to develop a safe cellular product for stroke cell therapy. Regen Med 2009; 4(2): 251–63.
68. Ratajzcak MZ, Kucia M, Reca R, Majka M et al, Stem cell plasticity revised:CXR4 positive cells expressing mRNA for earlu muscle, liver and neural cells "hide out" in the bone marrow. Leukemia 2004, 19(1), pp. 29–40.
69. BP Chen and KW Leong :Scafolding in tissue engineering :general approaches and tissue-specific considerations. Eur Spine J. 2008, 17, (Suppl 4)): 467–479.
70. J.G. Nemeno-Guanzon et al. Trends in Tissue engineering.J Biomjed, Biotech, 2012. Doi:1155/2012/956345.
71. J. I. Lee, M. Sato, H. W. Kim, and J. Mochida, "Transplantatation of scaffold-free spheroids composed of synovium-derived cells and chondrocytes for the treatment of cartilage defects of the knee", *European Cells and Materials Journal*, vol. 22, pp. 275–290, 2011.
72. Michael, A.K. Liebchner (Ed) Compter Aided Tissue Engineering. Humana Press 2012, Xi, ISBN 978-1-61779-764-4.
73. Sun W, Darkling A, Starly B, Nam J: Computer-aided tissue engineering :overview, scope and shallenges. Biotecnol Appl, Biochem 2004, 39 (Pt1):29–47.
74. Boland T, Xu T, Damon B, Cui X: Application of inkjet printing to tissue engineering. Biotechnol J. 2006 (9):910–7.
75. A. Atala, Bauer S, Soker S, Yoo JJ, Retik Ab: Tissue-engineered bladders for patients needing cytoplasty. The lancet, 367, 9518,:1241–1246, 2006.
76. Strauer BE, Schannwell CM, Brehm M. Therapeutic potentials of stem cells in cardiac diseases. Minerva Cardioangiol 2009; 57(2): 249–67.

Chapter 4
Innovations in 3D Interventional X-ray Imaging

Svitlana Zinger, Daniel Ruijters, Rudolph M. Snoeren, Chrysi Papalazarou and Peter H. N. de With

Abstract Minimal invasive interventions allow the treatment of lesions without the strain of full open surgery. Such image guided interventions and therapies fully rely on the guidance and navigation based on real-time peri-interventional imaging equipment, such as interventional X-ray and ultrasound. Since these imaging modalities are the 'eyes' of the treating physician, the associated image quality and imaging features are essential. The addition and further development of 3D imaging capabilities in recent years has broadened the possibilities and capabilities of such procedures, and enabled minimal invasive treatment that could only be performed by open surgery in the past. In this chapter we describe several recent innovations in the area of 3D interventional X-ray imaging in the areas of image quality, 3D model-based catheter reconstruction, multi-modal image fusion, and stereoscopic visualizations.

S. Zinger (✉) · R. M. Snoeren · C. Papalazarou · P. H. N. de With
Video Coding and Architectures research group, Eindhoven University of Technology,
Den Dolech 2, 5600 MB Eindhoven, The Netherlands
e-mail: s.zinger@tue.nl

R. M. Snoeren
e-mail: r.m.snoeren@tue.nl

P. H. N. de With
e-mail: p.h.n.de.with@tue.nl

D. Ruijters
Interventional X-Ray Innovation, Philips Healthcare,
Veenpluis 6, 5680 DA Best, The Netherlands
e-mail: danny.ruijters@philips.com

C. Papalazarou
Philips Research, Eindhoven, The Netherlands
e-mail: c.papalazarou@tue.nl, chrysi.papalazarou@philips.com

B. Furht and A. Agarwal (eds.), *Handbook of Medical and Healthcare Technologies*,
DOI: 10.1007/978-1-4614-8495-0_4, © Springer Science+Business Media New York 2013

Introduction

The volume of image guided interventions and therapy is rapidly increasing, because of associated better clinical outcome and reduced patient strain. One of the drivers of this development is the introduction of high quality 3D imaging in the cathlab. The innovations in this area enable more complex procedures, and reduce the need of moving the patient from the intervention room to diagnostic modalities, such as Computed Tomography (CT) and Magnetic Resonance Imaging (MRI), and therefore improving the patient workflow for the hospital and the clinical pathway for the patient.

X-ray imaging and associated forms of medical imaging are at the brink of a revolution in technology, particularly at the level of supplementary sensing combined with the induced signal analysis and at the level of advanced presentation of medical results. At the sensing level, the use multi-modal sensing is growing where the second signal supplements the primary signal. This leads to combinations with the above-mentioned CT and MR imaging signals. This trend has started already, but the emphasis is in the chapter on another aspect: three-dimensional (3D) imaging. The transition to three-dimensional capturing and associated processing is a process that is also taking place in the consumer electronics domain and e.g. professional geo-referenced and engineering imaging. It is evident that 3D imaging offers a potential wealth of enhancement possibilities for diagnostic and interventional medical imaging. For example, diagnostic details can better isolated and presented in 3D and the modeling and presentation of vital organs, disease development, and so on, are better intuitively presented and understood on a 3D display. The transition to larger scale deployment of 3D technology in medical imaging is emerging, both in laboratories and in novel applications in hospitals. This has motivated us to describe examples of these developments, selected such that they cover various stages of the X-ray image processing chain.

The selected 3D imaging examples in this chapter discuss recent scientific advancements regarding interventional 3D imaging. The following paragraphs summarize these examples briefly to present the overview for the whole image acquisition, processing and visualization chain.

Section "Hysteresis Reduction in 3D X-ray Flat Panel Imaging" concentrates on an improved detection of X-ray signals and will discuss the image quality aspects of 3D volumetric imaging with an interventional X-ray C-arm system. Current flat-panel detectors can have memory effects that deteriorate the image quality, thereby hampering the diagnostic capabilities of the images. This plays particularly a role in 3D cone-beam reconstructions with interventional X-ray systems. Various memory effects can occur such as residual signals (e.g. a gain hysteresis effect) and afterglow, each with specific decay properties. The section develops a microscopic model where positive Pb ions act as electron donor centers, created by specially imposed LED UV radiation on the scintillating layer. As a counterpart, Na+ ions limit the radiation damage and reduce the counter effect of trap depletion. It is shown that the above memory effects largely disappear and ring artifacts are reduced.

Section "Robotic Modeling for Non-rigid 3D Reconstruction of Steerable Catheters" describes the 3D reconstruction of steerable catheters in the cathlab. The 3D reconstruction of non-rigid catheters with a time-varying behavior caused by and during the intervention posed a formidable signal processing problem. The proposed solution adopts technology from outside the medical world and bridges to the computer vision domain and kinematic modeling in robotics. The catheter is modeled with non-rigid structure from motion techniques, relying on multiple views from the X-ray system by moving the beam capturing along the C-arm for a limited angle. With these structure from motion techniques, a model can be established that tracks the catheter and then allows a successful 3D reconstruction using projective geometry.

Section "Multi-modal Integration in the Cathlab" addresses the integration and fusion of pre-interventional 3D datasets such as fluoroscopic images and peri-interventional data as used with e.g. tomographic images. The purpose of this technique is to present the combined data in a fused image during the intervention, so that the physician optimally benefits from the improved presentation. A high-quality fusion is achieved by deploying an elastic co-registration algorithm that aligns the tomographic images with the interventional images. The algorithm is based on optimizing a similarity measure, while deforming the second signal according to organic principles using a uniform B-spline driven deformation field. Real-time performance is obtained by implementing this algorithm on a graphics processing unit.

Section "View Interpolation for Autostereoscopic Displays in the Cathlab" presents an efficient strategy for the transmission and visualization of clinical data on autostereoscopic 3D displays. Such displays offer depth perception, thereby facilitating a faster and better interpretation of the morphology and patient's pathology and contextual anatomy. The section describes an algorithm adopted from free-viewpoint rendering, where the camera parameters from surrounding reference views and the pixel-based depth information are jointly exploited. With a real-time rendering unit in the autostereoscopic display, multi-view 3D displaying is enabled. Details of the rendering algorithm disclose how imperfections of the image warping can be hidden with sophisticated signal processing techniques, such as filtering, special occlusion filling and mixed blending.

With the previously summarized sections, the chapter provides a state-of-the-art view into advanced signal processing concepts and algorithms and the corresponding modeling techniques from the vast world of signal processing theory and applications, existing both within the medical imaging domain and outside this domain in related professional and consumer fields. The deployment of 3D processing and modeling is a natural trend in signal processing, as the anatomy is of three dimensional nature, offering improved diagnostic and interventional features in medical X-ray imaging.

Hysteresis Reduction in 3D X-ray Flat Panel Imaging

Memory effects in X-ray Flat Panel (FP) imagery can be detrimental for Image Quality (IQ). The actual images are tainted by traces of former images (Siewerdsen [52]). Particularly, in 3D cone-beam reconstructions using a C-arc cardio-vascular system,

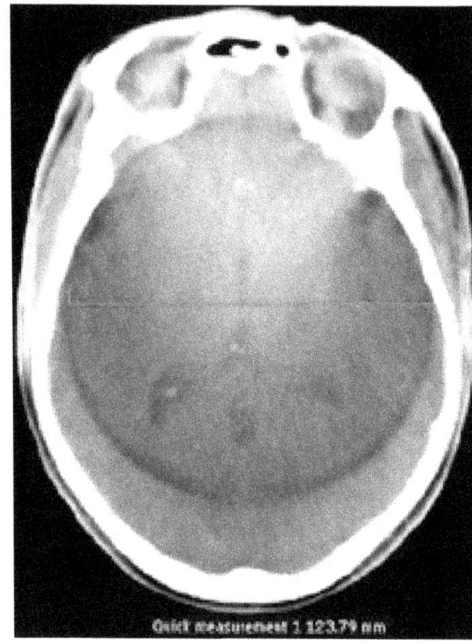

Fig. 4.1 Imprinted ring caused by a zoomed field edge transition inside the skull

low contrast imaging may suffer from this phenomenon. The effects in FP X-ray detection can be divided into two classes: *additive*, such as residual signals in the photodiodes and afterglow in the scintillator, or a hysteresis type of *multiplicative* effects in the photodiodes as well as in the scintillator (Wieczorek [61]). Each of the temporal effects has its characteristic decay scale: afterglow for the CsI:Tl scintillator may extend far in the seconds range, albeit at a very low level. The *hysteresis* or bright-burn effect will exist for days or weeks and depending on the Tl concentration and the history, its maximum level can accumulate to as high as 10 %. An example is given in Fig. 4.1 which displays a ring pattern that can be found upon reconstruction of a persistent X-ray-irradiation transition in an imaging field. As far as photodiodes are concerned, their residual (additive) signal can last for seconds and a gain effect of a few percent can be encountered, decaying in several minutes (Overdick [34]). These effects are based on a mechanism of trapping/de-trapping of charge carriers at crystal imperfections or impurities and their slow release thereafter. Depending on the imaging history, patterns may be imprinted superimposed on the acquired images in both gain and off-set. Attempts to reduce the effects by model-based cancelation prove to be difficult, so addressing the problem at its origin will be advantageous. The temporal gain effects in the photodiodes are properly reduced by existing back-lighting (Overdick [34]). For the scintillator, to avoid memory effects, we propose to fully populate traps by irradiating with an auxiliary light source of a proper wavelength.

Let us further detail this proposal. The combination of photo-induced electron transfer and X-ray excitation for medical imaging with flat detectors is not obvious (Snoeren [54]), since pure CsI:Tl scintillators will not exhibit such a behavior. A direct optical excitation of a wide band-gap material beyond the band edge, such as a regularly ordered CsI crystal, is impossible. For a Tl-activated material, which is a necessity for an efficient X-ray detection with Si photodiodes, an anomalous behavior is found in a commercially available detector. The photo-assisted trap-population effect, like we encountered, cannot be explained by a Tl dotation only and other elements should be in play, since we find a response in the near-UV/blue wavelength range. The very existence of such contaminating elements is revealed by chemical analysis. Complexation of excited foreign entities with a locally disordered crystal, will play a key role in the process of memory-effect reduction. We will describe the fundamental unraveling of the photo-electronic properties related to these contaminants, which eventually will yield a basis for a framework giving an optimal design. It will be shown that Pb^{++} ions act as perturbed V_K-electron centers, created by UV/blue photons. These centers are concurrently destroyed and subsequently release their electrons. Na^+ ions act as radiation-damage-limiting entities and reduce the counter effect of trap depletion through color centers. The validity of the proposed microscopic model is supported by various experiments and the relation between microscopic features and (macroscopic) IQ aspects is established. We will find an optimum procedure to reduce the memory effects below the visibility level at 3D reconstruction. In the following sections we will discuss a model, experimental results combined with a discussion and finalize with conclusions.

Modeling

We base our model hypothesis on an interpretation of an extensive analysis of chemical, optical, X-ray and IQ properties. CsI:Tl scintillating crystals show specific optical properties after irradiation, when the crystals are disordered by contaminants such as Pb and/or Na and refer to photochemical effects. First, we review the creation and destruction of traps and the effects on electron-transfer, followed by modeling of the gain and contrast properties.

Microscopic Model

Chemical analysis on various samples of CsI:Tl reveals that significant fractions of Pb and Na are present in the scintillator material under test. We expect these elements to play a key role in the hysteresis and afterglow properties of the material. We have distilled a physical model of the creation, destruction, population and depletion of charge-centers. Impurities and defects change the charge states of ions and their neighborhood. From closed-shell configurations, being typical for a stable crystal, the ions and their neighborhood therefore become able to absorb light (Lempicki [20]). Two competing phenomena can be discerned, which form a basis for a theory explaining the observations: (1) an electron donor supplying electrons for the population of electron traps and (2) color-center-capturing electrons (Rabin [38], Markham [26]). An explanation in the near-UV wavelength range and at room temperature, points at least at the impurity-induced absorption band of Pb-doted CsI at 3.39 eV (Radhakrishna [39, 40]), which has a sufficient bandwidth to respond to an optical irradiation of 3.42 eV, i.e. at the 362-nm LED emission that we used in our experiments.

Defects formation under UV irradiation in impurity-induced bands has been studied by Babin [2] for CsI:Pb crystals containing electron traps. Babin identifies an electron transfer from the impurity-perturbed halogen ion states, resulting in electrons and holes in the crystal. The electrons are trapped by lead ions and the holes are self-trapped.[1] Under optical irradiation in the absorption bands of Na-contaminated CsI:Pb, an electron transfer occurs from the I^- ion perturbed by a Pb^{2+} ion to this Pb^{2+} ion, or to a neighboring Pb^{2+} ion or a Na^+ ion. This results in the creation of an electron Pb^+ and a Pb^0 center, or a Na^0 center and the creation of self-trapped mobile holes in the valence band at different distances of the impurity, which migrate through the crystal. The electron centers can subsequently be destroyed by photostimulation and the electrons are available to populate Tl-related electron centers via the conduction band. The effect is an excitation of Pb^+ with an UV/blue photon to produce Pb^{2+} and an electron, or Na^0 to produce Na^+ and an electron. This process thus involves both the optical creation of centers and concurrent destruction by photons of the same energy. This leads to the conclusion that electrons are produced and move towards the conduction band and populate Tl-bound traps. The first (creation) process prevails, when there are more Pb^{2+} ions. The concentration of Pb^+ increases until saturation (equilibrium) is reached. The effectiveness of producing electrons strongly depends on the irradiation spectrum and is associated with an aggregate $CsPbI_3$ exciton absorption (Nikl [33]).

The above-mentioned population of deep traps is countered by electron scavenging through color centers. A first stage in producing color centers is found in X-ray-induced electron traps (X-ray radiation damage). A competing coloration is found in a second mechanism. This mechanism reveals itself as UV/blue-induced electron-trap creation caused by UV radiation. The corresponding damage is manifested as color centers in the host material CsI. The centers remove electrons from traps that diverted the electrons from the scintillation process. Both sensitivity and hysteresis are affected in this way.

Macroscopic Model

We propose an equilibrium model, based on the process of creation, destruction, population and depletion. Optical attenuation caused by color centers, can be described in a quantitative way by the Stern-Volmer [56] relation. This relation describes a ratio between input intensity I and output intensity I_0 for a luminescent specimen, which relies on the color-center density n_F, a depleting factor by scavenging k, yielding

[1] The holes constitute an "ion molecule" at two adjacent halogen anions in the host crystal.

$$\frac{I}{I_0} = \frac{1}{1 + kn_F}. \tag{4.1}$$

Following Quaranta et al. [37] for low fluences (number of photons per unit area), which is satisfied in our case, this equation holds and the scavenging factor k can be considered as a constant. The decrease in light output depends on the concentration n_F in the form of complementary F-H pairs (Frenkel pairs: anion vacancies and interstitial halogens). The process can be described by a linear differential equation, specified by

$$\frac{dn_F}{d\phi} = -n_0\sigma(1 - v_{RF}n_F), \tag{4.2}$$

where n_F is the defect concentration, ϕ the fluence and n_0 denotes the iodine cation-sublattice atomic concentration. Parameter σ represents the cross-section per interacting light-photon for the formation of a defect pair and v_{RF} the recombination volume for two complementary defects. Solving the previous differential equation yields

$$n_F(\phi) = \frac{1}{v_{RF}}(1 - \exp(-v_{RF}n_0\sigma\phi)). \tag{4.3}$$

Here, the fraction $1/v_{RF}$ can be interpreted as the maximum concentration of color centers in the limit of recombination versus annihilation. The color centers can scavenge electrons from deep Tl-associated traps. The *depletion rate* of the deep traps with respect to the irradiation flux can then be expressed as

$$\frac{I}{I_0} = \frac{1}{1 + \frac{k}{v_{RF}}(1 - \exp(-v_{RF}n_0\sigma\phi))}. \tag{4.4}$$

At this point, we elaborate on the Stern-Folmer relation, yielding an expression of the *trap-population* effect as an ameliorating effect on the scintillator-gain:

$$\frac{I}{I_0} = 1 + kn_e, \tag{4.5}$$

where n_e denotes the *generated electron* concentration. The k-factor should be interpreted as an electron population factor for the deep electron traps, which are responsible for the hysteresis effect. The differential equation for electron (donor) generation resembles the equation for the color center (electron acceptor) generation. The subscripts F and e will be used for electron scavenging and for electron production, respectively. The two effects can be combined, assuming independency of donor and acceptor generation.

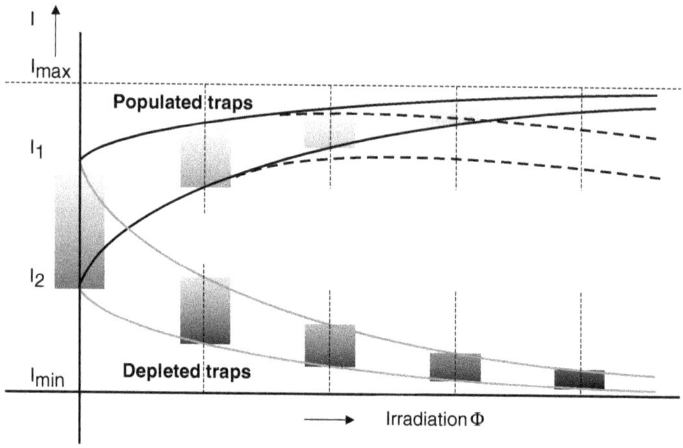

Fig. 4.2 Detector gain variation as a function of irradiating flux and the effect on contrast. *Solid lines* trap-population-only and trap-depletion-only. *Dashed lines* a combined effect

$$\frac{I}{I_0} = \frac{1 + \dfrac{k_e}{v_{Re}}\left[1 - \exp\left(-v_{Re}\, n_{0e}\, \sigma_e \phi\right)\right]}{1 + \dfrac{k_F}{v_{RF}}\left[1 - \exp(-v_{RF} n_{0F} \sigma_F \phi)\right]}, \tag{4.6}$$

Figure 4.2 explains the effect on contrast as a function of irradiance energy. The contrast is reduced until an equal effect of filling and emptying is attained. Beyond this point, the contrast increases , due to an equal depletion of the signal regions I_1 and I_2, (since the contrast definition is $C = (I_1 - I_2)/I_2$ and I_2 is lowered).

Results

Let us first briefly discuss the illumination system. An array of Surface Mounted Device (SMD) LEDs irradiates the CsI:Tl scintillation layer through the glass substrate. The LED pitch is chosen such that a maximally flat irradiation pattern on the scintillator layer is guaranteed. The results on contrast on the detector level will be discussed first, followed by the effect on actual reconstructions at the system level, using an optimal UV irradiation and LED wavelength. This wavelength has been chosen such that maximum trap population occurs, while minimizing trap depletion.

Detector Level

Figure 4.3 shows the results of the contrast measurement for an experiment with varying LED-pulse-width and constant current. The contrasts are generated by applying

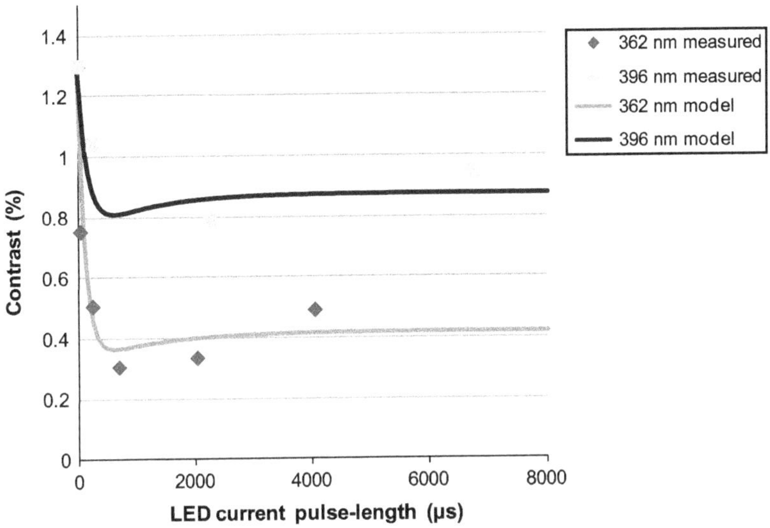

Fig. 4.3 Detector contrast as a function of LED pulse-length for a frame rate of 7.5 fr/s and a current of 10 mA. *Two cases are depicted* 362-nm peak wavelength and 396-nm peak-wavelength

a large dose on the detector (10 mGy), which is partly covered with a lead slab. The ghost imprint is subsequently read out by low-dose imaging. Two wavelengths are shown with their effects on ghost-contrast reduction. A steep decrease in remnant contrast, i.e. the contrast between the irradiated part and the non-irradiated part, can be observed for an increasing irradiation pulse-energy. The effect is countered at larger irradiation energies. The plot includes best-fit curves according to the first-order contrast model, using the combined gain expression. Clearly, the 362-nm wavelength is more effective than the 396-nm wavelength and equals an alternative ghost-reduction method based on flooding the detector with a large X-ray dose.

As important IQ parameters at the detector level are concerned, we find that (1) the noise spectral behavior for an UV-irradiated patch (362 nm) of the CsI(Tl,Na,Pb) layer, is virtually equal to that of a non-irradiated part. Moreover, (2) the MTF of the scintillator is invariant upon UV irradiation. As a consequence, (3) Detective Quantum Efficiency (DQE) calculations reveal no changes with respect to a non-irradiated layer. The (4) sensitivity of the scintillator increases with irradiation to a saturation level, which is consistent with the notion of saturated trap population. Finally, (5) the afterglow is improved as well, as the traps are kept populated and will not contribute to a delayed emission.

System Level

As an experiment, we have employed a modified detector in a commercial vascular imaging system, equipped with 3D imaging software. On the one hand, ghosts are imprinted by applying a small-format detector zoom mode (diagonal 22 cm), in order to create transitional ghosts at the field-limiting shutter edges and on the other hand, the zoom field is partially covered with a 1.8-mm Cu attenuator, thereby mimicking skull transitions. Using automatic exposure control for a number of runs distributed over time, we imitate a prolonged vascular intervention. The tube voltage is set at 80 kV. The un-attenuated integrated detector dose amounts to 10.3 mGy. Upon imprinting a ghost image, a 3D run with an empty volume is acquired using a proper beam attenuation, to ensure a correct detector working point. Finally, a 3D reconstruction of the empty volume is performed. Figure 4.4 displays the reconstruction result of the empty projection images after a ghost imprint. At the right part of (a), the scintillator is irradiated by UV at optimum irradiation, whereas the left part is not. The outer dark lines are due to ramp-filtered shutter transitions which are imprinted before the image acquisition sequence. The transitions become blurred by focus projection. The inner brighter lines are due to 1.8-mm Cu-to-air and [1.8-mm Cu]-to-[0.3-mm Cu] transitions. The improvement as shown at the right part of the image is obvious. Figure 4.4 b and c show transverse planes through the left and right parts of (a), respectively. After rendering the slices, the images are displayed at the same window width/window level.

Conclusions

We have studied the reduction of ghost images for FP X-ray systems by using near-UV irradiation on the scintillator. We have devised a method for reducing hysteresis effects by at least a factor of 4 for a CsI:Tl-doped scintillator contaminated with Pb and Na. This approach can be used in a commercially available large-area flat

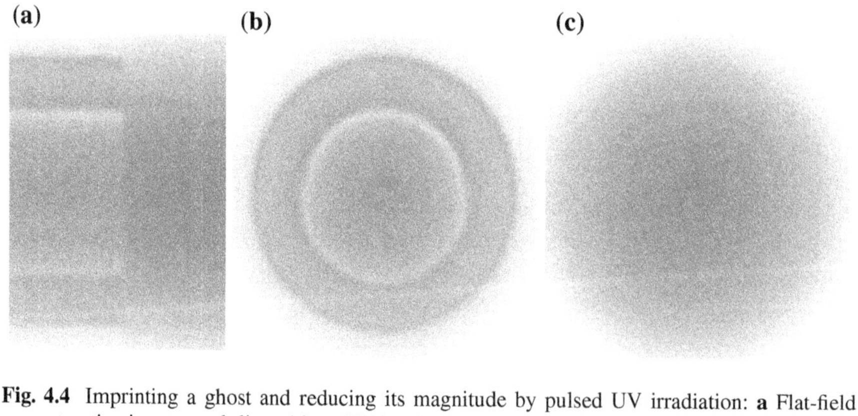

Fig. 4.4 Imprinting a ghost and reducing its magnitude by pulsed UV irradiation: **a** Flat-field reconstruction in a coronal slice without UV irradiation (*left part*) and optimal pulsed UV irradiation (*right part*). **b** Transverse slice through the *left part* of (**a**). **c** Transverse slice through the *right part* of (**a**)

X-ray detector. For reduction of the sensitivity for ghosting, we use back-lighting of the scintillator layer, employing LED arrays. Our proposal combats the ghosting problem at the root where it is generated: the sensitivity variations due to memory effects across the detector field are reduced by saturated trap filling through UV.

We have modeled the process on a microscopic qualitative level and on a macroscopic quantitative level and found that an *optimum UV-irradiation fluence* exists. In a competing mechanism, electron-scavenging color centers are activated along with electron-producing centers. An *optimum wavelength at 364 nm* has been found, which maximizes trap population and minimizes trap depletion. Based on our experiments and literature study, we assume a reduction of color centers by adding Na as a co-dopant, which effects a virtually population-only process by Pb as an electron donor. At the detector level, we find that the main IQ parameters in terms of noise, sharpness and sensitivity, are not affected by the proposed method. As a beneficial side effect, we find an improved afterglow performance. Our method for the reduction of ghost images is as efficient as de-ghosting by X-ray, thereby depriving the detector of its susceptibility to memory effects.

Robotic Modeling for Non-rigid 3D Reconstruction of Steerable Catheters

Minimally-invasive interventions typically have a dynamic nature, where object motion plays a crucial part. In this section, we examine such a dynamic scenario, namely that of steerable catheters (Fig. 4.5a) that deform during cardiac ablation procedures, guided by X-ray fluoroscopy. Catheters undergo both *rigid* motion (due to e.g. patient breathing), as well as *non-rigid* deformation, resulting from interaction with vessel walls, cardiac motion and manipulation by the surgeon. Correct catheter navigation is a difficult task, as the information of three-dimensional (3D) pose of the catheter is lost during the projection onto the 2D image plane. If such 3D information could be explicitly reconstructed from the available 2D data, it could greatly improve surgical insight.

The 3D reconstruction of the time-varying catheter shape is equivalent to attempting the reconstruction of *a moving object with a moving camera*, which is an inherently underconstrained problem. This problem can be regarded from the perspectives of two different fields: Medical Imaging and Computer Vision. Medical Imaging aims at achieving the goal of catheter localization within a clinical scenario, and solutions in that field often make use of different imaging or localization technologies, such as external sensors [25, 28, 32], biplane systemsl [3, 4]. In single-view imaging, Esthappan et al. [12] fit a (known) rigid 3D model of the catheter, while van Walsum et al. [59] and Bruckner et al. [6] have described deformable reconstruction using single-plane imaging for guidewires. In contrast to our work, these methods rely on a pre-existing segmented 3D volume to constrain the solution space, whereas our goal is to use only the available 2D projection data.

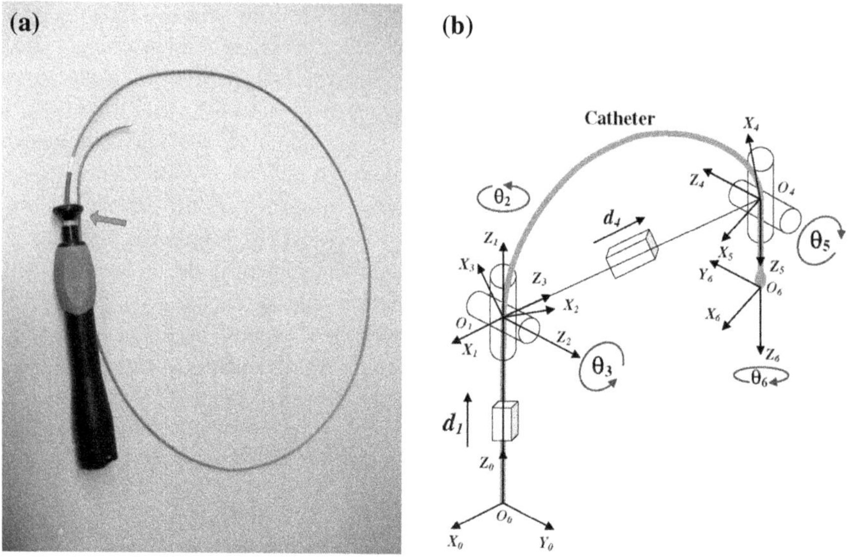

Fig. 4.5 **a** Ablation catheter where the control knob for the deflection is highlighted with the *arrow*. **b** Schematic of the catheter kinematic model (reproduced from [14] with permission. ©2009 IEEE)

By contrast, Computer Vision uses available multi-view camera technology and mathematical modeling to search for solutions for the problem of deformable 3D reconstruction. We aim at a solution using the current X-ray system, without additional equipment and with a limited view separation (such that the C-arm motion is not disruptive to the intervention), therefore we employ the Computer Vision approach. The problem of reconstructing a deforming object using views captured by a moving camera is termed *Non-Rigid Structure-from-Motion*(NRSfM), and is inherently underconstrained. Bregler et al. [5] first proposed to use a low-rank shape model, representing shape as a linear combination of a fixed number of basis shapes for orthographic cameras, while Hartley and Vidal [15] have given a closed-form solution for perspective cameras. Fayad et al. [13] use quadratic deformation models that can capture locally non-linear deformations, which can describe physical aspects such as bending, stretching and twisting. However, that approach requires the shape to be at rest for part of the sequence, while it is difficult to impose physical constraints to the model.

Robotics: Ganji and Janabi [14] have proposed a Robotics-based kinematic model for steerable catheters, which describes the kinematic properties of steerable catheters with a few parameters only. The main limitation of this model is that it does not deal with the interaction of the catheter with its surrounding tissue. Based on the above kinematic formulation, we have proposed in [36] an NRSfM framework to reconstruct the deformable 3D shape of catheters, using X-ray projections made with a small view separation. In this chapter, we extend the approach presented in [36] with the following contributions.

- The model of [14] is extended to describe interaction of the catheter with surrounding material; the performance of the extended model for catheter shape description as well as for 3D+T reconstruction is tested.
- Extensive simulations are performed, illustrating the accuracy and limitations of the proposed approach.
- The effect of rigid motion on successful initialization is analyzed, and an alternative initialization is proposed.
- Experiments are performed on a "stop-motion animation" phantom dataset, and 3D error evaluated.

Robotics Modeling of Catheters

Ganji et al. [14] first proposed to view the catheter as a *continuum robot*, which is a continuously curving manipulator, and described its kinematic properties in a model, shown in Fig. 4.5b. This approach aims at allowing the analysis of catheter position and control, as opposed to our goal of resolving its 3D shape using multi-view images. For manipulation of the catheter in free space, two assumptions have been made and validated in [14]. First, because of the catheter's pullwire mechanism, the deflection of the bending section is in-plane, thus the catheter bends with zero-torsion. Second, the bending occurs with constant curvature, such that the bending part takes the shape of a circular arc. From these assumptions, it can be derived that parameters d_4 and θ_5 are coupled to θ_3, while θ_6 is coupled to θ_2 (see Fig. 4.5b). Thus, the catheter model can be described with three free parameters in total, namely d_1, θ_2 and θ_3 (assuming the length of the distal shaft, d_7, is known).

A. Extension of the kinematic model.
The kinematic model presented above imposes parameter constraints, arising from a consideration of the pull-wire mechanism of the catheter. However, as the authors note in [14], these constraints do not allow modeling of the catheter's interaction with surrounding material. When the assumptions of planar deflection and constant curvature are violated, the model becomes inaccurate.

In the following, we extend the model to accommodate shape deformations that arise from the interaction with surrounding tissue. In the context of our NRSfM formulation, the most important consideration when attempting such an extension is to keep the parameter space as small as possible, such that a solution can be reached given the limited 2D information. Therefore, explicit modeling of the physical properties of tissue, as well as the dynamic behavior of the catheter (which would be crucial for e.g. robotic navigation), have not been considered.

Instead, we have limited ourselves to the kinematics only, as we are interested in retrieving the 3D pose of the catheter from its known 2D projections. Therefore, we take a simplified view of the problem, where the contact forces operate inside a "black box", and we observe only the resulting deformation. Our approach retains the simple kinematic formulation, but removes the geometric constraints, which are based on operation of the catheter in free space. Thus, instead of attempting to solve this complex problem by analyzing the dynamics of the interaction, we instead search for *a description of the deformations caused by such an interaction*. In the following, we will discuss individual adaptations to the original kinematic model, referring to the main model assumptions: (1) constant curvature, and (2) in-plane deflection.

Constant-curvature assumption. To relax the curvature constancy assumption, which describes that chord d_4 is a function of θ_3, we introduce a parameter θ_4 that expresses the deviation of the model from the coupled form described in [14]. This couples the chord d_4 to both θ_3 and θ_4, as $d_4 = 2R\sin(\pi/2 - \theta_3 - \theta_4)$ (see Fig. 4.6a), allowing the catheter to bend with a curvature larger or smaller (depending on the sign of θ_4) than the value predicted by the coupling. Note that we are still assuming that the bending part forms a circular arc, to allow a compact model representation.

In-plane deflection assumption. The other main assumption of the three-parameter, free-space model is that the catheter deflects in-plane, so that the proximal part O_0O_1, the bending section O_1O_4 and the distal shaft O_4O_6 remain on the same plane during deformation (see Fig. 4.5b). It is evident that when the catheter interacts with tissue, e.g. pressing against the endocardium, this assumption may be violated. The out-of-plane deflection is modeled as an angle θ_7, which acts on the catheter from point O_1 onwards and rotates it with respect to its rigid base O_0O_1. Figure 4.6b shows an example illustration.

By removing the two assumptions of constant-curvature and in-plane deflection, θ_5 and θ_6 are also decoupled. We introduce two new parameters, θ_5' and θ_6', which parameterize the difference of θ_5 and θ_6 from the values predicted in the original model: $\theta_5' = \theta_5 - \pi/2 + \theta_2$ and $\theta_6' = \theta_6 - \pi + \theta_2$. Thus, we have introduced a seven-parameter extended model, where the free parameters are $d_1, \theta_2, \theta_3, \theta_4, \theta_5', \theta_6', \theta_7$. The formulation of the extra parameters as differences with the original three-parameter model allows us to control the degree to which the assumptions are violated. It should be noted that the extended model proposed here does not comply anymore with the Denavit-Hartenberg convention. However, this is not a requirement for NRSfM and therefore, we have not reformulated our model according to this convention.

Deformable Reconstruction Using NRSfM

In the remainder, we follow the technique presented in [36]; we will here describe only additional elements relative to that work. The object shape consists of $N = \sum N_k$ 3D points $\mathbf{S}(\theta)$ (where $k = (1, \ldots, 3)$ for each of the three parts of the catheter), and is a function of the parameter vector $\theta = (d_1, \theta_2, \theta_3, d_4, \theta_5, \theta_6, d_7)$. We assume the 2D tracking data is available as a $2 \times N \times F$ tensor $\mathbf{x}$. For the implementation of the robotics model, we have used the toolbox of [7]. In the case of the extended model, the original model pose given by the toolbox is adapted according to the extra parameters, to create the final pose.

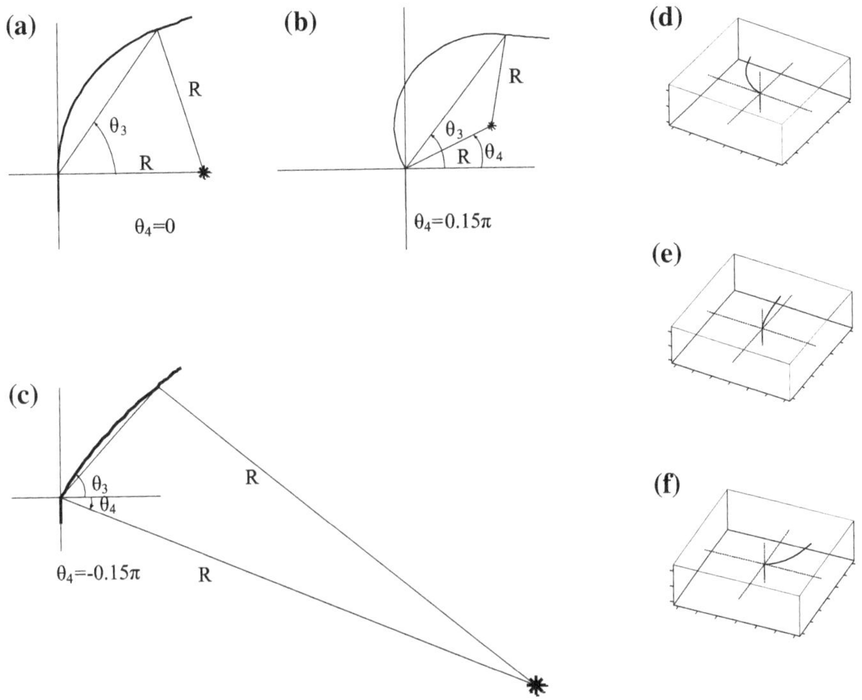

Fig. 4.6 Example of the effect of parameter θ_4 on the shape of the bending section. **a** $\theta_4 = -0.15\pi$, **b** $\theta_4 = 0$, **c** $\theta_4 = 0.15\pi$. Negative values cause the bending section to be "squeezed" ($R < L/(\pi - 2\theta_3)$), while positive values cause it to be "stretched" ($R > L/(\pi - 2\theta_3)$). (**d–f**) Example of the effect of the off-plane deflection parameter θ_7 on the shape of the bending section. **d** $\theta_7 = -0.3\pi$, **e** $\theta_7 = 0$, **f** $\theta_7 = 0.3\pi$. We have chosen large values of θ_7 for clarity

Non-rigid Structure-from-Motion

The catheter shape is observed by the X-ray camera, a projective camera with known calibration parameters, encapsulated in the $3 \times 4 \times F$ projection matrix $\mathbf{P}$. The model observations can be written as $\hat{\mathbf{x}}_i \sim \mathbf{P}_i\mathbf{S}i(\mathbf{p}_i)$, where $\sim$ denotes equality up to a non-zero scaling. The true 2D coordinates of the projected shape $\mathbf{x}$ are obtained by 2D tracking of the object. The NRSfM formulation then consists of solving for the shape parameters that minimize the reprojection error. We also add a temporal smoothness regularization term to ensure realistic deformation over time. The reprojection error term consists of the difference between model and tracked positions (reshaped to a $1 \times 2NF$ vector) $\mathbf{r}_{repr} = \hat{\mathbf{x}} - \mathbf{x}$, while the temporal smoothness term is introduced using the Sobolev functional $\mathbf{r}_t = \Delta\theta/\mathscr{R}_\theta$, where $\mathscr{R}_\theta$ denotes the range of parameter θ. The total cost function can thus be written as the concatenation of the two cost term vectors $\mathbf{r} = (\mathbf{r}_{repr}\|\lambda_t\mathbf{r}_t)$, where the parameter λ_t is used to control the amount of allowed temporal smoothness. In all experiments, $\lambda_t = 1$. The above formulation allows the Levenberg-Marquardt algorithm (LMA) to estimate the parameter vector

$\hat{\mathbf{p}}$ as $\hat{\mathbf{p}} = argmin(\sum_{i,j}^{F,N} \|\mathbf{r}\|^2)$. In this minimization, we consider all projection parameters known and fixed, since C-arm systems are calibrated very accurately.

Initialization and Rigid Registration

The crucial step in the above analysis is the model initialization: if the initialization is very far from the average 3D position of the catheter during its deformation, then the ensuing optimization can easily be trapped in a local minimum. Often, it is assumed that a subset of points on the object are rigid [8], or that the shape remains static for a few frames [13], which is an impractical assumption in the clinical scenario. In [36], it has been assumed that the *base* of the catheter does not move during the sequence, and only one overall rigid transformation is estimated. This may not hold when there is strong interaction with surrounding tissue. A straightforward solution would be to include the parameters of the rigid motion in the overall optimization. However, this would result in a severely underconstrained problem, since six extra parameters per frame (three for rotation and three for translation) would be needed. This is equivalent to the case of a system with unknown extrinsic calibration.

Therefore, instead of first performing a rigid reconstruction and then fitting the rigid transformation $\mathbf{T}$ to this reconstruction, as is done in [36], we calculate $\mathbf{T}$ directly from the 2D image measurements. Specifically, we seek a parameter vector $\mathbf{p}$, defining a rigid transformation $\mathbf{T}(\mathbf{p})$, that minimizes the reprojection error between the first N_1 points of the model and the tracked catheter points $\mathbf{x}_i$, $i = 1, \ldots, F$. The transform $\mathbf{T}$ acts on the original catheter model $\mathbf{S}_0(\theta_0)$, such that the transformed model can be written as $\mathbf{S} = \mathbf{T}\mathbf{S}_0$.

A sliding window is applied: for each frame $f = 1, \ldots, F$ of the sequence, with sub-sequence length F_0, the transformation is calculated using information from frames $f - \lfloor F_0/2 \rfloor$ to $f + \lceil F_0/2 \rceil$. For $f = 1, \ldots, \lfloor F_0/2 \rfloor$ and $f = \lceil F_0/2 \rceil, \ldots, F$, we repeat the solutions for $f = \lfloor F_0/2 \rfloor + 1$ and $f = \lceil F_0/2 \rceil - 1$, respectively. For each window, the result of the previous window is used as an initialization. In the first window, the rigid transformation parameters are initialized randomly.

A synthetic example illustrates the effect of rigid motion on the rigid initialization. We have constructed a synthetic catheter based on the kinematic model (using $d_1 = 40$ mm, $\theta_2 = 0$, $\theta_3 = 0.2\pi$), moving with a constant velocity, between 0.2–3.0 voxels per frame, and we use $F = 10$ frames. In Fig. 4.7, we show the difference between the above approach and the one described in [36]. It can be seen that the method described above achieves better rigid estimation. However, when the velocity increases significantly, the method fails: observing a moving point with a moving camera remains an inherently underconstrained problem. Adding more views for the reconstruction could even have a detrimental effect: introducing more unknown parameters per frame and thus increasing the uncertainty. Nonetheless, this small experiment shows that when the rigid motion is relatively constrained (to within a voxel per frame), we may expect to obtain a reasonable rigid registration result to initialize our algorithm.

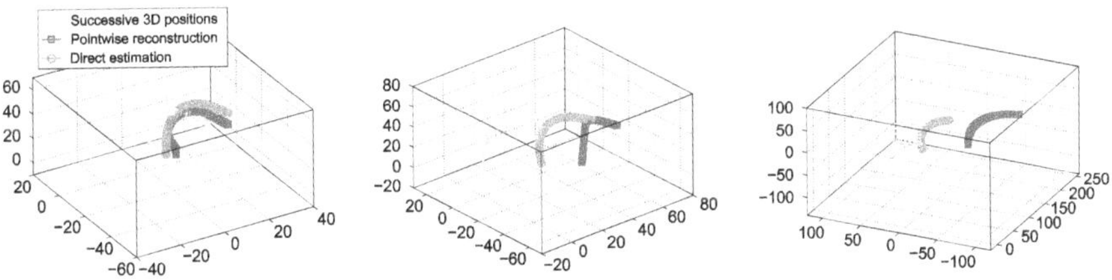

0.2 voxels/frame | 1 voxel/frame | 3 voxels/frame

Fig. 4.7 Comparison between the two methods of obtaining a rigid initial registration in case of rigid motion, for three different catheter velocities. The successive 3D position of the catheter are shown for different velocities, the pointwise reconstruction result according to [36], and a direct estimation of rigid transformation from 2D data, as in Sect. "Initialization and Rigid Registration". It can be seen that the error of the direct estimation is smaller, especially for a fast moving catheter

Experimental Results

In this section, we first describe the experiments performed for the validation of the two catheter models, the original kinematic model of [14] and the extended one proposed in Sect. "Robotics Modeling of Catheters", henceforth referred to as *order-3* and *order-7* models, respectively. Afterwards, we elaborate on a set of synthetic and phantom multi-view experiments.

Rigid Model Fitting

An industrially available cardiac ablation catheter[2] is placed inside a heart phantom with elastic walls filled with water. The catheter is manually manipulated into 36 different postures, for each of which a 3D volumetric reconstruction is obtained, capturing the ground-truth shape of the catheter. During its deformation, the catheter moves inside the phantom while pressing against its walls. The 3D shape of the catheter is manually annotated in each of the resulting 3D volumes and sampled at equidistant intervals. To fit the catheter model, first the overall rigid pose is retrieved by fitting a rigid 3D transformation to the annotated points of the catheter base. Next, the LMA is used to obtain the model parameters that minimize the error between the model and the 3D measurements.

Figure 4.8a shows some characteristic examples of the results, while in Fig. 4.8b, the error for both models is shown. It can be seen both from the qualitative as well as from the quantitative results that the order-7 model achieves a better fit (≈4.5 mm at the base and 4 mm at the tip) than the order-3 model (6 and 5 mm, respectively). The difference between the models is larger along the bending part of the catheter, because at this part, the order-3 model fails to capture the off-plane deflection of the catheter, which occurs in several frames of this sequence. The large standard

[2] Qwikstar 7F 26-pole catheter by Biosense Webster.

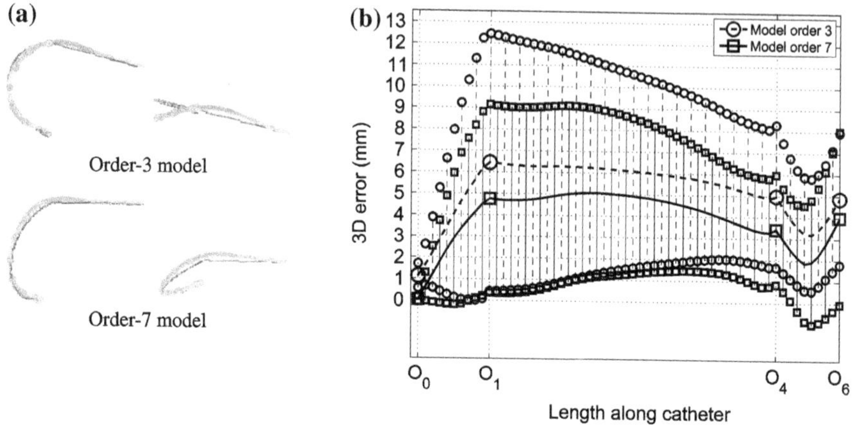

Fig. 4.8 **a** Example results of the rigid model fitting experiment, shown from two different viewpoints. Light thick curves denotes the ground-truth volumetric reconstruction, while the calculated model is shown as *dark thin curves*. **b** Error results in the rigid model fitting experiment. Mean and standard deviation are shown along the length of the catheter model. Points $O_1 \ldots O_6$ are as in Fig. 4.5b

deviation observed in these results is due to the fact that in 5 out of the 36 frames, the rigid transformation has not been estimated correctly. As a result, the model fitting also fails in these cases.

NRSfM Experiments

In [35], we have performed extensive simulation experiments to test the algorithm's accuracy bounds and convergence, as well as to compare between the two kinematic models. Here, we will describe a phantom experiment testing the proposed NRSfM algorithm on real data. As discussed in [36], it is difficult to design a multi-view X-ray experiment for deformable catheters, in which the ground-truth catheter shape is available for each frame. In that work, non-rigid catheter reconstructions of a manually manipulated catheter, with no ground-truth available, were shown to be repeatable to within 5 mm. To emulate a dataset where a 3D+T ground truth is known, we apply the technique of "stop-motion animation", where the catheter deformation is approximated by small discrete steps. In each step, the catheter is manipulated slightly using the control knobs, and a volumetric scan is performed. In this way, a 3D+T dataset is obtained, in which the catheter deforms while its position is known. From this dataset, 2D views from successive time steps form the input for the NRSfM algorithm. We have used a fixed view separation of 1.7°, taken from successive frames in each of the 36 scans. Both the order-3 and the order-7 model are evaluated.

Due to the discrete steps in the stop-motion experiment, the motion created in such an experiment cannot be smooth. The catheter controls do not have a linear

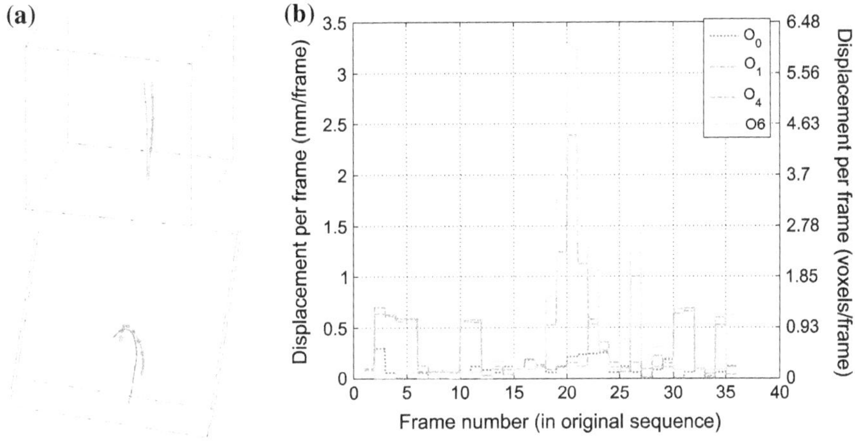

Fig. 4.9 **a** Some snapshot results of the "stop-motion" experiment (order-3 model). *Light thick curve* ground truth. *Dark thin curve* reconstructed result. **b** Average displacement per frame of the catheter points for the same dataset

response to the input applied, such that the motion often exhibits sudden jumps, which are not repeatable. This complicates the task of our NRSfM algorithm, which explicitly assumes temporal smoothness in the data. Figure 4.9b shows the average displacement per frame for this experiment. When juxtaposing this to the analysis of Sect. "Initialization and Rigid Registration", it can clearly be seen that the displacement per frame (velocity) between frames 17–30 of this sequence is quite large (>6 voxels/frame) and can be expected to limit the success of NRSfM.

Some snapshots of the results of the proposed Robotic-NRSfM algorithm, with automatic rigid registration as described in Sect. "initialization and rigid registration", are shown in Fig. 4.9, while the 3D error results are presented in Fig. 4.10. It can be noted that the error increases close to the catheter tip, which is expected, as the displacement at that point is maximal. We note the large error of the order-7 model (in the order of 60 mm), caused by erroneous estimation of the rigid transform. The wrong estimation is propagated through the sliding-window estimation until frame 30, where the error drops to a level lower than that of the order-3 model ($\approx$20 mm). With respect to the performance of the two different models, we have observed (Sect. "Rigid Model Fitting") that the extended model fits more accurately to 3D measurements of a catheter bending against an elastic wall. However, in the NRSfM experiments, it has been discovered that this 7-parameter model does not outperform the original 3-parameter model. Although the order-7 model is more suitable to *describe* catheter deformation, it is less useful in *retrieving* the 3D deformation from multiple 2D images, since the larger parameter space leaves the optimization underconstrained. Therefore, we conclude that for the present application, the original 3-parameter model is a better choice.

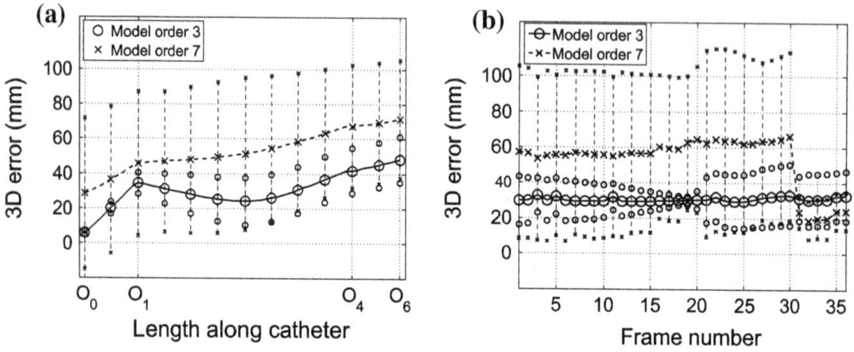

Fig. 4.10 (a) 3D error along the length of the catheter, averaged over the entire sequence. (b) Error for each frame of the sequence, averaged over the length of the catheter

Conclusions and Outlook

In this section, we have explored the potential of multi-view X-ray to recover the deformable 3D shape of a steerable catheter, using only multi-view information. To this end, we have adopted the framework of NRSfM, but instead of the models proposed in Computer Vision, we have selected a *kinematic* model from the field of Robotics. Based on this model, we have constructed an algorithm that recovers 3D+T shape, given the 2D catheter tracks and the system calibration as input. It has been shown in previous work that the proposed algorithm produces reconstructions that are reproducible up to 3–5 mm, in a catheter manually manipulated. We have now seen that even in a phantom experiment exhibiting pronounced rigid motion and significant abrupt deformation, the average error remains around 30 mm. In the context of the clinical application (RF ablation), where an accuracy of a few millimeters suffices for correct catheter guidance, these preliminary results show that Robotic-NRSfM can operate within or close to the accuracy requirements. To the best of our knowledge, these are the first experimental results reported on deformable 3D+T reconstruction of a catheter using only multi-view X-ray with non-simultaneous acquisition.

For the future deployment of this approach in clinical practice, a number of open issues remain. The first of these relates to the rigid registration step of the algorithm. We have proposed an initialization scheme that can handle some rigid motion, but its robustness is limited in cases of pronounced displacements; the exact limitations in estimating overall motion using limited X-ray views remain to be explored. Secondly, in the context of the clinical application, the factor of computational performance comes into play. Although our present implementation does not operate in real time, such a goal is achievable, as large parts of the processing can be parallelized. Finally, the clinical validation of this approach introduces challenges, mainly pertaining to two factors: the presence of cardiac motion (which increases the dimensionality of the problem), and the definition of an appropriate test bench in the absence of ground-truth 3D+T clinical data.

The above results and discussion show that the proposed technique can potentially provide live 3D guidance of catheter placement not only during a procedure, but even during the actual manipulation of the catheter. Additionally, the modularity of the robotic formulation allows many categories of man-made objects, including surgical instruments, to be expressed in terms of simple parameterized models. In this way, it can be applied in the context of a generic interventional system to several clinical applications, and provide invaluable insight in ambiguous situations that arise during surgical guidance.

Multi-modal Integration in the Cathlab

During minimally invasive medical treatment the clinician relies on radiological images, often produced in real-time, to guide the intervention. Prior to treatment, diagnosis and intervention planning is frequently performed using tomographical images, which provide a detailed representation of the patient's anatomy and pathology. In this section the fusion of those different types of images is presented, in order to provide the clinician with more relevant data to guide the procedure [46]. Since the fusion is performed during the clinical intervention, it is essential that the technical steps can be executed within limited time. Furthermore, it is vital that the resulting fused representations are easy to interpret. The technical approaches that are described here to achieve this goal comprise rapid co-registration of multiple image datasets, and intuitive visualization of the fused data.

In order to achieve an optimal performance the parallel computation power of the graphics processing unit (GPU) can be exploited in the registration and visualization algorithms. In the following sections a detailed strategy to map the processing capabilities of the GPU on an elastic co-registration algorithm is described [48]. The objective of a registration algorithm is to find a spatial mapping between two image datasets. Typically intensity-based registration algorithms consist of a similarity measure, indicating the quality of a given spatial mapping, and an optimization strategy, which iteratively searches the optimum of the similarity measure. The search space consists of the multi-dimensional control variables of the spatial mapping. Non-rigid registration algorithms employ a spatial mapping that allows to model local deformations. Such non-rigid spatial mappings typically are driven by a large number of parameters, increasing the computation times and therefore increasing the need for fast and efficient solutions.

Computational Methods and Theory

In this chapter we will restrain ourselves to the class of algorithms, in which the similarity measure can be expressed as a sum of contributions per spatial element (pixel for 2D, voxel for 3D, etc.). Sum of Squared Differences (SSD) and Cross-Correlation

(CC) are examples of members of this class. This class generally can be written as follows:

$$E = \frac{1}{\|I\|}\sum_{\mathbf{i}\in I} e(A(\mathbf{i}),\ B^{\tau}(\mathbf{i})) = \frac{1}{\|I\|}\sum_{\mathbf{i}\in I} e\,(A(\mathbf{i}),\ B(\boldsymbol{\tau}(\mathbf{i}))) \tag{4.7}$$

Whereby E represents the similarity measure, e the contribution to the similarity measure per spatial element, A the reference image, and B the floating image. $\boldsymbol{\tau}(\mathbf{i})$ denotes the deformation of the reference image coordinate system to the floating image coordinate system and B^{τ} is the deformed floating image. $\mathbf{i} \in I \subset \mathbb{Z}^N$ represents the set of N-dimensional discrete spatial positions (i.e pixel or voxel positions in the image).

The deformation is driven by a set of parameters $\mathbf{c}_j$. It is this set of parameters that is manipulated by the iterative optimization algorithm. A uniform B-spline driven deformation field is well suited to represent organic deformations. The uniform B-spline driven deformation field then can be described by the following equation [19]:

$$\tau(\mathbf{i}) = \mathbf{i} + \sum_{j\in J} \mathbf{c}_j \cdot \beta_3(\mathbf{i}/\mathbf{h} - j) \tag{4.8}$$

The control points are denoted by $\mathbf{c}_j \in \mathbb{Z}^N$, and J is the set of parameter indices. Vector $\mathbf{h}$ represents the spacing of the control points, which we require to be integer. Since $\mathbf{i}$ is added to the sum, the identity deformation corresponds to all control points being zero. $\beta_3(\mathbf{i})$ is the N-dimensional tensor product of a uniform cubic B-spline function.

In order to obtain a better prediction of the parameters used in the next iteration, the Jacobian matrix, containing the partial derivatives of the similarity measure to the parameter space $\delta E/\delta c_{j,m}$ is required [18], with m denoting the axis. The partial derivative can be decomposed into the following product:

$$\frac{\delta E}{\delta c_{j,m}} = \frac{1}{\|I\|}\sum_{\mathbf{i}\in I} \frac{\delta e(\mathbf{i})}{\delta B^{\tau}(\mathbf{i})}\ \frac{\delta B(\mathbf{x})}{\delta x_m}\bigg|_{\mathbf{x}=\boldsymbol{\tau}(\mathbf{i})} \frac{\delta \tau_m(\mathbf{i})}{\delta c_{j,m}} \tag{4.9}$$

The derivative of the first multiplicand in Eq. 4.9 depends on the used similarity measure. In Table 4.1 the derivatives for SSD and CC are given. In contrary to [19], we do not obtain the derivative $\delta B(\mathbf{x})/\delta x_m$ of the deformed floating image analytically. We rather use an image based approach, employing a convolution with Sobel-like kernels. As can be understood from Eq. 4.8, the derivative of the deformation field $\delta \tau_m(\mathbf{i})/\delta c_{j,m}$ simply is a constant term: $\beta_n(\mathbf{i}/\mathbf{h} - j)$.

Table 4.1 Similarity measures, and their derivative with respect to the deformed image

Similarity measure	Contribution per pixel	Derivative
Sum of squared differences (SSD)	$e(\mathbf{i}) = (A(\mathbf{i}) - B^{\tau}(\mathbf{i}))^2$	$\delta e/\delta B^{\tau} = 2 \cdot (A(\mathbf{i}) - B^{\tau}(\mathbf{i}))$
Cross-correlation (CC)	$e(\mathbf{i}) = A(\mathbf{i}) \cdot B^{\tau}(\mathbf{i})$	$\delta e/\delta B^{\tau} = A(\mathbf{i})$

Program Description

The derivative of the floating image $\delta B(\mathbf{x})/\delta x_m$ has to be calculated at $\boldsymbol{\tau}(\mathbf{i})$ for all $\mathbf{i} \in I$. In order to obtain this derivative, the gradient image of the floating image is pre-calculated. It should be noted that this gradient image is static during the optimization process, and therefore needs to be calculated only once for the entire registration procedure. The gradient image can be easily obtained on the GPU by convolving the floating image with Sobel-like derivative kernels of size 3^N.

The GPU implementation of the similarity measure and the first order derivatives is illustrated in Fig. 4.11, and works as follows: for every voxel in the reference image a thread is started, and its contribution to the similarity measure and derivatives is calculated. In the thread the corresponding location in the deformed floating data is obtained by adding the cubic B-spline driven deformation offset to the thread's voxel coordinate, see Eq. 4.8. Hereby, we can make efficient use from the fact that a cubic B-spline lookup can be decomposed into 8 linearly weighted interpolations, rather than 64 nearest neighbor lookups, which is much faster on the GPU [47, 53].

When the deformed coordinate has been established, the voxel intensities of the reference and floating datasets are fetched, and the similarity measure contribution of the thread can be established, see Eq. 4.7. The gradient of the floating dataset and

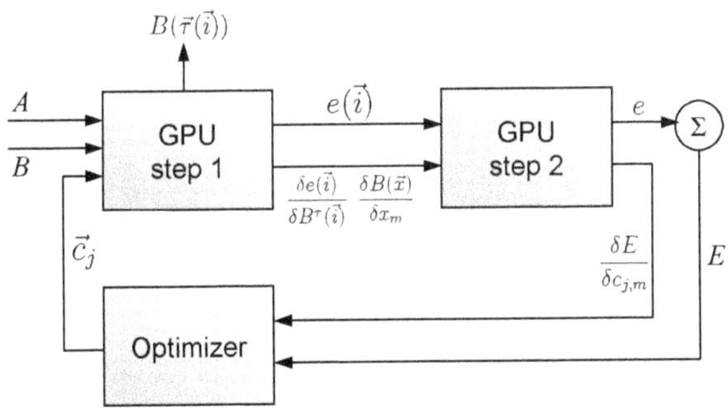

Fig. 4.11 Block diagram showing the overall dataflow in the algorithm. The first GPU pass takes the reference image A, the floating image B, and the set of deformation coefficients $\mathbf{c}_j$ as input. It calculates the contribution to the similarity measure per voxel and the first part of the derivative per voxel. This data is passed to the second GPU pass. This establishes the derivative of the similarity measure to the B-spline coefficients, and passes those to the optimizer. The optimizer determines the new set of B-spline coefficients, and the cycle repeats until the optimum of the similarity measure is found

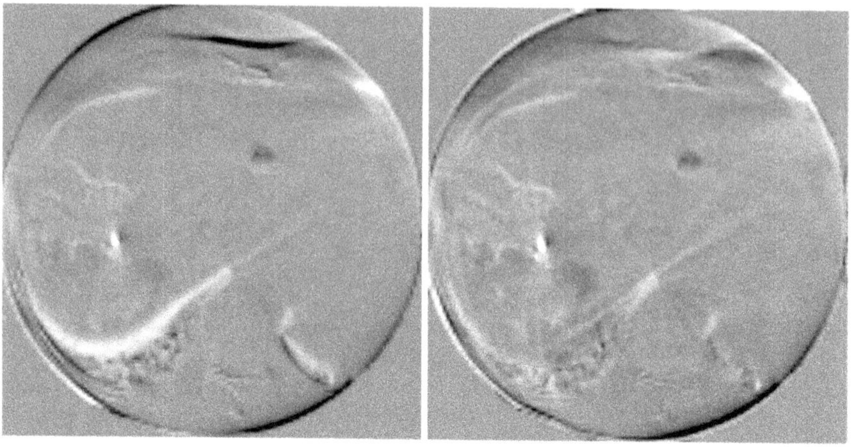

Fig. 4.12 A slice of a cone-beam CT reconstruction of the abdomen is taken at the beginning and during the course of interventional treatment. The *left image* shows the subtraction of both slices without any registration applied, whereby dark and light areas indicate the differences between the images. The *right image* illustrates the subtraction after the elastic registration has been performed

its intensities are stored in a single texture with four entries per voxel. In this way the interpolated lookup at the deformed coordinate simultaneously yields the intensity and the gradient of the floating data $\delta B(\mathbf{x})/\delta x_m$ at this particular location.

The derivative of the similarity measure to the control points consists of three multiplicands, see Eq. 4.9. Two of those can be established for each GPU thread; the gradient of the floating data $\delta B(\mathbf{x})/\delta x_m$, and the derivative of the similarity measure to the voxel space $\delta e/\delta B^{\tau}$. The similarity measure and first order derivatives contributions are stored in an intermediate 3D data array for each thread.

In the second pass, the first order derivatives $\delta E/\delta c_{j,m}$ are calculated by multiplying a subset of the previously stored derivative data with the B-spline weights $\beta_3(\mathbf{i}/\mathbf{h}-j)$. The B-spline weights are constant, and can be decomposed into a tensor product of three pre-computed 1D arrays of width $4 \cdot h_m$.

Results

Figure 4.12 illustrated the effect of the described registration algorithm, using real clinical data. The data concerned two cone-beam CT reconstruction of the same volume of interest of 256^3 voxels. The registration was performed by the GPU implementation in 14.2 s by downsampling the datasets to 128^3 voxels using 5 iterations with 8^3 control points and 30 iterations with 16^3 control points. As can be seen from the difference images, the deformation of the organs (the liver in this case) is largely corrected by the elastic deformation field.

Table 4.2 Distribution of the time per iteration over the passes, using datasets of 128^3 voxels and 16^3 control points

Implementation	Pass 1 (ms)	Pass 2 (ms)	Overhead (ms)
SSE	536.8	474.2	3.1
GPU	9.6	128.8	1.5

In order to characterize the calculation time of the proposed algorithm, the GPU implementation was compared to a straight-forward single threaded CPU implementation and a multi-threaded SSE optimized CPU version. We used a 2.33 GHz quad-core Intel Xeon with 2 GB memory and an NVIDIA GeForce GTX 260 with 896 MB memory to perform our measurements. As test data we used eight different cone-beam CT datasets of the head of patient with either arterio-venous malformations or aneurysms. The datasets consisted of 256^3 isotropic voxels, with voxel sizes ranging from 0.28 to 0.40 mm in each direction. The reference and floating data was obtained by deforming each CT dataset according to a B-spline field of 16^3 uniformly distributed control points, whereby their magnitude was randomly determined in the range $[-8,\ 8]$ and some white noise was added to the voxel values. The randomly deformed dataset then served as reference, and the original as floating data. We measured the time to obtain the similarity measure and first order derivatives by performing a quasi-Newton driven optimization in 40 iterations, and averaging the time per iteration. The dataset sizes ranged from 32^3 voxels to 256^3 voxels

The speedup factor of the GPU version compared to the other two implementations is illustrated in Fig. 4.13. It shows that the multi-threaded SSE implementation provides a speedup of approximately a factor 10 over the straight-forward CPU version, whereas the GPU implementation delivers an average speed improvement of approximately a factor 50.

When we dissected the time per iteration into the time used for the first and second pass (Table 4.2), we discovered that the GPU version spends considerably more time in the second pass than in the first pass.

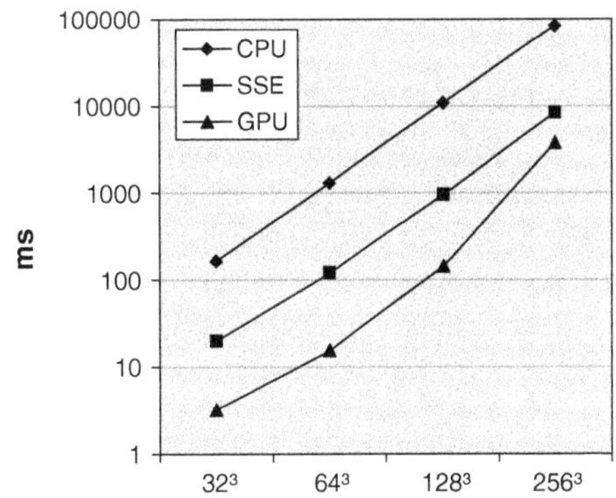

Fig. 4.13 The calculation time per iteration (y-axis, in milliseconds, logarithmic scale) for different dataset sizes (x-axis, in amount of voxels), using 16^3 B-spline control points, for the three implementations

Discussion

The application of elastic registration during interventional treatment demands that the registration can be obtained within a limited time frame. The number of iterations that has to be evaluated in the iterative optimization of a similarity measure can be reduced by more accurately predicting the next step towards the optimum, based on the derivative of the similarity measure with respect to the parameter space. In this section we have demonstrated how the similarity measure and its derivative can be calculated on the GPU, using a two pass algorithm. In the first pass the floating image is deformed, using an elastic uniform cubic B-spline deformation field, and the similarity measure and first order derivatives contribution are stored per voxel. The second pass yields the derivative of the similarity measure per control point. The calculation of the derivative was further accelerated by using a static gradient image of the floating image, that was obtained by a convolution with Sobel-like kernels.

In this section we focussed on the calculation time of the CPU and GPU implementations of the same basic algorithm. In practise, a good approach has proven to start the registration in low resolution with few control points to find large deformations, and to gradually refine the registration by moving to higher resolutions and more control points [41]. Lets consider e.g a registration that first performs 20 iterations at a resolution of 64^3 with 8^3 control points, then 10 iterations at 128^3 with 16^3 control points, and finally 5 iterations at 256^3 with 32^3 control points. The straight-forward CPU version would take 329 s (5.5 min) to perform this registration, the multi-threaded SSE version costs 31.2 s, and the GPU implementation takes 7.4 s. Five minutes is unacceptable for many interventional and surgical applications, 31.2 s becomes an issue when the registration has to be performed multiple times (to compensate for progressively deforming of the brain), while 7.4 s is considered to be quite acceptable.

Clinical Applications

Peri-interventional registration, as described in this section, can be very usefull in the cathlab. Here, a number of practical applications are listed. A more detailed description can be found in [45].

- The navigation of a catheter based on multiple image sources (MR, 3DRA and fluoroscopy) during the treatment of an arterio-veneous malformation (AVM) in the brain, see Fig. 4.14.
- The planning of a percurtaneous needle puncture path using fusion of diagnostic CT images and live X-ray fluoroscopy, see Fig. 4.15.

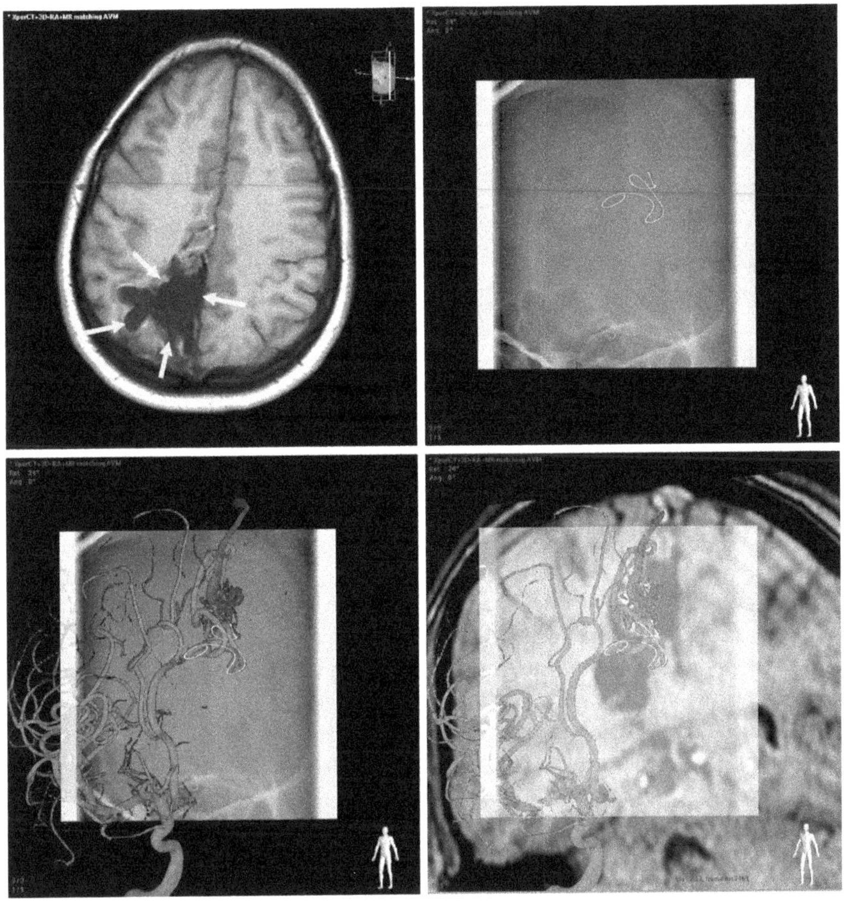

Fig. 4.14 *Upper row, left* An MR image shows an arterioveneous malformation (AVM) and the affected brain tissue (*arrows*). *Upper row, right* The live fluoroscopy image, without any contrast agent, shows the guidewire, but not the context of the vessels and soft tissue. *Lower row, left* The fluoroscopy image fused with the 3DRA vessel tree adds the vascular context to the live image. *Lower row, right* The fluoroscopy image, the 3DRA vessel tree and a cross-section of the MR data

View Interpolation for Autostereoscopic Displays in the Cathlab

The introduction of autostereoscopic displays to a clinical setting allows physicians to perceive depth in medical images. The addition of depth perception leads to a faster and better interpretation of the morphology of the patient's pathology and contextual anatomy. Stereoscopic images are being used in various clinical applications, such as surgical planning [55], surgical navigation [22–24], minimally invasive endoscopic surgery [42], autostereoscopic intracranial MRA visualization [1], etc. Autostereoscopic visualization of the patient's anatomy has the potential to be combined with

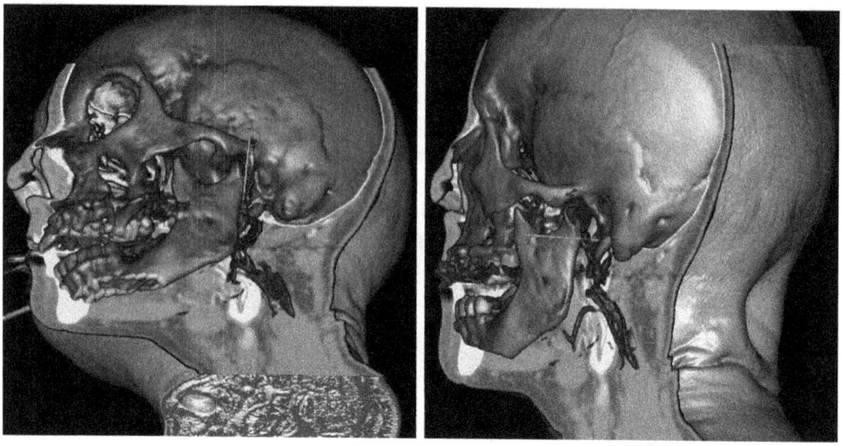

Fig. 4.15 The fused pre-operative CT data (skin) and the intra-operative C-arm cone-beam CT data (bone) are shown together with the planned needle path

augmented reality, which has been reported to increase the surgical instrument placement accuracy [22]. Displaying medical images in a clinical context imposes several restrictions on the image transmission chain. A digital imaging chain may contain errors and artifacts. Such errors involve image digitization, compression, transfer function limitations, dynamic range limitations, etc., which have to be kept below a stringent threshold. The obvious reason for this is the fact that medical decisions are taken based on these images, and flaws in the image may lead to misinterpretations.

The development of high-resolution LCD grids (such as QuadHD grids) has brought high-resolution autostereoscopic screens within reach. However, these screens introduce a new challenge, since the amount of the visualized data becomes enormous, while the images have to be rendered and conveyed to the display in real-time. To cope with this, we intend to transmit fewer views than the autostereoscopic display emits, and to render the missing views at the receiver side using 2D texture+depth information. To this end, the display unit in the operating room is extended with embedded receiver hardware.

Autostereoscopic Display

A stereoscopic display presents the viewer with different images for the left and the right eye. Provided that these images contain proper stereoscopic information, the viewer will have the sensation of seeing depth. Principally there are two kinds of stereoscopic displays: the first type requires the viewer to wear goggles or glasses, and the second type, called autostereoscopic display, allows stereoscopic viewing without any external aid. For the usage of such displays during medical interventions, the absence of goggles is a significant benefit, since there is no compromise of sterility by any external attributes and the goggles might be considered to be disturbing when the clinician is not looking at the stereoscopic display (which typically will be the case during a major part of the clinical procedure) [43]. In contrast to the binocular stereoscope, mutli-view autostereoscopic displays emit more than two views (which in principle would be enough for stereoscopy), in order to have a wider range where the observer can see a proper stereoscopic image, and to allow multiple viewers to perceive the stereoscopic image [22]. Especially in the operating room, where the observer is not fixed to a single spot, this is of relevance.

Popular techniques to achieve autostereoscopy are parallax barrier and lenticular displays. Both techniques can be used to implement multi-view displays. In parallax barrier displays, a raster of slits is placed at a small distance in front of the display, showing a different subset of pixels when viewing it from various angles. A multi-view autostereoscopic lenticular display consists of a cover sheet of cylindrical lenses (lenticulars) placed on top of an LCD, in such a way that the LCD image plane is positioned at the focal plane of the lenses [58]. As a consequence of this arrangement, different LCD pixels underneath the lenses become visible when viewed from a set of predetermined directions. The fact that mutually exclusive subsets of LCD pixels are assigned to different views (spatial multiplex), leads to a lower effective resolution per view than the intrinsic resolution of the LCD grid [11]. In order to distribute this loss of resolution over the horizontal and vertical axis, the lenticular cylindrical lenses are not placed vertically and parallel to the LCD column, but slanted at a small angle.

When the pixels of the autostereoscopic display are loaded with suitable stereo information, a 3D stereo effect is obtained, in which the left and right eye see different, but corresponding, information [44]. Most commercially available display lines offer eight or nine distinct views, but our technology will be applicable to any number of views. The stereoscopic views have to be loaded with the images corresponding to the angle they are emitted. The angle between the views is typically in the range of 1–5°, depending on the monitor setup. In clinical interventional applications, the screen is typically mounted at the opposite side of the patient table with respect to the surgeon. The viewing distance amounts from approximately 1.5 to 5 m. For example, assuming a 7-cm distance between the left and right eye, and 3 m from the viewer to the screen, delivers a 1.3° viewing angle between the view for the left and right eye.

Medical data typically consists of voxel data sets of several hundreds of Megabytes, which can be visualized through a technique called volume rendering [16, 21, 44]. The raw voxel data typically consists of 12-bit or 16-bit scalar data. Often a transfer function is used to zoom on a user-defined scalar range. This transfer function can also be used to map the scalar data on RGB colors and transparencies. The result of the volume rendering is typically stored as 24-bit RGB images. The individual views displayed on the autostereoscopic display are generated on the medical workstation. A naïve approach would be to simply generate an image for every view that is displayed. In case of displaying a scene at 25 frames per second on a 9-view autostereoscopic screen, this would require rendering 225 views per second. In case of a 256-MB 3D data set (512^3 voxels, 16-bit per voxel), the naïve approach would need to parse more than 56 GB/s. Alternatively, Hübner and Pajarola have proposed to generate the composed multi-view volume rendered data in a single pass [16]. Though this approach leads to a slightly better image quality, it does not reduce the strain on volume rendering bottleneck, nor on the transmission channel.

View Interpolation

Principle

In order to reduce the load of the 3D rendering on the workstation and the transmission channel, we create fewer views than those displayed on the lenticular screen. The missing views are interpolated after decoding the video stream at the receiver side, see Fig. 4.16 [49].

As a start, the concept of our interpolation is adopted from free-viewpoint rendering [31]. This method takes into account the camera parameters and the depth information per pixel. This depth quantifies the distance between the screen and the object displayed at a particular pixel. The camera focus point and the pixel location define a ray in a virtual ray space [57]. By using this information, more accurate interpolated views can be created than using a naïve interpolation method, such as linear interpolation. The conceptual chain for multi-view imaging from rendering to display is illustrated in Fig. 4.17.

A QuadHD LCD grid consists of 3840 × 2160 pixels. Assuming that a 9-view QuadHD autostereoscopic display is used, it would make sense to build up a single view in a resolution of 1280 × 720 pixels [44]. The views that are used for the interpolation algorithm can consist of 32 its per pixel, where 24 its are required for the RGB components and 8 bits for depth information. Usage in clinical interventions requires a minimum frame rate of 24 frames per second (fps). When for example four views are transmitted at 24 fps, and the others are interpolated, this would require a bandwidth of 4 views × 1280 × 720 pixels × 24 fps × 32 bits = 2.6 Gbit/s (for uncompressed video data) versus 4.4 Gbit/s for 9 views without depth information.

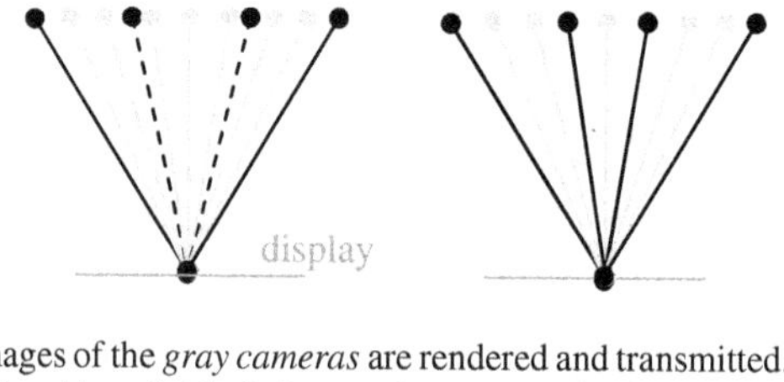

Fig. 4.16 Only the images of the *gray cameras* are rendered and transmitted. For the *white cameras* only their parameters (position, field of view, etc.) are transmitted. The missing views are interpolated at the receiver side. Finally all views are emitted to their respective angle by the lenticular display

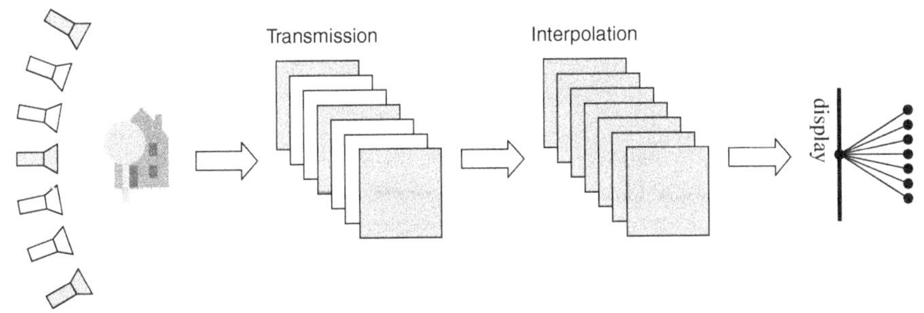

Fig. 4.17 Two possible configurations for 4 transmitted views, and 9 displayed views. *Solid black* transmitted views that can be mapped directly on an output view. *Dashed* transmitted views that cannot be mapped on an output view. *Gray* interpolated view

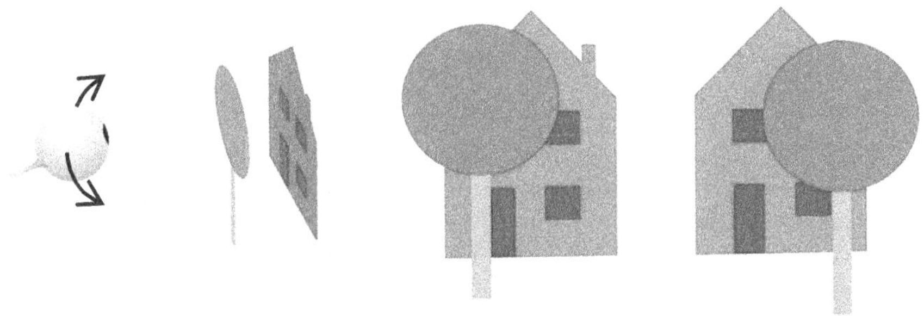

Fig. 4.18 Depending on the viewing position, different parts of a background object are occluded

Furthermore, the load on the volume rendering bottleneck on the medical workstation is reduced considerably, since only 4/9 of the data rendered in the naïve approach needs to be generated.

Artifacts Resulting from Rendering

A key artifact that may appear when using free-viewpoint interpolation is the occurrence of disocclusions [17, 60]. When this happens, a part of the scene becomes visible that was hidden in any of the transmitted views, see Fig. 4.18. Consequently, there is no proper information available that should be filled in at the affected pixels. Fortunately, the impact of this effect is very limited for our application, since the transmitted views and the interpolated views are very close to each other. Disocclusions mainly occur for views that are rather far apart, which is not the case for our setup.

Another related artifact of free-viewpoint interpolation concerns semi-transparent parts of the depicted scene. The free-viewpoint algorithm expects a single depth value per pixel. However, when the object that is being depicted is semi-transparent, a pixel can contain visible information that is composed of the light that is reflected by several objects. Once the reflected light has been blended into a single pixel color, it is impossible to dissect it. In the rendering of 3D medical data, this effect is even amplified, since the depicted data is often the result of a volume rendering process [43, 44], whereby a ray of light traverses through a continuous range of semi-transparent material. Therefore, the proposed technique is limited to representations whereby the majority of the volume consists of completely transparent data together with more or less opaque data.

Constraints of the Rendering Process

Since the medical context demands that there are no severe artifacts, the angle between the virtual cameras has to be small, because it will lead to high similarities between the interpolated and the original views, and thus fewer interpolation artifacts. Furthermore, the small angles will lead to fewer and smaller disoccluded areas. This is particularly important, as the content of the disoccluded areas has to be extrapolated from the surrounding information. Because the images are input to medical decisions, it is essential that the artifacts do not lead to misinterpretations of the interpolated images.

It is our aim to achieve a real-time hardware implementation of the proposed interpolation method. Therefore the complexity of the post-processing has to be limited. The rendering algorithm should be simple, while providing an acceptable quality of the rendering results.

Interpolation Algorithm

Image Warping

Depth Image Based Rendering (DIBR) algorithms are based on warping the image from a camera view to another view [27]. Let us specify this in some more detail. Consider a 3D point at homogeneous coordinates $P_w = (X_w, Y_w, Z_w, 1)^T$, captured by two cameras and projected onto the reference and synthetic image plane at pixel positions p_1 and p_2. The 3D position of the original point P_w in the Euclidean domain can be written as

$$P_w = (K_i R_i)^{-1}(\lambda_i p_i + K_i R_i C_i), \tag{4.10}$$

where matrix R_i describes the orientation of the camera i, K_i represents the 3×3 intrinsic parameter matrix of camera i, and C_i gives the coordinates of the camera center. Parameter λ_i represents the positive scaling factor defining the position of the 3D point on the ray through point p_i. Assuming that Camera 1 is located at the world coordinate system origin and looking into the Z direction, i.e., the direction from the origin to P_w, we can write the warping equation as

$$\lambda_2 p_2 = K_2 R_2 K_1^{-1} Z_w p_1 - K_2 R_2 C_2. \tag{4.11}$$

Equation (4.11) constitutes the 3D image warping equation that enables the synthesis of the virtual view from a reference texture view and a corresponding depth image. This equation specifies the computation for one pixel only, so that it has to be performed for the entire image. The depth map of the virtual view can be obtained in a similar manner, given the depth map of the real view.

Algorithm Backbone

The aforementioned warping forms the basis ingredient for our view interpolation algorithm [9]. The algorithm is illustrated in Fig. 4.19. In multi-view video, the information for warping is taken from the two surrounding camera views, I_L and I_R, to render a new synthetic view I_{new}. Typically, two warped images are blended to create a synthetic view at the new position:

$$I_{new} = Warp(I_L) \oplus Warp(I_R), \tag{4.12}$$

where *Warp* is a warping operation and the operation $\oplus$ denotes blending of the warped views. Such an approach requires several post-filtering algorithms, in order to improve the visual quality of the results and it is especially important to close the empty areas on the resulting image caused by occlusions. Initial images I_L and I_R may be divided into layers, prior to performing the warping as described in [64].

The latest research has shown that a better rendering quality is possible when we first create a depth map for a new image [29, 30], since it provides better handling of disoccluded areas. Using this depth map, we perform an "inverse mapping" in order to obtain texture values for I_{new} - the new image to be rendered. In this case, we have two main stages of the rendering algorithm: (1) create a depth map $Depth_{new}$ for I_{new}; (2) create a texture of the new image I_{new}.

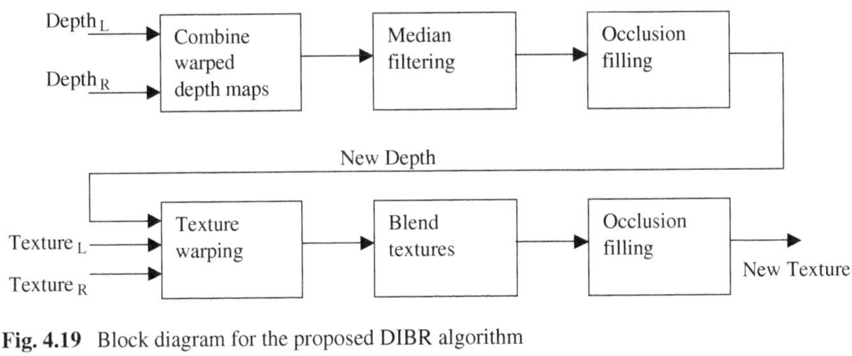

Fig. 4.19 Block diagram for the proposed DIBR algorithm

The above two stages, which form the backbone of the rendering algorithm, are similar to the approach of Morvan [30] and Mori et al. [29]. Our method additionally employs the surrounding depth information to fill in the disoccluded regions more reliably, avoiding cracks in the interpolated image. A detailed evaluation can be found in [62].

Depth Map Creation

The depth map creation consists of the following steps.

1. *Combine warped depth maps.* Combine the depth maps warped from the closest left and right cameras:

$$Depth_{comb} = C\left(Warp(Depth_L), Warp(Depth_R)\right), \tag{4.13}$$

where C defines the operation of combining two depth maps of both neighboring input cameras by taking the depth values that are closer to the virtual camera. For example, C is set to $Warp(Depth_L(x, y))$ when it is closer to the camera. In practice, combining warped depth maps means taking a maximum or minimum value of each couple of corresponding pixels.

2. *Median filtering.* The filtering function called $Median(Depth_{comb})$ involves applying median filtering to the depth map obtained at the previous step. We take a 3×3 window for the median filter, which allows us to find pixel values that occurred due to rounding of pixel coordinates during the warping. Typically, the rounding of pixel coordinates occasionally produces line-shaped gaps of one pixel width, and a 3×3 window is sufficient to close these gaps.

3. *Occlusion processing.* The resulting image still contains empty regions - disoccluded areas. The following operation finds values for filling in these regions by taking the closest found background value of the depth map obtained at the previous step. We perform search in eight directions from each empty pixel and take the value closest to the depth of the background:

$$Depth_{new} = Occ\_filling\left(Median(Depth_{comb})\right). \tag{4.14}$$

For a practical implementation, it means that we take a minimum or a maximum depth value (depending on which depth value represents the background). We aim at finding eight values around an empty pixel. If one of the surrounding eight pixels is also empty, which is often the case, then we move further in the same direction until we find a pixel containing a depth value.

Texture Creation

Besides the depth image, we need to compute the texture of the new view, which is the final objective. The texture I_{new} is created by the following operations.

1. *Warping textures for the new view.* The new texture image is based on pixels from the left and right texture images. We select the pixels from the left and right image according to the "inverse warping" of the intermediate depth image. This results in

$$Texture_i = Warp_i^{-1}(Depth_{new}) \tag{4.15}$$

where index i represents the left or right camera, and $Warp^{-1}$ is "inverse warping" - from the location of the new image to a position where the existing left (or right) view is located. When warping, we use the coordinates of the depth map to obtain the corresponding coordinates of the texture at the left (or right) view.

2. *Blending.* The textures obtained at the previous step are blended, specified by:

$$Texture_{blended} = Dilate(Texture_L) \oplus Dilate(Texture_R), \tag{4.16}$$

where *Dilate* is depth map-based filtering which aims at preventing ghosting artifacts. These artifacts result from warping the contours of objects that are often represented in the texture as a mixture of foreground and background pixels. We dilate the empty areas on the textures with a square 5×5 structural element. This removes the ghosting artifacts already present on the contours of these areas. Afterwards, the textures are blended. The drawback of this method is that it leads to larger empty areas in the textures, therefore requiring more occlusion filling operations. Experimental results have shown that the ghosting artifacts are typically two pixels wide, which means that at least a 5×5 structural element is needed to avoid them [62]. For computational efficiency we do not use a larger kernel.

3. *Occlusion filling.* Finally, the rendered image is created from the blended texture and by filling the occlusion holes:

$$I_{new} = Occ\_filling(Texture_{blended}). \tag{4.17}$$

In our optimized version of this rendering approach, both texture and depth are warped simultaneously but kept separated [10]. This leads to less warping operations, thereby increasing the execution speed of the algorithm.

Discussion

We have presented an approach for efficient rendering and transmitting views to a high-resolution autostereoscopic display for medical purposes. Stereoscopic vision can be introduced to medical imaging as it facilitates surgeon's knowledge about key objects in 3D during an intervention. The stereoscopic image allows interpreting the 3D shape, including the out-of-plane curvature (the curvature in the z-direction of the image), in a single glance without any additional input interaction. Therefore, it reduces the mental stress on the clinician during the intervention. Further, the stereoscopy reduces the risk of misinterpreting pathologies, due to a biased interpretation.

Autostereoscopic display requires a number of views of the same scene taken from a slightly different angle. These views have to be transported from the control room, where the views are rendered, to the display in the operating room. The contribution of this section is twofold. At first, it describes a setup of rendering fewer views by the medical workstation and interpolating the missing views at the receiver side. This is a considerable reduction of the load on the 3D rendering pipeline in the medical workstation, and therefore aids in reaching interactive frame rates. Furthermore, the fewer views also relieve the load on the transmission channel. Secondly, this section describes an efficient algorithm for the interpolation of the views, and examines its signal-to-noise characteristics.

In order to examine the artifacts introduced by the view interpolation, the errors that were caused by the interpolation approach can be quantified [63]. The quantitative measurements have shown that for the mesh models the PSNR is higher than 30 dB and the number of affected pixels is lower than 1 %, when the angle between the cameras is less than 2.5° . In order to analyze to which extend the observed results are valid for volume rendered medical data, we have also interpolated volume rendered images of the same real world data set. As can be seen from Fig. 4.20, the interpolated image and the ground truth image are very similar. Most pronounced differences can be observed at the edges of the vessels, which contain semi-transparent voxels. For volume rendering of clinical vascular data the PSNR was even considerably better than for triangulated mesh data (starting over 50 dB) for small angles, and comparable for larger angles. We have also investigated the effect of large volumes with very low (but non-zero) opacities. This can lead to severe artifacts, and therefore the described approach is not suitable for such visualizations. It should be noted though, that for realistic vascular data sets, these kind of transfer functions are rather uncommon.

The observed PSNR levels correspond approximately to a compression ratio of 20:1, when using JPEG compression [50]. The literature suggests that lossy compression ratios of 15:1 to 20:1 are still acceptable for medical images [51]. This leads us to conclude that a misdiagnosis in this range is unlikely to happen, and therefore our approach could be evaluated in a clinical trial. The experiments also point out that the behavior and quality degradation for an increased angle between the cameras shows a stable behavior and may be well modeled. The percentage of occluded pixels as a function of the angle between the cameras is smoothly increasing with the angle value. This enables us to ensure a sufficiently high quality for the clinical usage of our technique. Besides the previous discussion, it should be considered that 3D rendering in multi-view imaging is a quite novel research area which may show significant progress in performance and quality in the near future, as it is also a focal point in the introduction of 3D television. This progress can be readily exploited for the medical application discussed in this section. Future work can further evaluate the trade-off between lossy compression of the transmitted texture and depth maps in order to save bandwidth and its influence on the quality (PSNR) of the interpolated image [9], when applied in a medical context.

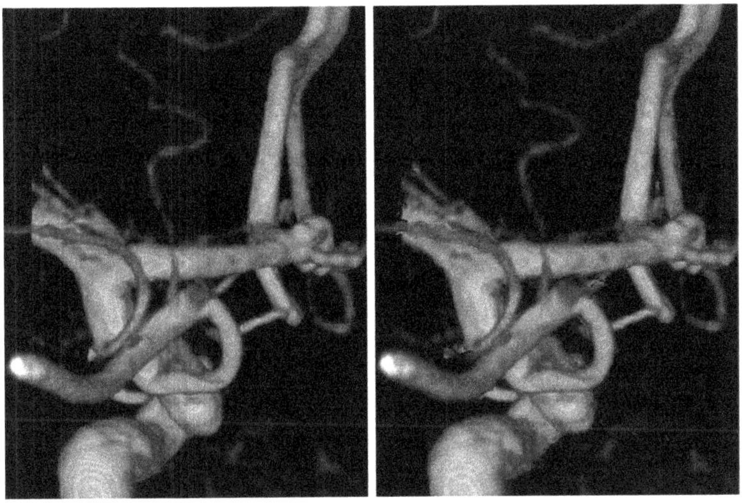

Fig. 4.20 *Left* ground truth reference volume rendering for a given camera position. *Right* interpolated image, using two neighboring volume rendered images, whereby the cameras are 2.5° apart

Conclusions

Interventional X-ray imaging provides excellent possibilities for minimally invasive surgery and image guided treatment and therapy. Minimally invasive procedures are highly desired in healthcare because they minimize the stress of the patient and make the recovery procedures shorter and easier. With the decreasing strain of the patient, the demands for underlying technology rise significantly. This chapter has discussed selected improvements for interventional X-ray imaging with solutions adopted from various fields of signal processing and progress in devices. The chapter has concentrated on four areas: image acquisition, catheter reconstruction, fusion of 3D pre-interventional datasets with the interventional data, and, finally, 3D visualization of clinical data. Let us briefly conclude and reflect on the current achievements and the future research in these areas.

For improving the X-ray image quality, the study on the reduction of ghost images for flat-detector X-ray systems by using near UV and blue-light irradiation, offers a beneficial path for generic image quality improvement. We have designed a method for reducing the hysteresis effects by at least a factor of four in a CsI:TI-doped scintillator. The detector is at the beginning of the image processing chain, thus improvements at that level contribute significantly for improving the overall quality of the chain.

During the intervention, it is of great value for the medical doctor to recognize and navigate the instruments inside the body of the patient. The section on 3D catheter reconstruction aims at progress on this area. Our presented algorithm of 3D catheter reconstruction using multi-view X-ray images, has shown that multi-view X-ray can provide 3D reconstructions of relevant objects with a sufficiently high accuracy for a number of interventions. Experiments provide the localization of catheters with an accuracy in the order of millimeters. We therefore conclude that multi-view X-ray, along with the techniques proposed in this chapter, can be employed in the near future for unambiguous 3D guidance in a real clinical scenario. In this area, several points of research do remain. First, the exact limitations in estimating overall motion using limited X-ray views remain to be explored. Second, for a real-time application of this technology, an in-depth study on fast algorithms is indispensable and efficient platform execution needs to be implemented. We are convinced that such solutions can be successfully performed in the upcoming years.

While interventional X-ray imaging allows us to see the patient during the operation, using different image modalities can clearly improve the insight in the pathology and add contextual information. If pre-operative 3D data of the patient is available, such as MR or CT scans, then data fusion can be performed. This can be very informative for planning of e.g., a needle path or for catheter navigation. At the same time, such fusion algorithms should be fast because the results are needed during interventional treatment and therefore the computation time for the co-registration must be relatively short. To address this issue, the solution proposed in this chapter addresses GPU programming and delivers processing times that are clinically acceptable while maintaining high quality of the registration result.

For better navigation and visualization of pathologies during an operation, we have proposed autostereoscopic visualization of the 3D data of the patient. Taking into account that a number of views are needed for an autostereoscopic screen, and that the views should be of a high quality for correct diagnosis, the problem of bandwidth should be solved for practical application of 3D visualization in a hospital settings. The proposed solution of this problem is based on a novel free-viewpoint algorithm. This algorithm makes it possible to transmit only a fraction of the necessary views and to interpolate the missing views at the receiver side. Our approach allows an efficient transmission and rendering of the views to the autostereoscopic screen. Interesting system issues remain for consideration. This solution is partly based on multiview 3D processing in R&D from professional broadcasting. The discussion in that field moves now to a new standard called MVC, which provides the most efficient algorithms known today for high-quality 3D multi-channel image communication. The application of such technology with high-quality medical application as a target would form an interesting and challenging case study.

In this chapter, we have touched upon several research areas in interventional X-ray imaging and have shown with our contributions that proven and new concepts from related areas such as computer vision and robotics can be successfully re-applied for medical imaging. The 3D medical imaging area is a rapidly developing domain which opens new research and development directions in several disciplines: physics, electrical engineering, computer vision etc. We expect that new exciting applications will soon enter our lives making healthcare more efficient and less invasive. Furthermore, we envision that those applications will grow increasingly from the hospital and care centers into the personal lives of the patient and at home.

References

1. A. Abildgaard, A. Kasid Witwit, J. Skaarud Karlsen, E. A. Jacobsen, B. Tennøe, G. Ringstad, and P. Due-Tønnessen. An autostereoscopic 3D display can improve visualization of 3D models from intracranial MR angiography. *International Journal of Computer Assisted Radiology and Surgery*, 5:549–554, 2010.
2. V. Babin. Charge-transfer processes in doped alkali halides. *Radiation Effects and Defects in Solids*, 158:227–230(4), Numbers 1–6/January-June 2003.
3. S. A. M. Baert, E. B. van de Kraats, T. van Walsum, M. A. Viergever, and W. Niessen. 3D guide wire reconstruction from biplane image sequences for integrated display in 3D vasculature. *IEEE Trans. on Medical Imaging*, 22(10):1252–1258, 2003.
4. H.-J. Bender, R. Männer, C. Poliwoda, S. Roth, and M. Walz. Reconstruction of 3D catheter paths from 2D X-ray projections. In *MICCAI*, volume 1679 of *LNCS*, pages 981–989, 1999.
5. C. Bregler, A. Hertzmann, and H. Biermann. Recovering non-rigid 3D shape from image streams. In *CVPR*, volume 2, pages 690–696, 2000.
6. M. Brückner, F. Deinzer, and J. Denzler. Temporal estimation of the 3D guide-wire position using 2D X-ray images. *In MICCAI*, pages 386–393, 2009.
7. P. Corke. A robotics toolbox for MATLAB. *IEEE Robotics and Automation Magazine*, 3(1):24–32, 1996.
8. A. Del Bue, X. Lladó, and L. Agapito. Non-rigid metric shape and motion recovery from uncalibrated images using priors. In *CVPR*, volume 1, 2006.
9. L. Do, S. Zinger, and P. H. N. de With. Quality improving techniques for free-viewpoint DIBR. In *IST / SPIE Electronic Imaging*, volume 7524, page 10 pages, San Jose, USA, Feb 2010.
10. L. Do, S. Zinger, Y. Morvan, and P. H. N. de With. Quality improving techniques in DIBR for free-viewpoint video. In *3DTV Conference: The True Vision—Capture, Transmission and Display of 3D Video*, page 4 pages, Potsdam, Germany, May 2009.
11. N. A. Dodgson. Autostereo displays: 3D without glasses. In *EID: Electronic Information Displays*, 1997.
12. J. Esthappan and K. Hoffmann. Estimation of catheter orientations from single-plane X-ray images. In *SPIE Medical Imaging*, volume 3976, pages 28–36, 2000.
13. J. Fayad, A. Del Bue, L. Agapito, and P. Aguiar. Non-rigid structure from motion using quadratic deformation models. In *BMVC*, 2009.
14. Y. Ganji and F. Janabi-Sharifi. Catheter kinematics for intracardiac navigation. *IEEE Transactions on Biomedical Engineering*, 56(3):621–632, 2009.
15. R. Hartley and R. Vidal. Perspective nonrigid shape and motion recovery. In *ECCV (I)*, pages 276–289, 2008.
16. T. Hübner and R. Pajarola. Single-pass multiview volume rendering. In *Proc. IADIS International Conference on Computer Graphics and Visualization (CGV'07)*, Lisbon, Portugal, July 2007.
17. S. Ince and J. Konrad. Geometry-based estimation of occlusions from video frame pairs. In *Proc. IEEE International Conference on Acoustics, Speech, and Signal Processing (ICASSP'05)*, volume 2, pages ii/933-ii/936, Philadelphia, USA, 2005.
18. S. Kabus, T. Netsch, B. Fischer, and J. Modersitzki. B-spline registration of 3D images with levenberg-marquardt optimization. In *SPIE Medical Imaging'04*, pages 304–313, 2004.
19. J. Kybic and M. Unser. Fast parametric elastic image registration. *IEEE Trans. Image Processing*, 12(11):1427–1442, Nov 2003.
20. A. Lempicki. The physics of inorganic scintillators. *Journal of Applied Spectroscopy*, 62:787–802, 1995. 10.1007/BF02606530.
21. M. Levoy. Effcient ray tracing of volume data. *ACM Transactions on Graphics*, 9(3):245–261, 1990.
22. H. Liao, T. Inomata, I. Sakuma, and T. Dohi. 3-D augmented reality for MRI-guided surgery using integral videography autostereoscopic image overlay. *IEEE Trans. Biomed. Eng.*, 57(6):1476–1486, June 2010.

23. H. Liao, H. Ishihara, H. H. Tran, K. Masamune, I. Sakuma, and T. Dohi. Fusion of laser guidance and 3-D autostereoscopic image overlay for precision-guided surgery. *Lecture Notes in Computer Science, Medical Imaging and Augmented Reality*, 5128:367–376, 2008.
24. M. Liévin and E. Keeve. Stereoscopic augmented reality system for computer-assisted surgery. *International Congress Series, Computer Assisted Radiology and Surgery*, 1230:107–111, June 2001.
25. Z. Lunwei, Q. Jinwu, S. Linyong, and Z. Yanan. Fbg sensor devices for spatial shape detection of intelligent colonoscope. In *Proceedings ICRA '04. 2004 IEEE International Conference on Robotics and Automation, 2004.*, volume 1, pages 834–840, 2004.
26. J. J. Markham. *F-centers in alkali halides*. Academic Press, 1966.
27. L. McMillan and R. S. Pizer. An image based approach to three-dimensional computer graphics. Technical Report TR97-013, University of North Carolina at Chapel Hill, 1997.
28. C. Merdes and P. Wolf. Locating a catheter transducer in a three-dimensional ultrasound imaging field. *IEEE Transactions on Biomedical Engineering*, 48(12):1444–1452, Dec 2001.
29. Y. Mori, N. Fukushima, T. Fujii, and M. Tanimoto. View generation with 3d warping using depth information for FTV. *Image Communication*, 24(1–2):65–72, 2009.
30. Y. Morvan. *Acquisition, compression and rendering of depth and texture for multi-view video*. Ph.D. thesis, Eindhoven University of Technology, 2009.
31. Y. Morvan, D. Farin, and P. H. N. de With. System architecture for free-viewpoint video and 3D-TV. *IEEE Transactions on Consumer Electronics*, 54:925–932, 2008.
32. M. Nagel, M. Hoheisel, R. Petzold, and W. A. K. U. H. W. Krause. Needle and catheter navigation using electromagnetic tracking for computer-assisted c-arm ct interventions. *In SPIE Medical Imaging*, volume 6509, page 6509J, 2007.
33. M. Nikl, K. Nitsch, F. Somma, P. Fabeni, G. Pazzi, and X. Feng. Luminescence of ternary nanoaggregates in CsI-PbI_2 thin films. *Journal of Luminescence*, 87–89:372–374, 2000.
34. M. Overdick, T. Solf, and H.-A. Wischmann. Temporal artifacts in flat dynamic X-ray detectors. volume 4320, pages 47–58. SPIE, 2001.
35. C. Papalazarou. *3D Object Reconstruction During Image-Guided Interventions Using Multi-view X-ray*. PhD thesis, University of Technology Eindhoven, 2012.
36. C. Papalazarou, P. M. Rongen, and P. H. N. de With. Deformable 3D catheter reconstruction using non-rigid structure-from-motion and a robotics model. In *SPIE Medical Imaging: Image-Guided Procedures, Robotic Interventions, and Modeling*, pages 8316–71, 2012.
37. A. Quaranta, F. Gramegna, V. Kravchuk, and C. Scian. Radiation damage mechanisms in CsI(Tl) studied by ion beam induced luminescence. *Nuclear Instruments and Methods in Physics Research Section B: Beam Interactions with Materials and Atoms*, 266(12–13):2723–2728, 2008. Radiation Effects in Insulators—Proceedings of the Fourteenth International Conference on Radiation Effects in Insulators, Fourteenth International Conference on Radiation Effects in Insulators.
38. H. Rabin and C. C. Click. Formation of F centers at low and room temperatures. *Phys. Rev.*, 117(4):1005–1010, Feb 1960.
39. S. Radhakrishna. Polarised luminescence from lead centers in cesium halides. *Journal of luminescence*, 12/13:409–411, 1976.
40. S. Radhakrishna and K. P. Pande. Lead centers in cesium halides. *Phys. Rev.* B, 7(1):424–431, Jan 1973.
41. T. Rehman, G. Pryor, J. Melonakos, and A. Tannenbaum. Multi-resolution 3D nonrigid registration via optimal mass transport on the GPU. In *Proc. Computational Biomechanics for Medicine-II, MICCAI*, pages 122–132, 2007.
42. S. Röhl, S. Speidel, G. Sudra, T. Gehrig, B. P. Müller-Stich, C. Gutt, and R. Dillmann. A surface model for intraoperative soft tissue registration. *International Journal of Computer Assisted Radiology and Surgery*, 4 Suppl. 1:S106–S107, June 2009.
43. D. Ruijters. Integrating autostereoscopic multi-view lenticular displays in minimally invasive angiography. In *Proc. MICCAI AMI-ARCS workshop*, pages 87–94, New York, USA, Sept 2008.

44. D. Ruijters. Dynamic resolution in GPU-accelerated volume rendering to autostereoscopic multiview lenticular displays. *EURASIP Journal on Advances in Signal Processing*, 2009:Article ID 843753, 2009.
45. D. Ruijters. *Multi-modal image fusion during minimally invasive treatment*. Ph.D. thesis, Katholieke Universiteit Leuven anad University of Technology Eindhoven, 2010.
46. D. Ruijters, R. Homan, P. Mielekamp, and P. van de Haarand Drazenko Babic. Validation of 3D multimodality roadmapping in interventional neuroradiology. *Physics in Medicine and Biology*, 56(16):5335–5354, Aug 2011.
47. D. Ruijters, B. M. ter Haar Romeny, and P. Suetens. Efficient GPU-based texture interpolation using uniform B-splines. *Journal of Graphics Tools*, 13(4):61–69, 2008.
48. D. Ruijters, B. M. ter Haar Romeny, and P. Suetens. GPU-accelerated elastic 3D image registration for intra-surgical applications. *Computer Methods and Programs in Biomedicine*, 103(2):104–112, Aug 2011.
49. D. Ruijters and S. Zinger. IGLANCE: transmission to medical high definition autostereoscopic displays. *In 3DTV Conference: The True Vision— Capture, Transmission and Display of 3D Video*, page 4, Potsdam, Germany, May 2009.
50. R. Shahnaz, J. F. Walkup, and T. F. Krile. Image compression in signal-dependent noise. *Appl Opt.*, 38(26):5560–5567, Sept 1999.
51. Y.-H. Shiao, T.-J. Chen, K.-S. Chuang, C.-H. Lin, and C.-C. Chuang. Quality of compressed medical images. *Journal of Digital Imaging*, 20(2):149–159, June 2007.
52. J. H. Siewerdsen and D. A. Jaffray. A ghost story: Spatio-temporal response characteristics of an indirect-detection flat-panel imager. *Medical Physics*, 26(8):1624–1641, 1999.
53. C. Sigg and M. Hadwiger. Fast third-order texture filtering. In M. Pharr, editor, *GPU Gems 2: Programming Techniques for High-Performance Graphics and General-Purpose Computation*, pages 313–329, 2005.
54. R. M. Snoeren, H. Steinhauser, L. Alving, H. Stouten, and P. H. N. de With. Flat detector ghost image reduction by UV irradiation. volume 7258, page 72583J. SPIE, 2009.
55. A. T. Stadie, R. A. Kockro, R. Reisch, A. Tropine, S. Boor, P. Stoeter, and A. Perneczky. Virtual reality system for planning minimally invasive neurosurgery. *Journal of Neurosurgery*, 108:382–394, 2008.
56. O. Stern and M. Volmer. Über die Abklingungszeit der Fluoreszenz. *Physikalische Zeitschrift*, 20:183–188, 1919.
57. M. Tanimoto. FTV (free viewpoint TV) and creation of ray based image engineering. *ECTI Trans. Electrical Eng., Electronics, Communications*, 6(1):3–14, Feb 2008.
58. C. van Berkel. Image preparation for 3D-LCD. In *Proc. SPIE, Stereoscopic Displays and Virtual Reality Systems VI*, volume 3639, pages 84–91, 1999.
59. T. van Walsum, S. Baert, and W. Niessen. Guide Wire Reconstruction and Visualization in 3DRA using Monoplane Fluoroscopic Imaging. *IEEE Trans. on Medical Imaging*, 24(5):612–624, 2005.
60. C. Vázquez and W. J. Tam. 3D-TV: Coding of disocclusions for 2D+depth representation of multiview images. In *Proc. Tenth IASTED International Conference on Computer Graphics and Imaging (CGIM)*, pages 26–32, Innsbruck, Austria, 2008.
61. H. Wieczorek and M. Overdick. Afterglow and hysteresis in CsI:Tl. volume 1, pages 385–390. Moscow State University, 2000.
62. S. Zinger, L. Do, and P. H. N. de With. Free-viewpoint depth image based rendering. *Journal Visual Communication and Image Representation*, 21(5–6):533–541, 2010.
63. S. Zinger, D. Ruijters, L. Do, and P. H. N. de With. View interpolation for medical images on autostereoscopic displays. *IEEE Transactions on Circuits and Systems for Video Technology*, 22(1):128–137, Jan 2012.
64. C. L. Zitnick, S. B. Kang, M. Uyttendaele, S. Winder, and R. Szeliski. High-quality video view interpolation using a layered representation. *In ACM SIGGRAPH '04*, pages 600–608, 2004.

Chapter 5
Automated Classification of Echo-Cardiography Images Using Texture Analysis Methods

Jyotismita Chaki and Ranjan Parekh

Introduction

Medical imaging has been undergoing a revolution in the past decade with the advent of faster, more accurate and less invasive devices [1]. This has driven the need for corresponding software development which in turn has provided a major impetus for new algorithms in signal and image processing. Imaging technology in medicine enabled doctors to view internal portions of the body for easy diagnosis. This is also helpful for keyhole surgeries to reach the interior parts without really opening too much of the body. CT scanning, echocardiography, ultrasound and magnetic resonance imaging took over X-ray imaging by enabling doctors model the body in 3-D. While the CT scanner is used to identify the diseased areas without causing discomfort or pain to the patient, MRI picks up signals from the body's magnetic particles and converts the magnetic sources into revealing pictures of internal organs. In recent times digital image processing techniques are being used to modify and analyze the digital outputs of medical imaging systems for automated detection of symptoms and diseases.

Mathematical models are the foundation of biomedical computing. Basing those models on data extracted from images continues to be a fundamental technique for achieving scientific progress in experimental, clinical, biomedical, and behavioral research. Today, medical images are acquired by a range of techniques across all biological scales, which go far beyond the visible light photographs and microscope images of the early tweenth century. Modern medical images may be considered to be geometrically arranged arrays of data samples which quantify such diverse physical phenomena. A key research area is the formulation of biomedical engi-

J. Chaki · R. Parekh (✉)
School of Education Technology, Jadavpur University, Calcutta, India
e-mail: ranjan_parekh@yahoo.com

J. Chaki
e-mail: jyotismita.c@gmail.com

B. Furht and A. Agarwal (eds.), *Handbook of Medical and Healthcare Technologies*,
DOI: 10.1007/978-1-4614-8495-0_5, © Springer Science+Business Media New York 2013

neering principles based on rigorous mathematical foundation in order to develop general purpose software methods that can be integrated into complete therapy delivery system. Such systems support the more effective delivery of many image guided procedures such as biopsy, minimally invasive surgery and radiation therapy.
The advantages of Digital Processing for Medical Applications [2] include the following :

- Digital data may be reproduced any number of times without perceptible degradation
- Images can be immediately displayed after acquisition
- Images can be enhanced using imaging software for better detection of features. This includes transformations like scaling and rotating specific parts for better viewing as well as improving visual clarity by adjusting brightness, contrast, color etc.
- Easy search over a huge dataset of images using textual and non-textual search patterns
- Easy to detect changes over a period of time and quick comparison of several images using specific criteria.

Additionally the following terms pertain to advantages in using digital image processing techniques in medical imaging systems:

- Image enhancements.
- Changing density dynamic range of B/W images.
- Color correction in color images.
- Manipulating of colors within an image.
- Contour detection.
- Area calculations of the cells of a biomedical image.
- Display of image line profile.
- Restoration of images.
- Smoothing of images.
- Registration of multiple images and mosaicing.
- Construction of 3-D images from 2-D images.
- Generation of negative images.
- Zooming of images.
- Pseudo coloring.
- Point to point measurements.
- Getting relief effect.
- Removal of artifacts from the image.

The current work provides a set of studies to demonstrate the advantages in employing digital image processing techniques combined with pattern recognition methods in detecting and identifying disease patterns from digital medical images in an automated way. It uses a number of techniques applied to echocardiograms of the human heart for detection of diseases. Echocardiography is a painless technique that uses sound waves to create moving pictures of the heart. The pictures show the size and shape of the heart as well as how the heart's chamber and valves are working in real-time. The current work studies the efficacy of a number of techniques to identify and classify heart diseases from the echocardiograms and attempts to find out which method is best suited for the purpose. The organization of the paper is as follows: "Related Works" provides an overview of the previous works, "Proposed Approaches" outlines the proposed approaches, "Experimentations and Results" details the experimentations done and results obtained, "Analysis" analyses the current work vis-à-vis contemporary works, "Conclusions and Future Directions" brings up the overall conclusions and future scopes.

Related Works

A number of techniques and methods have been proposed in extant literature for automated medical image analysis . In [3] a comparison of several texture analysis methods such as Integrated Cortical Model (ICM), Autocorrelation Function (ACF), Coding Method (CM), Edge Frequency (EF), Law's Mask (LM), Run Length (RL), Binary Stack Method (BSM), Texture Spectrum (TS) are used to classify the pulse images of mammalian visual cortex. K-nearest neighbor is used for classification. In [4] the authors proposed a novel registration method between two chest X-ray images with different rotation angles around an axis parallel to X-ray films. Automatic recognition of rib images and detection of abnormal shadows in lung images have been discussed in [5]. In [6] grid formation, local thresholding, threshold value interpolation, segmentation using fuzzy index measure, background removal and morphological filtering is done for the X-ray images for revealing cracks of bones. In [7] the authors proposed a method of analysis of patient dose and image quality for chest digital radiology. Patient dose indices, i.e. entrance surface dose and dose area product (DAP) are measured during routine chest examination, and analysis are performed for adult Chinese patients. In [8] a color management framework for medical applications is proposed. The framework is based on color science developed by the CIE and covers multispectral imaging in addition to conventional 3-channel imaging. In [9] a 3-D display system for medical imaging is developed, each point in 3-D space is reconstructed by the convergence of rays from many pixels on the computer display through a lens array, only the coordinate of the best point is computed for each pixel on the display. In [10] a review of medical imaging techniques with emphasis on X-ray detectors is presented. Developments and perspectives on X-ray imaging is also discussed in [11]. Paper [12] presents the role of transthoracic 3-D echocardiography in adult patients with congenital heart disease. Advantages of additional information obtained when compared with standard 2-D, is emphasized. In [13] medical image recognition based on line feature and neural network is proposed. Here ten types of medical images are taken onto account, and a comparison is made between the line moment and area moment. In [14] the medical image recognition is done by Fuzzy Morphological Associative Memories. Recognition of useful signals from badly populated image is discussed. In [15] the recognition of medical images is done by Local Binary Pattern (LBP) with Image Euclidean Distance (IMED). To improve recognition, several methods using local binary pattern (LBP) have been utilized. In [16] a comparison is made between two methods for medical image segmentation i.e. the color set back propagation algorithm and segmentation using hexagonal structure. The experimental results were made on a database with 400 medical images from digestive area captured by an endoscope. Paper [17] proposes an ultrasound medical image recognition system with artificial intelligence for Parkinson's disease classification. The main goal of this work is classification of ROI substantia nigra in midbrain. In [18] the oral medical image recognition is done by top-hat morphology. Different gray value is used for different oral disease detection.

Proposed Approaches

This paper proposes a scheme for automated classification of echocardiography images depicting three medical conditions of the heart by analyzing the textural information contained within them. Techniques discussed involve using Gabor filter, Hu's invariant moments and Law's texture energy. The objective is to find out whether these methods provide reliable ways to classify such images and which techniques provide the best results.

The Idea of Texture

Textures are characteristic intensity variations that typically originate from roughness of object surfaces. For well defined textures, intensity variations will normally exhibit both regularity and randomness. In practice, a surface is taken to be textured if there are large numbers of texture elements (or 'texels'). In general the components of a texture, the 'texels', are uniform micro objects which are placed in a specific orientation to form a particular texture. Texture may vary according to randomness, regularity, directionality and orientation.
There are two main approaches of texture based classification:

- Structural approach, which assumes that texture consists of a set of primitive texels in some regular or repeated relationship.
- Statistical approach, which assumes that texture is a quantitative measure of the variation of intensities in an image region.

Gabor Filter

A complex Gabor filter is defined as the product of a Gaussian kernel times a complex sinusoid. The Gaussian function is called the envelope and the complex sinusoid is called the carrier. A 2D Gaussian curve with a spread of σ in both x and y directions, is represented as below:

$$g(x, y, \sigma) = \frac{1}{2\pi\sigma^2} \cdot \exp\left(-\frac{x^2 + y^2}{2\sigma^2}\right) \quad (5.1)$$

The complex sinusoid is defined as follows, where u denotes spatial frequency, θ denotes the orientation and φ the phase shift ($j = \sqrt{-1}$).

$$s(x, y, u, \theta, \varphi) = \exp\{j\,2\pi(x \cdot u\cos\theta + y \cdot u\sin\theta) + \varphi\} \quad (5.2)$$

The complex Gabor function can therefore be represented as follows

$$\boldsymbol{h}(x, y, \sigma, u, \theta, \varphi) = g(x, y, \sigma) \cdot s(x, y, u, \theta, \varphi) \quad (5.3)$$

A grayscale image $I(x, y)$ is convolved with a Gabor filter with experimentally determined filter parameters to produce a set of complex signals.

$$J(x, y) = I(x, y) \otimes \boldsymbol{h}(x, y, \sigma, u, \theta, \varphi) \quad (5.4)$$

The real and imaginary parts of the signal are separated out and converted to binary values using an appropriate threshold.

$$P(x, y) = \mathrm{Re}\,\{J(x, y)\}$$

$$Q(x, y) = \mathrm{Im}\,\{J(x, y)\} \quad (5.5)$$

The distributed signal is converted to a scalar representation by summing over all the discrete signal values.

$$R = \sum_x \sum_y P(x, y)$$

$$I = \sum_x \sum_y Q(x, y) \quad (5.6)$$

The feature used for texture recognition is generated by subtracting the imaginary portion from the real portion

$$F = |R - I| \quad (5.7)$$

Invariant Moments

Hu [19] proposes 7 moment features that can be used to describe images and are invariant to rotation, translation and scaling. For a digital image, the moment of a pixel $P(x, y)$ at location (x, y) is defined as the product of the pixel value with its coordinate distances i.e. $m = x \cdot y \cdot P(x, y)$. The moment of the entire image is the summation of the moments of all its pixels. More generally the moment of order

(p, q) of an image $I(x, y)$ is given by

$$m_{pq} = \sum_x \sum_y \{x^p \cdot y^q \cdot I(x, y)\} \tag{5.8}$$

Based on the values of p and q the following can be defined :

$$\begin{aligned}
m_{00} &= \sum_x \sum_y \{x^0 \cdot y^0 \cdot I(x, y)\} = \sum_x \sum_y \{I(x, y)\} \\
m_{10} &= \sum_x \sum_y \{x^1 \cdot y^0 \cdot I(x, y)\} = \sum_x \sum_y \{x.I(x, y)\} \\
m_{01} &= \sum_x \sum_y \{x^0 \cdot y^1 \cdot I(x, y)\} = \sum_x \sum_y \{y.I(x, y)\} \\
m_{11} &= \sum_x \sum_y \{x^1 \cdot y^1 \cdot I(x, y)\} = \sum_x \sum_y \{xy.I(x, y)\} \\
m_{20} &= \sum_x \sum_y \{x^2 \cdot y^0 \cdot I(x, y)\} = \sum_x \sum_y \{x^2 \cdot I(x, y)\} \\
m_{02} &= \sum_x \sum_y \{x^0 \cdot y^2.I(x, y)\} = \sum_x \sum_y \{y^2 \cdot I(x, y)\} \\
m_{21} &= \sum_x \sum_y \{x^2 \cdot y^1 \cdot I(x, y)\} = \sum_x \sum_y \{x^2 y \cdot I(x, y)\} \\
m_{12} &= \sum_x \sum_y \{x^1 \cdot y^2 \cdot I(x, y)\} = \sum_x \sum_y \{xy^2 \cdot I(x, y)\} \\
m_{30} &= \sum_x \sum_y \{x^3 \cdot y^0 \cdot I(x, y)\} = \sum_x \sum_y \{x^3.I(x, y)\} \\
m_{03} &= \sum_x \sum_y \{x^0 \cdot y^3 \cdot I(x, y)\} = \sum_x \sum_y \{y^3 \cdot I(x, y)\}
\end{aligned} \tag{5.9}$$

The invariant moments which are invariant to rotation, are then defined as follows :

$$\begin{aligned}
\varphi_1 &= m_{20} + m_{02} \\
\varphi_2 &= (m_{20} - m_{02})^2 + (2m_{11})^2 \\
\varphi_3 &= (m_{30} - 3m_{12})^2 + (3m_{21} - m_{03})^2 \\
\varphi_4 &= (m_{30} + m_{12})^2 + (m_{21} + m_{03})^2 \\
\varphi_5 &= (m_{30} - 3m_{12})(m_{30} + m_{12})\{(m_{30} + m_{12})^2 - 3(m_{21} + m_{03})^2\} \\
&\quad + [(3m_{21} - m_{03})(m_{21} + m_{03})\{3(m_{30} + m_{12})^2 - (m_{21} + m_{03})]^2\} \\
\varphi_6 &= (m_{20} - m_{02})\{(m_{30} + m_{12})^2 - (m_{21} + m_{03})^2\} + 4m_{11}(m_{30} + m_{12})(m_{21} + m_{03})
\end{aligned} \tag{5.10}$$

$$\varphi_7 = (3m_{21} - m_{03})(m_{30} + m_{12})\{(m_{30} + m_{12})^2 - 3(m_{21} + m_{03})^2\}$$
$$- (m_{30} - 3m_{12})(m_{21} + m_{03})\{3(m_{30} + m_{12})^2 - (m_{21} + m_{03})^2\}$$

To make the moments invariant to translation the image is shifted such that its centroid coincides with the origin of the coordinate system. The centroid of the image in terms of the moments is given by :

$$x_c = \frac{m_{10}}{m_{00}}, \qquad y_c = \frac{m_{01}}{m_{00}} \tag{5.11}$$

Then the central moments are defined as follows:

$$\mu_{pq} = \sum_x \sum_y \{(x - x_c)^p \cdot (y - y_c)^q \cdot I(x, y)\} \tag{5.12}$$

To compute μ moments using central moments the m terms in Eq. 5.10 need to be replaced by μ terms. It can be verified that

$$\mu_{00} = m_{00}, \qquad \mu_{10} = 0 = \mu_{01} \tag{5.13}$$

To make the moments invariant to scaling the moments are normalized by dividing by a power of μ_{00}.

$$\gamma_{pq} = \frac{\mu_{pq}}{(\mu_{00})^{\omega}}, \quad \text{where } \omega = 1 + \frac{p+q}{2} \tag{5.14}$$

The normalized central moments are defined by substituting m terms in Eq. 5.10 by γ terms and φ terms by M terms.

Laws Texture Detection Method

Laws Texture detection method [20] uses local masks to detect various types of textures. Laws developed a texture energy approach that measures the amount of variation within a fixed-size window. The 2-D convolution kernels typically used for texture discrimination are generated from the following set of 1-D convolution kernels of length five:

$$\begin{aligned} L &= [1 \quad 4 \quad 6 \quad 4 \quad 1] \\ E &= [-1 \quad -2 \quad 0 \quad 2 \quad 1] \\ S &= [-1 \quad 0 \quad 2 \quad 0 \quad -1] \\ W &= [-1 \quad 2 \quad 0 \quad -2 \quad 1] \\ R &= [1 \quad -4 \quad 6 \quad -4 \quad 1] \end{aligned} \tag{5.15}$$

These mnemonics stand for Level, Edge, Spot, Wave, and Ripple. All kernels except L are zero-sum. From these1-D convolution kernels, 25 different 2-D kernels are generated by convolving a vertical 1-D kernel with a horizontal 1-D kernel. As an example, the LE kernel is created by convolving a vertical L kernel with a horizontal E kernel.

$$LE = \begin{bmatrix} -1 & -2 & 0 & 2 & 1 \\ -4 & -8 & 0 & 8 & 4 \\ -6 & -12 & 0 & 12 & 6 \\ -4 & -8 & 0 & 8 & 4 \\ -1 & -2 & 0 & 2 & 1 \end{bmatrix} \qquad (5.16)$$

Of these 25 2-D convolution kernels, 24 are zero-sum, except LL. A listing of all 5 × 5 kernel names is given below:

LL	EL	SL	WL	RL
LE	EE	SE	WE	RE
LS	ES	SS	WS	RS
LW	EW	SW	WW	RW
LR	ER	SR	WR	RR

Given a sample image with N rows and M columns, each of the 25 convolution kernels are convolved with the image. The result is a set of 25 N × M grayscale images, which form the basis for the textural analysis of the original image.
Now every pixel $p(x, y)$ in the 25 N × M separate grayscale images is replaced with a Texture Energy Measure (TEM) $p'(x, y)$ calculated from the neighbourhood around the pixel. This is done by looking in a local neighborhood of 15 × 15 square around each pixel and summing together the absolute values of the neighborhood pixels.

$$p'(x, y) = \sum_{i=-7}^{7} \sum_{j=-7}^{7} p(x + i, y + j) \qquad (5.17)$$

A new set of images are generated, which will be referred to as the TEM images. At this point 25 TEM images from the original image have been generated. The TEM images are named as follows:

LLT	ELT	SLT	WLT	RLT
LET	EET	SET	WET	RET
LST	EST	SST	WST	RST
LWT	EWT	SWT	WWT	RWT
LRT	ERT	SRT	WRT	RRT

All convolution kernels used thus far are zero-mean with the exception of the LLT kernel. In accordance with Laws' suggestions, this can be used as a normalization image i.e. normalizing any TEM image pixel-by-pixel with the LLT image will

normalize that feature for contrast. After this is done, the LLT image is typically discarded and not used in subsequent textural analysis.
In the final step, similar features are combined to remove a bias from the features from directionality. For example, LET is sensitive to vertical edges and ELT is sensitive to horizontal edges. If these TEM images are added together, a single feature, sensitive to simple 'edge content' can be achieved.

$$LE = \begin{bmatrix} -1 & -2 & 0 & 2 & 1 \\ -4 & -8 & 0 & 8 & 4 \\ -6 & -12 & 0 & 12 & 6 \\ -4 & -8 & 0 & 8 & 4 \\ -1 & -2 & 0 & 2 & 1 \end{bmatrix} \qquad EL = \begin{bmatrix} -1 & -4 & -6 & -4 & -1 \\ -2 & -8 & -12 & -8 & -2 \\ 0 & 0 & 0 & 0 & 0 \\ 2 & 8 & 12 & 8 & 2 \\ 1 & 4 & 6 & 4 & 1 \end{bmatrix}$$

$$LE + EL = \begin{bmatrix} -2 & -6 & -6 & -2 & -0 \\ -6 & -16 & -12 & 0 & 2 \\ -6 & -12 & 0 & 12 & 6 \\ -2 & 0 & 12 & 16 & 6 \\ 0 & 2 & 6 & 6 & 2 \end{bmatrix} \tag{5.18}$$

Following this example, features that were generated with transposed convolution kernels are added together. These new features are denoted with an appended 'R' for 'rotational invariance'.

ELTR = ELT + LET
SLTR = SLT + LST
WLTR = WLT + LWT
RLTR = RLT + LRT
SETR = SET + EST
WETR = WET + EWT
RETR = RET + ERT
WSTR = WST + SWT
RSTR = RST + SRT
RWTR = RWT + WRT

To keep all features consistent with respect to size, the remaining features can be scaled by 2:

EETR = EET * 2
SSTR = SST * 2
WWTR = WWT * 2
RRTR = RRT * 2

The result, if LLT is deleted altogether, is a set of 14 texture features which are rotationally invariant. If these images are stacked up, a data set can be obtained where every pixel is represented by 14 texture features.

Image Classification

Image classification for all above methods, is done by dividing the dataset into a training set T and a testing set S each consisting of n samples. The ith training class T_i is represented by the mean of the feature values of all its component samples.

$$T_i = \frac{1}{n}\{T_{i1}^F + T_{i2}^F + \cdots + T_{in}^F\} \tag{5.19}$$

The jth test sample S_j with feature value S_j^F is classified to class k if the absolute difference $D_{j,i}$ between the jth test sample and ith training class is minimum for $i = k$ i.e.

$$S_j \rightarrow k, \quad if\ D_{j,i} = |S_j^F - T_i|\ is\ minimum\ for\ i = k \tag{5.20}$$

Experimentations and Results

Experimentations are performed by using echo-cardiography videos showing the left-ventricle of the heart, downloaded from YouTube [21, 22]. The total media set consist of 240 images divided into three classes 1, 2, 3, corresponding to three cardiac conditions : (1) normal (2) dilated cardiomyopathy (3) hypertrophic cardiomyopathy. The images are scaled to standard dimensions of 265×194 and stored in JPEG format. Among the 80 images used for each class, 40 are used for training the system and the remaining 40 for testing. Samples of both training and testing set images are shown in Figs. 5.1 and 5.2. The top row shows samples for class-1 images labeled 1(1), 1(2), ..., 1(21), 1(22),..., the middle row shows samples for class-2 images labeled 2(1), 2(2), ..., 2(21), 2(22),..., and the bottom row shows samples for class-3 images labeled as 3(1), 3(2), ..., 3(21), 3(22),....

Invariant Moments

The percentage recognition accuracies using Moments Invariant features are listed in Table 5.1. It shows that best recognitions are achieved using M_6 (74.2 %).
The variation of the M_6 feature values for training and testing samples for each of the 3 classes are indicated in Fig. 5.3.
Figure 5.4 indicates the classification plots for the M_6 feature. The figure shows the differences of the testing samples of each class with the training samples of the three classes. The symbols have the following meaning : *dmn* indicates difference between testing samples of class-*m* with the mean of the training samples of class-*n*. The top sub-figure shows results for class-1, the middle sub-figure for class-2 and the bottom sub-figure for class-3.

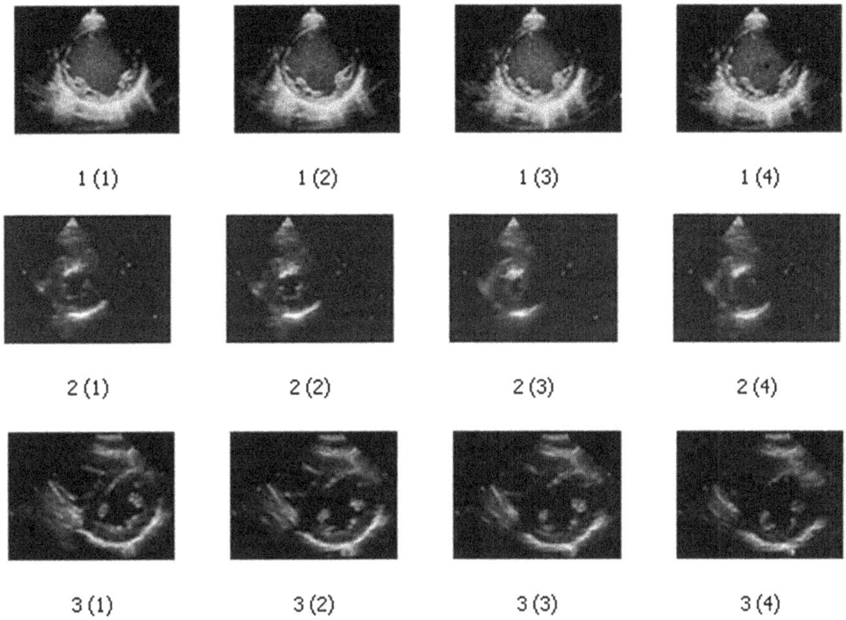

Fig. 5.1 Samples of training set images

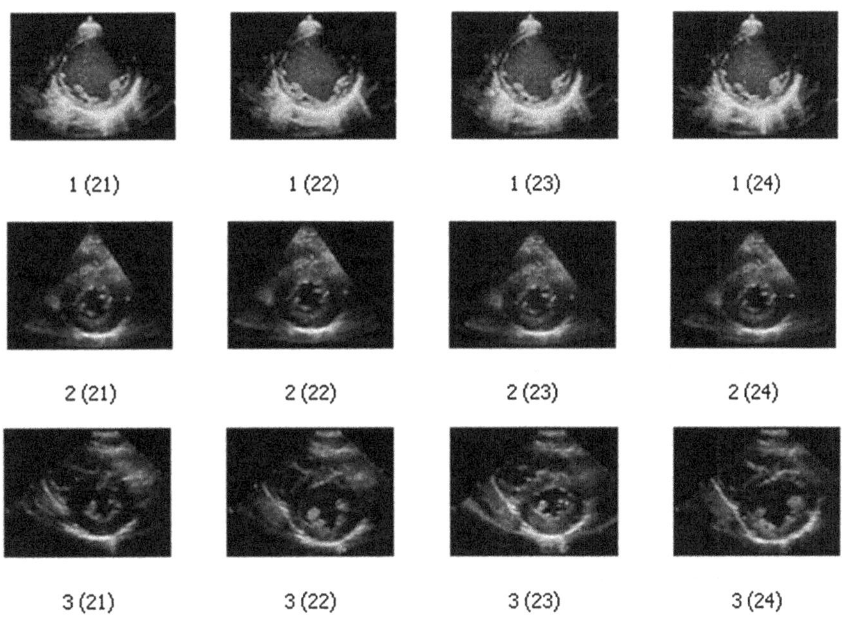

Fig. 5.2 Samples of testing set images

Table 5.1 Percentage accuracy values using moment invariant features

Feature	Class 1	Class 2	Class 3	Overall accuracy
M_1	100	30	40	56.7
M_2	100	42.5	30	57.5
M_3	100	52.5	57.5	70
M_4	100	10	47.5	52.5
M_5	100	40	45	61.7
M_6	100	45	77.5	74.2
M_7	100	37.5	42.5	60

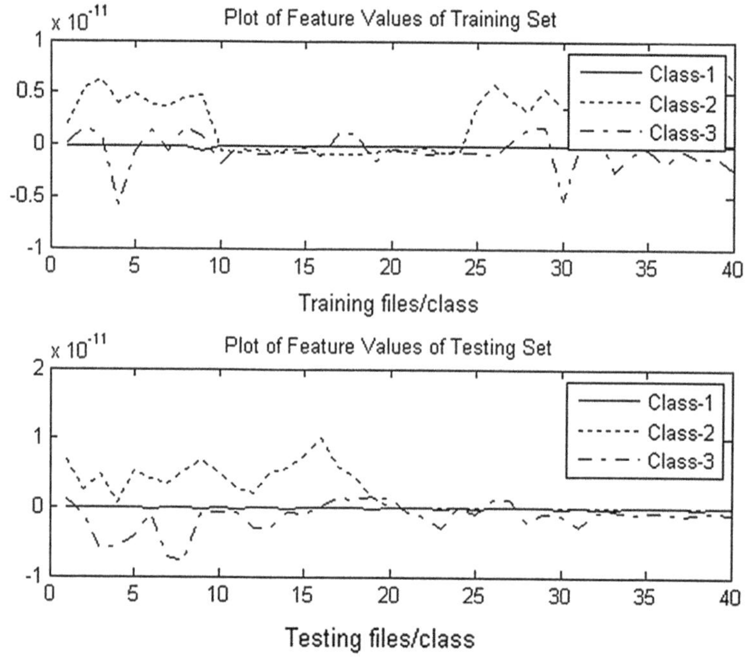

Fig. 5.3 Variation of M_6 feature values for training and testing files

Gabor Filter

Each image is convolved with a 2-D Gabor filter with specific values of $x, y, \sigma, \theta, \varphi$. The real and imaginary part of the output are separated out and converted into binary values using an appropriate threshold. The 2-D distributed signal is converted to a scalar by summing over all the discrete signal values. The feature value is generated by subtracting the imaginary portion from the real portion. Table 5.2 indicates accuracies obtained by varying the parameters of the Gabor filter. The size is varied from 1 to 10, φ from 0 to in steps of $\frac{\pi}{8}$, and θ from 1 to 10. The best results are obtained for the combination of $x = y = 3, \varphi = \frac{\pi}{4}, \theta = 2$ which is 82.5 %.

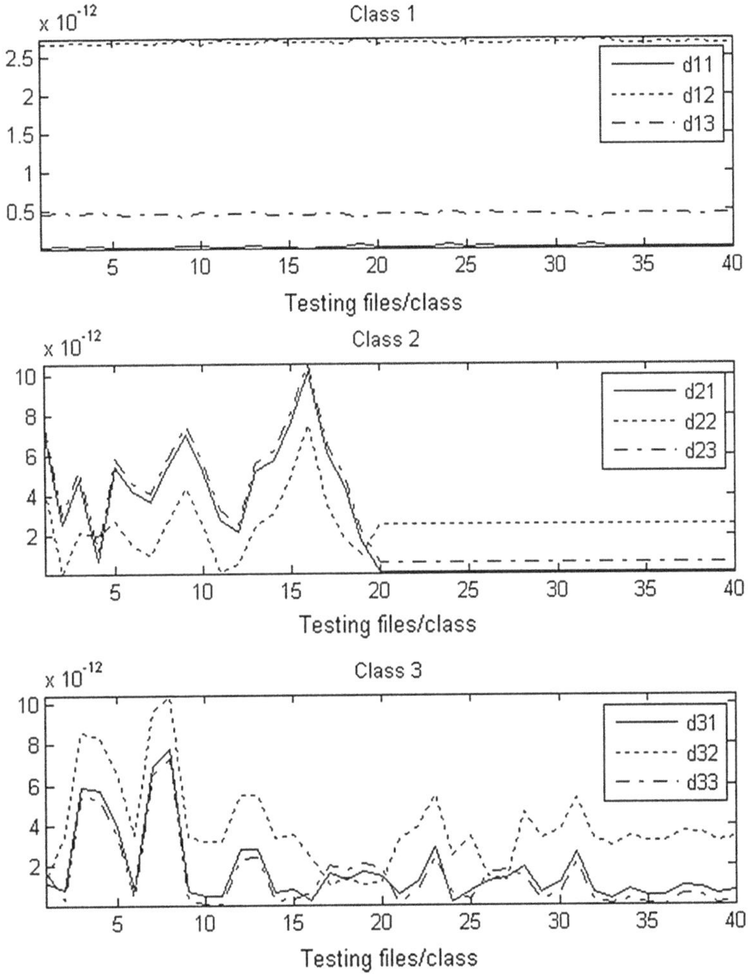

Fig. 5.4 Classification using M_6 feature values

Figure 5.7 indicates the classification plots for the feature F. The figure shows the differences of the testing samples of each class with the training samples of the three classes. The symbols have the following meaning : dmn indicates difference between testing samples of class-m with the mean of the training samples of class-n. The top sub-figure shows results for class-1, the middle sub-figure for class-2 and the bottom sub-figure for class-3. The variations of the real (R), imaginary (I) and feature values (F) of the training and testing samples for all 3 classes are shown in and Figs. 5.5 and 5.6 respectively.

Table 5.2 Percentage accuracy values by varying Gabor filter parameters

Parameter	Overall accuracy	Parameter	Overall accuracy	
$x = y = 1$	55.8	$x = y = 2$	63.3	
$x = y = 3$	79.2	$x = y = 4$	49.2	
$x = y = 5$	70.0	$x = y = 6$	73.3	
$x = y = 7$	69.2	$x = y = 8$	56.7	
$x = y = 9$	48.3	$x = y = 10$	44.2	
		x = y = 3		
$\varphi = 0$	62.5	$\varphi = \frac{\pi}{8}$	60	
$\varphi = \frac{2\pi}{8}$	82.5	$\varphi = \frac{3\pi}{8}$	66.7	
$\varphi = \frac{4\pi}{8}$	51.7	$\varphi = \frac{5\pi}{8}$	77.5	
$\varphi = \frac{6\pi}{8}$	74.2	$\varphi = \frac{7\pi}{8}$	79.2	
$\varphi = \frac{8\pi}{8}$	79.2	$\varphi = \frac{9\pi}{8}$	77.5	
$\varphi = \frac{10\pi}{8}$	75.0	$\varphi = \frac{11\pi}{8}$	75.8	
$\varphi = \frac{12\pi}{8}$	76.7	$\varphi = \frac{13\pi}{8}$	62.5	
$\varphi = \frac{14\pi}{8}$	54.2	$\varphi = \frac{15\pi}{8}$	73.3	
$\varphi = \frac{16\pi}{8}$	62.5			
		x = y = 3, $\varphi = \frac{\pi}{4}$		
$\theta = 1$	67.5	$\theta = 2$	82.5	
$\theta = 3$	57.5	$\theta = 4$	42.5	
$\theta = 5$	65	$\theta = 6$	81.6	
$\theta = 7$	52.2	$\theta = 8$	75	
$\theta = 9$	78.3	$\theta = 10$	80.8	
Feature	**Class 1**	**Class 2**	**Class 3**	**Overall accuracy**
Gabor filter				
$x = y = 3, \varphi = \frac{\pi}{4}, \theta = 2$	100	47.5	100	82.5

The variations of the real (R), imaginary (I) and feature values (F) of the training and testing samples for all 3 classes are shown in and Figs. 5.5 and 5.6 respectively

Laws Texture Detection Method

A total of 14 features as explained in section on "Proposed Approach" are computed from each image of each class. Each feature is in the form of a 2-D matrix and as such can be represented pictorially as an image. Figure 5.8 provides an indicative view of the pictorial representation of each feature. The first sub-image at the top left corner is the original medical image.

The results of classification accuracy based on these 14 features are tabulated below in Table 5.3. The SL feature is seen to provide the best accuracy of 100 % while 11 of the others are seen to correctly classify 119 out of the 120 test images providing an accuracy of 99.2 %.

Figure 5.9 indicates the pictorial representation of the linearized SL feature vector averaged over all the training and testing samples of each class. Based on the size

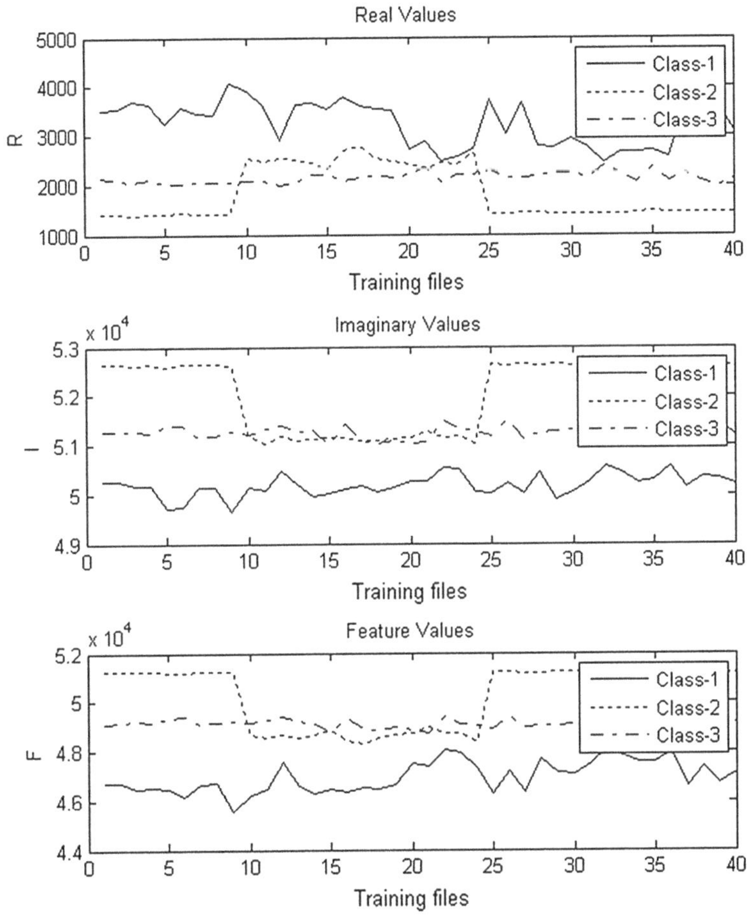

Fig. 5.5 Variation of feature values of Gabor filter for training files

of each image the feature vector consists of around 52000 elements. The top three sub-figures show the average vector of each of the three classes of the training set, while the lower three sub-figures indicate the same for the testing set.

Figure 5.10 indicates the classification plots for the feature SL which provides the highest accuracy. The figure shows the differences of the testing samples of each class with the training samples of the three classes. The symbols have the following meaning : *dmn* indicates difference between testing samples of class-*m* with the mean of the training samples of class-*n* . The top sub-figure shows results for class-1, the middle sub-figure for class-2 and the bottom sub-figure for class-3.

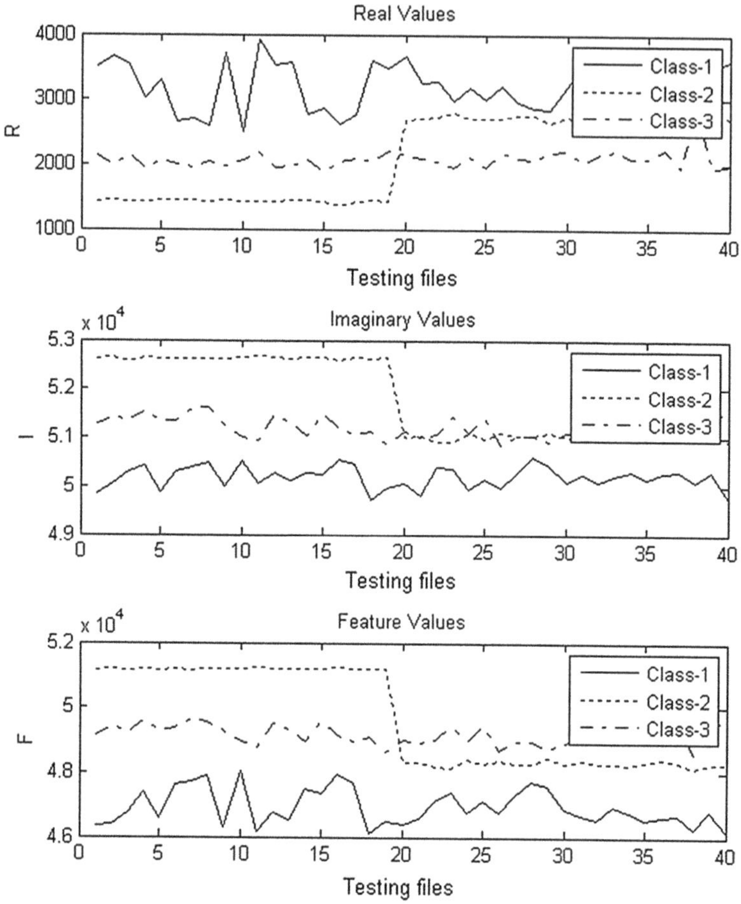

Fig. 5.6 Variation of feature values of Gabor filter for testing files

Analysis

Classification of echocardiography images depicting three medical conditions of the heart is demonstrated using texture recognition techniques. The best accuracies obtained range from 74.2 % for Hu Moment Invariant to 82.5 % with Gabor filter and 100 % for Law's Texture Detection method. To put the above results in perspective with the state of the art, the best results reported is 94 % for identification of mammalian visual cortex [3], 80 % for identification of bone X-ray image and 77 % for chest X-ray images [6], 96 % for the recognition of medical images using area moments [13], 90 % for the recognition of brain images [14], while in [15] the correct recognition rate of medical images is reported to be 92 %. Hence, it may be concluded that the proposed method in the current work has recognition rates comparable to

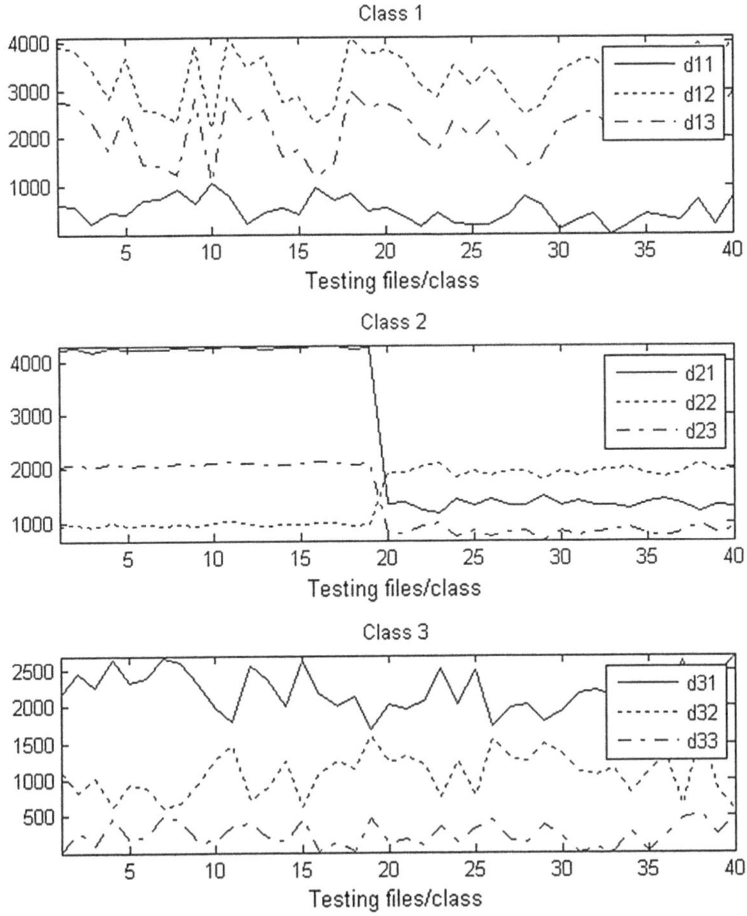

Fig. 5.7 Classification using Gabor filter feature values

those in related works. In [18] the oral medical images are recognized by the top-hat morphological operator. For direct comparisons, the top-hat method is applied to the current dataset. The variation of the feature values for training and testing samples for each of the 3 classes are indicated in Fig. 5.11.

Figure 5.12 indicates the classification plots for the top-hat feature. The figure shows the differences of the testing samples of each class with the training samples of the three classes. The symbols have the following meaning : *dmn* indicates difference between testing samples of class-*m* with the mean of the training samples of class-*n*. The top sub-figure shows results for class-1, the middle sub-figure for class-2 and the bottom sub-figure for class-3.

The correct recognition rate for the testing samples using top-hat method is found to be 100 % (Class-1), 42.5 % (Class-2), 97.5 % (Class-3) and 80 % (overall).

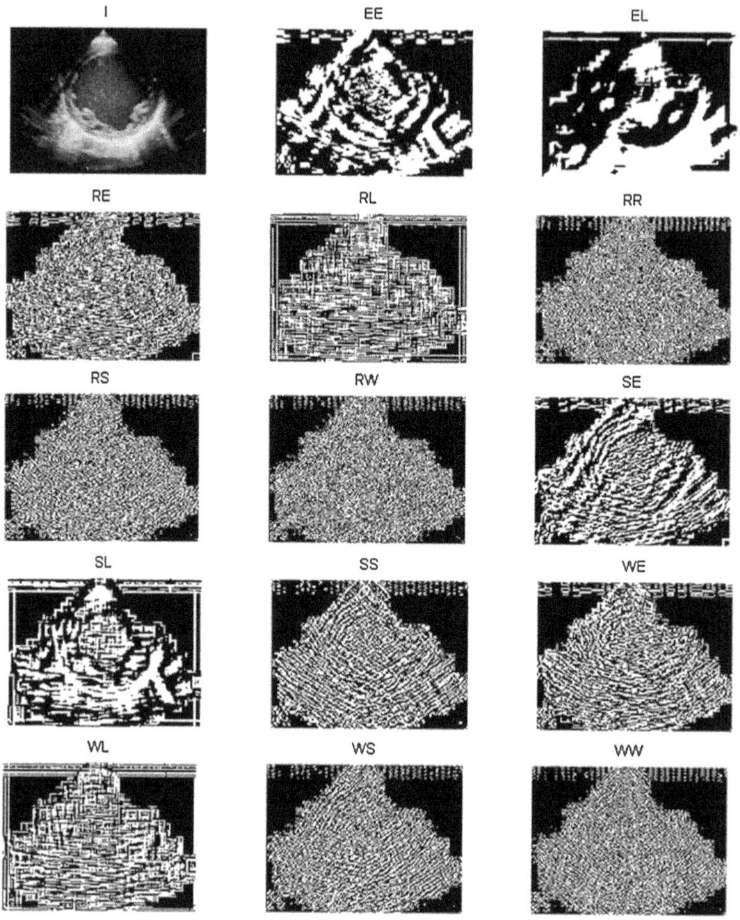

Fig. 5.8 Original image (I) and its Law's feature representations

Table 5.4 provides a summary of results obtained using the various techniques discussed.

The clock time and processing time required for executing each of the methods for all training and testing samples of the 3 classes are tabulated below in Table 5.5. The system configuration is Pentium-4, 2.4 GHz, 1 GB RAM.

Conclusions and Future Directions

This paper proposes an automated system for recognition of the images of echocardiography pertaining to three medical conditions, using texture detection methods.

Table 5.3 Percentage accuracy values by using laws texture detection method

Feature	Class 1	Class 2	Class 3	Overall accuracy
EE	100	82.5	97.5	93.3
EL	100	52	100	84.2
RE	100	100	97.5	99.2
RL	100	100	97.5	99.2
RR	100	100	97.5	99.2
RS	100	100	97.5	99.2
RW	100	100	97.5	99.2
SE	100	100	97.5	99.2
SL	100	100	100	100
SS	100	100	97.5	99.2
WE	100	100	97.5	99.2
WL	100	100	97.5	99.2
WS	100	100	97.5	99.2
WW	100	100	97.5	99.2

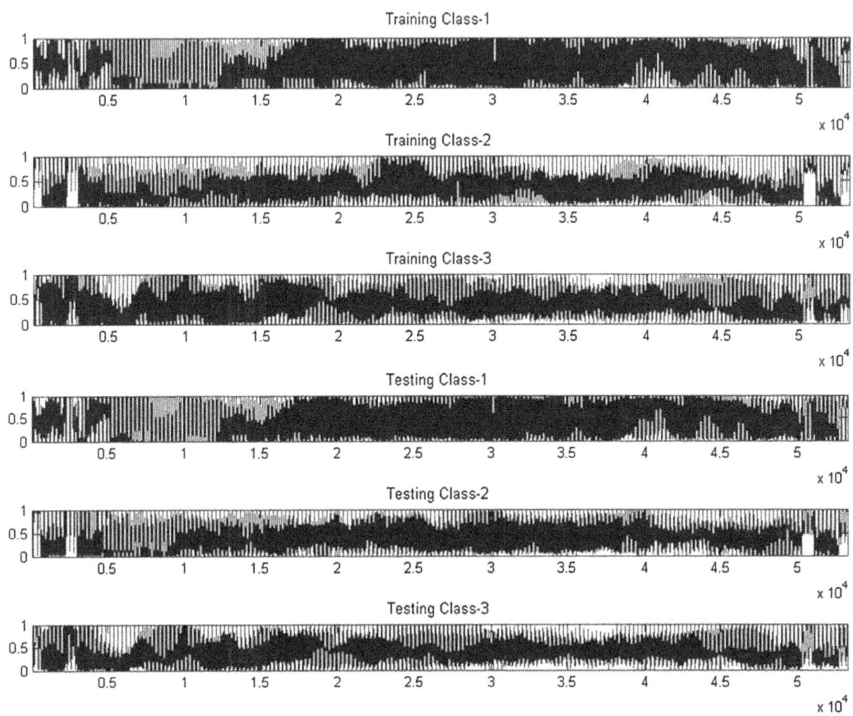

Fig. 5.9 Average Law's feature vector for each class of training and testing sets

Four different techniques were studied and recognition accuracies for each on a dataset of 240 images were computed. Best results of 100 % for each class were

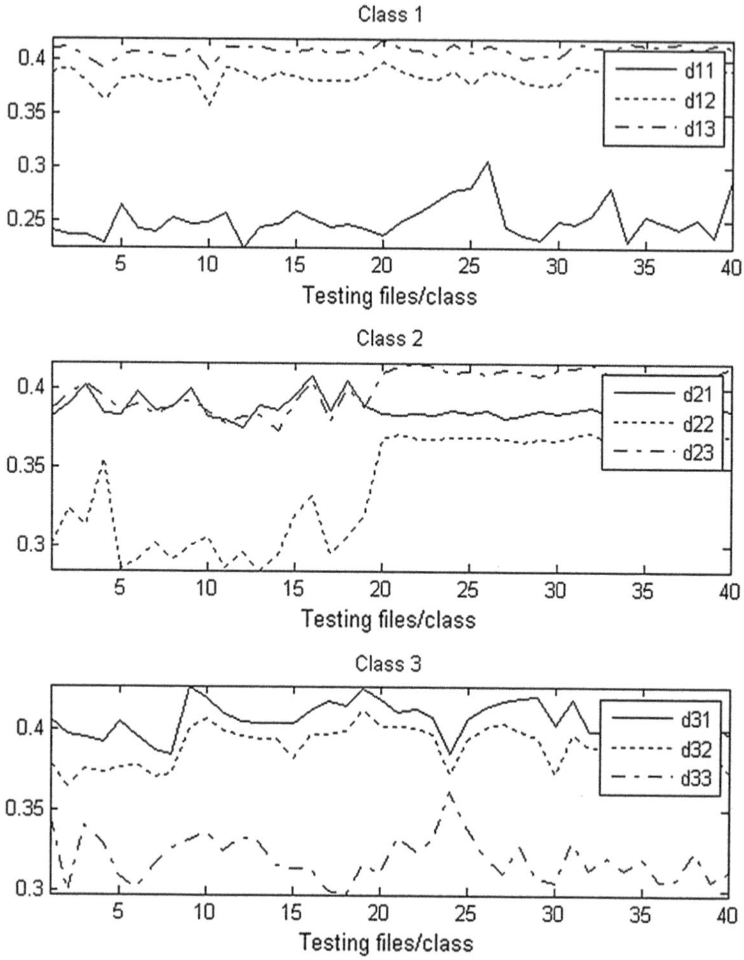

Fig. 5.10 Classification of testing samples by Law's feature SL

achieved using Law's texture detection method and such results were found to be comparable or better than those reported in contemporary literature. Time complexity of proposed methods does not exceed 200 s for 240 images and as such these are variable to be carried out in real-time. In contrast to systems like ASSERT [23] that require physicians to manually specify regions of interest, this system is fully automated and hence more accurate, less costly and easily scalable with increasing size of datasets. Finally unlike systems like Archimedes [24] which use relational databases for storing images implying the need for textual descriptors for storing and searching, the proposed system works entirely based on non-textual metadata extracted directly from the images for searching and retrieval of relevant images.

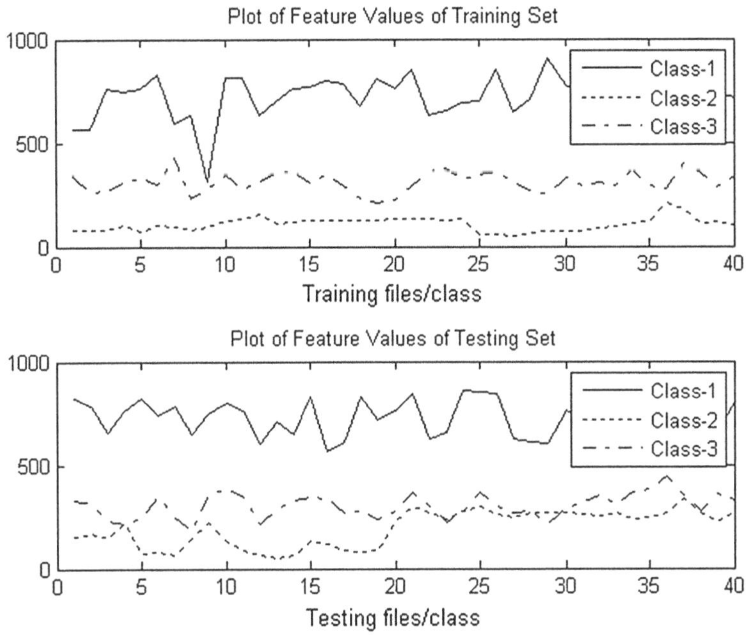

Fig. 5.11 Variation of top-hat feature values for training and testing files

Table 5.4 Comparison between three techniques

Feature	Best accuracy (%)
Hu moment invariant	74.2
Top-hat morphology	80
Gabor filter	82.5
Laws texture detection method	100

Table 5.5 Processing overheads

Feature	Clock time (min:s)	CPU time (s)
Hu moment invariant	1:35	89.6094
Top-hat morphology	0:07	4.9688
Gabor filter	0:06	6.5938
Laws texture method	3:35	200.1875

Such automated classification system can prove useful for quick and efficient classification of heart disease, at least to an initial level, especially where adequate medical personnel are absent. Future work for improving the system would be focused on : (1) including more classes and improving the feature vector by combining several

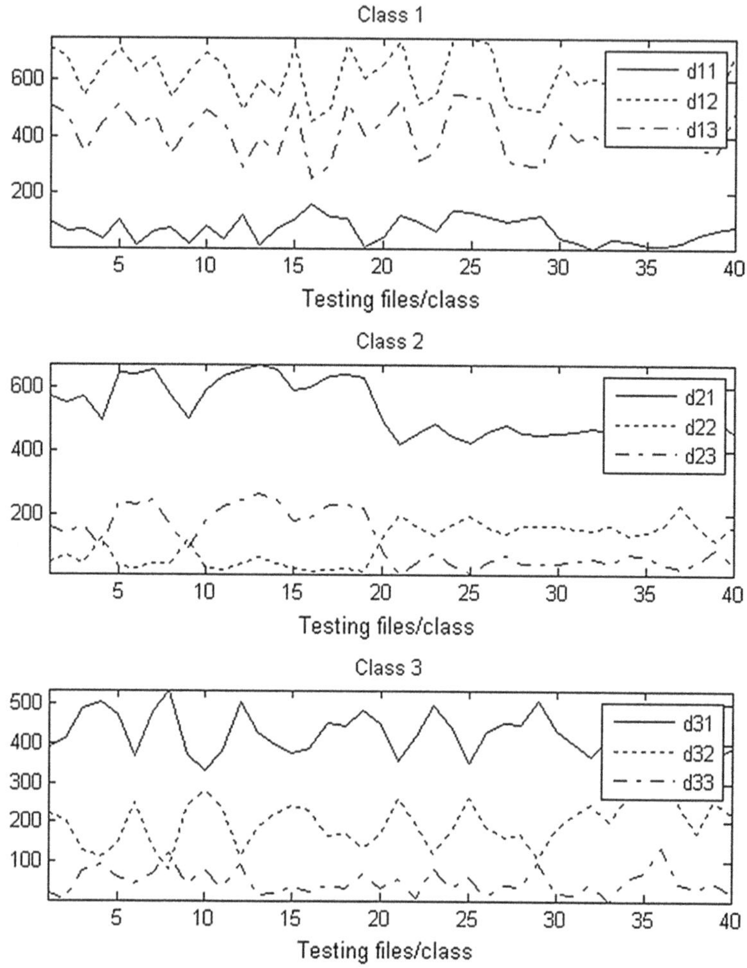

Fig. 5.12 Classification of testing samples using top-hat method

techniques together (2) using a statistical classifier like a neural network for classification (3) handling images which may be rotated or skewed.

References

1. S. Angenent, E. Pichon, A. Tannenbaum, "Mathematical Methods in Medical Image Processing", Bulletin of the American Mathematical Society, Vol. 43, 2006, pp. 365–306.
2. K.M.M. Rao, V.D.P. Rao, "Medical Image Processing", e-book, 2006 [www.drkmm.com/resources/MEDICAL_IMAGE_PROCESSING_25sep06.pdf].

3. J. M. Kinser and G. Wang, "Texture recognition of medical images with the ICM method," ELSEVIER, Nuclear Instruments and Methods in Physics Research, 2004, pp. 387–391.
4. A. Shimizu, Y. Matsuo and H. Kobatake, "Registration method for interval change detection between two chest X-ray images with different rotation angles," ELSEVIER International Congress Series 1268, 2004, pp. 917–922.
5. J. Tomwaki, Y. Suenaga, T. Negoho and T. Fukumura, "Pattern Recognition of Chest X-Ray Images," Computer Graphics and Image Processing, 1973, pp. 252–271.
6. C. H. Linda and G. Wiselin Jiji, "Crack detection in X-ray images using fuzzy index measure," ELSEVIER, Applied Soft Computing, 2011, pp. 3571–3579.
7. H.Y. Tsai, C.H. Yang, K.M. Huang, M.J. Li and C.J. Tung, "Analyses of patient dose and image quality for chest digital radiography," ELSEVIER, Radiation Measurements, 2010, pp. 722–725.
8. M. R. Luo, "A colour management framework for medical imaging applications", ELSEVIER, Computerized Medical Imaging and Graphics, 2006, pp. 357–361.
9. S. Nakajima, K. Nakamura, K. Masamune, I. Sakuma and T. Dohi, "Three-dimensional medical imaging display with computer-generated integral photography", ELSEVIER, Computerized Medical Imaging and Graphics, 2001, pp. 235–241.
10. M. Hoheisel, "Review of medical imaging with emphasis on X-ray detectors", ELSEVIER, Nuclear Instruments and Methods in Physics Research, 2006, pp. 215–226.
11. J. Freudenberger, E. Hell and W. Kn.upfer, "Perspectives of medical X-ray imaging," ELSEVIER Nuclear Instruments and Methods in Physics Research, 2001, pp. 99–104.
12. A. Salustri, S. Spitaels, J. Mcghie, W. Vlet-Fer, Jos R. T. C. Roelandt, Facc "Transthoracic Three-Dimensional Echocardiography in Adult Patients With Congenital Heart Disease," JACC Vol. 26, No. 3, 1995, pp. 759–767.
13. F. Linan, T. Dan, Y. Lujia, "Medical Image Recognition Based on Line Moment and the BP Neural", IEEE International Conference on Electronic Measurement and Instruments, 2007, pp. 747–751.
14. H. Ping, T. Yu-bo, "Medical Image Recognition Based on the Fuzzy Morphological Associative Memories", IEEE, 2009, pp. 1101–1103.
15. X. Xianchuan, Z. Qi, "Medical Image Retrieval Using Local Binary Patterns with Image Euclidean Distance", IEEE, 2009, pp. 1–4.
16. Liana Stanescu, Dumitru Dan Burdescu, "Medical Image Segmentation - A Comparison of Two Algorithms", IEEE International Workshop on Medical Measurement and Applications, 2010, pp. 165–170.
17. J. Blahuta, T. Soukup, P. Čermák, J. Rozsypal, M. Večerek, "Ultrasound medical image recognition with Artificial intelligence for Parkinson's disease classification", IEEE MIRPO, 2012, pp. 958–962.
18. Wang Yingli Zhao Xueli Wang Ming, "Based on the top-hat algorithm of oral medical image information recognition and data processing", IEEE International Conference on Measurement, Information and Control, 2012, pp. 158–162.
19. M-K Hu, "Visual pattern recognition by moment invariants", IRE Transactions on Information Theory, 1962, pp. 179–187.
20. K. Laws, "Textured Image Segmentation", Ph.D. Dissertation, University of Southern California, January 1980.
21. Normal echo [http://www.youtube.com/watch?v=7TWu0_Gklzo]
22. Obstruction midcavity hypertrophic cardiomyopath[http://www.youtube.com/watch? EFCYu5QLBvU]
23. C. R Shyu, A. Kak, A. Kosaka, "ASSERT : A Physician in the Loop CBRS for HRCT Image Databases", Computer Vision and Image Understanding, Vol. 75, No. 1, 1999, pp. 111–132.
24. D. Tahmoush and H. Samet, "A Web Collaboration system for Content based Retrieval of Medical Images", Proceedings of SPIE Medical Imaging PACS and Medical Informatics, Vol. 6516, SPIE, 2007.

Chapter 6
Innovative Soft Computing Methodologies for Evaluating Risk Factors of Atherosclerosis

M. Naresh Kumar and V. Sree Hari Rao

Introduction

Cardiovascular disease is a major health concern as more than 17.3 million deaths per year were reported as per the statistics of WHO report 2008 [1, 2]. The distribution of the deaths across the regions of the world is shown in Fig. 6.1. The cardiovascular disease caused by thickening of the walls of the arteries known as atherosclerosis has a long sub-clinical incubation period ranging from 30 to 50 years. The physicians would like to assess the risk of patients having a severe clinical event such as stroke or heart attack and predict the same if possible. Some of the major known risk factors that eventually lead to the development of atherosclerosis are as follows: (i) family history of premature coronary heart disease or stoke in a first degree relative under the age of 60, (ii) tobacco abuse, (iii) type 2 diabetes, (iv) high blood pressure, (v) left ventricular hypertrophy (thickened heart muscle), (vi) high triglycerides, (vii) high low-density lipoprotein (LDL) cholesterol, and (viii) low high-density lipoprotein (HDL) cholesterol. Large number of factors influence the onset of atherosclerosis making it a difficult task for the physicians to diagnose in its early stages. Though main risk factors are identified, development of automated effective risk prediction models using data mining techniques becomes essential for better health monitoring and prevention of deaths due to cardiovascular diseases [3, 4]. Establishing a diagnostic procedure for early detection of atherosclerosis is very important as any delay would increase the risk of serious complications or even disability. Determining the conditions (risk factors) predisposing the development of atherosclerosis can lead to

M. Naresh Kumar (✉)
National Remote Sensing Centre (ISRO), Hyderabad, Andhra Pradesh 500037, India
e-mail: nareshkumar_m@nrsc.gov.in

V. Sree Hari Rao
Foundation for Scientific Research and Technological Innovation, Alakapuri, Hyderabad, Andhra Pradesh 500035, India
e-mail: vshrao@gmail.com

B. Furht and A. Agarwal (eds.), *Handbook of Medical and Healthcare Technologies*, DOI: 10.1007/978-1-4614-8495-0_6,

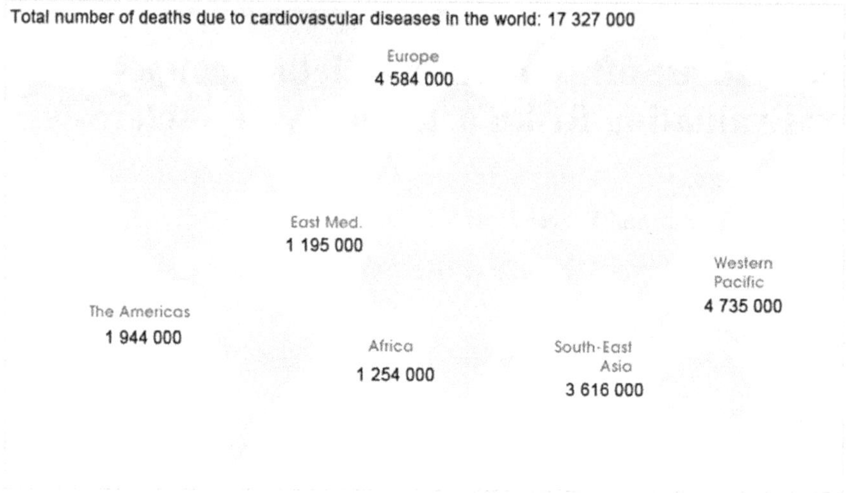

Fig. 6.1 Total number of deaths due to cardiovascular disease in the world. Data Source: WHO, adapted from http://www.world-heart-federation.org/cardiovascular-health/global-facts-map/

tests for identifying the disease in its early stages. Presently, stenosis severity is the current mark for surgical decisions.

The observations on patients are available as data in different formats. The attributes in the medical data sets include demographic details (i.e.age, sex), medical history (i.e. diabetes, obesity) and laboratory examinations (e.g. creatinine, triglyceride) having both categorical and/ or integer and real types. In addition the biomedical signals such as Electrocardiography (ECG), Electromyography (EMG) form an important dimension in the prognosis of the disease. Though the clinical risk factors of CHD are identified, there is a need for additional understanding on the disease progression for effective management of clinical cases [5]. Researchers have been focusing on techniques for quantifying atherosclerosis plaque morphology, composition, mechanical forces etc., hoping for better patient screening procedures. Imaging of atherosclerotic plaques helps in both diagnosis and monitoring of the progression for future management [6, 7, 91].

Machine learning approaches have been employed in a variety of real world problems to extract knowledge from data for predictive tasks [8, 9]. In [10] a test for predicting atherosclerosis is proposed using genetic algorithm and a fitness function that depends on area under the curve (AUC) of receiver operator characteristics (ROC). In [11] a three step approach based on clustering, supervised classification and frequent itemsets search is adopted to predict whether atherosclerosis can develop in individuals based on the correlation between his or her habits and the social environment. Support vector machines were employed in [12] for discriminating patients between coronary and non-coronary heart diseases. Supervised classifiers such as Naive Bayes (NB), Multi Layer Perceptron (MLP), Decision Trees (DT) utilize the associations among the attributes for predicting future cardiovascular disorders in the individuals [13]. A correlation based feature selection with C4.5 decision tree is applied in [14] for risk prediction of cardiovascular diseases. There are many other studies wherein machine learning techniques have also been employed for predicting the risk of CHD due to atherosclerosis using ultrasound and other imaging methods [15, 16]. Community based studies help in understanding the risk factors of atherosclerosis in different social strata [17, 18].

The presence of large number of attributes in medical databases affects the decision making process as some of the factors may be redundant or irrelevant. Also, the presence of missing values and highly skewed value distributions in the attributes of medical datasets require development of new preprocessing strategies. Feature selection methods are aimed at identifying feature subsets to construct models that can best describe the dataset. The other advantages in using feature selection methods include: identifying and removing of redundant/irrelevant features [19], reducing the dimensionality of the dataset, and improving the predictive capability of the classifier. The present study attempts to identify risk factors causing atherosclerosis and the possible risk that the individuals are running at.

The salient features of this chapter are:

- identifying the missing values (MV) in the dataset and imputing them by using a newly developed non-parametric imputation procedure;
- determining factors that would help in the prediction of the risk of developing atherosclerosis among the different groups in the community;
- description of a predictive model that has the capability of rendering effective prediction of risk factors in realtime;
- comparing the performances of the state-of-the-art methods used in the identification of risk factors of atherosclerosis;
- computing time complexity and scalability of the soft computing algorithms;
- discussing other diagnostic methods used by doctors.

This chapter is organized as follows: A brief introduction to the biology, the pathogenesis and pathophysiology of atherosclerosis are presented in section "Biology, Pathogenesis, and Pathophysiology". The sign, symptoms and diagnosis is presented in section "Symptoms and Diagnosis", imaging techniques for identification of the plaque morphology and its quantification are discussed in section "Imaging Methods" and the soft computing techniques being employed in identifying the risk factors are discussed in section "Soft Computing Methods for Predictive Modeling". The description of the datasets and the experimental results are presented in section "Experiments and Results". Conclusions and discussion are deferred to section "Conclusions and Discussion".

Biology, Pathogenesis, and Pathophysiology

Atherosclerosis is an inflammatory disease of arteries due to deposition of lipids and smooth muscle cells. The onset of this disease may result in coronary heart diseases or heart stroke (Fig. 6.2). Atherosclerosis is a progressive disease with a long phase without visible symptoms. For the molecular biology and other details of this chronic disease, we refer the readers to [20, 21, 92]. The disease starts with an inflammatory response that encourages cell migration and finally develops in to a plaque. The plaque obstructs the blood flows in the arterial vessels causing obstruction the blood flow in arterial vessels.

Molecular risk factors, such as elevated plasma lipids and glucose levels, represent major risk factors for atherosclerosis and cardiovascular disease; the latter risk factors have been implicated in atherosclerosis appearance and progression by starting a cascade of molecular events leading to plaque instability and cardiovascular events.

Atherosclerosis is a progressive disease caused by multiple factors that remain asymptomatic for many years before serious complication arise in the cardiovascular health of individuals. Understanding the pathogenesis of atherosclerosis first requires knowledge of the structure and biology of the normal artery and its indigenous cell types. Normal arteries have a well-developed trilaminar structure (Fig. 6.3). The innermost layer, the tunica intima, is thin at birth in humans and many nonhuman species. The structure of the adult human intima is actually much more complex and heterogeneous. The endothelial cell of the arterial intima constitutes the crucial contact surface with blood. Arterial endothelial cells possess highly regulated mechanisms that gets disturbed during the pathogenesis of the arterial diseases.

From the pathophysiological point of view, atherosclerosis is a single systemic disease caused by a common process, regardless of the vascular territory involved [22]. Atherosclerosis begins with the dysfunction of the endothelium (the natural barrier

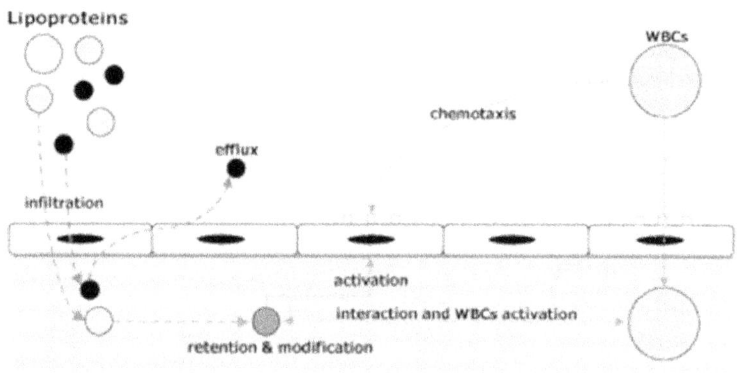

Fig. 6.2 Mechanisms of lipoprotein mediated atherogenesis. Intermediate size lipoproteins (*grey circles*) are those that are preferentially retained into the artery wall and activate the atherosclerosis cascade. Small size lipoproteins (*black circles*) infiltrate the artery wall, but may be also cleared away from the artery. *WBCs* white blood cells. Adapted from Elmo and Matteo [21]

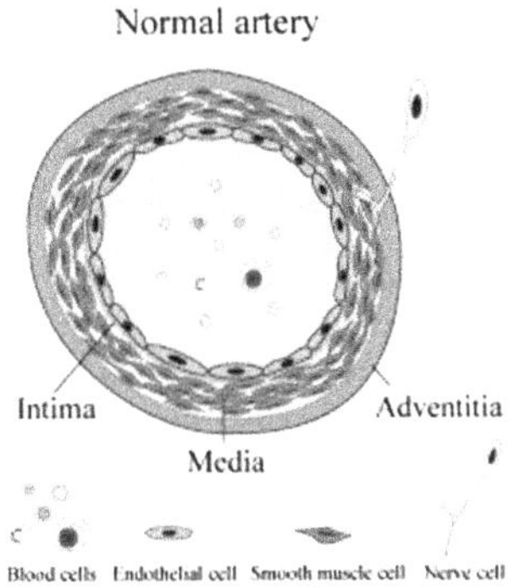

Fig. 6.3 Trilaminar structure of a normal artery. Adapted from http://www.inflammation.dk/iir/14athero/_intro.htm

between the blood flow and the arterial wall). Its main function is to render the wall nonadhesive besides capable of adapting to the rheological needs of the arterial vessel. The initial lesions are fatty streaks, which consist of the subendothelial accumulation of cholesterol-loaded macrophages (foam cells) that appear very early in the aorta, subsequently in the coronary arteries and, later, in the cerebral circulation. Once the endothelium becomes dysfunctional, it allows low-density lipoprotein (LDL) cholesterol molecules to penetrate the arterial wall through the endothelium. In an attempt to contain this invasion, monocytes/macrophages phagocytose the previously oxidized LDL cholesterol and become cholesterol-loaded cells. When the macrophages are replete with cholesterol, they become foam cells. Due to the fact that cholesterol is not easily metabolized outside the liver, its continuous accumulation within the cells, which fail to thrive, leads them to commit suicide (apoptosis or programmed cell death), with the resulting release of prothrombotic substances, such as tissue factor. Following the death of the macrophage foam cells, the cholesterol is again released into the arterial wall, thus perpetuating the process.

Symptoms and Diagnosis

The signs and symptoms of atherosclerosis may develop gradually and sometimes may be totally asymptomatic, as the plaque builds up in the artery. Symptoms may also vary depending on the affected artery. However, when a major artery is blocked, signs and symptoms may be severe, such as those occurring with heart attack, stroke, aneurysm, or blood clot. The symptoms of atherosclerosis may resemble other cardiac conditions. It is always advised to consult a physician for a final diagnosis [23].

The diagnostic procedures for atherosclerosis may include any, or a combination of, the following:

1. physical examination of the individuals is the first procedure adopted by doctors by listening to the arteries using a stethoscope. Abnormal whooshing sound called

a bruit may indicate poor blood flow due to build of plaque. Also, a weak or absent pulse indicate a blocked artery.

2. basic tests on the blood sample of the individual for fats, cholesterol, sugar and protein levels would help in determining the risk of atherosclerosis.
3. electrocardiogram tests record the electrical activity of heart. The strength and timing of the electrical signals would help in diagnosis of CHD and can show signs of a previous or current heart attack.
4. chest X-ray shows the organs and structure of the chest such as heart, lungs and blood vessels which helps in identifying the signs of CHD.
5. the blood pressure between the lower legs and the arm serves as an indicator (Ankle Brachial Index) that would help in diagnosis of peripheral arterial disease.

Imaging Methods

The ECG is noninvasive procedure to record the electrical activity of the heart through signals received from the metal electrodes connected to the chest wall and the extremities. Despite the advances in computer interpretation of ECGs one of the limitations is the interpretation of the incomplete or inaccurate readings which may be most likely due to arrhythmias and complex abnormalities [24].

Recent developments in imaging methods have given new insights on the molecular and metabolic activity of atherosclerotic plaques [25–27, 91]. There are two modes of imaging atherosclerosis (i) invasive and (ii) non-invasive. Among the invasive methods X-ray angiography is the most prominent imaging technique even though it has certain limitations in providing information on plaque composition [28]. The invasive procedures such as intravascular ultrasound (IVUS) [29] and Angioscopy [30] help in understanding the plaque size and to a limited extent its composition. The intravascular thermography [31] aids in monitoring the changes in plaque composition and metabolism. The non-invasive procedures such as B-mode ultrasound [32], computerized tomography (CT) [33] and magnetic resonance imaging (MRI) [26], can provide information on plaque composition on vascular beds but they fail to provide the metabolic activity of the plaque inflammatory cell. Also, the medical images generated in digital form using functional magnetic resonance imaging (FMRI), positron emission tomography (PET), single photon emission computed tomography (SPECT) etc., are important sources for identifying the markers of the disease. Though nuclear imaging techniques such as single photon emission computed tomography (SPECT) and positron emission tomography (PET) [34] have the potential for 2D and 3D surface reconstruction of thrombus using radio labels to provide information on molecular, cellular and metabolic activity of plaques [35], they lack the required resolution, quality for detection and functional assessment in medium-to-small arteries found in coronary circulation. The modalities used in the acquisition of the atherosclerotic plaque images can be expensive and it is difficult in practice to obtain these measurements accurately in comparison to other methods such as serum biomarker. In addition, depending on the plaque anatomic location, one needs to select an appropriate imaging technique which may range from the simple, quick and cost effective use of ultrasound to the expensive magnetic resonance technology [36].

Keeping in view the limitations of imaging techniques there is still a greater need for developing automated methods for predicting the risk factors of atherosclerosis in individuals which would be of great help in reducing the disease related deaths.

Soft Computing Methods for Predictive Modeling

The observations on the real world processes are collected using sensors and these datasets are prone to issues such as noise that gets manifested in terms of missing entries and redundant values which affects the capabilities of the predictive models. Soft computing is an interdisciplinary area of computational intelligence which aids in building solutions to the NP complete problems by using inexact methods to give useful but inexact answers to intractable problems. In the following sections we discuss the methods for handling missing values, feature selection and building classification models.

Missing Values: Issues

The missing values in databases may arise due to various reasons such as value being lost (erased or deleted) or not recorded, incorrect measurements, equipment errors, or possibly due to an expert not attaching any importance to a particular procedure. The incomplete data can be identified by looking for null values in the data set. However, this is not always true, since missing values can appear in the form of outliers or even wrong data (i.e. out of boundaries) [37]. Especially in medical databases, most data are collected as a by product of patient care activities rather than from an organized research point of view [38].

There are three main strategies for handling missing data situations. The first consists of eliminating incomplete observations, which has major limitations namely loss of substantial information, if many of the attributes have missing values in the data records [39] and this renders introduction of biases in the data [40]. The second strategy is to treat the missing values during the data mining process of knowledge discovery and data mining (KDD) as envisaged in C4.5. The third method of handling missing values is through imputation, replacing each instance of the missing value with a probable or predicted value [41] which is most suitable for KDD applications, since the completed data can be used for any data mining activity.

There are numerous methods for predicting or approximating missing values. Single imputation strategies involve using the mean, median or mode [42] or regression-based methods [43] to impute the missing values. Traditional approaches of handling missing values like complete case analysis, overall mean imputation and missing-indicator method [44] can lead to biased estimates and may either reduce or exaggerate the statistical power. Each of these distortions can lead to invalid conclusions. Statistical methods of handling missing values consist of using maximum likelihood and expectation maximization algorithms [45, 46]. Some of these methods would work only for certain types of attributes either nominal or numeric. Machine learning approaches like neural networks with genetic algorithms [47], neural networks with particle swarm optimization [48] have been used to approximate the missing values. The use of neural networks comes with a greater cost in terms of computation and training. Methods like radial basis function networks, support vector machines and principal component analysis have been utilized for estimating the missing values.

A missing value imputation method developed in [9] for predicting the risk factors of the atherosclerosis disease is presented in section "Imputation Method".

Feature Selection

Decision making in databases is based on the attributes or features that form the data set. The set of attributes that contribute to better decision making are termed as influential attributes. The presence of features that do not contribute much to the decision making degrades the performance accuracies of the supervised machine learning algorithms. The severity of this problem can be felt if one needs to search for patterns in large databases with out considering the correlations between the attributes and the influence of such attributes on the decision attribute. The selection of influential features that maximizes the gain in the knowledge extracted from the data set is an important question in the field of machine learning, knowledge discovery, statistics and pattern recognition.

The machine learning algorithms including the top down induction of decision trees such as classification and regression trees (CART), and C4.5 suffer from attributes that may not contribute much to decision making, thus affecting the performance of classifiers. A good choice of features would help reduce the dimensionality of the data set resulting in improved performance of the classifier in terms of accuracies and the size of the models, resulting in better understanding and interpretation.

We may categorize the feature selection algorithms as supervised, unsupervised and semi-supervised based on whether the data set is labeled, unlabeled or partially labeled. Supervised feature selection [49, 50] determines feature relevance by evaluating the correlation of the features with the class, and without labels. Unsupervised feature selection exploits data variance and separability to evaluate feature relevance [51]. Semi-supervised feature selection algorithms [52] can use both labeled and unlabeled data, and their motivation is to use small amount of labeled data as additional information to improve the performance of unsupervised feature selection.

Feature selection algorithms can be broadly classified into three categories (i) filter, (ii) wrapper, and (iii) embedded models. Filter methods utilize the intrinsic properties of the data to select subsets of features as a preprocessing step, independently of the chosen classifier. Features are assessed by their relevance or discriminant powers with regard to targeted classes. The wrapper model requires a predetermined learning algorithm and uses its performance as evaluation criterion to select features. Wrappers can often find small feature subsets with high accuracy because the features are well correlated with the learning methods. However, wrappers typically require extensive computation. It is argued that filters have better generalization properties as they are independent of any specific learning method. A survey on the filter and the wrapper model for feature selection is discussed in [53]. Algorithms with embedded models such as C4.5 [54] and least angle regression (LARS) [55], incorporate variable selection as a part of the training process, and feature relevance is obtained analytically from the objective of the learning model. Feature selection algorithms with filter and embedded models may return either a subset of selected features or the weights (measuring feature relevance) of all features.

In wrapper based approach [56, 57] the feature subset selection algorithm exists as a wrapper around the induction algorithm (classifier) (Fig. 6.4). The feature subset selection algorithm conducts a search for a good subset using the induction algorithm itself as part of the function evaluating feature subsets. In the wrapper approach the induction algorithm is regarded as a black box and is run on the data sets usually partitioned into internal training and holdout sets with different sets of features removed from the data. The feature subset with the highest evaluation is chosen as the final set on which the induction algorithm is applied. The resulting classifier is then evaluated on an independent test set that is not used during the search.

The identification of feature subset is of utmost importance in real world problems. The presence of large number of clinical symptoms and laboratory features requires one to search large sub spaces for optimal feature subsets. These issues unless addressed appropriately would hinder the development of accurate and computationally effective diagnostic system.

The risk factors that may influence the onset of atherosclerosis may not always be known a priori. Also, sometimes there may be too many factors that need to be evaluated for diagnosing the patients. Hence features that are redundant or those that are weakly participating in the decision making must be identified and appropriately handled. The feature selection procedures can be categorized as random or sequential. The sequential methods such as forward selection, backward elimination and bidirectional selection employ greedy procedures and hence may not often be successful in finding the optimal features subsets. In comparison to genetic algorithms (GA) employed for feature selection in [8] particle swarm optimization (PSO) search offers advantages over other methods in terms of its ability in handling optimization problems with multiple local optima reasonably well and its simplicity of implementation. Sree Hari Rao and Naresh Kumar [9] identified the risk factors of atherosclerosis diseases by adopting an approach based on wrapper subset based feature evaluation model where in an alternating decision tree (ADT) classifier is used to determine the importance or fitness of the feature subset identified by the PSO.

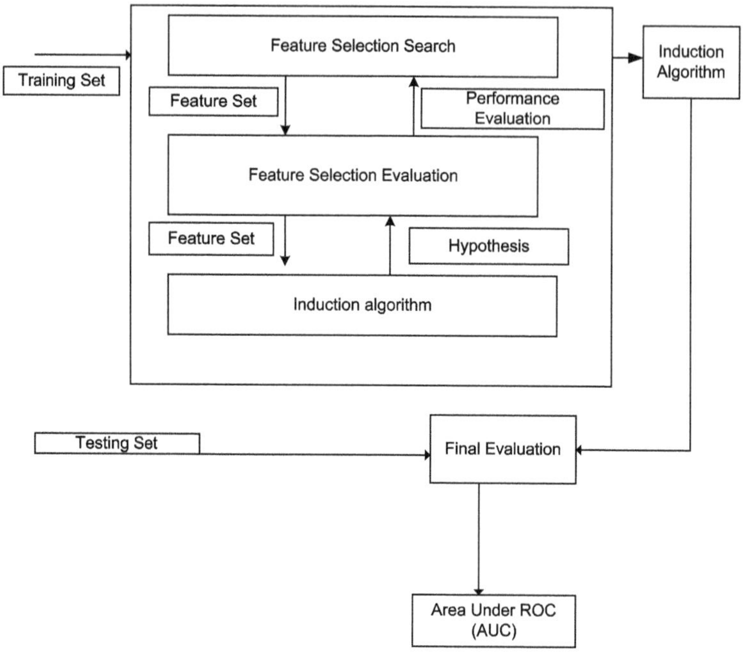

Fig. 6.4 Wrapper method of subset evaluation for selecting influencing attributes

Correlation Based Feature Selection

The goal of feature selection is to obtain a set of features that are highly correlating with the decision/class attribute and uncorrelated with other attributes in the dataset. The above heuristic can be formalized as

$$M_S = \frac{n * \bar{F_c}}{\sqrt{n + n * (n-1)\bar{F_f}}} \tag{6.1}$$

where M_S denotes the merit of the feature subset S and n is the number of features in the subset S, $\bar{F_c}$ denotes the mean correlation between the features and the class attribute and $\bar{F_f}$ denotes the average or mean correlation among the features of the subset S.

The numerator gives an indication on how predictive is a group of features on the class attribute whereas the denominator shows how much redundancy there is among the features in the subset. The above heuristic handles irrelevant features as they will be poor predictors of the class and redundant attributes as they will be highly correlated with one or more of the other features [58].

The first step in CFS method involves converting the continuous attributes to nominal attributes using a discretization method [59]. To estimate the degree of association between the nominal features a measure known as information gain is generally employed. If X and Y are two random discrete variables then the entropy of Y given X is computed as

$$I(Y) = -\sum_{y \in Y} p(y) \log_2 p(y) I(Y|X) = -\sum_{x \in X} p(x) \sum_{y \in Y} p(y|x) \log_2 p(y|x) \quad (6.2)$$

A decrease in the entropy of Y indicates an additional information about Y provided by X and is called as Information gain [54] given by

$$G = I(X) + I(Y) - I(X, Y) \quad (6.3)$$

The information gain (G) is biased in favor of features with more values (attributes with greater numbers of values) will appear to gain more information than those with fewer values even if they are actually not more informative. So a standardization procedure based on symmetrical uncertainty is adopted in CFS to compensate the bias towards attributes with more values and normalizes its value to the range [0, 1] [58].

$$U = 2 * \frac{G}{I(X) + I(Y)} \quad (6.4)$$

CFS starts from the empty set of features and uses a forward best fist search with a stopping criterion of five consecutive fully expanded non-improving subsets. The subsets are evaluated using the measure given in Eq. 6.1. The steps involved in the CFS method is shown in the Fig. 6.5.

Due the reason that the correlations are estimated globally over all training instances CFS tends to select a core subset of features that have low redundancy and is strongly predictive of the class. However, in some cases there may be subsidiary features that are locally predictive in a small area of the instance space. The CFS method includes a heuristic to consider locally predictive features and avoid re-introduction of redundancy.

Genetic Algorithms

Genetic Algorithms (GA) are stochastic optimization methods, inspired by the principle of natural selection. The search algorithms based on GA are capable of effectively exploring large search spaces [60]. GAs performs a global search as compared to many search algorithms, which perform a local or a greedy search.

A genetic algorithm is mainly composed of three operators: reproduction, crossover, and mutation. Reproduction selects good string; crossover combines good strings to try to generate better offsprings; mutation alters a string locally to attempt to create a better string. In each generation, the population is evaluated and tested for termination of the algorithm. If the termination criterion is not satisfied, the population is operated upon by the above GA operators and then re-evaluated. This

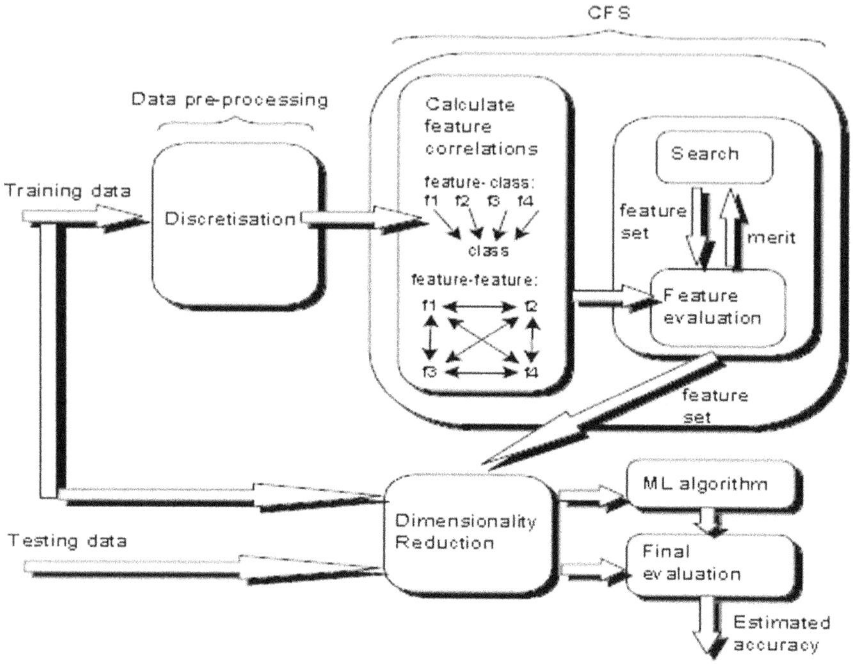

Fig. 6.5 Steps involved in the correlation based feature selection: reproduced with permission [58]

Table 6.1 Parameter values for genetic search

Attribute	Value
Start set	No attributes
Population size	20
Number of generations	20
Probability of crossover	0.6
Probability of mutation	0.033
Report frequency	20
Random number seed	1

procedure is continued until the termination criterion is met. The default parameters for GA search [8, 61] are given in Table 6.1.

Particle Swarm Optimization

A PSO search consists of a set of particles initialized with a candidate solution to a problem. Each particle is associated with a position vector and a velocity vector. The particles evaluate the fitness of the solutions iteratively and store the location where they had their best fit known as the local best (L). The particles change their position and velocity iteratively in a suitable manner with respect to the best fit solution to

Table 6.2 PSO search parameters

Attribute	Value
η_1	2.0
η_2	20
Max generations	50
Number of particles (N)	100

reach a global optimal solution. The best fit solution among the particles is called the global best (G). We represent the position vector of the particle as a binary string and accuracy of the learning algorithm as the fitness function for evaluation. The velocity and position vectors of the particles are modified using the procedure suggested in [62].

Let x_{id}^t denote the dth element of the ith particle position vector in a k-dimensional space at time t, then x_{id}^t takes values iteratively as follows,

$$v_{id}^t = v_{id}^{t-1} + c_1(L_{id} - x_{id}^{t-1}) + c_2(G_d - x_{id}^{t-1}),$$
$$Sigmoid(v_{id}^t) = \frac{1}{1+e^{-v_{id}^t}},$$
$$if\ \kappa_{id} < Sigmoid(v_{id}^t)\ then\ x_{id}^t = 1\ else\ x_{id}^t = 0,$$

$$Sigmoid(v_{id}^t) = \frac{1}{1+e^{-v_{id}^t}},$$

$$if\ \kappa_{id} < Sigmoid(v_{id}^t)\ then\ x_{id}^t = 1\ else\ x_{id}^t = 0,$$

where v_{id}^t and v_{id}^{t-1} are velocities of dth element of ith particle in time t and $t-1$ respectively, L_{id}, G_d denote the local best and global best of the particles, $Sigmoid(v_{id}^t)$ function maps the values of v_{id}^t between [0.0, 1.0]. The term κ_{id} denote the random values between 0.0 and 1.0 chosen from a normal distribution. The terms c_1, c_2 represent the cognitive and social factors respectively and are chosen as 2.0 in the experiments. A standard PSO search parameters are given in Table 6.2.

Machine Classifiers

Machine classifiers are supervisory learning methods that are widely employed in knowledge extraction from medical datasets. We present in the following sections some of the popular techniques that are being used in identifying the risk factors of the atherosclerosis disease.

Decision Trees

Decision trees are machine learning methods that can solve the problems of labeling or classifying data items out of a given finite set of classes using the features in the data items. Decision trees such as C4.5 [54], Classification and Regression trees (CART), Alternating decision trees (ADTree) [63] have been used in computational biology, bio-informatics and clinical diagnosis [8, 64–67]. The C4.5 decision tree handles the missing values during the model induction phase of generating the tree.

Alternating decision trees are based on AdaBoost algorithm which generates rules based on the majority votes over simple weak rules [63, 67]. An alternating decision tree consists of decision nodes (splitter node) and prediction nodes which can be either an interior node or a leaf node. The tree generates a prediction node at the root and then alternates between decision nodes and further prediction nodes. Decision nodes specify a predicate condition and prediction nodes contain a single number denoting the predictive value. An instance can be classified by following all paths for which all decision nodes are true and summing any prediction nodes that are traversed. A positive sum implies membership of one class and negative sum corresponds to the membership of the opposite class.

To generate an alternating decision tree we apply the algorithm proposed by Sree Hari Rao and Naresh Kumar [67] on the data set given in Table 6.3 specifically chosen for the purpose of demonstration. The data set has three attributes namely Attribute1 $\in \{A, B, C\}$, Attribute2 $\in \{true, false\}$ and a decision attribute $\in \{class1, class2\}$. There in total $n = 14$ instances out of which $n_1 = 9$ belong to class1 and $n_2 = 5$ belong to class2.

We designate the instances belonging to class1 as negative (-ve) and those belonging to class2 as positive (+ve). The weights of each of these instances ($w_{i,t}$ $i = 1 \ldots n$ denotes the instances and t denotes the boosting iteration) is initialized to 1 i.e, set $w_{i,0} = 1 \forall i = 1 \ldots n$ as shown by attribute $W0$ in Table 6.3. We designate the condition before the split (precondition) as P_t and rule that is being currently considered for the split (condition) as C. The initial (boosting iteration $t = 0$) sum of the weights of the instances with a precondition $P_0 = T$ and condition $C = T$ where T denotes *true* is given by $\sum_{j=1, j \in class1}^{n_1} w_{j,0}$ represented as $W_-(T) = 9$ for class1 and $\sum_{k=1, k \in class2}^{n_2} w_{k,0}$ represented as $W_+(T) = 5$ for class2. For the first boosting iteration ($t = 1$) the initial prediction value at the root node is computed as $a = \frac{1}{2}\ln(\frac{W_+(T)+1}{W_-(T)+1}) = \frac{1}{2}\ln\frac{5+1}{9+1} = -0.255$. The weights associated with each of these instances are then updated as $w_{j,1} = w_{j,0}e^{a}$ $\forall j = 1 \ldots n_1 \wedge j \in class1$ for negative instances (class1) and $w_{k,1} = w_{k,0}e^{-a}$ $\forall k = 1 \ldots n_2 \wedge k \in class2$ for positive instances (class2). Based on the above step the weights of the instances belonging to class1 are updated as $w_{j,1} = 1 * e^{-0.255} = 0.7749$ $\forall j = 1 \ldots n_1 \wedge j \in class1$ and the instances of class2 are re-weighted as $w_{k,1} = 1 * e^{0.255} = 1.2904$ $\forall k = 1 \ldots n_2 \wedge k \in class2$. The symbol $\wedge$ indicates that both the conditions to be satisfied for the entire condition to be true. The updated weights are shown as $W1$ in the Table 6.3.

The next step is to identify the rules for splitting the dataset. The Attribute1 is of nominal type and has three values $\{A, B, C\}$ where as the Attribute2 is having only two values $\{true, false\}$. One can identify weak rules (c_2) based on the attribute values such as $Attribute1 = A$, $Attribute1 = B$, $Attribute1 = C$, $Attribute2 = false$. To find the best split we compute a measure $Z_t(c_1, c_2)$ value where $c_1 \in P_t$ and $c_2 \in C$ as follows

$$\begin{aligned} Z_t(c_1, c_2) = 2 * (&\sqrt{(W_+(c_1 \wedge c_2) + 1.0) * (W_-(c_1 \wedge c_2) + 1.0)} + \\ &\sqrt{(W_+(c_1 \wedge \neg c_2) + 1.0) * (W_-(c_1 \wedge \neg c_2) + 1.0)}) \\ &+ W(\neg c_2) \end{aligned}$$

For $Attribute1 = A$ there are 3 instances in class2 (+ve) with weight of each instance being 1.2904 and 2 instances in class1 (-ve) with weight of each instance being 0.7749. The $Z_t(c_1, c_2)$ is computed as

$$\begin{aligned} Z_1(c_1, c_2) &= 2 * (\sqrt{4.8712 * 2.5498} + \sqrt{3.5808 * 6.4243}) + 0.5739 \\ &= 2 * (3.524 + 4.796) + 0.5739 \\ &= 17.2139 \end{aligned}$$

For $Attribute1 = B$ there are 0 instances in class2 (+ve) with weight of each instance being 1.2904 and 4 instances in class1 (-ve) with weight of each instance being 0.7749. The $Z_t(c_1, c_2)$ is computed as

$$\begin{aligned} Z_1(c_1, c_2) &= 2 * (\sqrt{1.0 * 4.0996} + \sqrt{7.452 * 4.8745}) + 0.5739 \\ &= 2 * (2.024 + 6.027) + 0.5739 \\ &= 16.6759 \end{aligned}$$

For $Attribute1 = C$ there are 2 instances in class2 (+ve) with weight of each instance being 1.2904 and 3 instances in class1 (-ve) with weight of each instance being 0.7749. The $Z_t(c_1, c_2)$ is computed as

$$\begin{aligned} Z_1(c_1, c_2) &= 2 * (\sqrt{3.58 * 3.3247} + \sqrt{4.872 * 5.6494}) + 0.5739 \\ &= 2 * (3.4499 + 5.246) + 0.5739 \\ &= 17.9657 \end{aligned}$$

For $Attribute2 = false$ there are 2 instances in class2 (+ve) with weight of each instance being 1.2904 and 6 instances in class1 (-ve) with weight of each instance being 0.7749. The $Z_t(c_1, c_2)$ is computed as

$$\begin{aligned} Z_1(c_1,c_2) &= 2*(\sqrt{2.5808*4.6494}+\sqrt{5.8712*4.3247})+0.5739 \\ &= 2*(3.4639+5.0389)+0.5739 \\ &= 17.5795 \end{aligned}$$

Therefore, the minimum $Z_1(c_1, c_2)$ value is 16.6759 for the split $Attribute1 = B$. So the first split is based on $Attribute1 = B$ resulting in two branches having prediction values $a = \frac{1}{2}\ln\frac{W_+(T \wedge Attribute1 = B)+1}{W_-(T \wedge Attribute1 = B)+1} = 0.5*\ln\frac{(0*1.2904)+1}{(4*0.7749)+1} = -0.705$ and $b = \frac{1}{2}\ln\frac{W_+(T \wedge Attribute1 \neq B)+1}{W_-(T \wedge Attribute1 \neq B)+1} = 0.5*\ln\frac{(5*1.2904)+1}{(5*0.7749)+1} = 0.213$. The precondition is updated as P_{t+1} to be P_t with addition of $c_1 \wedge c_2$ and $c_1 \wedge \neg c_2$. So the precondition is set as $P_2 = (T \wedge Attribute = B, T \wedge Attribute \neq B)$.

The weights are then updated using the formula $w_{j,t+1} = w_{j,t}e^{r_1(x_j)}\ \forall j = 1\ldots n_1 \wedge j \in class1$ and $w_{k,t+1} = w_{k,t}e^{-r_1(x_k)}\ \forall k = 1\ldots n_2 \wedge k \in class2$ where $r(x_i)$ denotes the rule associated with instance x_i i.e the weights $w_{j,2} = 0.7749*e^{0.213}$ $\forall j = 1\ldots n_1 \wedge j \in class1 \wedge Attribute1 \neq B \Rightarrow 0.958849366$, $w_{j,2} = 0.7749*e^{-0.705}$ $\forall j = 1\ldots n_1 \wedge j \in class1 \wedge Attribute1 = B \Rightarrow 0.382884734$ and $w_{k,2} = 1.2904 * e^{-0.213}\ \forall k = 1\ldots n_2 \wedge k \in class2 \wedge Attribute1 \neq B \Rightarrow 1.042844679$. The updated weights are shown in the Table 6.3 as attribute $W2$.

Since the prediction value for the node $Attribute1 \neq B$ is higher than for the node $Attribute1 = B$ in the next boosting iteration the new node is attached to $Attribute1 \neq B$. The prediction value a for $Attribute1 \neq B \wedge Attribute2 = true$ is computed as $a = \frac{1}{2}\ln(\frac{W_+(T \wedge Attribute1 \neq B \wedge Attribute2 = true)+1}{W_-(T \wedge Attribute1 \neq B \wedge Attribute2 = true)+1}) = \frac{1}{2}\ln\frac{(3*1.042845)+1}{(1*0.9588)+1} = 0.373$ and the prediction value b for $Attribute1 \neq B \wedge Attribute2 = false$ is computed as $b = \frac{1}{2}\ln(\frac{W_+(T \wedge Attribute1 \neq B \wedge Attribute2 = false)+1}{W_-(T \wedge Attribute1 \neq B \wedge Attribute2 = false)+1}) = \frac{1}{2}\ln\frac{(2*1.042845)+1}{(4*0.9588)+1} = -0.224$.

An alternating decision tree for the data set given in Table 6.3 is shown in Fig. 6.6. The root node indicates a predictive value of the decision tree before the splitting takes place. If the sum of all prediction values is positive then the instance belongs to the labeled class1, otherwise it is placed in class2. The prediction nodes are shown as ellipses and decision nodes as rectangles. The number in the ellipse indicates the boosting iteration. The dotted line connects the prediction nodes and the decision nodes; where as a solid line connects the decision nodes with the prediction nodes.

To classify an instance having attribute values $Attribute1 \neq B$ and $Attribute2 = true$ we first consider the root prediction value and based on the each instance value traverse the tree and add the prediction value of the particular node traversed. We derive the following sum by going down the appropriate path in the tree collecting all the prediction value encountered: $-0.255 + 0.213 + 0.373 = 0.331$ indicating that the instance belongs to class2.

Table 6.3 An example data set for generating alternating decision tree

Attribute1	Attribute2	Decision	W0	W1	W2
A	true	class1	1	0.7749	0.958849366
A	false	class1	1	0.7749	0.958849366
B	true	class1	1	0.7749	0.382884734
B	false	class1	1	0.7749	0.382884734
B	true	class1	1	0.7749	0.382884734
B	false	class1	1	0.7749	0.382884734
C	false	class1	1	0.7749	0.958849366
C	false	class1	1	0.7749	0.958849366
C	false	class1	1	0.7749	0.958849366
A	true	class2	1	1.2904	1.042844679
A	false	class2	1	1.2904	1.042844679
A	false	class2	1	1.2904	1.042844679
C	true	class2	1	1.2904	1.042844679
C	true	class2	1	1.2904	1.042844679

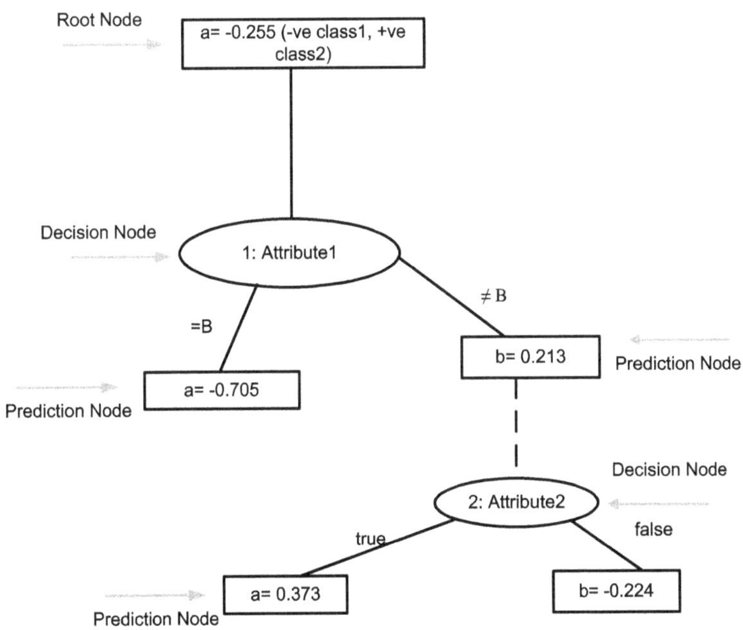

Fig. 6.6 Alternating decision tree for the toy example dataset in Table 6.3

Support Vector Machine

Support Vector Machines (SVMs) are the newest supervised machine learning techniques [68]. An excellent survey on SVMs may be found in [69]. SVMs revolve around the notion of a margin either side of a hyperplane that separates two data classes. Maximizing the margin and thereby creating the largest possible distance between the separating hyperplane and the instances on either side of it has been proven to reduce an upper bound on the expected generalization error.

Naive Bayes

Naive Bayesian networks (NB) are very simple Bayesian networks which are composed of directed acyclic graphs with only one parent (representing the unobserved node) and several children (corresponding to observed nodes) with a strong assumption of independence among child nodes in the context of their parent. Thus, the independence model (Naive Bayes) is based on estimating:

$$R = \frac{P(i|X)}{P(j|X)} = \frac{P(i)P(X|i)}{P(j)P(X|j)} = \frac{P(i)\prod P(X,i)}{P(j)\prod P(X,j)}.$$

Comparing these two probabilities, a large probability indicates that the class label value that is more likely to be the actual label (if $R > 1$: predict i else predict j). Since the Bayes classification algorithm uses a product operation to compute the probabilities P(X, i), it is especially prone to being unduly impacted by probabilities of 0. This can be avoided by using Laplace estimator or m-estimate, by adding one to all numerators and adding the number of added ones to the denominator [70].

Performance Metrics and Evaluation Methods

To evaluate the models generated by the decision trees, a k-fold cross validation algorithm ($k = 10$) is considered a powerful methodology to overcome data overfitting [71]. The data set is divided into k subsets, and the holdout method is repeated k times. Each time, one of the k subsets is used as the test set and the other $k - 1$ subsets are put together to form a training set. Then the average error across all k trials is computed. To compare and evaluate the decision trees popular performance measuressuch as sensitivity, specificity, receiver operator characteristics (ROC) and area under ROC (AUC) [72, 73] have been employed. The definitions of the above measures are discussed briefly for the benefit of the readers. The classification task generates a set of rules which can be used for classifying individuals to different classes/groups. This may result in the following situations:

(1) False positive (FP): The rules may predict the diagnosis of the patient as positive (presence of the disease) where as the actual diagnosis is negative (absence of the disease).
(2) False negative (FN): The rules may predict the diagnosis of the patient as negative (absence of the disease) where as the actual diagnosis is positive (presence of the disease).

(3) True positive (TP): When the prediction of the classifier matches with the actual diagnosis as positive.
(4) True negative (TN): When the prediction of the classifier matches with the actual diagnosis as negative.

Based on the above situations the performance of the classifiers can be compared using the following standard measures:

(i) Sensitivity: The proportion of the people who are predicted as positive of all the people who are actually positive $\frac{TP}{(TP+FN)}$.
(ii) Specificity: The proportion of the people who are predicted as negative of all the people who are actually negative $\frac{TN}{(TN+FP)}$.
(iii) Positive predictive value: The proportion of the people whose predictions matches with the actual diagnosis as positives $\frac{TP}{(TP+FP)}$.
(iv) Negative predictive value: The proportion of the people whose predictions matches with the actual diagnosis as negatives $\frac{TN}{(TN+FN)}$.

A theoretical, optimal prediction can achieve 100 % sensitivity (i.e. predict all people from the sick group as sick) and 100 % specificity (i.e. not predict anyone from the healthy group as sick).

ROC is a plot between (1-specificity) on x-axis and sensitivity on y-axis. The AUC is a measure of overall performance of the algorithm. The accuracy of the decision tree algorithms can be evaluated using the AUC measure as given in Table 6.4.

The trade off between the sensitivity and specificity is better captured by an ROC curve, which shows how sensitivity and specificity of a model vary with some tuneable parameter, is related in a direct and natural way to cost/benefit analysis [74, 75] of diagnostic decision making. ROC curves allow one to distinguish among different models, depending on what model characteristics we need, and to determine which parameter values will give us the best performance for a given application.

By measuring the area under the ROC curve (AUC) [76, 77] one can obtain the accuracy of the test. The larger the area, the better the diagnostic test is. If the area is 1.0, we have an ideal test because test achieves 100 % sensitivity and 100 % specificity. If the area is 0.5, we have a test which has effectively 50 % sensitivity and 50 % specificity. In short the area measures the ability of the test to correctly classify those with and without the disease.

$$AUC = \int_0^1 ROC(t)dt \tag{6.5}$$

where t = 1-specificity (false positive rate) and ROC (t) is sensitivity (true positive rate). We can establish the classification given in Table 6.4 for the test.

Generally two approaches are employed for computing AUC. A non-parametric method based on constructing trapezoids under the curve as an approximation of area and a parametric method using a maximum likelihood estimator to fit a smooth curve to the data points. Huang et al. [78] demonstrated that AUC is a better evaluation measure than accuracy or error rate. A nonparametric method based on Mann-Whitney U

Table 6.4 AUC based classification for assessing accuracy of the test results

Range	Class
0.9 < AUC < 1.0	Excellent
0.8 < AUC < 0.9	Good
0.7 < AUC < 0.8	Worthless
0.6 < AUC < 0.7	Not good
0.5 < AUC < 0.6	Failed

statistic (actually the p statistic from the U statistic) has been applied for evaluating the classifiers [67].

The standard definitions of performance measures such as the specificity (SP), sensitivity (SE), receiver operator characteristics (ROC) and area under ROC (AUC) based on number of true positives, true negatives, false positives and false negatives as described in [8] are employed by Sree Hari Rao and Naresh Kumar [9] for comparing the performances of the machine classifiers utilized in identifying the risk factors of atherosclerosis.

Predictive Modeling

The predictive modeling strategy adopted by Sree Hari Rao and Naresh Kumar [9] in identifying the risk factors of atherosclerosis is presented in the following sections.

Data Representation

In general the medical datasets can be represented as a set S having row vectors $(R_1, R_2, \ldots, R_m)$ and column vectors $(C_1, C_2, \ldots, C_n)$. Each record can be represented as an ordered n-tuple of clinical and laboratory attributes $(A_{i1}, A_{i2}, \ldots, A_{i(n-1)}, A_{in})$ for each $i = 1, 2, \ldots, m$ where the last attribute (A_{in}) for each i, represents the physician's diagnosis to which the record $(A_{i1}, A_{i2}, \ldots, A_{i(n-1)})$ belongs and without loss of generality we assume that there are no missing elements in this set. Each attribute of an element in S that is A_{ij} for $i = 1, 2, \ldots, m$ and $j = 1, 2, \ldots, n-1$ can either be a categorical (nominal) or numeric (real or integer) type. Clearly all the sets considered are finite sets. These databases may have missing values which needs to be treated as discussed in section "Missing Values: Issues" before the extraction of knowledge in terms of diagnostic rules from them.

Imputation Method

The imputation algorithm proposed by Sree Hari Rao and Naresh Kumar [9] is now presented in this section. The following were the salient features of their algorithm:

- takes incomplete datasets as input and returns the completed datasets with all instances of missing attribute values filled with possible values;
- handles datasets with attributes of different types for example nominal or numeric;
- considers the higher order statistics of the data before computing the indexing measure;
- values to be imputed are obtained by using the data from within the dataset;
- a weighted average technique for Real attribute type was adopted to impute the missing values.

The first step in any imputation algorithm is to compute the proximity measure in the feature space among the clinical records to identify the nearest neighbors from where the values can be imputed. The most popular metric for quantifying the similarity between any two records is the Euclidean distance. Though this metric is simpler to compute, it is sensitive to the scales of the features involved. Further it does not account for correlation among the features. Also, the categorical variables can only be quantified by counting measures which calls for the development of effective strategies for computing the similarity [79]. Considering these factors we first propose a new indexing measure $I_{C_l}(R_i, R_k)$ between two typical elements R_i, R_k for $i, k = 1, 2, \ldots, m$, $l = 1, 2, \ldots, n-1$ belonging to the column C_l of S which can be applied on any type of data, be it categorical (nominal) and/or numeric (real). We consider the following cases:

Case I: $A_{in} = A_{kn}$

Let A denote the collection of all members of S that belong to the same decision class to which R_i and R_k belong. Based on the type of the attribute to which the column C_l belongs, the following situations arise:

(i) Members of the column C_l of S i.e $(A_{1l}, A_{2l}, \ldots, A_{ml})^T$ are of nominal or categorical or integer type: We now express A as a disjoint union of non-empty subsets of A, say $B_{\gamma_{p_{1l}}}, B_{\gamma_{p_{2l}}}, \ldots, B_{\gamma_{p_{sl}}}$ obtained in such a manner that every element of A belongs to one of these subsets and no element of A is a member of more than one subset of A. That is $A = B_{\gamma_{p_{1l}}} \bigcup B_{\gamma_{p_{2l}}} \bigcup, \ldots, \bigcup B_{\gamma_{p_{sl}}}$, in which $\gamma_{p_{1l}}, \gamma_{p_{2l}}, \ldots, \gamma_{p_{sl}}$ denote the cardinalities of the respective subsets $B_{\gamma_{p_{1l}}}, B_{\gamma_{p_{2l}}}, \ldots, B_{\gamma_{p_{sl}}}$ formed out of the set A, with the property that each member of the same subset has the same first co-ordinate and members of no two different subsets have the same first co-ordinate. We define an index $I_{C_l}(R_i, R_k)$ for each $l = 1, 2, \ldots, n-1$

$$I_{C_l}(R_i, R_k) = \begin{cases} \min\{\frac{\gamma_{p_{il}}}{\gamma}, \frac{\gamma_{q_{kl}}}{\gamma}\}, & \text{for } i \neq k; \\ 0, & \text{otherwise.} \end{cases}$$

where $\gamma_{p_{il}}$ represents the cardinality of the subset $B_{\gamma_{p_{il}}}$, all of whose elements have first co-ordinates A_{il}, $\gamma_{q_{kl}}$ represents the cardinality of that subset $B_{\gamma_{q_{kl}}}$, all of whose elements have first co-ordinates A_{kl} and $\gamma = \gamma_{p_{1l}} + \gamma_{p_{2l}} + \ldots, +\gamma_{p_{sl}}$ represents the cardinality of the set A.

(ii) Members of the column C_l of S i.e $(A_{1l}, A_{2l}, \ldots, A_{ml})^T$ are of real (fractional or non-integer numbers): We consider the set P_l for $l = 1, 2, \ldots, n-1$ which is a collection of all the members of the column C_l. We then compute the skewness measure $sk(P_l) = \frac{\frac{1}{m}\sum_{i=1}^{m}(A_{il}-\overline{A_{il}})^3}{(\sqrt{\frac{1}{m}\sum_{i=1}^{m}(A_{il}-\overline{A_{il}})^2})^3}$ where $\overline{A_{il}}$ denote the mean of A_{il} for each $l = 1, 2, \ldots, n-1$. Define the sets $M_l = \{a \in P_l | a \leq A_{il}$, for $sk(P_l) < 0\}$ or, $M_l = \{b \in P_l | b > A_{il}$, for $sk(P_l) \geq 0\}$ and similarly $N_l = \{a \in P_l | a \leq A_{kl}$, for $sk(P_l) < 0\}$ or, $N_l = \{b \in P_l | b > A_{kl}$, for $sk(P_l) \geq 0\}$. Let τ_l and ρ_l be the cardinalities of the sets M_l and N_l respectively. Construct the index $I_{C_l}(R_i, R_k)$,

$$I_{C_l}(R_i, R_k) = \begin{cases} \min\{\frac{\tau_l}{\gamma}, \frac{\rho_l}{\gamma}\}, & \text{for } i \neq k; \\ 0, & \text{otherwise.} \end{cases}$$

In the above definition γ represents the cardinality of the set P_l.

Case II: $A_{in} \neq A_{kn}$

Clearly R_i and R_k belong to two different decision classes. Consider the subsets P_i and Q_k consisting of members of S that share the same decision with R_i and R_k respectively. Clearly $P_i \bigcap Q_k = \emptyset$. Based on the type of the attribute of the members, the following situations arise:

(i) Members of the column C_l of S i.e $(A_{1l}, A_{2l}, \ldots, A_{ml})^T$ are of nominal or categorical type:
Following the procedure discussed in Case I item (i) we write P_l and Q_l for each $l = 1, 2, \ldots, n-1$ as a disjoint union of non-empty subsets of $P_{\beta_{1l}}, P_{\beta_{2l}}, \ldots, P_{\beta_{rl}}$ and $Q_{\delta_{1l}}, Q_{\delta_{2l}}, \ldots, Q_{\delta_{sl}}$ respectively in which $\beta_{1l}, \beta_{2l}, \ldots, \beta_{rl}$ and $\delta_{1l}, \delta_{2l}, \ldots, \delta_{sl}$ indicate the cardinality of the respective subsets. We define the indexing measure between the two records R_i and R_k as

$$I_{C_l}(R_i, R_k) = \begin{cases} \max\{\frac{\beta_{rl}}{\delta_{sl}+\beta_{rl}}, \frac{\delta_{sl}}{\delta_{sl}+\beta_{rl}}\}, & \text{for } i \neq k; \\ 0, & \text{otherwise.} \end{cases}$$

where β_{rl} represents the cardinality of the subset $P_{\beta_{rl}}$ all of whose elements have first co-ordinates A_{il} in set P_l and δ_{sl} represents the cardinality of that subset $Q_{\delta_{sl}}$, all of whose elements have first co-ordinates A_{kl} in set Q_l.

(ii) Members of the column C_l of S i.e $(A_{1l}, A_{2l}, \ldots, A_{ml})^T$ are of numeric type:
If the type of the attribute is an integer we follow the procedure discussed in Case II item (i). For fractional numbers we follow the procedure discussed in Case I item (ii) and we define the set P_l as the members of column C_l that belong to decision class A_{in} and Q_l as the members of column C_l that belong to decision class A_{kn}. We then compute the skew-

ness measure $sk(P_l) = \frac{\frac{1}{m}\sum_{i=1}^{m}(A_{il}-\overline{A_{il}})^3}{(\sqrt{\frac{1}{m}\sum_{i=1}^{m}(A_{il}-\overline{A_{il}})^2})^3}$ where $\overline{A_{il}}$ denote the mean of A_{il} for each $l = 1, 2, \ldots, n-1$ and $sk(Q_l) = \frac{\frac{1}{m}\sum_{i=1}^{m}(A_{kl}-\overline{A_{kl}})^3}{(\sqrt{\frac{1}{m}\sum_{i=1}^{m}(A_{kl}-\overline{A_{kl}})^2})^3}$ where $\overline{A_{kl}}$ denote the mean of A_{kl} for each $l = 1, 2, \ldots, n-1$. We then construct the sets T_l and S_l as follows: $T_l = \{a \in P_l | a \leq A_{il}, \text{for } sk(P_l) < 0\}$ or, $T_l = \{b \in P_l | b > A_{il}, \text{for } sk(P_l) \geq 0\}$ and similarly $S_l = \{a \in P_l | a \leq A_{kl}, \text{for } sk(P_l) < 0\}$ or, $S_l = \{b \in P_l | b > A_{kl}, \text{for } sk(P_l) \geq 0\}$. We now define the index $I_{C_l}(R_i, R_k)$ between the two records R_i, R_k as

$$I_{C_l}(R_i, R_k) = \begin{cases} \min\{\frac{\beta_l}{\lambda}, \frac{\delta_l}{\lambda}\}, & \text{for } i \neq k; \\ 0, & \text{otherwise.} \end{cases}$$

In the above definition β_l and δ_l represents the cardinalities of the sets T_l and S_l respectively. The sum of the cardinalities of the sets P_l and Q_l is represented by λ

The proximity or distance scores between the clinical records in the data set S can be represented as $D = \{\{0, d_{12}, \ldots, d_{1m}\}; \{d_{21}, 0, \ldots, d_{2m}\}; \ldots; \{d_{m1}, d_{m2}, \ldots, 0\}\}$ where $d_{ik} = \sqrt{\sum_{l=1}^{n-1} I_{C_l}^2(R_i, R_k)}$. For each of the missing value instances in a record R_i our imputation procedure first computes the score $\alpha(x_k) = \frac{(x_k - median(x))}{median|x_i - median(x)|}$ where $\{x_1, x_2, \ldots, x_n\}$ denote the distances of R from R_k. We then pick up only those records (nearest neighbors) which satisfy the condition $\alpha(x_k) \leq 0$ where $\{d_{i1}, d_{i2}, \ldots, d_{im}\}$ denote the distances of the current record R_i to all other records in the data set S. If the type of attribute is categorical or integer, then the data value that has the highest frequency (mode) of occurrence in the corresponding columns of the nearest records is imputed. For the data values of type real we first collect all non zero elements in the set D and denote this set by B. For each element in set B we compute the quantity $\beta(j) = \frac{1}{B(j)}$ $\forall j = 1, \ldots, \gamma$ where γ denote the cardinality of the set B. We compute the weight matrix as $W(j) = \frac{\beta_j}{\sum_{i=1}^{\gamma}\beta(i)}$ $\forall j = 1, \ldots, \gamma$. The value to be imputed may be taken as $\sum_{i=1}^{\gamma} P(i) * W(i)$.

A Methodology for Predicting the Risk factors of Atherosclerosis

The mean value imputation proposed in [8] can be employed only when the attribute values are normally distributed. In case of highly skewed attribute values the above method may result in biased estimates as mean value is not a true representative of a non-normal distribution. Motivated by the above issues in [9] a methodology comprising of a novel nonparametric missing value imputation method that can be applied on (i) data sets consisting of attributes that are of the type categorical (nominal) and/or numeric (integer or real), and (ii) attribute values that belong to highly skewed distri-

Algorithm 1 An Algorithm for Generating Decision Rules to Predict the Risk Factors of Atherosclerosis[9]

Require: (a) Data sets for the purpose of decision making $S(m, n)$ where m and n are number of records and attributes respectively and the members of S may have MV in any of the attributes except in the decision attribute, which is the last attribute in the record.
(b) The type of attribute C of the columns in the data set.
Ensure: (a) Classification accuracy for a given data set S.
(b) Performance metrics AUC, SE, SP.
Algorithm

(1) Identify and collect all records in a data set S
(2) Impute the MV in the data set S using the procedure discussed in section "Imputation Method".
(3) Extract the influential features using a wrapper based approach with particle swarm optimization search for identifying feature subsets and ADT for its evaluation.
(4) Split the dataset in to training and testing sets using a stratified a k fold cross validation procedure. Denote each training and testing data set by T_k and R_k respectively.
(5) For each k compute the following
    (i) Build the ADT using the records obtained from T_k.
    (ii) Compute the predicted probabilities (scores) for both positive and negative diagnosis of CHD from the ADT built in Step (5)-(i) using the test data set R_k. Designate the set consisting of all these scores by P.
    (iii) Identify and collect the actual diagnosis from the test data set R_k in to set denoted by L.
(6) Repeat the Steps (5)-(i) to Step (5)-(iii) for each fold.
(7) Obtain the performance metrics AUC, SE and SP utilizing the sets L and P.
(8) RETURN AUC, SE, SP.
(9) END.

bution. The methodology proposed in [63] ignores missing values while generating the decision tree, which renders lower prediction accuracies. We have embedded our present imputation strategy (section "Imputation Method") into an alternating decision tree (ADT) which has been found to improve the performance of the classifier on datasets having missing values. Also, the authors in [9] develop an effective wrapper based feature selection algorithm utilizing particle swarm optimization (PSO) search to identify the most influential feature subset. This methodology comprises in utilizing the new imputation embedded ADT and the wrapper based features subset selection algorithm and can predict the diagnosis of CHD in real time. In fact the decision rules obtained by employing their novel methodology will be useful to diagnose other individuals based on the risk factors of the individuals.

Experiments and Results

In [9] a stratified ten-fold cross validation ($k = 10$) methodology was adopted wherein the dataset is split into subsets consisting of training and testing datasets such that the samples in the training datasets do not appear in the testing dataset. A standard implementation SVM with radial basis function kernel using LibSVM package [80] is employed for comparison. The following standard parameter values for PSO (i) number of particles $Z = 50$, (ii) number of iterations $G = 100$, (iii) cognitive factor $c_1 = 2$, and (iv) social factor $c_2 = 2$ are considered for simulation. The standard implementation of C4.5, Naive Bayes (NB), Multi Layer Perceptron (MLP) algorithms in Weka© [61] are considered for evaluating the performance of our algorithm. An implementation of correlation based feature selection (CFS) [81] algorithm with genetic search has been considered for comparing with our methodology. The authors in [9] have implemented the Algorithm 1 and the performance evaluation methods in Matlab©. A non-parametric statistical test proposed by Wilcoxon [82] is used to compare the performance of the algorithms. The Algorithm 1 is compared with the state-of-the-art methodologies employed in the prediction of risk factors for atherosclerosis using different performance measures discussed in section "Performance Metrics and Evaluation Methods".

Dataset

The authors in [9] have utilized STULONG dataset [83] which is a longitudinal primary preventive study of middle-aged men lasting twenty years for assessing the risk of atherosclerosis and cardiovascular health depending on the personal and family history of individuals collected at IKEM and the Medicine Faculty at Charles University. The STULONG dataset is divided into four sub-groups namely Entry, Letter, Control and Death. The Entry dataset consists of 1417 patient records with 64 attributes having either codes or results of size measurements of different variables or results of transformations of the rest of the attributes during the first level examination. The Entry, Control and Death datasets are utilized for predictive modeling. The Entry level dataset is divided into three groups (a) normal group (NG), (b) pathological group (PG), (c) risk group (RG), and (d) not alloted (NA) group, based on KONSKUP attribute value in (1, 2), (5), (3, 4), (6) respectively. We form a new dataset by joining Entry, control and Death datasets as follows: (i) we write the identification number of a patient (ICO) based on the selection criteria suggested in [84] and determine the susceptibility of a patient to atherosclerosis based on the attributes recorded in Control and Death tables. An individual is considered not having a cardiovascular disease if he or she had other disease(s) in his or her history (i.e., he or she has at least one positive value on attributes angina pectoris found in (HODN1), diabetes mellitus found in (HODN4), finding of an ischaemic heart disease without stating (HODN11), finding of claudications (HODN12), finding of a tumour disease (HODN15), coronary artery by pass graft/percoutaneus transluminal coronary angioplasty carried out (HODN21), and operation/plastic of lower limbs arteries (HODN23) in the Control group) or the patient died by other disease(s) (i.e., the record appears in the Death group with cause of death (PRICUMR) attribute equal to 08 (other causes), 09 (sudden death), 10 (cause of the death unknown), or 16 (tumorous disease)), (ii) also, an individual is considered to have cardiovascular disease if he or she has heart disease in the history (i.e., he or she has at least one positive value on attributes such as finding of myocardial infarction (HODN2), cerebrovascular accident found (HODN3), finding of silent myocardial ischaemia (HODN13), finding of silent myocardial infarction (HODN14)), or died by heart disease (i.e., the record appears in the Death table with PRICUMR attribute equal to

05 (myocardial infarction), 06 (coronary heart disease), 07 (stroke), or 17 (general atherosclerosis)), (iii) otherwise, the individuals are considered healthy and have no cardiovascular disease. We introduce a new decision attribute in the Entry dataset based on the Step (ii) and Step (iii) having values positive and negative based accordingly as the presence or absence of cardiovascular. Now we divide the Entry dataset in to four datasets DS1, DS2, DS3 and DS4 based on whether the patients are in NG, RG, PG, NA respectively.

The authors in [14] observed that some attributes have a large number of missing values or highly skewed value distributions and removed these attributes from their considerations. In our approach we deleted only those attributes that do not have values for any of the records in the dataset. In dataset DS1 we removed 12 attributes namely drinking of 7 beer (PIVO7), medicines in myocardial infarction (IML), diet in hyper tension (HTD), medicines in hyper tension (HTL), medicines in ictus found (ICTL), diet in diabetes found (DIABD), medicines in diabetes found (DIABL), before how many year myocardial infarction has appeared (IMTRV), before how many years hyper tension has appeared (HTTRV), before how many years ictus has appeared (ICTTRV), before how many years diabetes has appeared (DIABTRV), and before how many years hyperlipidemia has appeared (HYPLTRV). In DS2 two attributes IML and ICTL are deleted. In DS3 two attributes PIV07, ICTL are dropped. In DS4 11 attributes PIV07, IML, ICTL, DIABD, DIABL, therapy by a diet for hyperlypoproteinemia (HYPLD), therapy by medicines for hyperlypoproteinemia (HYDLL), IMTRV, ICTTRV, DIABTRV, HYPLTRV are ignored. The datasets DS1, DS2, DS3 and DS4 now contain 49, 51, 57, 48 attributes and the number of patient records being 51, 366, 53, and 53 records respectively.

Results

The performance of the Algorithm 1 is compared with other methodologies (C4.5, SVM, MLP and NB) on the data sets used in the present study and the classification accuracies are presented in Table 6.5. A hundred percent accuracy is reported by Algorithm 1 in dataset DS4 and higher percentage in other datasets.

The imputation strategy and the PSO search employed in [9] has improved the classification accuracies over correlation based feature selection (CFS) and mean value imputation strategy with C4.5, SVM, MLP and NB classifiers.

The feature subsets identified by the Algorithm 1 are shown in Table 6.6.

In risk group dataset DS2 the Algorithm 1 could identify the patients with an accuracy of 99.73 % who are affected by atherosclerosis using only 13 out of 51 attributes. The wrapper based feature selection using PSO and ADT could identify the influential factors such as alcohol (ALKOHOL), daily consumption of tea (CAJ), hypertension or ictus (ICT), hyperlypoproteinemia (HYPLIP), since how long hyper tension (HT) has appeared (HTTRV), before how many years hyperlipidemia has appeared (HYPLTRV), blood pressure II systolic (DIAST2), cholesterol in mg % (CHLST), sugar in urine (MOC), obesity (OBEZRISK), hypertension (HTRISK)

Table 6.5 Performance comparison of the Imputation Method with other methodologies (C4.5, SVM, NB, MLP) on the data sets used in the present study

Dataset	Method	Accuracy (%)	SE	SP	AUC
DS1	**Algorithm 1**	**98.04**	**93.75**	**100.00**	**0.94**
	C4.5	70.59	6.25	100.00	1.00
	NB	52.94	56.25	51.43	0.53
	SVM	35.29	100.00	5.71	0.53
	MLP	66.67	0.00	97.14	0.97
DS2	**Algorithm 1**	**99.73**	**99.35**	**100.00**	**1.00**
	C4.5	50.00	55.48	45.97	0.52
	NB	61.20	48.39	70.62	0.58
	SVM	45.63	92.26	11.37	0.56
	MLP	57.92	0.65	100.00	1.00
DS3	**Algorithm 1**	**90.57**	**85.19**	**96.15**	**0.86**
	C4.5	49.06	3.70	96.15	0.98
	NB	58.49	55.56	61.54	0.53
	SVM	52.83	55.56	50.00	0.53
	MLP	47.17	0.00	96.15	0.98
DS4	**Algorithm 1**	**100.00**	**100.00**	**100.00**	**1.00**
	C4.5	66.04	31.58	85.29	0.46
	NB	62.26	63.16	61.76	0.69
	SVM	49.06	94.74	23.53	0.62
	MLP	69.81	63.16	73.53	0.61

which are in conformity with other studies related to cardiovascular diseases [85–87]. We have identified a new fact that even in normal group DS1 individuals who mostly confine to sitting positions without any physical activity (AKTPOZAM=1) may lead to atherosclerosis [88].

The ADT generated for the risk group (DS2) is shown in Fig. 6.7.

The following decision rules are extracted from the decision tree shown in Fig. 6.7:

1. A high predictive value of -2.098 for positive diagnosis of atherosclerosis is observed if hyperlipidemia has appeared 1.5 years back;
2. If hypertension has appeared recently (<3.5 years) has a predictive value of -1.348 for positive diagnosis of the disease;
3. If a patient has hyperlipidemia has appeared 1.5 years back and below 4 years ($HYPLTRV \geq 1.5$ and <4.0), hypertension has appeared within 3.5 years, cholesterol levels are below 166, sugar in urine is present and hyperlypoproteinemia is present then the predictive probability is $-2.098 - 1.348 - 2.849 - 0.966 - 0.43 - 0.249 = -7.94$ which indicates a positive diagnosis for atherosclerosis.

The ROC curves comparing the performance of the algorithm discussed in section "Performance Metrics and Evaluation Methods", with other methodologies are shown in Fig. 6.8. The operating point or cut off point ($p < 0.001$) is shown as

Table 6.6 Influential features subsets identified by Algorithm 1

Data set	# Orignal features	# Influential features	Accuracy (%)	Features identified
DS1	47	11	98.04	ZODPOV, AKTPOZAM, ALKOHOL, PIVO10, PIVO12, PIVOMN, ICT, HYPLL, DIAST1, RARISK, HTRISK
DS2	51	13	99.73	STAV, VZDELANI, ALKOHOL, CAJ, ICT, HYPLIP, HTTRV, HYPLTRV, DIAST2, CHLST, MOC, OBEZRISK, HTRISK
DS3	57	3	90.57	ICT, HYPLTRV, CHOLRISK
DS4	48	3	100.00	HTTRV, BOLHR, SYST1

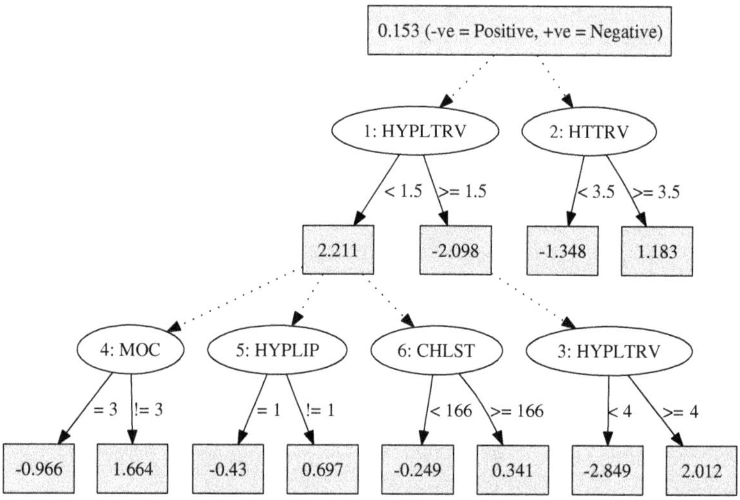

Fig. 6.7 Alternating decision tree generated for dataset DS2 [9]

a pentagon on each of the ROC curves. The ROC curves clearly demonstrate the superior performance of Algorithm 1 over other methods used in the diagnosis of atherosclerosis.

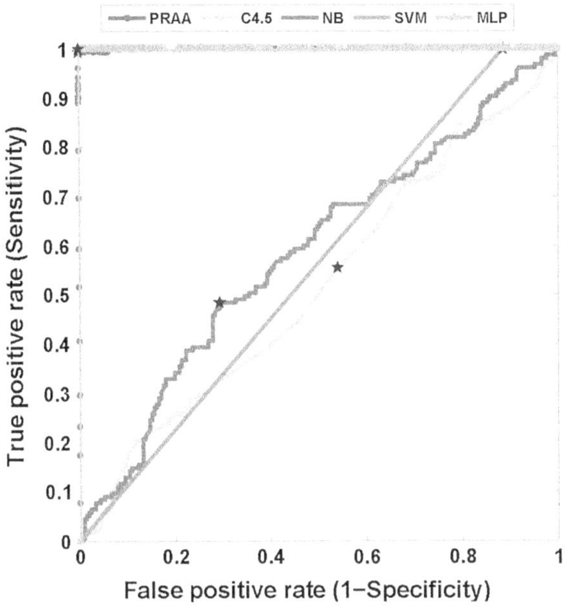

Fig. 6.8 ROC curve DS2 [9]

Table 6.7 Wilcoxon sign rank statistics for matched pairs comparing the new imputation algorithm with other imputation methods using C4.5 decision tree

Method	Rank sums (+, −)	Test statistics	Critical series	Series p-value
FKMI	28.0, 0.0	0.0	3	0.02
KMI	28.0, 0.0	0.0	3	0.02
KNNI	15.0, 0.0	0.0	0	0.06
WKNNI	21.0, 0.0	1.0	18	0.03

Performance Comparison of the Imputation Algorithm on Benchmark Datasets

Since no specific studies on imputation of missing values in cardiovascular disease data sets are not available in the literature the authors in [9] utilized some bench mark data sets obtained from Keel and University of California Irvin (UCI) machine learning data repositories [89, 90] to test the performance of the new imputation algorithm. The Wilcoxon statistics in Table 6.7 is computed based on the accuracies obtained by the new imputation algorithm with the accuracies of those obtained by other imputation algorithms using a C4.5 decision tree. The results in Table 6.7 clearly demonstrate that our algorithm is superior to other imputation algorithms as the positive rank sums are higher than the negative rank sums ($p < 0.05$) in all cases.

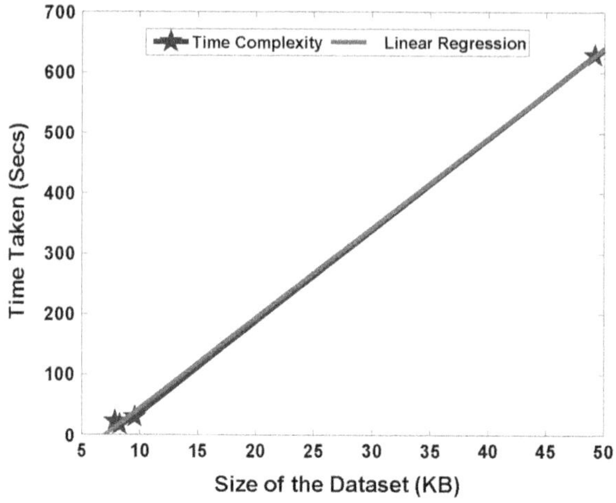

Fig. 6.9 Computational complexity of the Algorithm 1 [9]

Computational Complexity and Scalability

The computational complexity is a measure of the performance of the algorithm which can be measured in terms of the number of CPU clock cycles elapsed in seconds for performing the methodology on a dataset. For each data set having n attributes and m records, the authors in [9] selected only those subset of records $m_1 \leq m$, in which missing values are present. The distances are computed for all attributes n excluding the decision attribute. So, the time complexity for computing the distance would be $O(m_1 * (n - 1))$. The time complexity for computing skewness is $O(m_1)$. The time complexity for selecting the nearest records is of order $O(m_1)$. For computing the frequency of occurrences for nominal attributes and weighted average for numeric attributes the time taken would be of the order $O(m_1)$. Therefore, for a given data set with k-fold cross validation having n attributes and m records, the time complexity of our new imputation algorithm would be $k * (O(m_1 * (n-1) * m) + 3 * O(m_1))$ which is asymptotically linear. Our experiments were conducted on a personal computer having a Intel(R) core (TM) 2 Duo, CPU @2.93 GHZ processor with 4 GB RAM and the time taken by Algorithm 1 for varying database sizes is shown Fig. 6.9. A linear regression was employed on the above results to obtained a relation between the time taken (T) and the data size (D) as $T = 14.909D - 104.655, \alpha = 0.05, p = 0.0003, r^2 = 0.994$. The presence of the linear trend (red line in Fig. 6.9) between the time taken and the varying database sizes ensures the numerical scalability of the performance of Algorithm 1 in terms of asymptotic linearity.

Table 6.8 Evaluation of Algorithm 1 with other related methodologies on atherosclerosis [9]

State-of-the-art	Records with missing values	Method	Accuracy (%)	SE (%)	SP (%)
Tsang-Hsiang et al. [14]	Deleted	CFS (Best first), C4.5	67.26	35.3	84.8
Tsang-Hsiang et al. [14]	Deleted	CFS (Genetic), C4.5	65.81	39.4	82.8
Tsang-Hsiang et al. [14]	Deleted	CFS (Exhaustive), C4.5	64.85	32.10	84.8
Hongzong et al. [12]	-	SVM	90.57	95	90
Kukar et al. [3]	-	NB	80	92	53
Kukar et al. [3]	-	MLP	80	82	76
Algorithm 1 on DS2	New imputation	PSO, ADT	99.73	99.35	100.0

Performance Comparison of Softcomputing Methodologies

The authors in [9] compared their results (Table 6.8) with those obtained in [3, 12, 14] on the risk group dataset DS2. As compared to [14] where in CFS with genetic search and C4.5 is employed a SE of 39.4 % and SP of 82.8 % is observed. In [12] SVM was used to classify the patients with a SE of 95 % and SP of 90 %. In [3] both NB and MLP were used for classification with an accuracy of 80 % and the could obtain SE of 92 and 82 %, SP of 53 and 76 % respectively. In comparison the new methodology when applied on the dataset DS2 resulted in an accuracy of 99.73%, SE of 99.35 % and SP of 100 % which is regarded as to be a good classification model since both SE and SP are higher than 80%. In case of DS4 the new methodology has resulted in an accuracy of 100 %, SE of 100 % and SP of 100 %.

From these comparisons it is concluded that the Algorithm 1 methodology is better than the methods in [3, 12, 14] in terms of the performance measures.

Conclusions and Discussion

In the present chapter biology, pathogenesis and pathophysiology of the atherosclerosis disease is discussed. The diagnostic procedures including the advanced imaging methods such as computed tomography, MRI, SPECT and PET have been presented in the chapter. Soft computing methods, performance metrics and their evaluation methods for predictive modeling are discussed. An algorithm with built in features for imputation of missing values that can be applied on datasets wherein the attribute values are either normal and/or highly skewed having either categorical and/or numeric attributes and identification of risk factors using wrapper based feature selection is discussed. The Algorithm 1 has outperformed over the state-of-the-art methodologies in determining the risk factors associated with the onset of atherosclerosis disease. The Algorithm 1 has generated a decision tree with an accuracy of 99.7 % for dataset DS2. Based on the performance measures we conclude that the use of the new imputation strategy and feature selection methods with wrapper based subset evaluation including particle swarm optimization search have improved the accuracies of the predictions. We hold the view that more intensive and introspective studies of this kind will pave way for effective risk prediction and diagnosis of atherosclerosis. Further, we are of the view that developing soft computing techniques for identification of biomarkers using imaging sensors would be of much help in early detection and quantification of the atherosclerosis disease.

Acknowledgments This research is supported by the Foundation for Scientific Research and Technological Innovation (FSRTI)—A Constituent Division of Sri Vadrevu Seshagiri Rao Memorial Charitable Trust, Hyderabad-500035, India.

References

1. Lloyd-Jones, Donald, Adams, and R. J. et al., "Heart disease and stroke statistics2010 update," Circulation, Vol. 121, No. 7, 2010, pp. e46–e215. [Online]. Available: http://circ.ahajournals.org/content/121/7/e46.short
2. CDC, "Heart disease and stroke: The nation's leading killers," National Center for Chronic Disease Prevention and Health Promotion, Tech. Rep., 2011.
3. M. Kukar, I. Kononenko, and C. Groselj, "Analysing and improving the diagnosis of ischaemic heart disease with machining learning," Artificial Intelligence in Medicine, Vol. 16, No. 1, 1999, pp. 25–50.
4. N. Lucas, J. Azé, M. Sebag, "Atherosclerosis risk identification and visual analysis," Proceedings of the Discovery Challenge PKDD (PKDD2002), 2003. http://lisp.vse.cz/challenge/ecmlpkdd2002/proceedings/Lucas.pdf. Cited 28 Mar 2013
5. B. Natasha, G. Melanie, N. Mads et al, "Abdominal aortic calcification quantified by the morphological atherosclerotic calcification distribution (macd) index is associated with features of the metabolic syndrome," BMC Cardiovascular Disorders, Vol. 11, No. 75, 2011, pp. 1–9.
6. J. R. Davies, J. H. Rudd, and P. L. Weissberg, "Molecular and metabolic imaging of atherosclerosis," Journal of Nuclear Medicine, Vol. 45, No. 11, 2004, 1898–1907.
7. J.-C. Tardif, F. Lesage, F. Harel, et al., "Imaging biomarkers in atherosclerosis trials," Circulation. Cardiovascular Imaging. Vol. 4, No. 3, 2011, pp. 319–333.
8. V. Sree Hari Rao and M. Naresh Kumar, "A new intelligence based approach for computer-aided diagnosis of dengue fever," IEEE Transactions on Information Technology in, BioMedicine, Vol. 16, No. 1, 2011, pp. 112–118.
9. V. Sree Hari Rao and M. Naresh Kumar, "Novel approaches for predictive modeling and machine diagnosis of atherosclerosis," IEEE Journal of Biomedical and Health Informatics, Vol. 17, No. 1, 2012, pp. 183–189.
10. J. Azé, N. Lucas, M. Sebag, "A new medical test for atherosclerosis detection Geno," Proceedings of Discovery Challenge PKDD (2003), 2003. http://lisp.vse.cz/challenge/ecmlpkdd2003/proceedings/Aze.pdf. Cited 28 Mar 2013
11. O. Couturier, H. Delalin, H. Fu, et al., "A three-step approach for stulong database analysis: Characterization of patients groups," Proceedings of the 9th European Conference on, Machine Learning (2004), 2004.

12. S. Hongzong, W. Tao, Y. Xiaojun, et al., "Support vector machines classification for discriminating coronary heart disease patients from non-coronary heart disease," West Indian Medical Journal, Vol. 56, No. 5, 2007, 451–457.
13. S. Jose Ignacio, T. Marie, and Z. Jana, "Machine learning methods for knowledge discovery in medical data on atherosclerosis," European Journal for Biomedical Informatics, Vol. 2, No. 1, 2006, 6–33.
14. C. Tsang-Hsiang, W. Chih-Ping, and S. T. Vincent, "Feature selection for medical data mining: Comparisons of expert judgment and automatic approaches," Proceedings of the 19th IEEE Symposium on Computer-Based Medical Systems (CBMS'06) (2006), 2006.
15. S. Mougiakakou, S. Golemati, I. Gousias et al., "Computer-aided diagnosis of carotid atherosclerosis based on ultrasound image statistics, laws' texture and neural networks," Ultrasound Med. Biol., Vol. 33, No. 1, 2007, 26–36.
16. C. Christodoulou, C. Pattichis, M. Pantziaris, and A. Nicolaides, "Texture-based classification of atherosclerotic carotid plaques," IEEE Trans Med Imaging, Vol. 22, No. 7, 2003, 902–912.
17. L. Chambless, "Coronary heart disease risk prediction in the atherosclerosis risk in communities (aric) study," Journal of Clinical Epidemiology, Vol. 56, No. 9, 2003, pp. 880–890.
18. E. Selvin, J. Coresh, S. H. Golden, et al., "Glycemic control, atherosclerosis, and risk factors for cardiovascular disease in individuals with diabetes," Diabetes Care, Vol. 28, No. 8, 2005, pp. 1965–1973.
19. H. Liu, E. R. Dougherty, J. G. Dy, K. Torkkola, E. Tuv, H. Peng, C. Ding, F. Long, M. Berens, L. Parsons, Z. Zhao, L. Yu, and G. Forman, "Evolving feature selection," IEEE Intelligent Systems, Vol. 20, 2005, pp. 64–76.
20. John R. Davies, James H. Rudd, and Peter L. Weissberg, "Molecular and Metabolic Imaging of Atherosclerosis," J Nucl Med., Vol. 45, 2004, pp. 1898–1907.
21. Elmo Mannarino and Matteo Pirro Clin, "Molecular biology of atherosclerosis," Cases Miner Bone Metab., Vol. 5, No. 1, 2008, pp. 57–62.
22. Borja Ibez, Antonio Pinero, Miguel Orejas, and Juan J. Badimna, "Novel Imaging Techniques for Quantifying Overall Atherosclerotic Burden," Rev Esp Cardiol, Vol. 60, No. 3, 2007, pp. 299–309.
23. J. Breslow, "Cardiovascular disease myths and facts," Cleveland Clinic Journal of Medicine, Vol. 65, No. 6, 1998, pp. 286–287.
24. Ary L. Goldberger, "ELECTROCARDIOGRAPHY," Harrison's Cardiovascular Medicine, Mc Graw Hill, 2010.
25. J. Crouse, "Imaging atherosclerosis: state of the art," Journal of Lipid Research, Vol. 47, 2006, 1677–1699.
26. R. Corti and V. Fuster, "Imaging of atherosclerosis: magnetic resonance imaging," European Heart Journal, 2011. doi:10.1093/eurheartj/ehr068
27. B. Ibaez, J. J. Badimon, and M. J. Garcia, "Diagnosis of atherosclerosis by imaging," The American Journal of Medicine, Vol. 122, No. 1, 2009, S15–S25.
28. H.-D. Liang, J. A. Noble, and P. N. T. Wells, "Recent advances in biomedical ultrasonic imaging techniques," Interface Focus, Vol. 1, No. 4, 2011, 475–476.
29. H. M. Garcia-Garcia, M. A. Costa, and P. W. Serruys, "Imaging of coronary atherosclerosis: intravascular ultrasound," European Heart Journal. Vol. 31, No. 20, 2010, 2456–2469.
30. Y. Ueda, A. Hirayama, and K. Kodama, "Plaque characterization and atherosclerosis evaluation by coronary angioscopy," Herz, Vol. 28, No. 6, 2003, 501–504.
31. J. Belardi, M. Albertal, F. Cura, et al., "Intravascular thermographic assessment in human coronary atherosclerotic plaques by a novel flow-occluding sensing catheter: a safety and feasibility study," J. Invasive Cardiol., Vol. 17, No. 12, 2005, pp. 663–666.
32. C. Magnussen, R. Thomson, M. Juonala, et al., "Use of b-mode ultrasound to examine preclinical markers of atherosclerosis: image quality may bias associations between adiposity and measures of vascular structure and function," J. Ultrasound Med, Vol. 30, No. 3, 2011, 363–369.
33. M. Wintermark, S. Jawadi, J. Rapp, et al., "High-resolution ct imaging of carotid artery atherosclerotic plaque," American Journal of Neuroradiology, Vol. 29, No. 5, 2008, 875–882.

34. E. Laufer, H. Winkens, M. Corsten, et al, "Pet and spect imaging of apoptosis in vulnerable atherosclerotic plaques with radiolabeled annexin a5," Q J Nucl Med Mol Imaging, Vol. 53, No. 1, 2009, 26–34.
35. R. P. Choudhury and E. A. Fisher, "Molecular imaging in atherosclerosis, thrombosis, and vascular inflammation," Arteriosclerosis, Thrombosis, and Vascular Biology, Vol. 29, No. 7, 2009, 983–991.
36. Triantafillos G Giannakopoulos, Efthimios D Avgerinos, Konstantinos G Moulakakis, Nikolaos P Kadoglou, Ourania Preza, Anastasios Papapetrou, Christos Papasideris, Christos D LiapisDisclosures, "Biomarkers For Diagnosis of the Vulnerable Atherosclerotic Plaque" Interv Cardiol., Vol. 3, No. 2, 2011, pp. 223–233.
37. Pearson R, "Mining Imperfect Data: Dealing with Contamination and Incomplete Records," SIAM, Philadelphia, 2005.
38. Cios KJ, Mooree W, "Uniqueness of medical data mining," Artificial Intelligence in Medicine, Vol. 26, 2002, pp. 1–24.
39. Kim JO, Curry J, "The treatment of missing data in multivariate analysis" Sociological Methods & Research, Vol. 6, No. 2, 1977, pp. 215–240.
40. Little R and Rubin D, "Statistical analysis with missing data," Wiley, New York, 1987.
41. Dixon J, "Pattern recognition with partly missing data," IEEE Transactions on Systems, Man, and Cybernetics, Vol. 9, No. 10, 1979, pp. 617–621.
42. Schafer J, "Analysis of Incomplete Multivariate Data," Chapman & Hall, 1997.
43. Horton N and Lipsitz S, "Multiple imputation in practise:comparison of software packages for regression models with missing variables," The American Statistician, Vol. 55, No. 3, 2001, pp. 244–254.
44. Heijden G, Donders A, Stijnen T, Moons K, "Imputation of missing values is superior to complete case analysis and the missing-indicator method in multivariable diagnostic research: a clinical example," Journal of Clinical Epidemiology, Vol. 59, No. 10, 2006, pp. 1102–1109.
45. Allison P, "Missing data Thousand Oaks," Sage publications, 2002.
46. Roderick JL and Donald BR, "Statistical Analysis with Missing Data," 2nd Edition, Wiley, 2002.
47. Mussa A, Tshilidzi M, "The use of genetic algorithms and neural networks to approximate missing data in database," Computing and Informatics, Vol. 24, 2006, pp. 1001–1013.
48. Qiao W, Gao Z, Harley R, "Continuous online identification of nonlinear plants in power systems with missing sensor measurements," Proceedings of IEEE International Joint Conference on Neural Networks, Montreal, 2005, pp. 1729–1734.
49. M. R. Šikonja and I. Kononenko, "Theoretical and empirical analysis of relieff and rrelieff." Machine Learning, Vol. 53, 2003, pp. 23–69.
50. J. Weston, A. Elisseeff, B. Schölkopf, and M. Tipping, "Use of the zero norm with linear models and kernel methods," J. Mach. Learn. Res., Vol. 3, 2003, pp. 1439–1461.
51. G. D. Jennifer, "Feature selection for unsupervised learning," Journal of, Machine Learning, Vol. 5, 20004, pp. 845–889.
52. Z. Zhao and H. Liu, "Semi-supervised feature selection via spectral analysis," Proceedings of the 7th SIAM International Conference on Data Mining, 2007.
53. I. n. Inza, P. Larrañaga, R. Blanco, and A. J. Cerrolaza, "Filter versus wrapper gene selection approaches in dna microarray domains," Artificial intelligence in medicine, Vol. 31, No. 2, 2004, pp. 91–103.
54. J. R. Quinlan, "C4.5: programs for machine learning," San Francisco, CA, USA: Morgan Kaufmann Publishers Inc., 1993.
55. B. Efron, T. Hastie, I. Johnstone, and R. Tibshirani, "Least angle regression," Annals of Statistics, Vol. 32, No. 2, 2004, pp. 407–499.
56. R. Kohavi and G. H. John, "The wrapper approach," Feature Extraction, Construction and Selection: a data mining perspective, Kluwer, 1998, pp. 33–49.
57. K. Ron and H. J. George, "Wrappers for feature subset selection," Artificial Intelligence, Vol. 97, 1997, pp. 273–324.

58. Mark A Hall, Lloyd A Smith, "Feature Selection for Machine Learning: Comparing a Correlation based Filter Approach to the Wrapper," American Association for, Artificial Intelligence, 1998.
59. Fayyad, U and Irani, K, "Multi interval Discretisation of Continuous valued Attributes for Classification learning," Proceedings of the Thirteenth International Joint Conference on Artificial Intelligence, Morgan Kaufmann, 1993.
60. Goldberg DE, "Genetic algorithms in search, optimization and machine learning," Addison-Wesley, 1989.
61. I. Witten and E. Frank, "Data Mining: Practical machine learning tools and techniques," Morgan Kaufmann, San Francisco., 2005.
62. J. Kennedy and R. Eberhart, "Swarm Intelligence," Morgan Kaufmann, San Francisco, 2001.
63. Y. Freund and L. Mason, "The alternating decision tree learning algorithm," Proceeding of the Sixteenth International Conference on Machine Learning Bled, Slovenia, ACM, 1999.
64. Wong SL, Zhang LV, Tong AHY, Li Z, Goldberg DS, King OD, Lesage G, Vidal M, Andrews B, Bussey H, Boone C, Roth FP, "Combining biological networks to predict genetic interactions," Proceedings of the National Academy of Sciences of the United States of America, Vol. 101, No. 44, 2004, pp. 682–687.
65. Middendorf, "Predicting genetic regulatory response using classification," Bioinformatics, Vol. 20, 2004, pp. 232–240.
66. L. Tanner, M. Schreiber, J. Low, A. Ong, and T. Tolfvenstam, "Decision tree algorithms predict the diagnosis and outcome of dengue fever in the early phase of illness," PLoS Negl Trop Dis, Vol. 2, No. 3, 2008.
67. V. Sree Hari Rao and M. Naresh Kumar, "Predictive Dynamics: Modeling for Virological Surveillance and Clinical Management of Dengue", Dynamic Models of Infectious Diseases, V. Sree Hari Rao and Ravi Durvasula Eds., Vol. I, ISBN: 978-1-4614-3960-8, Springer Verlag, New York, 2013.
68. V. N. Vapnik, "The nature of statistical learning theory," Springer-Verlag, New York, 1995.
69. N. Cristianini and J. Shawe-Taylor, "An Introduction to Support Vector Machines and Other Kernel-based Learning Methods," Cambridge University Press, First edition, 2000.
70. B. Cestnik, I. Kononenko, I. Bratko, "A knowledge elicitation tool for sophisticated users," Proceedings of the Second European Working Session on, Learning, 1987, pp. 31–45.
71. Kothari R, Dong M, "Decision trees for classification: A review and some new results," World Scientific, 2000.
72. Metz C, "Basic principles of roc analysis," Sem Nuc Med, Vol. 8, 1978, pp. 283–298.
73. Crichton N, "Receiver operating characteristic (roc) curves," Journal of Clinical Nursing, Vol. 11, 2002, pp. 134–136.
74. Zweig M, Campbell G, "Receiver-operating characteristic (roc) plots: a fundamental evaluation tool in clinical medicine," Clinical chemistry, Vol. 9, No. 8, 1993, pp. 561–577.
75. Pepe MS, "The Statistical Evaluation of Medical Tests for Classification and Prediction," Oxford University Press, 2003.
76. Liu H, Wu T, "Estimating the area under a receiver operating characteristic curve for repeated measures design," Journal of Statistical Software, Vol. 8, 2003, pp. 1–18.
77. Hanley JA, McNeil BJ, "The meaning and use of the area under a receiver operating characteristic (roc) curve," Radiology, Vol. 143, 1982, pp. 29–36.
78. Huang J, Ling C, "Using auc and accuracy in evaluating learning algorithms," IEEE Trans Knowledge and Data, Engineering, 17(3), 2005, pp. 299–310.
79. U. Tadashi, M. Yoshihide, K. Daichi, et al., "Fast multidimensional nearest neighbor search algorithm based on ellipsoid distance," International Journal of Advanced, Intelligence, Vol. 1, No. 1, 2009, pp. 89–107.
80. C.-C. Chang and C.-J. Lin, "LIBSVM: A library for support vector machines," ACM Transactions on Intelligent Systems and Technology, Vol. 2, No. 3, 2001, pp. 1–27.
81. H. Liu and R. Setiono, "A probabilistic approach to feature selection - a filter solution," Proceedings of 13th International Conference on, Machine Learning, 1996.

82. F. Wilcoxon, “Individual comparisons by ranking methods,” Biometrics Bulletin, Vol. 1, No. 6, 1945, pp. 80–83.
83. Project STULONG, “Stulong study,”, 2004. [Online]. Available: http://euromise.vse.cz/stulong
84. N. S. Hoa and N. H. Son, “Analysis of stulong data by rough set exploration system (rses),” Proceedings of the 8th European Conference on, Machine Learning, 2003.
85. H. C. McGill, C. A. McMahan, E. E. Herderick, et al., “Obesity accelerates the progression of coronary atherosclerosis in young men,” Circulation, Vol. 105, No. 23, 2002, pp. 2712–2718.
86. M. Drechsler, R. T. Megens, M. van Zandvoort, et al., “Hyperlipidemia-triggered neutrophilia promotes early atherosclerosis/clinical perspective,” Circulation, Vol. 122, No. 18, 2010, pp. 1837–1845.
87. E. V. Lydia, O. Anath, U. Cuno, et al., “Adolescent blood pressure and blood pressure tracking into young adulthood are related to subclinical atherosclerosis: the atherosclerosis risk in young adults (arya) study,” Am J Hypertens, Vol. 16, No. 7, 2003, pp. 549–555.
88. P. D. Thompson, D. Buchner, I. L. Pina, et al., “Exercise and physical activity in the prevention and treatment of atherosclerotic cardiovascular disease,” Circulation, Vol. 107, No. 24, 2003, pp. 3109–3116.
89. J. Alcal-Fdez, A. Fernandez, J. Luengo, J. Derrac, S. Garca, L. Snchez, F. Herrera, “KEEL Data-Mining Software Tool: Data Set Repository, Integration of Algorithms and Experimental Analysis Framework,” Journal of Multiple-Valued Logic and Soft Computing, Vol. 17, No. 2–3, pp. 255–287, 2011.
90. A. Frank and A. Asuncion, “UCI machine learning repository,” 2010. [Online]. Available: http://archive.ics.uci.edu/ml
91. J. Farouc, A, L. Peter, and R. Weissleder, “Molecular and cellular imaging of atherosclerosis: Emerging applications,” Journal of the American College of Cardiology, Vol. 47, No. 7, 2006, pp. 1328–1338.
92. Libby P, “Inflammation in atherosclerosis” Nature, Vol. 420, 2002, pp. 868–874.

Chapter 7
Nanotechnology and Its Application in Medicine

Mirjana Pavlovic, John Mayfield and Bela Balint

Introduction

Nanotechnology is a field of science that controls the manipulation of atomic properties so as to make the functional systems and other materials acquire exclusive capabilities [1]. The amazing approach of nanotechnology has been developed within chemical engineering as an explosive response and inevitable consecutive inspiration caused by original development of fullerenes, designed and created by Sir Harry Kroto who was awarded Nobel Prize for his invention of the methodology for engineering and separation of members of fullerene family in1996 [1].

The prefix "nano" stems from the ancient Greek which stands for "dwarf". Nature (Figs. 7.1, 7.2 and 7.3) clearly indicates differences in size between macro, micro and nano-worlds. These figures have emphasized first of all, the structures developed in nature of the nano-size that have also geometric character/microarchitecture, ranging from viruses and nano-bacteria [1] to the wide spectrum of natural nanoparticles all over the nature surrounding our planet (especially ocean) of infinite structural forms. The scale of things in Fig. 7.3 is showing the shapes and architecture of many different entities from all levels, indicating that similar shapes can be formed not only at visible, but also at invisible parts of the scale.

Nanotechnology is generally defined as "the engineering of functional systems at the molecular scale" [1]. In other words, it is manipulation of matter at the atomic and molecular scale to create materials with remarkably varied and new properties with huge potential in many sectors, ranging from healthcare to construction of

M. Pavlovic (✉) · J. Mayfield
Department of Computer and Electrical Engineering and Computer Science,
Florida Atlantic University, Boca Raton, FL, USA
e-mail: mpavlovi@fau.edu

B. Balint
Military Medical Academy Belgrade, Belgrade, Serbia

B. Furht and A. Agarwal (eds.), *Handbook of Medical and Healthcare Technologies*,
DOI: 10.1007/978-1-4614-8495-0_7, © Springer Science+Business Media New York 2013

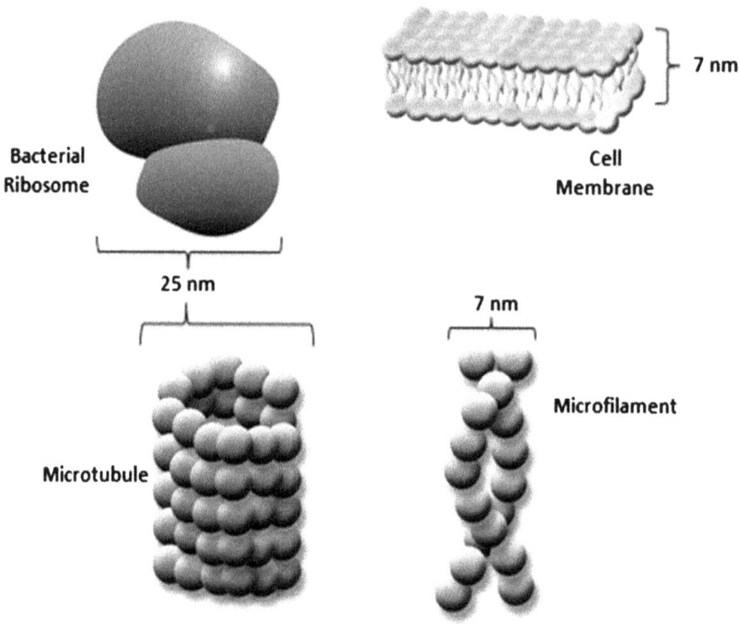

Fig. 7.1 The world of micrometer

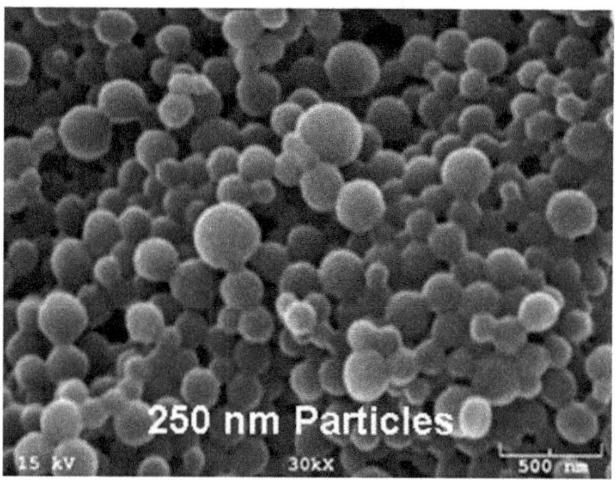

Fig. 7.2 The world of nanometer

electronics. In medicine, it promises to revolutionize drug delivery, gene therapy, diagnostics and many areas of research, development and clinical application.

The term "**nanotechnology**" has become much more popular and is often used to describe any type of manufacturing or research that takes place at dimensions less than 1000 nm [2]. Since in making the new molecules atoms have to collide with enough energy and under correct angle, [2] the idea is that we should soon be able to manipulate individual atoms and molecules to construct devices that are more powerful, more precise, lighter, smaller and despite all, stronger [2]. Here are proposed three main aims of devices manufactured using nanotechnology which reflect the perspective of this fascinating developing field:

1. we should be able to place every atom in exactly the right position;
2. we should be able to build anything that complies with the laws of physics, as long as we can understand it at a molecular or atomic level;
3. and perhaps, the one that drives most research in this field is the idea that the costs of manufacture should not be much higher than the costs of only the materials and energy required to put the product together.

Geometry and minimization are at the heart of nanotechnology. Look only into viruses! As of known nano-size, they have mostly stable icosahedron geometric shapes while in non-living state (out of the host) with their crystal DNA within the nano-particle, becoming alive during interaction with the host cells [3]. The interaction involves their DNA/RNA replication which involves the "borrowing" of enzymes for that particular procedure within the host cell.

There are also certain names already given to the particular structures emerging from nano-technological approaches [1, 4–12] such as:

Nanotubes which are elongated carbon forms with one or more concentric polygonal cylinders. They are grown from carbon under high-temperature, electrically-charged conditions. Due to their geometric similarity to the geodesic domes designed by the greatest thinker of twentieth century, R. Buckminster Fuller, nanotubes are furthermore called "**Bucky tubes**".

Nanohexagons are nanotubes with hexagonal ends. **Nanoctagons** are nanotubes with octagonal ends.

Nanocircles are circular nanostructures and nanospheres are spherical nanostructures. **Nanoshells** are hollow nanospheres, and lately used in medical purposes.

Within last decade, nanotechnology has moved from abstraction to reality with the development of tools such as the:

- Atomic Force Microscope (AFM),
- Scanning Tunneling Microscope (STM), and the
- Virtual Surface Profiling Microscope (VSPM). These microscopes do more than just let people view little materials. They also enable manipulation of matter on a perspective of nanometers in a vacuum, liquid or gas.

FM has a probe that creates three-dimensional images of specific atoms and molecules at the nano-scale dimension as it moves across an object's outside.

STMs may etch surfaces and move particles on dimension of nanometers.

VSPM digitizing the whole slide at high resolution, so that the viewer can zoom in-to areas and structures of interest on the slide. It creates what we call a digital slide, or a virtual slide, meaning that the user sees the same image in the screen

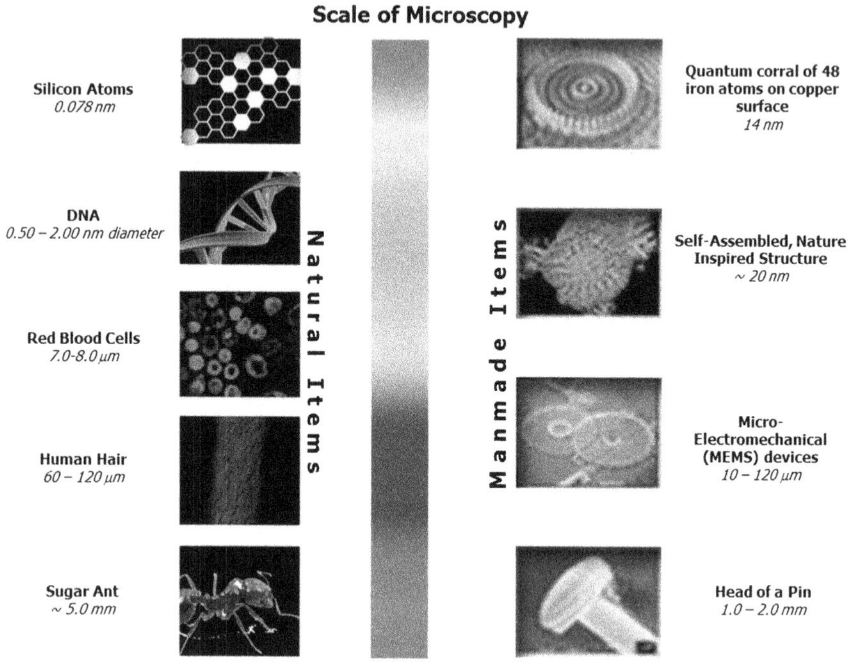

Fig. 7.3 The scale of things : architectonic parallelism

as they would get if they projected the microscope image onto the screen, but it's an electronic file. All of these methods help us to visualize invisible at the "nano" level.

How did the "Adventure in Nano-Space" Start and Who are the Facilitators of This Event?

The Adventure in Nanospace and the Synthesis and Separation of Sir Harry Kroto's "Fullerenes"

The discovery of fullerenes in 1985 led to a new field of study and a New Material Class of pure carbon that is significantly different from other forms of carbon, diamond and graphite [1]. Carbon Fullerenes are the third allotropes of carbone beside graphite and diamond, spherical, caged molecules with carbon atoms located at the corner of the polyhedral structure consisting of pentagons and hexagons, much like the shape of a Soccer ball. Carbon Fullerenes come in many forms. The most abundant form is Carbon 60 (which has a soccer ball shape), Carbon 70 (which has more of a rugby ball shape) and Carbon 84 (spherical). Fullerene get the name from the geodesic dome shape which was researched and promoted at macro-level by the most prominent thinker of twentieth century, Buckminster Fuller [1]. They need an carbon arc discharge (high pressure/temperature) in order to be created/synthesized.

Several interesting and important developments took place at the University of Sussex in UK between September 1985, when C_{60} was discovered by the Rice Group, and September 1990 when the brilliant paper on its extraction was submitted to *Nature* by Wolfgang Krätschmer, Lowell Lamb, Kostas Fostiropoulos and Donald Huffman [1]. During this period a parallel series of experiments to those of Krätschmer et al., was carried out at Sussex, by H. Crotto's group. A key reason for carrying out the experiment at Rice in the first place was an intriguing set of results obtained by Hintenberger and colleagues between 1958 and 1963 that showed, by mass spectrometry, that carbon species with as many as 33 carbon atoms were produced in a carbon arc discharge [1]. At Sussex, after the initial C_{60} discovery in 1985, Crotto had a hole drilled in an old carbon-arc evaporator they had, so that they could deposit carbon on a silica wafer at various argon pressures [1]. The idea was to follow up the Hintenberger et al. experiments [1] by recreating roughly the same conditions, that the group had achieved with the Rice nozzle as cheaply, as simply as possible with an electric arc discharge. At this point Crotto conjectured that as the argon pressure was increased he might be able to use the electron microscope that was available at Sussex to see the formation of roundish carbon particles which they conjectured might provide some circumstantial evidence for C_{60} formation. The group thought that the assembly processes that created C_{60} might also lead to the formation of large spheroidal soot-like carbon particles. What they found was that the smooth carbon coating obtained under very low pressure changed, more-or-less suddenly, at 70–80 μm pressure of argon creating an undulating blistered rough surface of the kind they vaguely expected.

This observation was encouraging as it seemed to be some sort of confirmation that the idea might be valid and that C_{60} might be forming. Here Crotto says he made a fundamental mistake—and not for the first time! He assumed that C_{60} would only be formed in minuscule amounts and only detectable, if at all, by the most sensitive analytical technique available i.e. mass spectrometry. After all, how could C_{60} be easily made when it had avoided detection until nearly the end of the twentieth century, and then only fleetingly, when it's two more famous siblings, diamond and graphite had been known since time immemorial. It is now hard, more than twenty five years later, when C_{60} is in every school science textbooks to realize that C_{60} was, prior to 1990, considered by some to be highly suspicious character and indeed by some even an imposter.

This "maneuvers" have helped them to completely isolate C_{60} and show that it exists in pure form, by using NMR. Since then, many fullerenes-based compounds have been synthesized, displaying a range of biological activities potentially useful in anticancer or antimicrobial therapy, cytoprotection, enzyme inhibition, controlled drug delivery and contrast- or radioactivity-based diagnostic imaging [1].

Discovery of the Structure of Graphene and Significance of Its Impact on Nanotechnology: Gaim and Novoselov

What is graphene? Graphene is a single layer of carbon packed in a hexagonal (honeycomb)-lattice, with a carbon–carbon distance of 0.142 nm and the angle between the 2 of 120° ( ). It is the first truly natural two-dimensional crystalline material and it is representative of a whole class of 2D materials including for example single layers of Boron-Nitride (BN) and Molybdenum-disulphide (MoS_2), which have both been produced after 2004 [4, 5].

As mentioned, fullerenes, the large carbon cage molecules represent third carbon allotrope beside graphite and diamond [1]. The most abundant form of fullerenes is buckminsterfullerene (C60) with 60 carbon atoms arranged in a spherical structure. As indicated, the shape of the molecule, known as truncated icosahedron, resembles that of a soccer ball, containing 12**C60** fullerene molecules. Carbon nanotubes, and graphite can all be thought of as being formed from graphene sheets, i.e. single layers of carbon atoms arranged in a honeycomb lattice .How is it obtained from the nature? It is interesting to consider that everyone who has used an ordinary pencil has probably produced graphene-like structures without knowing it. A pencil contains graphite, and when it is moved on a piece of paper, the graphite is cleaved into thin layers that end up on the paper and make up the text or drawing that we are trying to produce. A small fraction of these thin layers will contain only a few layers or even a single layer of graphite, i.e. graphene. Thus, the difficulty was not to **fabricate** the graphene structures, but to **isolate sufficiently large individual sheets in order to identify and characterize the graphene** and to verify its unique two-dimensional (2D) properties. This is what Geim, Novoselov, and their collaborators from Manchester group succeeded in doing and got in 2010 Nobel Prize, for [4, 5, 13–15] (Figs. 7.4, 7.5, 7.6).

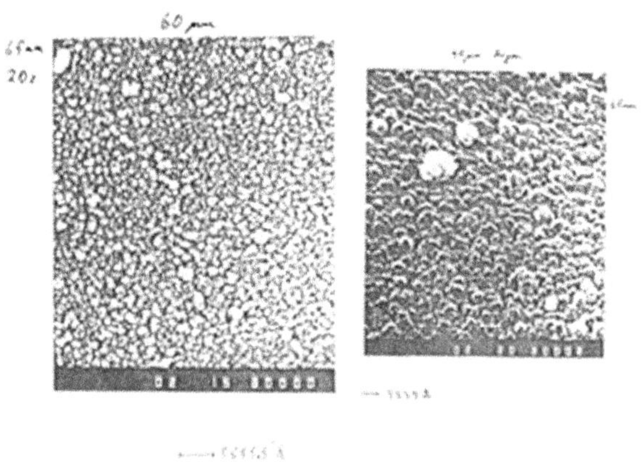

Fig. 7.4 Scanning electron microscope images showing morphological change in the deposit from carbon arc generated vapor condensed under 60 and 95 μm argon pressure

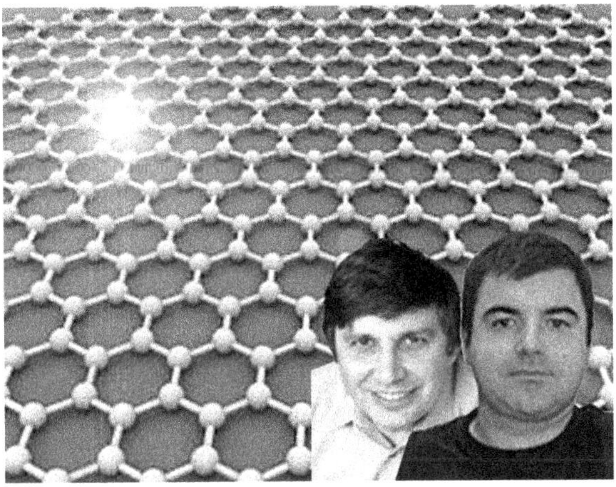

Fig. 7.5 Geim and Novoselov who got the NP in 2010

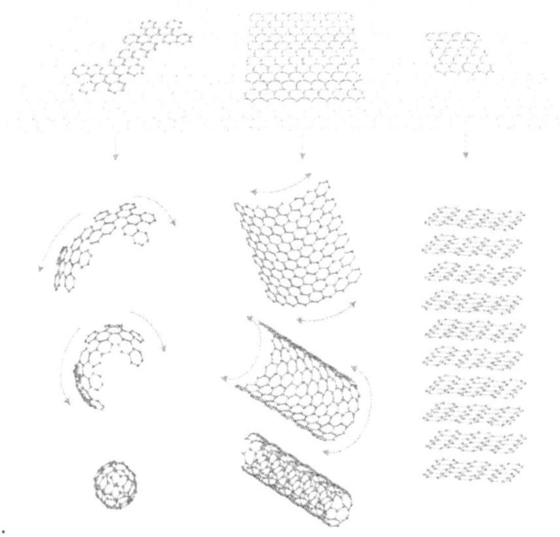

Fig. 7.6 Nanotubes and nanoshells

Essentials of technical approach are actually very simple. They used a simple but effective mechanical exfoliation method for extracting thin layers of graphite from a graphite crystal with Scotch tape and then transferred these layers to a silicon substrate. The development of this new material, opens new exiting possibilities. It is the first crystalline 2D-material with unique properties, which makes it interesting both for fundamental science and for future applications. The Manchester group succeeded by using an optical method, an Atomic Force Microscope (AFM) with which they were able to identify fragments made up of only a few layers, or even monolayer—that's how graphene was identified [4, 5].

Nanoparticles in the Nature and How Long the Adventure in the Nanospace Was?

It was Democritus in ancient Greece who first told that the matter must have smallest, invisible particle retaining all properties of that matter [2]. Democritus' model was a small, invisible non-particulated sphere. Athomos in Greek's means: non-dividable. In his vision it contained no electrons or nucleus.

He drew his model to show that all atoms are indestructible and unchangeable. Democritus also knew that atoms are different in size. He thought they were different in shape and temperature, as well. This was the first atomic model ever designed. Much later on, in modern era it has been determined that radius of He atom for example is in the range of nano-values [2].

John Dalton in 1803 was the first to seriously revise Democritus's theory [2]. He stated that atom is particulated and gave the first taw model which was then modified with work of many scientists such as: Rutherford, Bohr, Luis De Brogli, etc. [2] (Figs. 7.7, 7.8, 7.9).

However, Ernst Rutherford has proved that the nuclei of certain light elements, such as nitrogen, could be 'disintegrated' by the impact of particles arising from a radioactive source, and that during this process fast protons were emitted. It was

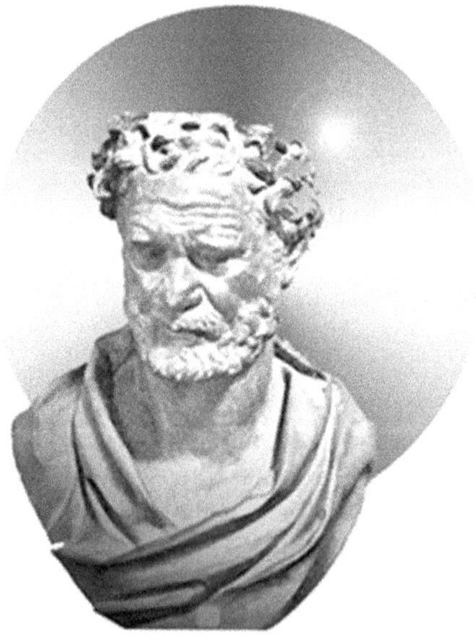

Fig. 7.7 Democritus of Abdera and his model of non-particulated atom (atoms-undividable)

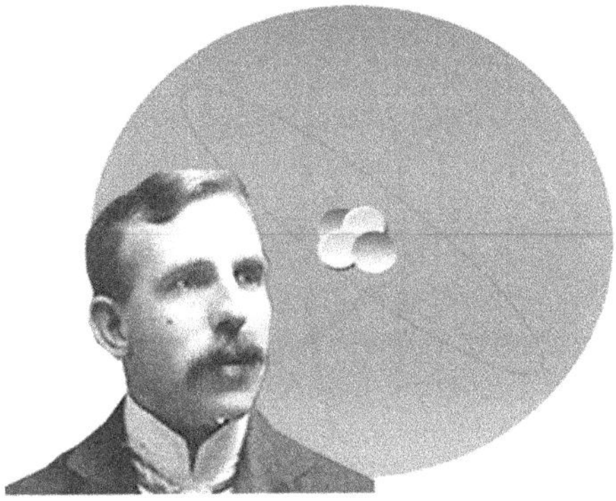

Fig. 7.8 Ernest Rutherford and his model of atom after Dalton

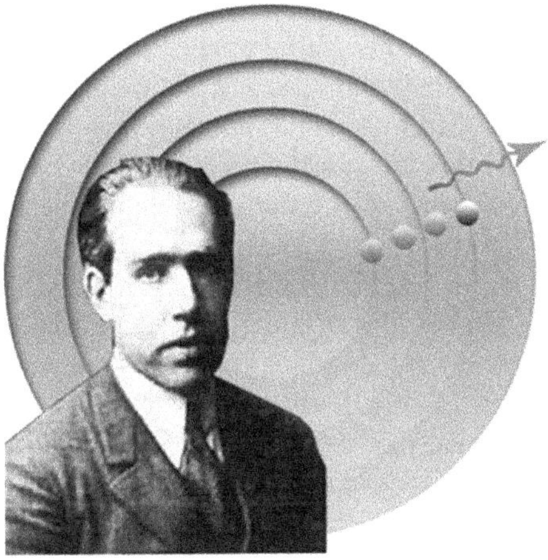

Fig. 7.9 Niels Bohr and Rutherford have given corrected model known as Rutherford–Bohr's model of atom used even today for certain explanation of atomic behavior

the first artificially induced nuclear reaction and it would change the world forever. Along with the eventual founding of CERN in 1954, it would lead to nuclear power and the atomic bombs that devastated Hiroshima and Nagasaki in World War Two.

What did Bohr improve on atomic structure? Rutherford's atomic theory described an atomic model with all the mass concentrated in a nucleus with electrons circling the nucleus in a fixed orbit. This theory was shown incorrect by using Maxwell's equations, which states since the electrons are moving in a circular motion, they are accelerating. Accelerating electrons means they are emitting radiation and therefore losing energy and would eventually spiral in motion toward the nucleus and collapse [2].

Bohr's insight was that he declared an electron could orbit the nucleus but only in discrete orbits which didn't emit radiation. An electron moves to a higher orbit, with a larger radius, by absorbing radiation (a photon) and in contrast will emit a photon of energy when the electron moves to a lower orbit with a smaller radius. Each orbit corresponds to an angular momentum value relating to Planck's constant (h) divided by 2pi. Insights regarding radiation and atoms were taken from Planck's Quantum Theory [2].

Bohr proposed that the outer orbits could accommodate more electrons than the inner orbits. In total, the atomic structure theory that Bohr proposed included an atom which was 1/10,000 the size of the atoms proposed by other scientists.

Somewhat before World War II Italian atomic scientist Enrico Fermi was invited to USA. What was Fermi's contribution to the development of atomic science? Within ten years of research he discovered that when an element is bombarded by a slow moving neutron, it becomes radioactive and starts emitting radiations. The result is one element changes into another element, very attractive idea suggesting the evolution of the Universe reflected in the periodic chart of elements as rather a dynamic system evolving with his time. In 1933 he discovered a neutral particle called neutrino [2]. He also produced eighty new artificial nuclei by neutron bombardment. Thus, Fermi opened the field of elemental particles and atomic manipulation through bombarding and radiation of elements (atoms of elements) and their changes from one into another, that will later on be elaborated by Gel Man who stated that this world is relying upon atoms that are based upon matter/antimatter co-existence of the particles within the atom, meaning that each particle has an anti-particle.

Fermi (Fig. 7.10) was instrumental in developing of an atom bomb during the Second World War, but his great contribution was also to the roots of nanotechnology. The roots of the idea of graphene's emergence from carbon atoms are in his work. It has been shown that the two-dimensional nature of graphene leads to many interesting electronic, thermal and elastic properties that could be used in different fields of human life, including medicine.

Fig. 7.10 Enrico Fermi

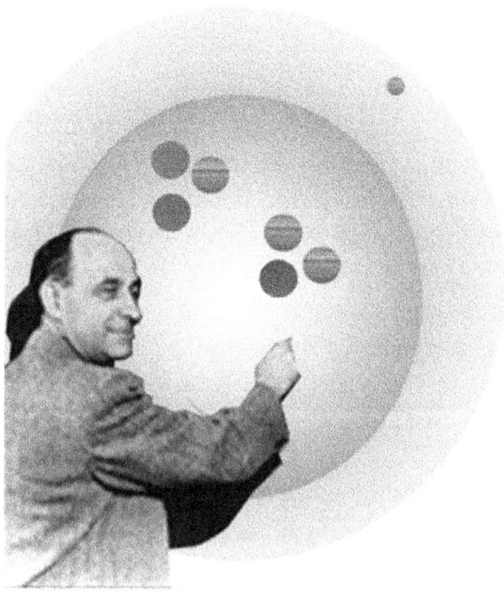

Fermi Level and Graphene. Fermi showed by bombarding atoms with neutrons under optimal conditions that they can become different elements. He also defined **Fermi level**—a measure of the energy of the least tightly held electrons within a solid (i.e. the valence electrons, which are in the outermost orbit of the atoms of a solid). The value of the Fermi level at absolute zero (−273.15°C) is called the **Fermi energy** and is a constant for each solid. The Fermi level changes as the solid is warmed and as electrons are added to or withdrawn from the solid (Figs. 7.11, 7.12).

Fermi–Dirac Statistics

The Fermi energy showed the temperature-dependent behavior similar to any other one-dimensional device in non-degenerate regime. However, in the degenerate regime, the normalized Fermi energy with respect to the band edge shown to be a function of carrier concentration [14]. In other words, modeling of Graphene Nanoribbon Fermi Energy is possible and has been developed into alternative approach to carbon nanotube (CNT) in order to show that different banding of tube is possible under different conditions opening possibilities for semiconducting electronic properties as well as for the nanoshells capable of distributing targeted drug delivery [15–20].

The breakthrough done by Geim, Novoselov and their co-workers with their paper from 2004 [4] which ignited the development of graphene-like materials brought them the Nobel Prize in Physics 2010.

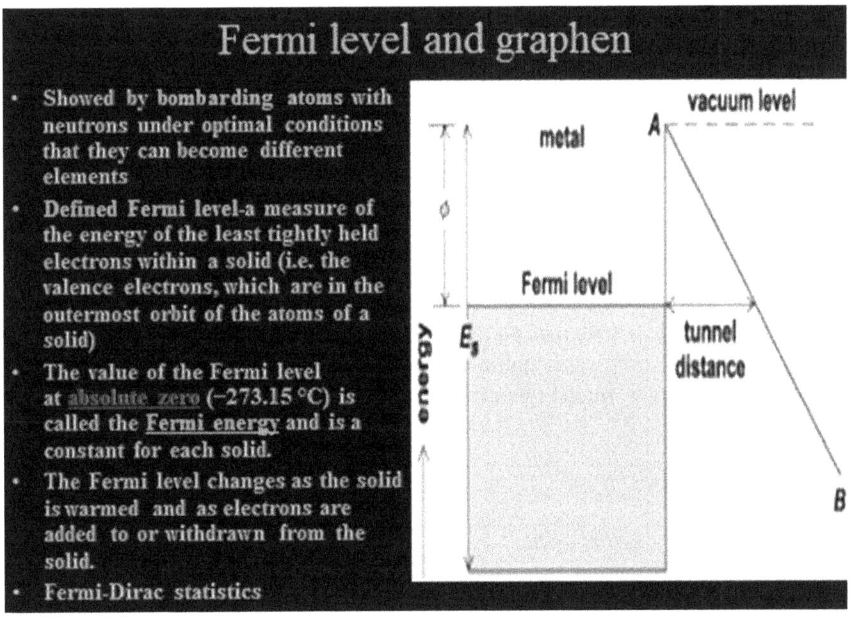

Fig. 7.11 Fermi level and graphene

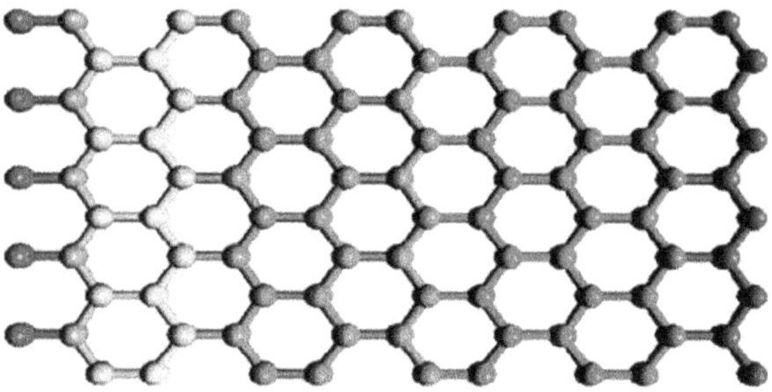

Fig. 7.12 Armchair of graphene nanoribbon (GNR) minimum energy band structure based on numerical solution of Fermi–Dirac integrals for nonparabolic region [14]

Electrical and Thermal Conductivity of Graphene

Electrical Conductivity

Using the layer thickness we get a bulk conductivity of $0.96 \times 10^6\,\Omega^{-1}\,\text{cm}^{-1}$ for graphene. This is somewhat higher than the conductivity of copper which is $0.60 \times 10^6\,\Omega^{-1}\,\text{cm}^{-1}$ [15].

Thermal Conductivity

The thermal conductivity of graphene is dominated by phonons and has been measured to be approximately $5000\,\text{W}\,\text{m}^{-1}\,\text{K}^{-1}$. Copper at room temperature has a thermal conductivity of $401\,\text{W}\,\text{m}^{-1}\,\text{K}^{-1}$. Thus, graphene conducts heat 10 times better than copper.

Graphene: Other Features

In contrast to low temperature 2D systems based on semiconductors, graphene maintains its 2D properties at room temperature. Graphene also has several other interesting properties, which it shares with carbon nanotubes. It is substantially stronger than steel, very stretchable and can be used as a flexible conductor. Its thermal conductivity is much higher than that of silver or cooper [21, 22] (Figs. 7.13, 7.14).

Nanotechnology Concepts

Here are two important concepts related to nanotechnology that are necessary if we are going to achieve the three aims mentioned before.

The first is known as "**positional assembly**", which is how we would get all of the molecules or atoms in the right place. This can be achieved through the use of

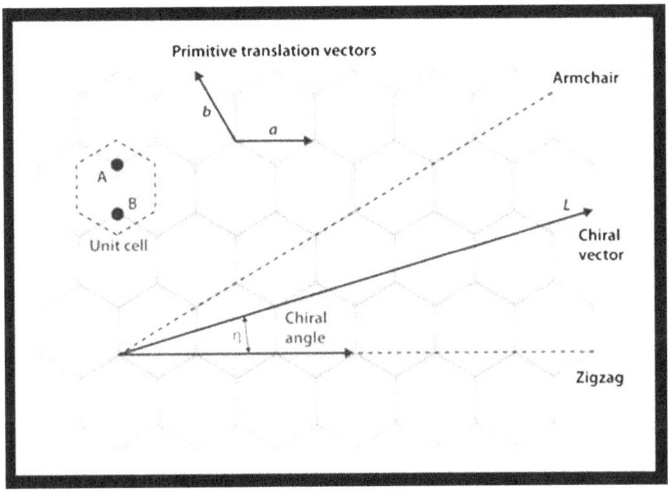

Fig. 7.13 Honeycomb lattice structure of graphene [21]

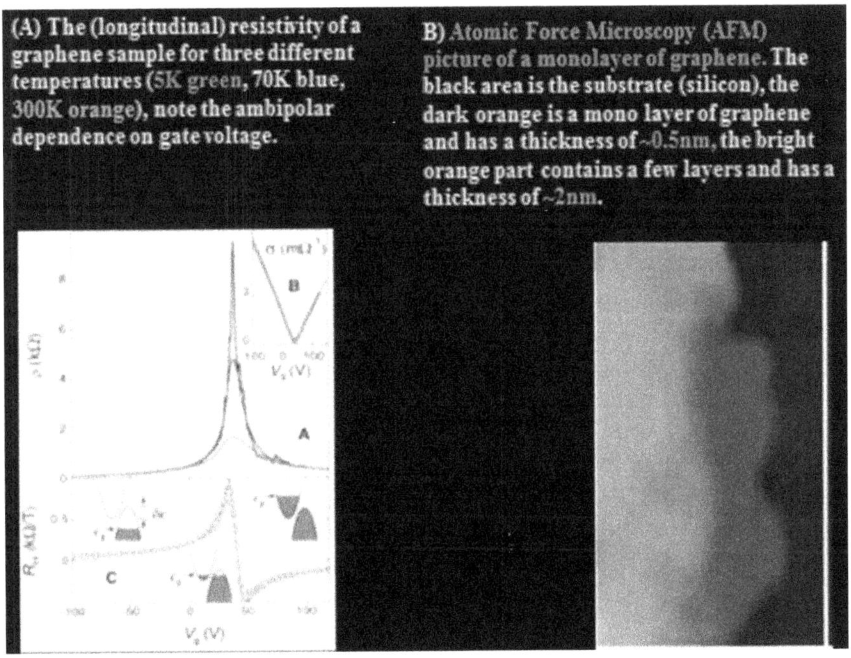

Fig. 7.14 Physicochemical aspects of nanoparticles

tiny robots, molecular in size and produced using nanotechnology themselves. A second concept is "**massive parallelism**", which is a way to reduce the costs of manufacturing. Because one molecule-sized robot is going to take a very long time to build anything of substantial size, the idea is to have many robots that work in a production line, getting larger at each stage until the process is completed.

Aspects of Nanotechnology Important for Medicine

Although in essence nanotechnology has emerged as a revolution in the field of computer technology, it is no more confined to just computers. The success of nanotechnology in curing fatal diseases is reaching new horizons.The ability to manipulate structures and properties at the nanoscale in medicine is like having a sub-microscopic lab bench on which you can handle cell components, viruses or pieces of DNA using a range of tiny tools, robots and tubes. Scientists are working now to create nanostructures that serve as new kinds of drugs for treating cancer, to engineer nanomaterials for use as artificial tissues that would replace diseased kidneys and livers, and even repair nerve damage, and to integrate nano-devices with the nervous system to create implants that restore vision and hearing, and build new prosthetic limbs [22–34].

The Current Use of Nanoparticles in Medicine

Considering the rapid progress in this field it is hoped that nanotechnology will soon be a huge force against diseases in the coming days and it will help in wiping away the most lethal diseases in the current era. Nano medicine is the science of things smaller than 1000 nms in size, applied to the field of medicine. As we have seen from only potential of graphene, there are a wide variety of uses in this area, ranging from the use of biosensors for detection of anomalies in the body, such as high blood sugar concentration, which would suggest diabetes, to the concept of nanorobots. Currently, nano medicine has applications in: drug delivery, cancer stem cell diagnosis and treatment, use in combination with laser beam as nanoshells in order to destroy cancerous tissue (Figs. 7.15, 7.16, 7.17).

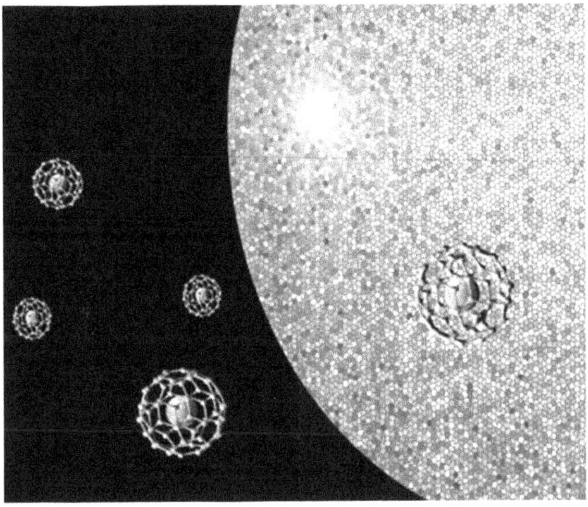

Fig. 7.15 The concept of drug delivery in bucky-ball

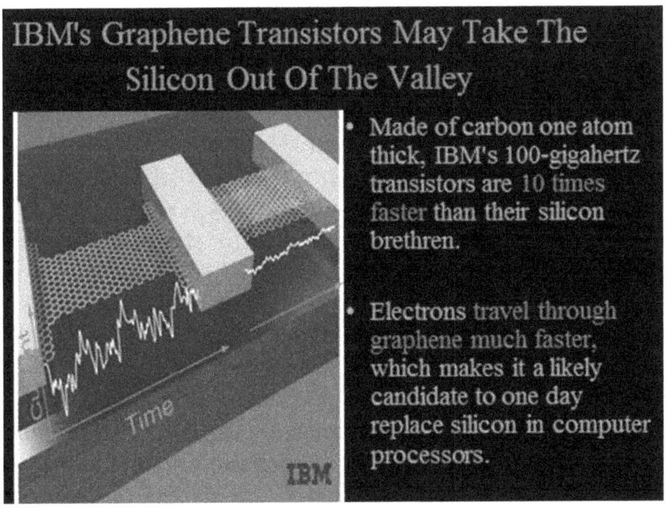

Fig. 7.16 Graphene as the conductor

- Concept of drug delivery

Pharmaceutical companies have started using nanotechnologies to develop genetically targeted drugs. This allows for much more precise drug development, and makes it faster to decide whether or not a substance is suitable for use in a drug delivery [22–27].

These systems are already working in some medical diseases. Originally the idea is coming from Robert Langer [22] who has synthesized drug-delivery systems based

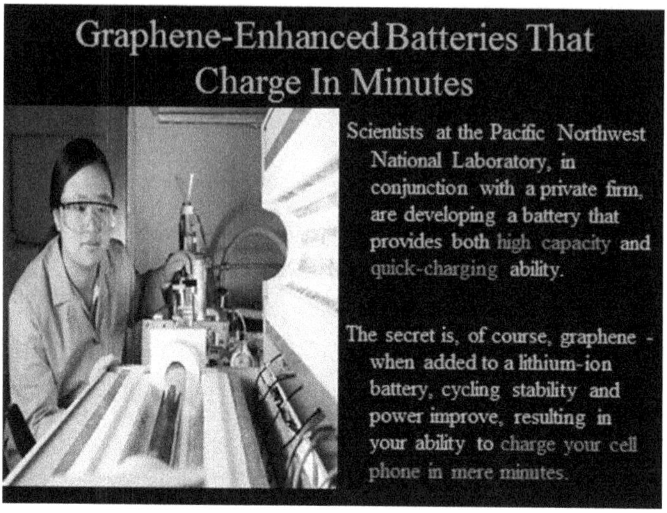

Fig. 7.17 Graphene as a battery stabilizer

upon different materials. They are so far known as controlled drug delivery systems-a slow-releasing cancer (for example) medications that can be administered directly where the cancerous tumor had been removed. He also pioneered a variety of remotely controlled drug delivery systems that vary the amount of drug released through electric impulse, ultrasound and magnetic field. *Polymers* are incredibly versatile and one can use them to make them into all kinds of shapes and forms, including nanoparticles.

How does the polymer work in developing a targeted drug delivery system? First, one has to inject the nanoparticle into the body-that can travel around the body for a long time, and ultimately find the target (diseased cells). A number of breakthroughs have facilitated this control, coming from material science and life science, as well. The integral thinking of bioengineering principles has enabled that event. Polymer delivery systems have a great impact currently in making of transdermal patches, but they are also in the pills, different implants, stents, etc. They are expected to have a huge impact after clinical studies in next 10 years. Some of them have antibodies for the targeted diseased cells surface molecules and in that way they are attached to it. The patents are numerous (about 300) and protected. So, controlled drug delivery has two important mechanisms : one is the attachment of the drug exclusively for the target (for example cancer cell and not the healthy one) while the other means that the dosage is controlled and individualized/personalized which will avoid the side effects sometimes critically detrimental and fatal [27–29].

- Nanorobot concept

Nanotech medical robots ("nano-medi-bots") is the concept which might develop into the nano-device that might be able to: monitor body function; repair damaged tissue at the nanoscopic level; deconstruct pathologic or abnormal matter or tissue such as cancer or plaque; and refine human health and functioning.

Although nanomedibots have not been developed, there are ongoing advances in nanofluidics and carbon nanotube flow sensors that could become their building blocks. As nanotechnology and biotechnology advance, nanomedibots and engineered useful microorganisms might be integrated.

Carbon is the element the most suitable for medical nanorobots, probably as diamond or fullerene allotropic modification, probably due to extraordinary strength and chemical inertia of diamond. Most of other light elements such as: hydrogen, sulfur, oxygen, nitrogen, fluor, silicon, etc, will be used in special purposes in nano-zupcanik and other components. It is impossible to say exactly how does the typical nanorobot looks like? Their purpose would have been to travel through the blood toward their target with precision of 500–3000 nm. Nanorobot can be 500–3000 nm in size and can be ingested with food or aerosol. Each kind of Nano robot would be designed to do a specific role.

Finally, maybe the most important: the nanorobot is being designed currently [35].There is a lot of theoretical designs which look well on the paper, but they can be fundamentally changed after development and testing. However, it seems to be possible and this tendency to minimization will facilitate a lot of medical procedures and approaches.

Beside nanorobot idea, where graphene could be potentially used, there are also other options like the one shown in Figs. 7.18, 7.19, and 7.20. The antibacterial effect of the grapheme has been discovered as well, and could be potentially used in hospitals, sterile labs and other facilities that require it (Figs. 7.18, 7.19).

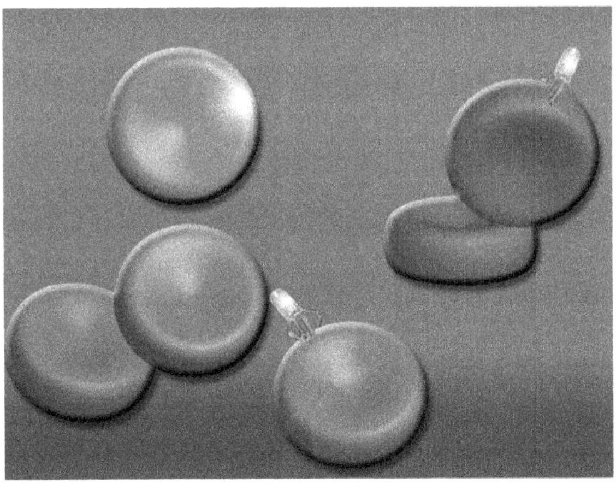

Fig. 7.18 precursor of nanorobot-microscopic machine roaming throughout the body

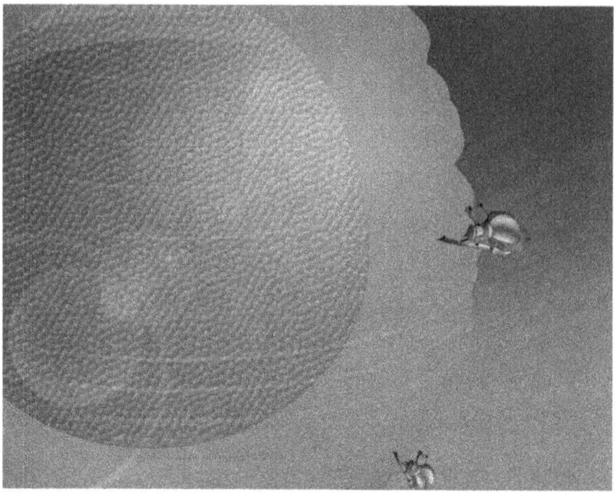

Fig. 7.19 The idea of nanorobot and comparable nanoparticles in the cell

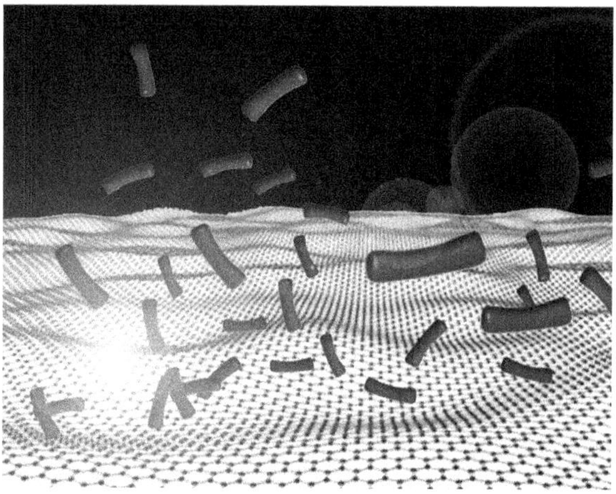

Fig. 7.20 Possible use of grapheme as antibacterial bandage

As technological advancement creates new opportunity in other realms of science, so too does it in the world of medicine (Fig. 7.21). Two new treatment modalities are on the forefront of oncological intervention: nanoparticle therapy and alternating magnetic fields on replicating cancer stem cells. Although in the early phases of testing, the two show promise of accomplishing limited-to-no side-effects as well as being as non-invasive as possible. These novel treatments could be used in combination with chemotherapy or radiotherapy, as indicated (Fig. 7.22).

The nanoparticle model has had difficulty from its inception with the use of quantum dots, later proven to be toxic.

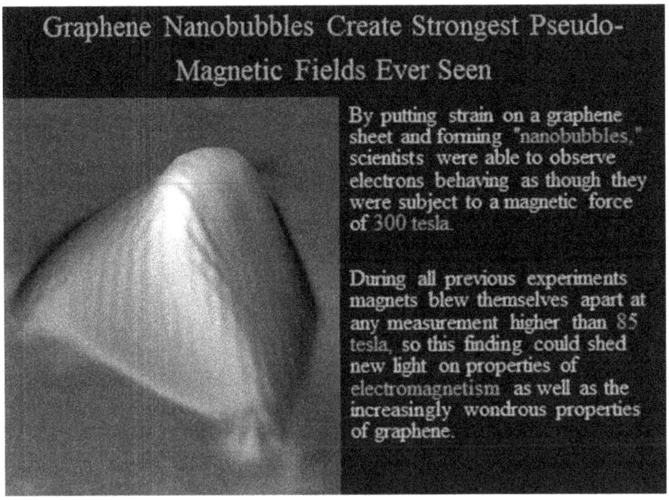

Fig. 7.21 Creation of pseudomagnetic fields by graphene

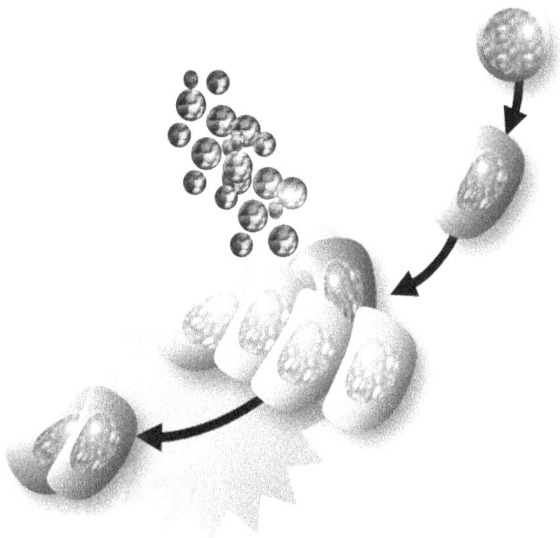

Fig. 7.22 Nanoparticles in drug-delivery systems in cancer treatment

- New concepts developed under strong influence of nanotechnology

However, recent models have proven dramatically more effective *as anti-cancer agents* through various methods of delivery [30–32]. The model proposes that nanoparticles that are composed of *silicon and can be coated with antibodies specific for stem cell markers found on cancer stem cells,* or similar molecular conjugates.

Through enhanced permeation retention, vascularized tumors would become infiltrated by these nanoparticles. Infrared radiation is then applied to the tumor, wherein the cancer stem cells that now contained these particles would increase in heat at a much greater rate than cells not containing the particles, thus killing the targeted cells. Studies have been carried out for a variety of cancer types including, breast, prostate and liver cancer [32].

Dynamic effects of therapeutic strategies directed against cancer stem cells (CSCs) are also a part of nanotechnology development. A tumor tissue is a complex mix of cancer cells at various stages of differentiation, from uncommitted CSCs through various stages of cancer progenitor cells to matured cancer cells, with a concomitant decrease in the levels of proliferative and/or metastatic potential. Both the CSC niche with supporting cell types and the matured cancer cell compartment create an intricate network of inter-dependency. Cancer therapy should ideally address both the CSCs and the matured cancer cells by slowing down proliferation and production of differentiated cancer cells and increasing apoptosis in both CSCs and matured cancer cells. In a fast-growing cancer, tumor therapy might come too late and/or be ineffective, or reduce tumor mass by killing matured cancer cells without targeting the CSC niche.

The latter effect might stimulate CSC proliferation and increase the CSC pool, which would consequently result in a resurgence of even larger numbers of matured cancer cells. In another scenario, therapeutic intervention itself might provoke an enlargement of the CSC pool by selecting for more radio- and chemoresistant CSC clones.

These CSCs will have a superior ability to repair DNA damage upon radiotherapy and/or overexpress members of the ABC transmembrane pumps, resulting in the swift efflux of certain chemotherapeutics. Over time, this new generation of CSCs could also include new mutant CSCs with even more aggressive signatures. CSC therapy targets the CSC niche itself by attenuating the self-replicating potential of CSCs and disturbing cellular crosstalk within the CSC niche. Increased apoptosis of CSCs will result in a significantly smaller number of matured cancer cells, which can then be addressed successfully with common anticancer therapies [33–35]. Thus, anticancer therapy that only results in apoptosis of the matured cancer cells and/or only inhibits the proliferation of CSCs provides a potential window of opportunity for new and more aggressive CSC mutants to occur and might be unsuccessful if not dangerous. It is expected that the elimination of cancer should target the CSC pool, and successful treatment regimens would need to be the result of an orchestrated "target and destroy" effect.

While the promise of reduced cross-effect oncological treatment via CSC targeting gives great hope to the future of oncology and the patients that suffer from cancer, a great deal of work still remains. CSCs are a moving target and exist in such a small population that effective use of treatment modalities, although more promising than some miRNA studies and the like, still does not, in its current state, exist as a viable treatment option for all cancers. Much as microbiologists have difficulty in the world of fighting an ever-adapting organism, so to shall the oncologist and researchers that pursue this path. In combination with other therapies, however, it does appear that

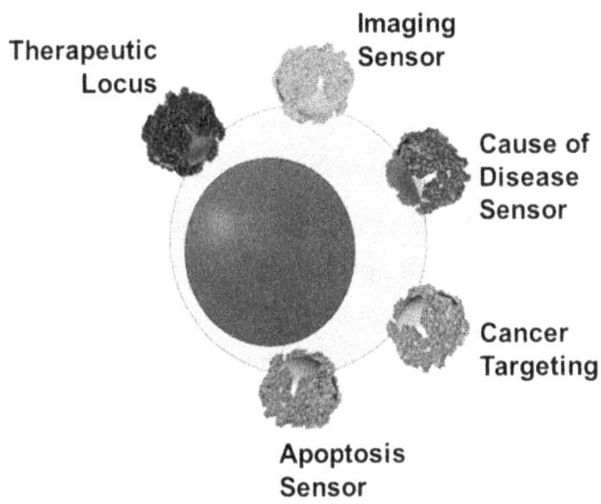

Fig. 7.23 Cellular nanosensors with diverse potentials: the future events?

a reduction in risk associated with current treatment modalities would be evident. In light of the difficulty of the manipulation of the CSC model, the research that has been done thus far is providing a solid framework upon which a new, improved paradigm of oncological treatment will be established (Fig. 7.23).

Viruses, parasites and bacteria are continuously mutating causing new diseases of our natural immune system [3]. Theoretically, nanorobot could protect our body from both current and future diseases. This would exclude the needed for vaccines in order to acquire immunity against certain diseases. Imagine the world without flu, or AIDS or other difficult viral or bacterial diseases!

- The future of nanotechnology in medical arena

As drugs get smaller, they will be able to easily "sneak" past the body's defense mechanisms and will be able to reach places that the drugs available today, cannot. Because smaller compounds have a large surface area to volume ratio, these new drugs should also be more reactive.

Tiny nanoparticles known as "quantum dots" can be made to give off different colors depending on their size, and so used for cellular disease detection [34]. They can also be made to attach to different biological components, such as certain proteins in certain colors, making it much easier to analyze blood for specific components.

Nano technology used for destruction of diseased tissues makes use of Nano shells, microscopic balls of glass coated in gold. Nano shells can also be designed to bind to specific components in the body, and can then be heated by lasers to destroy damaged tissue without causing any more damage to skin or other close by tissue.

It has already been said that the successful development of a medical nanorobot would "change the world of medicine forever" (Figs. 7.23, 7.24).

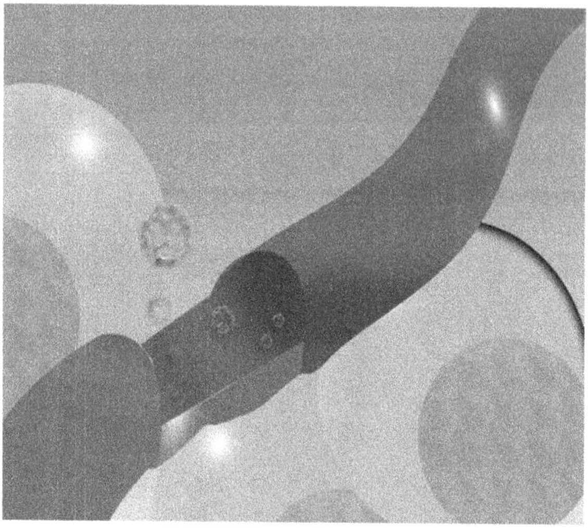

Fig. 7.24 Nanoparticles permeating BB

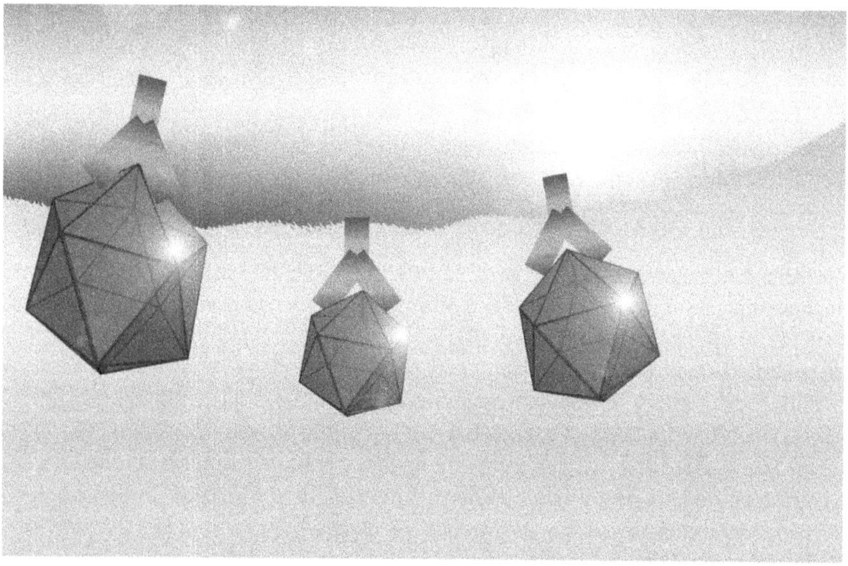

Fig. 7.25 Dendrimer as medically applied nanoparticle preventing the entrance of viruses into the cell

Conclusions and Future Directions

This chapter has taken in consideration the fundamental features of nanotechnology (geometry and minimization), the structure of the atom (as particulate entity), the synthesis of buckminsterfullerene's, discovery of graphene structure and its possible application in medical fields of drug-delivery, nano-robotics, anti-cancer therapy, anti-aging preparations, etc. It does comprehend the most fundamental physico-chemical aspects of this matter discovered and classified within last decade.

Nanotechnology for sure prepare us to looking in the future with optimism: In addition to innovation in other fields, nanotechnology will prompt the medicine to remove obstruction in the circulatory system, kill cancer cells, or take over the function of sub cellular organelles.

Killing viruses or bacteria, dissolving cholesterol or blood clots is very close to be done on nanotechnology basis.

Discovering the earliest signs of the diseases, even before the actual symptoms appear, is not a dream anymore.

We will be able to produce hearing aids that are actually a computer in each ear, artificial retinas to restore sight and many other medical wonders[35].

Nanotechnology would allow the gene combinations take place at the levels of molecules, rather than the larger gene. That would mean creating whole new organs for people, organs which their bodies won't reject as they do with transplanted human organs. Some of these will come within the next ten years, for sure. These persistent growing ideas will completely revolutionize the medical approach in sense of diagnosis, treatment and even prevention, minimizing equipment, space and errors that are inevitable today. Let it flourish, while we are creating and dreaming!

References

1. R. F. Curl Jr., H. Kroto, E. Autobiography, Nobelprize.org. 13 April, 2013.
2. Brown and Holme, 2011: Chemistry for engineering students.Edition 2. Print ISBN-13: 978–1439047910.
3. M.D. Pavlovic: Biomineralization and nanobacteria: at the door of the new concept? MD-Med Data Rev: 1, 2: 21–24, 2009.
4. A. K. Geim and K. S. Novoselov, "The rise of graphene", Nature Materials, vol. 6, no. 3, pp. 183–191, 2007.
5. K. S. Novoselov, A. K. Geim, S. V. Morozov, et al., "Electric field in atomically thin carbon films", Science, vol. 306, no.5696, pp. 666–669, 2004.
6. .C. Berger, Z. Song, X. Li, et al., "Electronic confinement and coherence in patterned epitaxial graphene", Science, vol. 312, no. 5777, pp. 1191–1196, 2006.
7. Y. Zhang, Y.-W. Tan, H. L. Stormer, and P. Kim, "Experimental observation of the quantum Hall effect and Berry's phase ingraphene", *Nature*, vol. 438, no. 7065, pp. 201–204, 2005.
8. K. S. Novoselov, A. K. Geim, S. V. Morozov, et al., "Two dimensional gas of massless Dirac fermions in graphene", *Nature*, vol. 438, no. 7065, pp. 197–200, 2005.
9. C. Berger, Z. Song, T. Li, et al., "Ultrathin epitaxial graphite: 2D electron gas properties and a route toward graphene-based nanoelectronics", *Journal of Physical Chemistry B*, vol. 108, no. 52, pp. 19912–19916, 2004.
10. .Y.-W. Son, M. L. Cohen, and S. G. Louie, "Energy gaps in graphene nanoribbons", *Physical Review Letters*, vol. 97, no. 21, Article ID 216803, 4 pages, 2006.
11. H. Xiang, E. Kan, S.-H. Wei, M.-H. Whangbo, and J. Yang, "Narrow" Graphene Nanoribbons Made Easier by Partial Hydrogenation", *Nano Letters*, vol. 9, no. 12, pp. 4025–4030, 2009.
12. M. Y. Han, B. Özyilmaz, Y. Zhang, and P. Kim, "Energy bandgap engineering of graphene nanoribbons", *Physical Review Letters*, vol. 98, no. 20, Article ID 206805, 4 pages, 2007.

13. D. A. Areshkin, D. Gunlycke, and C. T. White, "Ballistic transport in graphene nanostrips in the presence of disorder: importance of edge effects", *Nano Letters*, vol. 7, no. 1, pp. 204–210, 2007.
14. Zaharah et al, 2010 Z. Chen, Y.-M. Lin, M. J. Rooks, and P. Avouris, "Graphene nano-ribbon electronics", *Physica E*, vol. 40, no. 2, Article ID 0701599, pp. 228–232, 2007.
15. K. Nakada, M. Fujita, G. Dresselhaus, and M. S. Dresselhaus, "Edge state in graphene ribbons: nanometer size effect and edge shape dependence", *Physical Review B*, vol. 54, no. 24, pp. 17954–17961, 1996.
16. V. Barone, O. Hod, and G. E. Scuseria, "Electronic structure and stability of semiconducting graphene nanoribbons", *Nano Letters*, vol. 6, no. 12, pp. 2748–2754, 2006.
17. G. Liang, N. Neophytou, D. E. Nikonov, and M. S. Lundstrom, "Performance projections for ballistic graphene nanoribbon field-effect transistors", *IEEE Transactions on Electron Devices*, vol. 54, no. 4, pp. 677–682, 2007.
18. K. Wakabayashi, "Electronic and Magnetic Properties of Nanographite", in *Carbon-Based Magnetism–n Overview of the Magnetism of Metal Free Carbon-Based Compounds and Materials*, pp. 279–304, Elsevier, Amsterdam, The Netherlands, 2006.
19. Q. Yan, B. Huang, J. Yu, et al., "Intrinsic current-voltage characteristics of graphene nanoribbon transistors and effect of edge doping", *Nano Letters*, vol. 7, no. 6, pp. 1469–1473, 2007.
20. J. W. G. Wildoer, L. C. Venema, A. G. Rinzler, R. E. Smalley, and C. Dekker, "Electronic structure of atomically resolved carbon nanotubes", *Nature*, vol. 391, no. 6662, pp. 59–62, 1998.
21. R. A. Jishi, D. Inomata, K. Nakao, M. S. Dresselhaus, and G. Dresselhaus, "Electronic and lattice properties of carbon nanotubes", *Journal of the Physical Society of Japan*, vol. 63, no.6, pp. 2252–2290, 1994.
22. T. M. Fahmy, P. M. Fong, J. Park, T. Constable, and W. M. Saltzman : Nanosystems for Simultaneous Imaging and Drug Delivery to T Cells. *The AAPS Journal* 2007; 9 (2) Article 19.
23. NV Katre. The conjugation of proteins with polyethylene glycol and other polymers altering properties of proteins to enhance their therapeutic potential. *Adv Drug Deliv Rev*. 1993; 10 : 91–114.
24. H. Kobayashi, MW Brechbiel : Dendrimer-based nanosized MRI contrast agents. *Curr Pharm Biotechnol*. 2004; 5 : 539–549.
25. Kobayashi H, Brechbiel MW. Nano-sized MRI contrast agents with dendrimer cores. *Adv Drug Deliv Rev*. 2005; 57 : 2271–2286.
26. JM Anderson, MS Shive. Biodegradation and biocompatibility of PLA and PLGA microspheres. *Adv Drug Deliv Rev*. 1997; 28: 5–24.
27. R Langer, J Folkman. Polymers for the sustained release of proteins and other macromolecules. *Nature*. 1976; 263 : 797–800.
28. "Name-It: Naming and Detecting Faces in News Videos", IEEE MultiMedia, Vol. 6, No. 1, January-March (Spring), 1999, pp. 22–35.
29. Stupp, Roger, et al. "NovoTTF-100A versus physician's choice chemotherapy in recurrent glioblastoma: a randomised phase III trial of a novel treatment modality." European Journal of Cancer (2012).
30. Brannon-Peppas, Lisa, and James O. Blanchette. "Nanoparticle and targeted systems for cancer therapy." Advanced drug delivery reviews 56.11 (2004): 1649–1659.
31. Davis, Mark E. "Nanoparticle therapeutics: an emerging treatment modality for cancer." Nature Reviews Drug Discovery 7.9 (2008): 771–782.
32. Gagliardi, G., et al. "Long-term cardiac mortality after radiotherapy of breast cancer–application of the relative seriality model." British journal of radiology 69.825 (1996): 839–846.
33. Gaitanis, Alexander, and Stephen Staal. "Liposomal doxorubicin and nab-paclitaxel: nanoparticle cancer chemotherapy in current clinical use." Cancer Nanotechnology. Humana Press, 2010. 385–392.

34. Gil, Justyna, et al. "Cancer stem cells: the theory and perspectives in cancer therapy." Journal of applied genetics 49.2 (2008): 193–199.
35. http://www.bionano.neu.edu/NanoRobotics_in_Medicine.pdf

Chapter 8
Anomaly Detection Scheme for Medical Wireless Sensor Networks

Osman Salem, Alexey Guerassimov, Ahmed Mehaoua, Anthony Marcus and Borko Furht

Abstract Wireless Sensor Networks are vulnerable to a plethora of different fault types and external attacks after their deployment. We focus on sensor networks used in healthcare applications for vital sign collection from remotely monitored patients. These types of personal area networks must be robust and resilient to sensor failures as their capabilities encompass highly critical systems. Our objective is to propose an anomaly detection algorithm for medical wireless sensor networks, able to raise alarms only when patients enter in emergency situation and to discard faulty measurements. Our proposed approach firstly classifies instances of sensed patient attributes as normal and abnormal. Once we detect an abnormal instance, we use regression prediction to discern between a faulty sensor reading and a patient entering into a critical state. Our experimental results on real patient datasets show that our proposed approach is able to quickly detect patient anomalies and sensor faults with high detection accuracy while maintaining a low false alarm ratio.

O. Salem (✉) · A. Guerassimov · A. Mehaoua
LIPADE, University of Paris Descartes, Paris, France
e-mail: osman.salem@parisdescartes.fr

A. Guerassimov
e-mail: alexey.guerassimov@parisdescartes.fr

A. Mehaoua
Division of IT Convergence Engineering, POSTECH, Gyeongsangbuk-do, Korea

A. Mehaoua
LaBRI, Centre National de la Recherche Scientifique (CNRS), Bordeaux, France

A. Marcus · B. Furht
Department of Computer Science, Florida Atlantic University, Boca Raton, USA
e-mail: amarcu10@fau.edu

B. Furht
e-mail: bfurht@fau.edu

B. Furht and A. Agarwal (eds.), *Handbook of Medical and Healthcare Technologies*,
DOI: 10.1007/978-1-4614-8495-0_8,

Introduction

With the rise and precision of current medical procedures and the healthy lifestyles of many individuals turning towards a healthier lifestyle, the average lifetime expectancy is ever increasing [1]. Doctors are able to better diagnose and treat patients while the ability of individuals to cope and recover from illnesses is staggering. Technological advances incorporated with vast and accurate knowledge of the human anatomy have allowed healthcare professionals the ability to handle almost any scenario they encounter in individuals at hospitals and emergency treatment facilities [1, 2]. As the average individual lifetime expectancy has increased, this has also directly impacted our planets population and as such, a shortage of qualified healthcare professionals to treat the sick and needy has become an issue.

Scientists and researchers have developed numerous solutions to this problem, one of which allows patients to be remotely monitored utilizing networks of wireless sensors which relay, in real time, patient information to doctors and healthcare providers. Advances in sensor technologies and high throughput networks continue to refine the accuracy and increase the integrity and public trust of these systems. As a direct result, more individuals elect to utilize these systems as they allow greater freedom and mobility while maintaining the quality of care equivalent to direct medical interaction and attention found previously only in hospitals, clinics, and other specialized care facilities.

In medical applications, implementations of specialized Wireless Sensor Networks (WSN), known as Personal Area Networks (PAN) and Wireless Body Area Networks (WBAN), are comprised of numerous small devices attached to or implanted in the body of a patient. At present, many existing medical wireless devices are used to collect various patient metrics and vital signs, such as Heart Rate (HR), pulse, oxygen saturation (SpO2), Respiration Rate (RR), Body Temperature (BT), Electro Cardio Gram (ECG), Electro Myo Gram (EMG), Blood Pressure (BP), Blood Glucose Levels (BGL) and Galvanic Skin Response (GSR).

These networked medical sensors accumulate and transmit collected data to a central device (i.e., base station, PDA, smart phone) for processing and storage, This data may be then reevaluated and used to trigger medical alarms for caregivers or healthcare professionals, upon detection of anomalies in the physiological data, or clinical deterioration of monitored patients, to quickly react [2–4] by taking the appropriate actions.

The use of PANs and WBANs has been extended to monitor individuals having chronic illnesses (i.e., cardiovascular, Alzheimer's, Parkinson's, Diabetes, Epilepsy, Asthma) where these networks have enhanced the quality of life by: (i) reducing the healthcare costs (overcapacity, waiting, sojourn time, number of nurses, etc.), and (ii) providing mobility, while continuously collecting and relaying critical physiological data to their associated healthcare providers, e.g., long-term monitoring of patient recovery from surgical procedure after leaving the hospital, kinematic and rehabilitation assessment.

These types of Personal Area Networks (PAN), while extremely useful, are not without problems such as faulty measurements, hardware failure, and security issues. These networked small, lightweight wireless sensing devices also have additional drawbacks such as reduced computational power and limited capacity and energy resources. Sensor measurements from these networks are prone to a variety of other types of anomalies including environmental noise, constant faults resulting from bad sensor connections, energy depletion, badly placed sensors, malicious attacks through data injection, modification or replay attacks which may cascade and directly affect the collection point leading to unexpected results, faulty diagnosis, and a reduction in public trust of these systems.

Medical sensors with wireless capabilities are available in the market (MICAz, TelosB, Imote2, Shimmer [5], etc.). For example, ECG wireless sensor is connected to three electrodes attached to the chest for real time monitoring of heart problems. The pulse oximeter is used to measure the pulse and blood oxygenation ratio (SpO2), through the use of infrared light and photosensor. These valuable information can be exploited to detect asphyxia, insufficient oxygen (hypoxia) or pneumonia. A normal SpO2 ratio typically exceeds 95 %. When this ratio is lower than 90 %, an emergency alarm must be triggered due to possible lung problems or respiratory failure.

Sensor readings are unreliable and inaccurate [6, 7], due to constrained sensor resources and wireless communication interferences, which make them susceptible to various sources of errors. An improperly attached pulse oximeter clip or an external fluorescent light may cause inaccurate readings. In [3], the authors found that the sensing components were the first source of unreliability in medical WSNs, not networking issues. Faulty measurements from sensors negatively influence the measured results and lead to diagnosis errors. Furthermore, this may threaten the life of a patient after alerting emergency personnel for a code blue.

There may be many reasons for abnormal readings in WSNs [8], such as hardware faults, corrupted sensors, energy depletion, calibration, electromagnetic interference, disrupted connectivity, compromised sensors, data injection, patient with sweating, detached sensor, and heart attacks or some other health degradation, etc. Therefore, an important task is to detect abnormal measurements that deviate from other observations, and to distinguish between sensor faults and emergency situations in order to reduce the false alarm rate.

Over time, these networks accumulate vast amounts of historical data about an individual. Due to the enormity of information, it often becomes difficult to observe and extract sensor metric correlations and to distinguish between a patient entering a critical health state and a faulty sensor component. Therefore, an anomaly detection mechanism is required to identify abnormal patterns and to detect faulty data.

In contrast to signature based intrusion detection systems, where signatures are required to detect attacks, anomaly based systems [9] look for unexpected patterns in data measurements received from sensors. The abnormal pattern is a deviation from a dynamically updated normal model for sensed data, and is more adequate for WSNs given the lack of attack signatures. It is also important to note that anomaly based systems face challenges related to the training phase as it is difficult to find normal data in order to establish an appropriate normal profile.

Various anomaly-based detection techniques for sensor fault identification and isolation have been proposed and applied [9–12]. Distributed detection techniques identify anomalous values at individual sensors to prevent the transmission of erroneous values and reduce energy consumption. These techniques require resources that are not available in the sensors, and their accuracy is lower than centralized approaches, which have global view for spatio-temporal analysis.

Physiological parameters are correlated in time and space, and correlation must be exploited to identify and isolate faulty measurements, in order to ensure reliable operation and accurate diagnosis result. Usually, there is no spatial or temporal correlation among monitored attributes for faulty measurements.

In this chapter, we focus on anomaly detection in medical wireless sensor readings, and we propose a new approach based on machine learning algorithms to detect abnormal values. First we use J48 [13] decision tree algorithm to detect abnormal records, and when detected, we apply linear regression [14] to pinpoint abnormal sensor measurements in an abnormal record. However, physiological attributes are heavily correlated, and changes occur typically in at least two or more parameters, e.g., in Atrial Fibrillation (AF) and Asthma disease, the heart rate and respiration ratio increase simultaneously.

Our proposed solution is intended to provide reliability in medical WSNs used for continuous patient monitoring, where we detect anomalies in a patient's health, and differentiate between the individual entering a critical health state and faulty readings (or sensor hardware). We seek to reduce the false alarm rate triggered by inconsistent sensors readings.

The rest of this chapter is organized as follows. In section "Related Work", we review related work on anomaly detection and machine learning algorithms used in medical WSN. Section "Background" describes briefly linear regression and decision tree algorithm (J48) used in our detection system. The proposed approach is explained in section "Proposed Approach". In section "Experimental Results", we present our results from experimental evaluation, where we conduct a performance analysis of the proposed solution over medical dataset. Finally, section "Conclusion" concludes the chapter with a discussion of the results and future work.

Related Work

WSNs are becoming a major center of interest as they provide a viable solutions to avoid unnecessary casualties in many fields such as military, civil protection or medicine. Various vital sign monitoring systems have been proposed, developed and deployed, such as MEDiSN [4] and CodeBlue [15, 16] for monitoring HR, ECG, SpO2 and pulse, LifeGuard [17] for ECG, respiration, pulse oximeter and BP, AlarmNet [18] and Medical MoteCare [19] for physiological (pulse and SpO2) and environmental parameters (temperature and light), Vital Jacket [20] for ECG and HR. A survey of medical applications using WSNs is available in [21, 22].

However, collected data by WSNs have low quality and poor reliability. Many approaches for anomaly detection in WSNs have been proposed to detect abnormal deviation in collected data, and to remove faulty sensor measurements. Authors in [23] propose an algorithm for the identification of faulty sensors using the minimum and the maximum values of the monitored parameters. Any received measurement outside the [min-max] interval is considered an outlier or inconsistent data. In medical applications, we can not assume that all patients will have the same attribute interval ranges as the min-max values depend on sex, age, weight, height, health condition, etc.

Authors in [24] propose a hierarchical (cluster based) algorithm to detect outliers from compromised or malicious sensors. The proposed method is based on transmission frequency, and KNN distance between received values from different sensors. However, it is impractical in medical applications to put redundant sensors for monitoring the same parameters. A simple prediction and fault detection method for WSNs was proposed in [25]. The proposed algorithm is based on the detection of deviations between the reference and the measured time series. The proposed approach uses a predefined threshold and has been evaluated on the 3 types of faults: short time, long time and constant fault.

Authors in [11] propose a distance based method to identify insider malicious sensors, while assuming neighbor nodes monitoring the same attributes. Each sensor monitors its one hop neighbors and uses Mahalanobis distance between measured and received multivariate instances from neighboring sensors to detect anomalies in a distributed manner. Authors in [26] propose a voting based system to detect such events. Authors in [10] propose a failure detection approach for WSNs, which exploits metric correlations to detect abnormal sensors and to uncover failed nodes.

Authors in [27] explore four classes of methods for fault detection: rule-based, estimation-based, time series analysis, and learning based methods. They investigate fixed and dynamic threshold, linear least squares estimation, Auto Regressive Integrated Moving Average (ARIMA), Hidden Markov Model (HMM), etc. The authors found no best class of detection methods suitable for every type of anomaly.

Data mining techniques and machine learning algorithms have also used in WSNs to detect anomalies in multidimensional data. For example, Naïve Bayes [28], Bayesian network [29], Support Vector Machine (SVM [30]), etc. Authors in [31] propose an approach based on Support Vector Machine (SVM) and k-nearest neighbor (KNN) for anomaly detection in WSNs. Authors in [32] use an unsupervised approach for anomaly detection in WSNs, which is based on Discrete Wavelet Transform (DWT) and Self-Organizing Map (SOM). The DWT is used to reduce the size of input data for SOM clustering.

Authors in [33] propose the use of logistic regression modeling with a static threshold to evaluate the reliability of a WSN in the industrial field with a large number of sensors, and without updating the training model to be able to identify the cause of a potential loss of reliability. On the same scale of large sensor networks, authors in [13] propose a diagnosis method based on the enhanced *C*4.5 (*J*48 or decision tree algorithm) which merges the local classifiers into a large spanning tree to answer for the whole network accuracy. Another type of WSN deployment is presented in [28], which shows how to monitor the physical activity of a person using Sun SpOT sensors attached to the thighs. Authors use naïve Bayes based machine learning algorithm to determine if the person is sitting, standing, lying or walking. However, they do not consider that the values may be corrupted due to faulty hardware. Similarly, the authors in [34] present a system capable of discerning between mental stress states from relaxation states using logistic regression based on the heart rate variability.

In this chapter, we will use decision tree (J48) and linear regression algorithms to detect abnormal records and to pinpoint abnormal sensors reading. J48 is used to classify records and to reduce temporal complexity, and linear regression is used to predict current values. As physiological parameters are correlated, if only one monitored attribute deviates from estimated value, we classify the reading as faulty and perform data cleaning, and in the other cases, we trigger an alarm for patients entering into a critical state.

Background

In this chapter, we consider N medical wireless motes $(S_1, \ldots, S_N)$ attached to patient in order to monitor specific physiological parameters, as depicted in Fig. 8.1. These sensors transmit the collected data to the base station (smart phone) for real time analysis and alerting healthcare professionals when required. The base station may also transmit collected data to a remote/local DB for storage. The base station has higher computational power, memory storage and a greater transmission range than sensors. Collected data is analyzed at the base station before transmission to detect anomalies and raise alarms when a patient enters a critical state.

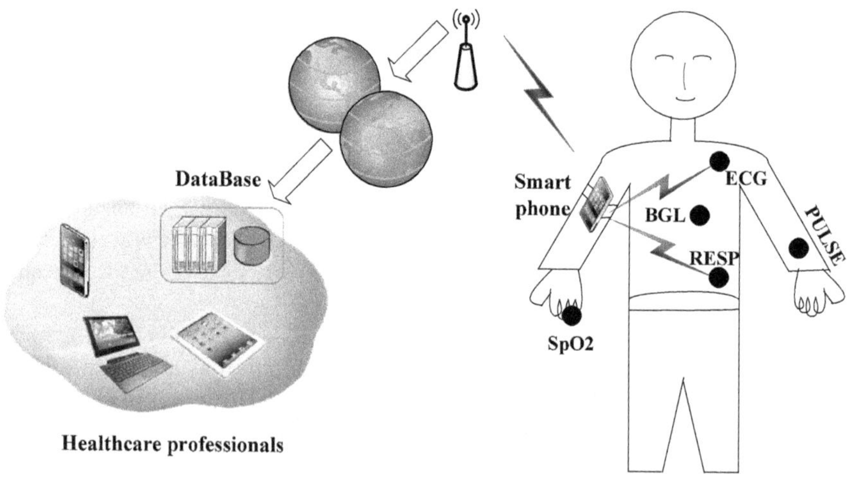

Fig. 8.1 WSN for collecting vital signs and raising alarms

The collected measurements for physiological parameters are represented by the data matrix $X = (X_{ij})$ where i is the time instance, j represents the monitored parameter. We denote by $X_k = (X_{1k}, X_{2k}, \ldots, X_{tk})$ the time series associated with each parameter. X_k is a column in the data matrix X given in Eq. 8.1.

$$X = \begin{matrix} \\ t_1 \\ t_2 \\ \vdots \\ t_m \end{matrix} \begin{matrix} X_1 & X_2 & X_3 & \cdots X_n \\ \left[\begin{matrix} x_{11} & x_{12} & x_{13} & \cdots & x_{1n} \\ x_{21} & x_{22} & x_{23} & \cdots & x_{2n} \\ \vdots & \vdots & \vdots & \ddots & \vdots \\ x_{m1} & x_{m2} & x_{m3} & \cdots & x_{mn} \end{matrix}\right] \end{matrix} \tag{8.1}$$

The collected data on the smart phone must be processed in real time for online anomaly detection. These measurements are probably of low quality and reliability, due to the constrained resources of sensors and the deployment context (sweat, detached, damaged sensor, interrupted communications, etc.). The accuracy of this monitoring system relies on the received data, where faulty measurements trigger false alarms for caregiver. Therefore, to increase the accuracy of diagnosis result, faulty observations must be detected and isolated to reduce the false alarms and to prevent faulty diagnosis.

To detect abnormal values, we use decision tree algorithm (J48) to classify records (or line) as normal or abnormal. When an abnormal record is detected, the linear regression algorithm is used to predict current measurements for each parameter, and when the difference between predicted and current value is larger than the predefined threshold, a correlation analysis is conducted to differentiate between faulty sensor and patient health degradation.

In the rest of this section, we briefly review decision tree (J48) and linear regression algorithms used in our approach. For detailed information about these algorithms, please refer to [14].

Decision Tree J48

J48 [13] is an implementation of the decision tree algorithm C4.5 (proposed by Ross Quinlan), and belongs to the family of the supervised machine learning approaches. Like other decision tree algorithms used in classification, J48 uses training set to generate an optimal tree structure, which will be used to classify the arriving data flow (test set).

The decision tree classification is a process starting at the root of the tree, where each node of the tree is an independent decision that leads to another node, and continues until a leaf node is reached. The leaf nodes represent the outcome of the classification. In our model, the tree nodes are the monitored physiological attributes and the leaf nodes are the class (normal and abnormal).

The decision process in J48 is based on the information carried by each attribute. This information is used by the algorithm to establish a hierarchical classification from root to leafs of the decision tree, and it is represented by the Information Gain $IG(X,X_k)$ in Eq. 8.4:

$$IG(X,X_k) = H(X) - \sum_{x_{ik} \in X} \frac{|x_{ik}|}{|X|} H(x_{ik}) \tag{8.2}$$

Where $H(X)$ is the entropy of the association between a training record (r_i) and the nominal class (normal or abnormal) given in Eq. 8.3, and x_{ik} are the values taken by the attribute X_k.

$$H(X) = \sum_{r_i \in X} p(r_i) \log_2 (\frac{1}{r_i}) \tag{8.3}$$

The attributes with higher Information Gain are placed on the top of the tree, as the most relevant decisions are taken on early for faster classification and to optimize the calculation time. The Information Gain does not take into account the distribution of attribute values between the classes. The Gain Ratio (*GR*) is used to take into account the class splitting factor of each attribute :

$$GR(X,X_k) = \frac{IG(X,X_k)}{SI(X,X_k)} \tag{8.4}$$

Where the Splitting Information is given by:

$$SI(X,x_{ik}) = -\sum_{c=1}^{n} \frac{|x_{ik}|}{|X|} \log_2 \frac{|x_{ik}|}{|X|} \tag{8.5}$$

Where n is the number of classes, and $SI(X,x_{ik})$ is the entropy of the apparition of the x_{ik} within each class. Therefore, by calculating the gain ratio for each attributes, we will be able to hierarchically distribute those attributes into the tree nodes.

Linear Regression

Linear regression is a statistical method which models a dependent variable y_{ik} using a vector of independent variables x_{ik} called regressors. The goal is to predict the value of y_{ik} at time instant t_i given the value of other attributes. The model itself is represented by the following relationship:

$$y_{ik} = C_0 + C_1 x_{i1} + C_2 x_{i2} + \cdots + C_n x_{in} \tag{8.6}$$

Where y_{ik} is the dependent variable, x_{ik} are the regressors and C_n are the coefficients of the regressors (weights). These coefficients are calculated in the training phase as the covariance of X_k and Y_k is divided by the variance of X_k.

$$C_k = \frac{Cov(X_k, Y_k)}{Var(X_k)} = \frac{\sum \left(x_{ik} - \bar{X}_k\right)\left(y_{ik} - \bar{Y}_k\right)}{\sum (x_{ik} - \bar{X}_k)} \tag{8.7}$$

The linear regression is used to predict the value of y_{ik} by using the other attributes in the same instance $x_{ij|j \neq k}$, and to compare the predicted (y_{ik}) with the actual value of x_{ik} to find if it fits within a small margin of error.

Proposed Approach

We consider a general scenario for remote patient monitoring, as shown in Fig. 8.1, where many wireless motes with a restricted resources are used to collect data, and a portable collection device (e.g., smart phone) with higher resources and greater transmission capability than WSN motes, is used to analyze collected data, and to raise alarms for emergency team when abnormal patterns are detected. We seek to detect abnormal values, in order to reduce false alarms resulted from faulty measurements, while differentiating faults from a patient's health degradation.

The proposed approach is based on decision tree and linear regression. It builds a decision tree and looks for linear coefficients from normal vital signs that fall inside restricted interval range of monitored attributes. In the rest of this chapter, we focus only on the following vital signs: HR $\in$ [80 – 120], pulse $\in$ [80 – 120], respiration rate $\in$ [12 – 30], SpO2 $\in$ [90 – 100], T° $\in$ [36.5 – 37.5]. Attributes values that fall outside these (restricted) normal intervals are considered abnormal. HR and pulse reflect the same attribute from different sensors, where pulse is obtained from the pulse oximeter and HR is measured as the number of interbeat intervals (R-R) in ECG signal.

Algorithm 1 Anomaly detection approach

for all received record R_i during T **do**
  Classify R_i using J48;
  if Class(R_i) == '*ABNORMAL*' **then**
    for all x_{ik} **do**
      $\hat{x}_{ik} = \sum_{j=1, j \neq k}^{n} C_j x_{ij}$
      $ctr += \left(\left|x_{ik} - \hat{x}_{ik}\right| \geq 0.1 * \hat{x}_{ik}\right) ?\ 1 : 0$
    end for
    if $ctr \geq 2$ **then**
      Raise alarm for healthcare;
    end if
  end if
end for

Equation 8.8 shows the residual threshold used to detect abnormal measurement:

$$e_i = \left|x_{ik} - \hat{x}_{ik}\right| \geq 0.1 * \hat{x}_{ik} \tag{8.8}$$

The proposed approach is based on two phases: training and detection. In the training phase, machine learning methods generate a model to classify data, and in the testing phase, inputs are classified as abnormal if they deviate from the established model. The J48 decision tree model (built using training data within restricted intervals) is used in our approach to classify each received record as normal or abnormal. In our experiments, the decision tree was the most efficient classification algorithm. The tree model is a set of rules (if-then) which is inexpensive to build, robust, and fast in processing as it is based on numerical comparisons for classification. Furthermore, abnormal instances detected by J48 will only trigger the forecasting with linear regression, and this is why we use restricted small intervals for monitored attributes in the training phase.

If a record is classified as abnormal by J48, we recursively assume that an attribute (x_{ik}) is missing, and the coefficients of linear regression are used to estimate the current value for this attribute ($\hat{x}_{ik}$) with respect to the others ($x_{ij|j \neq k}$), as given in Eq. 8.9 for heart rate estimation:

$$\hat{HR}_i = C_0 + C_1 Pulse_i + C_2 RESP_i + \cdots + C_5 T_i \tag{8.9}$$

If the Euclidian distance between current (HR_i) and estimated ($\hat{HR}_i$) values is larger than the predefined threshold (10 % of estimated value) for only one attribute, the measurement is considered faulty and replaced by estimated value with linear regression. However, if at least two readings are higher than the threshold, we trigger an alarm for response caregiver emergency team to react, e.g., heavy changes in the HR and reduced rate of SpO2 are symptoms of patient health degradation and requires immediate medical intervention. The majority voting is the optimal decision to detect events and correct faults, as the probability of many attributes (2 or more in our experiments) being faulty is very low.

J48 is used to reduce the computation complexity, and to prevent the estimation of each attribute for each instance on the base station. J48 is based on few comparisons for classification, and the combination of both approach for fault detection and classification is used. Sliding windows are not used in our experiments to reduce the complexity. When the model is well specified within the training data, updating or rebuilding the models requires additional complexity (temporal and spatial) without a large impact to the performance.

Experimental Results

In this section, we present the performance analysis results of the proposed approach for anomaly detection in medical WSNs. Afterwards, we conduct an analysis to study the impact of the decision threshold on true positive and false alarm ratios. We used real medical data from the Physionet database [35], which contains 30392 records, and each record contains 12 attributes (ABPmean, ABPsys, ABPdias, C.O., HR, PAPmean, PAPsys, PAPdias, PULSE, RESP, SpO2, T°). We only focus on 5

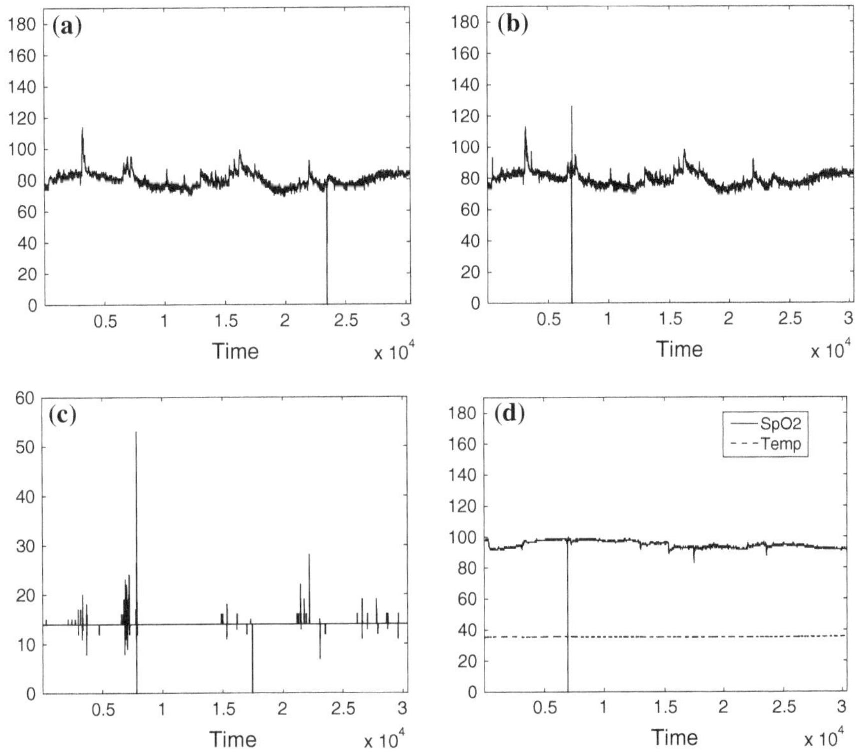

Fig. 8.2 **(a)** Heart Rate (HR), **(b)** Pulse, **(c)** Respiration rate, **(d)** Oxygenation ratio and body temperature

attributes: HR, PULSE, RESP, SpO2 and T°. The variations of Heart Rate (in beat per minute - bpm), Pulse and respiration rate are presented in Fig. 8.2a, b and c respectively. Figure 8.2d shows the variations of SpO2 (oxygenation ratio) and the body temperature (constant value: 37°C).

Figure 8.3a, b shows the predicted and error (difference between actual and predicted) values for HR with linear regression. The measured values of HR (actual) are presented in Fig. 8.2a. To test the efficiency of the used algorithms, we compare the results (predicted and error) with different classifiers using the WEKA [36] toolkit: Decision Table, Additive Regression and KNN for $K = 3$.

Figure 8.3c, d shows the same results (predicted and error respectively) with additive regression tree, where the error is higher than linear regression. Figure 8.4a, b shows the results for KNN which is more computationally expensive (slow) and has an error higher than additive regression. Figure 8.4c, d shows the results of the decision table classifier, which had the worst results of all the classifiers used. Figure 8.5c shows the mean absolute error for each of these classifiers, where decision table achieves the prediction with the highest mean error rate, followed in descending order by KNN, additive and linear Regression. Linear regression had the lowest error

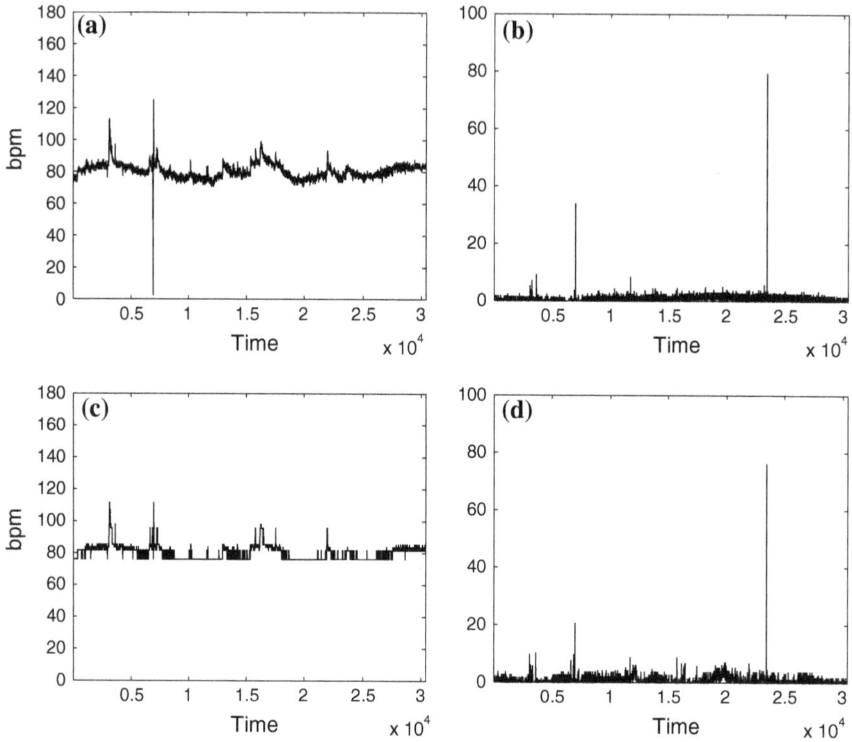

Fig. 8.3 (**a**) Predicted HR using linear regression, (**b**) Errors of prediction, (**c**) Predicted HR using additive regression, (**d**) Errors of prediction

percentage and the best overall performance out of the three classifiers, which is also why we use this classifier in the rest of this chapter.

Figure 8.5a shows the variations of the pulse and the respiration rate. Figure 8.5b shows the raised alarms by our proposed approach. The first alarm is raised when reported values for pulse and SpO2 (Fig. 8.5a) are abnormal in the same instant (both attributes are measured by the same sensor). The second alarm is triggered by the abnormal values of the HR attribute. These abnormal values are visible in Fig. 8.2a, b, c, and d when corresponding attributes suddenly fluctuate or decrease to zero.

To evaluate the performance of the proposed approach, we used the ROC (Receiver Operating Characteristic) to show the relationship between the true positive rate (Eq. 8.10) and the false positive rate (Eq. 8.11).

$$TPR = \frac{TP}{TP + FN} \tag{8.10}$$

Where *TP* is the number of true positives, and *FP* is the number of false positives. The false positive rate (FPR) is defined as:

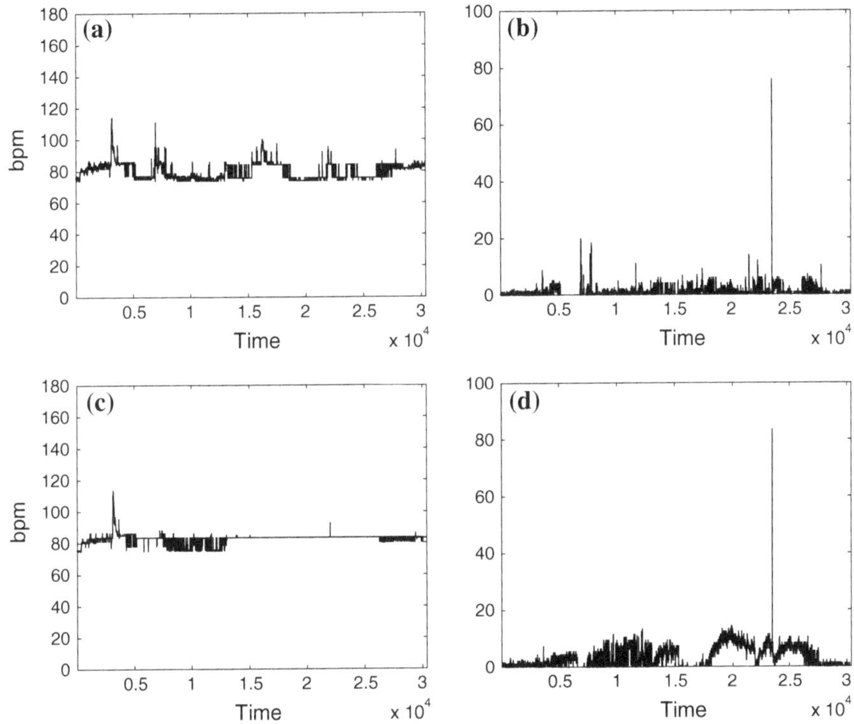

Fig. 8.4 (**a**) Predicted HR using KNN (k=3), (**b**) Errors of prediction, (**c**) Predicted HR using decision table, (**d**) Errors of prediction

$$FPR = \frac{FP}{FP + TN} \tag{8.11}$$

The ROC curve is used for accuracy analysis. A ROC curve is a graphical representation of the true positive rate versus the false positive rate when varying the value of the decision threshold. In general, a good detection algorithm must achieve a high detection ratio with the lowest false alarm rate. Figure 8.5d shows the ROC for the proposed approach where the first nominal classifier is J48, Logistic regression, NaïveBayes and Decision Table respectively. The J48 classifier achieves the best performance with TPR = 100 % and FPR = 7.4 %. These results demonstrate that our proposed approach can achieve very good accuracy for detecting motes anomalies.

Conclusion and Perspectives

In this chapter, we proposed a new framework which integrates decision tree and linear regression for anomaly detection in medical WSNs. The proposed approach achieves both a spatial and temporal analysis for anomaly detection. We have

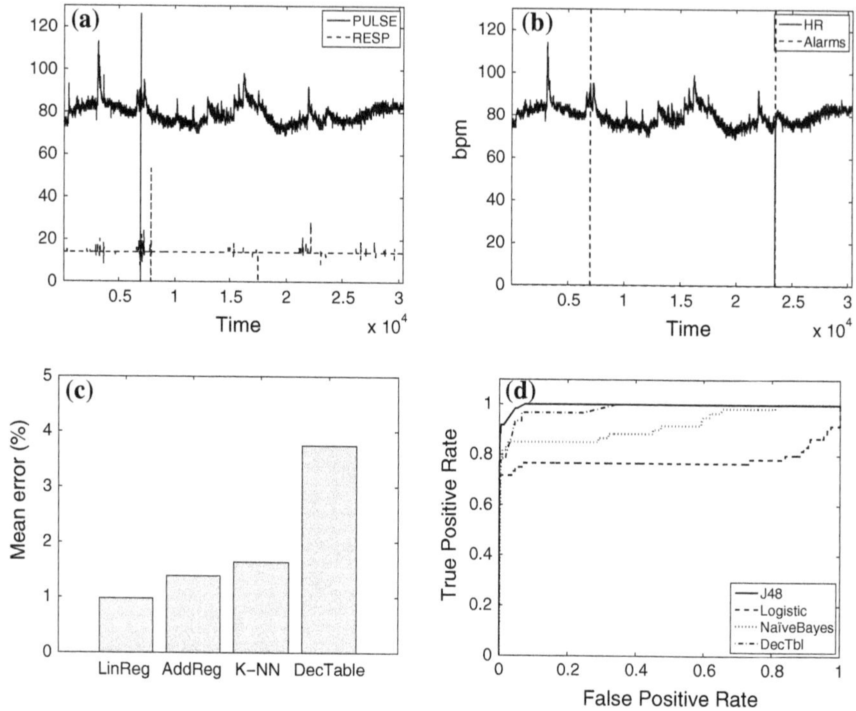

Fig. 8.5 **(a)** Pulse and respiration rate, **(b)** Raised alarms, **(c)** Mean error rate with # classifiers, **(d)** ROC

evaluated our approach on real medical data with many (both real and synthetic) anomalies. Our experimental results demonstrated the capability of the proposed approach to achieve a low false alarm rate with high detection accuracy.

We are currently investigating the performance of the proposed approach on real medical wireless sensor traffic using Shimmer platinum development kit [5]. In the future, knowing that most collected sensor measurements are normal, we look to experiment with data aggregation locally on the sensor motes to reduce the amount of exchanged data between the wireless sensors and the sink node without sacrificing accuracy.

Acknowledgments This research was supported by Korea Science and Engineering Foundation, under the World Class University (WCU) program with additional support from NSF grants CCF-0545488 and OISE-0730065 and the National Science Research Center (CNRS) LaBRI, France.

References

1. Pardeep Kumar and Hoon-Jae Lee. Security Issues in Healthcare Applications Using Wireless Medical Sensor Networks: A Survey. *Sensors*, 12(1):55–91, 2012.
2. JeongGil Ko, Chenyang Lu, Mani B. Srivastava, John A. Stankovic, Andreas Terzis, and Matt Welsh. Wireless Sensor Networks for Healthcare. *Proceedings of the IEEE*, 98(11):1947–1960, 2010.
3. Octav Chipara, Chenyang Lu, Thomas C. Bailey, and Gruia-Catalin Roman. Reliable Clinical Monitoring using Wireless Sensor Networks: Experiences in a Step-down Hospital Unit. In *Proceedings of the 8th ACM Conference on Embedded Networked Sensor Systems (SenSys'10)*, pages 155–168, 2010.
4. JeongGil Ko, Jong Hyun Lim, Yin Chen, Rvazvan Musvaloiu-E, Andreas Terzis, Gerald M. Masson, Tia Gao, Walt Destler, Leo Selavo, and Richard P. Dutton. MEDiSN: Medical Emergency Detection in Sensor Networks. *ACM Transactions on Embedded Computing Systems (TECS)*, 10(1):1–29, 2010.
5. Adrian Burns, Barry R. Greene, Michael J. McGrath, Terrance J. O'Shea, Benjamin Kuris, Steven M. Ayer, Florin Stroiescu, and Victor Cionca. SHIMMER™- A Wireless Sensor Platform for Noninvasive Biomedical Research. *IEEE Sensor Journal*, 10(9):1527–1534, 2010.
6. Honggang Wang, Hua Fang, Liudong Xing, and Min Chen. An Integrated Biometric-based Security Framework Using Wavelet-Domain HMM in Wireless Body Area Networks (WBAN). In *IEEE International Conference on Communications (ICC'11)*, pp. 1–5, 2011.
7. Yang Zhang, N. A. S. Hamm, N. Meratnia, A. Stein, M. van de Voort, and P. J. M. Havinga. Statistics-based outlier detection for wireless sensor networks. *International Journal of Geographical Information Science (GIS)*, 26(8):1373–1392, 2012.
8. Yang Zhang, Nirvana Meratnia, and Paul J. M. Havinga. Outlier Detection Techniques for Wireless Sensor Networks: A Survey. *IEEE Communications Surveys and Tutorials*, 12(2):159–170, 2010.
9. Raja Jurdak, X. Rosalind Wang, Oliver Obst, and Philip Valencia. *Wireless Sensor Network Anomalies: Diagnosis and Detection Strategies*, volume 10, chapter 12, pages 309–325. Springer, 2011.
10. Xin Miao, Kebin Liu, Yuan He, Yunhao Liu, and Dimitris Papadias. Agnostic Diagnosis: Discovering Silent Failures in Wireless Sensor Networks. In *IEEE INFOCOM'11*, pages 1548–1556, 2011.
11. Fang Liu, Xiuzhen Cheng, and Dechang Chen. Insider Attacker Detection in Wireless Sensor Networks. In *IEEE INFOCOM'07*, pages 1937–1945, 2007.
12. Yu-Chi Chen and Jyh-Ching Juang. Outlier-Detection-Based Indoor Localization System for Wireless Sensor Networks. *International Journal of Navigation and Observation*, 2012, 2012.
13. Xu Cheng, Ji Xu, Jian Pei, and Jiangchuan Liu. Hierarchical distributed data classification in wireless sensor networks. *Computer Communications*, 33(12):1404–1413, 2010.
14. Ian H. Witten, Eibe Frank, and Mark A. Hall. *Data Mining: Practical Machine Learning Tools and Techniques (Third Edition)*. Morgan Kaufmann Publishers Inc., 2011.
15. David Malan, Thaddeus Fulford-jones, Matt Welsh, and Steve Moulton. CodeBlue: An Ad Hoc Sensor Network Infrastructure for Emergency Medical Care. In *Proceedings of International Workshop on Wearable and Implantable Body Sensor Networks*, 2004.
16. Havard Sensor Networks Lab. CodeBlue: Wireless Sensors for Medical Care. http://fiji.eecs.harvard.edu/CodeBlue, Last visited January 2013.
17. K. Montgomery, C. Mundt, G. Thonier, A. Thonier, U. Udoh, V. Barker, R. Ricks, L. Giovangrandi, P. Davies, Y. Cagle, J. Swain, J. Hines, and G. Kovacs. Lifeguard - A personal physiological monitor for extreme environments. In *Proceedings of the IEEE 26th Annual International Conference on Engineering in Medicine and Biology Society*, pages 2192–2195, 2004.
18. A. Wood, G. Virone, T. Doan, Q. Cao, L. Selavo, Y. Wu, L. Fang, Z. He, S. Lin, and J. Stankovic. ALARM-NET: Wireless sensor networks for assisted-living and residential monitoring. Technical report, University of Virginia, 2006.

19. Karla Felix Navarro, Elaine Lawrence, and Brian Lim. Medical MoteCare: A Distributed Personal Healthcare Monitoring System. In *International Conference on eHealth, Telemedicine, and Social Medicine (eTELEMED'09)*, pages 25–30, 2009.
20. Jolla P. Silva Cunha, Bernardo Cunha, A. S. Pereira, W. Xavier, N. Ferreira, and L. Meireles. Vital-Jacket®: A wearable wireless vital signs monitor for patients' mobility in cardiology and sports. In *International Conference on Pervasive Computing Technologies for Healthcare, PervasiveHealth*, 2010.
21. Krešimir Grgic, Drago Žagar, and Višnja Križanovic. Medical applications of wireless sensor networks - current status and future directions. *Medicinski Glasnik*, 9(1):23–31, 2012.
22. Hande Alemdar and Cem Ersoy. Wireless sensor networks for healthcare: A survey. *Computer Networks*, 54(15):2688–2710, 2010.
23. Torsha Banerjee, Bin Xie, and Dharma P. Agrawal. Fault tolerant multiple event detection in a wireless sensor network. *Journal of Parallel and Distributed Computing*, 68(9):1222–1234, 2008.
24. Yiying Zhang, Han-Chieh Chao, Min Chen, Lei Shu, Chul hyun Park, and Myong-Soon Park. Outlier Detection and Countermeasure for Hierarchical Wireless Sensor Networks. *IET Information Security*, 2009.
25. Yuan Yao, Abhishek Sharma, Leana Golubchik, and Ramesh Govindan. Online Anomaly Detection for Sensor Systems: A Simple and Efficient Approach. *Performance Evaluation*, 67(11):1059–1075, 2010.
26. Sung-Jib Yim and Yoon-Hwa Choi. An Adaptive Fault-Tolerant Event Detection Scheme for Wireless Sensor Networks. *Sensors*, 10(3):2332–2347, 2010.
27. Abhishek B. Sharma, Leana Golubchik, and Ramesh Govindan. Sensor Faults: Detection Methods and Prevalence in Real-World Datasets. *ACM Transactions on Sensor Networks*, 6(3):1–39, 2010.
28. Xiuxin Yang, Anh Dinh, and Li Chen. Implementation of a Wearerable Real-Time System for Physical Activity Recognition based on Naïve Bayes Classifier. In *International Conference on Bioinformatics and Biomedical Technology (ICBBT'10)*, 2010.
29. Alfonso Farruggia, Lo Re Giuseppe, and Marco Ortolani. Probabilistic Anomaly Detection for Wireless Sensor Networks. In *Proceedings of the 12th international conference on Artificial intelligence around man and beyond*, pages 438–444, 2011.
30. Ajay Singh Raghuvanshi, Rajeev Tripathi, and Sudarshan Tiwari. Machine Learning Approach for Anomaly Detection in Wireless Sensor Data. *International Journal of Advances in, Engineering and Technology*, 1(4):47–61, 2011.
31. Miao Xie, Jiankun Hu, Song Han, and Hsiao-Hwa Chen. Scalable Hyper-Grid k-NN-based Online Anomaly Detection in Wireless Sensor Networks. *IEEE Transactions on Parallel and Distributed Systems*, PP(99):1–11, 2012.
32. Supakit Siripanadorn, Wipawee Hattagam, and Neung Teaumroong. Anomaly Detection in Wireless Sensor Networks using Self-Organizing Map and Wavelets. *International Journal of Communications*, 4(3):74–83, 2010.
33. Fei Huang, Zhipeng Jiang, Sanguo Zhang, and Suixiang Gao. Reliability Evaluation of Wireless Sensor Networks Using Logistic Regression. In *Proceedings of the 2010 International Conference on Communications and Mobile, Computing (CMC'10)*, pp. 334–338, 2010.
34. Jongyoon Choi, Beena Ahmed, and Ricardo Gutierrez-Osuna. Developpement and Evaluation of an Ambulatory Stress Monitor Based on Wearable Sensors. *IEEE Transaction and Information Technology in Biomedicine*, 16(2):279–286, 2012.
35. Physionet. http://www.physionet.org/cgi-bin/atm/ATM.
36. Weka data mining tool. http://www.cs.waikato.ac.nz/~ml/weka/.

Chapter 9
Predicting the Outcome of Antihypertensive Therapy Using Knowledge Mining

Srdjan Sladojevic, Miroslava Sladojevic, Katica Pavlovic, Nada Cemerlic-Adjic and Dubravko Culibrk

Introduction

Arterial hypertension represents the most common non-communicable disease of our time. The prevalence of hypertension varies according to gender and age criteria, but also depends on the geographical, ethnic and racial factors and has the character of an epidemic [1]. Among the adult population, arterial hypertension is considered as one of leading risk factors for the development of atherosclerosis. In a number of epidemiological studies, elevated blood pressure has been identified as a risk factor for heart failure, cerebrovascular disease, peripheral artery disease, renal failure, and, more recently, atrial fibrillation [2, 3].

Observational evidence is also available in support of the fact that blood pressure levels correlate negatively with cognitive function and that hypertension is associated with an increased incidence of dementia [4].

According to the latest data from the World Health Organization (WHO), one in three adults worldwide has raised blood pressure, a condition that causes around half of all deaths from stroke and heart diseases. An estimated 75 million Americans have hypertension. However, blood pressure is controlled and reduced to a healthy level in less than one in three [5]. Globally, hypertension is an even greater problem, with 13.5 % of all deaths attributed to blood-pressure-related diseases. Majority of those who suffer from this affliction belong to lower economic strata [6].

It should be noted that 30 % of adults are not aware that they suffer from hypertension, 40 % of patients with proven hypertension do not follow prescribed therapies, while

S. Sladojevic · D. Culibrk (✉)
Faculty of Technical Sciences, University of Novi Sad, Novi Sad, Serbia
e-mail: dculibrk@uns.ac.rs

M. Sladojevic · K. Pavlovic · N. Cemerlic-Adjic
Clinic of Cardiology, Institute of Cardiovascular Diseases Vojvodina, Sremska Kamenica, Serbia

B. Furht and A. Agarwal (eds.), *Handbook of Medical and Healthcare Technologies*,
DOI: 10.1007/978-1-4614-8495-0_9,

67 % of those undergoing treatment fail to keep the blood pressure values below 140/90 mmHg [7].

The continuous relationship between the blood pressure level and cardiovascular risk makes for a somewhat arbitrary definition of hypertension.

Optimal blood pressure is lower than 120/80 mmHg. Hypertension is defined as a systolic blood pressure of 140 mmHg or higher, or a diastolic blood pressure of 90 mmHg or higher, measured at least twice on separate days [7]. Hypertension is associated with changes in different organ systems of the body, such as left ventricular hypertrophy (LVH), proteinuria and renal failure, retinopathy and vascular dementia, jointly referred to as "target organ damage" (TOD). Although the majority of patients with hypertension remain asymptomatic for decades, a careful early evaluation identifies those with, or at risk of, target organ damage. Early identification of these patients and achieving blood pressure goals could potentially reverse early target organ damage and improve outcome in these patients. The effective management of hypertension is therefore an important primary health care objective in managing cardiovascular and renal disease [1].

In hypertensive patients, the primary goal of treatment is to achieve the maximum reduction in the long-term total risk of cardiovascular morbidity and mortality. This requires treatment of all the reversible risk factors identified, including smoking, dyslipidaemia, abdominal obesity or diabetes, and the appropriate management of associated clinical conditions, as well as treatment of the raised blood pressure *per se* [8]. Latest recommendations suggest that blood pressure should be lowered to <140/90 mmHg at least, and more aggressive antihypertensive treatment should be pursued in diabetic patients, for whom a target blood pressure of <130/80 mmHg appears to be a reasonable one.

Regarding antihypertensive therapy, standard major classes of antihypertensive agents used are:

- Thiazide diuretics,
- Beta-blockers,
- Calcium channel blockers (CCBs),
- ACE inhibitors and
- Angio-tensin-receptor blockers (ARBs).

These agents are suitable for the initiation and maintenance of antihypertensive treatment, whether used separately or combined. A not listed class, Alpha-blockers, could be considered as a therapeutic option, particularly for combination therapy [9].

Knowledge discovery and data mining have achieved numerous successful applications in the domain of medicine over the last 30 years. However, there has not been a widespread adoption of the practice in some fields, such as cardiology, regardless of the potential benefits this could lead to.

This chapter provides a detailed description of a novel study aimed at the development of a predictive model that is able to estimate the success of antihypertensive therapy using data mining techniques. In addition, an extensive overview of the different applications of data mining tools to the domain of cardiology is provided. Using the study as an example, we discuss the particularities involved with the data collection, preprocessing, domain expert involvement and knowledge mining in cardiology.

The study at the focus of this treatise is based on data that has been accumulated during clinical treatments of 388 patients, both men and women (equally distributed), aged 23–86 years. The patients were hospitalized between 2004 and 2008 and were diagnosed with hypertension. Control examinations were performed within the average period of around 6 months after hospitalization by ambulatory, 24 h, blood-pressure monitoring.

The exams yielded a balanced training and testing dataset, containing nearly the same number of successfully and unsuccessfully treated patients. The set contains the same number of men and women, where 58 % of patients regulated blood pressure and 42 % of patients did not. Each instance in the set is described by 385 attributes, which represent patients' personal data, anamnesis, laboratory tests and medical history.

Using a well known, open source data mining tool Waikato Environment for Knowledge Analysis (WEKA) [10], various machine learning algorithms have been applied in order to build a model, which can predict the results of antihypertensive therapy.

Of the various classifiers evaluated, C4.5 decision trees, in the grafted basic version, exhibited the best performance. Thus, a predictive model able to predict success of antihypertensive therapy with over 80 % accuracy has been developed. This level of accuracy justifies the implementation of predictive models in medical practice as this would increase the success of therapy when it comes to patients with hypertension.

The rest of the chapter is organized as follows: Sect. "Related Work" provides an overview of the related work, Sect. "Methodology" presents the methodology, Sect. "Experimental and Results" describes the experiments conducted and the results achieved. Section "Conclusions and Future Directions" holds our conclusions and provides some possible directions for future work.

Related Work

Predicting the outcome of a disease is one of the most interesting and challenging tasks in the field of data mining applications. Very few works have been published on the topic of comparison of classification techniques in different areas before 2002 [11]. Today, there is growing interest of researchers in this area.

Researchers in other fields may not be aware of the particular constraints and difficulties associated with the use of privacy-sensitive, heterogeneous, but voluminous data in medicine. Kryzstof et al. in their paper [12] describe the uniqueness of medical data mining. Ethical and legal aspects of medical data mining are discussed, including data ownership, fear of lawsuits, expected benefits, and special administrative issues. They noticed that medicine is primarily directed at patient-care activity, and only secondarily as a research resource. Thus, it is not easy to collect useful material for research. Also, in the medical data mining, often, one can get unpredictable results because human medical data are at once the most rewarding and difficult of all biological data to mine and analyze. As the authors state: "For an appropriately formulated medical question, finding an answer could mean extending a life, or giving comfort to an ill person. These potential rewards more than compensate for the many extraordinary difficulties along the pathway to success".

In 2008, Sumit Bhatia et al. [13] presented a decision support system for heart disease classification based on Support Vector Machines (SVM) [14] and an integer-coded Genetic Algorithm (GA) [15]. Simple Support Vector Machine (SSVM) algorithm has been used to determine the support vectors in a fast, iterative manner. The integer-coded genetic algorithm was used to select important and relevant features and discard those irrelevant and redundant, in order to maximize SVM's classification accuracy. Genetic algorithms are a family of computational models inspired by evolution. These algorithms encode a potential solution to a specific problem on a simple chromosome like data structure and apply recombination operators to these structures so as to preserve critical information. The heart disease database used in the study included 303 cases and only 13 diagnostic features from the University of California, Irvine (UCI) dataset. This database contains four data sets from the Cleveland Clinic Foundation, Hungarian Institute of Cardiology, V.A. Medical Center and University Hospital of Switzerland. In the Cleveland dataset used in this research, the problem of prediction can be treated as a 2-class problem, where one should predict whether a patient suffers from heart disease or not, or a 5-class problem, where one should predict whether a patient suffers from heart disease, as well as the type of disease. The integer coded genetic algorithm is able to find the optimal feature subset, which maximizes the SVM's classification accuracy and reduces the number of features used for classification. The SSVM algorithm is implemented using the simpleSVM toolkit and the performance of SVM is fine tuned by carrying out a detailed experimentation to determine the effect of different parameters provided with the toolkit. The maximum accuracy is obtained using 'one against one' multi-class SVM with a Radial Basis Function [16] kernel, with a width of 0.025 and penalty factor of 150. The application of the genetic algorithm for feature selection enhanced the performance of the SVM as a 5-class classifier to 72.55 % accuracy, indicating the potential for using the system as a practical decision support system. As a two class problem, the proposed method achieves 90.57 % accuracy, which surpasses that of any other published method on the dataset.

The applications of data mining in this domain are not always restricted to classification. Jinyan Li it et al. [17] tried to find rules in the dataset which could be useful to medical practitioners. They used association rule mining to capture significant dependences between items in transactional datasets. For the Cleveland heart disease dataset they identified a large number of rules with significant support and confidence. Two of the rules found were of particular interest. The first indicated that if the two symptoms, ST-T wave abnormality [18] and exercise-induced angina, appear, then the patients definitely suffer from heart disease of some degree (either slight or serious). The second rule showed that regardless of being male or female and whether suffering from heart disease or not, once the left-hand side symptoms appear, the patients must suffer from a typical angina and their fasting blood sugar is lower than 120 mg/dl. Rules such as this can be of great help to medical practitioners.

Sladojevic et al. [19] used data mining to find relationships and patterns within medical data and to develop new predictive models that are able to estimate the post-therapeutic ECG status of the patient based on the prescribed therapy. Several techniques of data mining have been used to search for relationships in a sample extracted from the clinical database of the Institute of Cardiovascular Diseases, Vojvodina, Serbia, in order to find new useful knowledge which could aid the therapy of patients with hypertension. A predictive model was developed which is able to predict the ECG status of a patient at the control test stage. The best prediction results are achieved by boosting C4.5 [20] decision tree classifiers. They were able to predict the status with 87.52 % accuracy.

Vaithiyanathan et al. [21] proposed a medical decision support system for heart disease risk classification, which is also based on a decision tree classifier. Standard UCI benchmark database of heart disease, literature from journals and expert discussions have contributed to the design of an attribute set for Ischemic Heart disease for the population in India. Their dataset was collected from the Cardio Thoracic Department, Medical College, Chennai, India from January to April 2011. A total of 712 patients examined were classified into 4 classes using a C4.5 decision tree classifier. Pre-processing steps were used to select a dataset pertinent to 662 patients. Their classification problem could be formulated as a 2-class or a 4-class problem, in order to predict whether the disease exists or not, or predict the exact type of disease. The authors conducted their experiments using WEKA and evaluated the performance of their methodology using10-fold cross validation. The achieved accuracy of the 4-cass classifier is 82.33 %. An accuracy of 92.56 % is achieved, when the problem is reduced to 2-class prediction. When evaluated on the UCI Cleveland dataset, their methodology achieved accuracy of 78.91 %.

The application of data mining to the problem of predicting hypertension-related issues has not been explored extensively in the literature. Michael Wozniak in the paper [22] used base and boosted decision trees to achieve diagnosis of the type of hypertension (essential hypertension and five types of secondary ones: fibroplastic renal artery stenosis, atheromatous renal artery stenosis, Conn's syndrome, renal cystic disease and pheochromocystoma). The model based its decision solely on blood pressure values, general information and basic biochemical data. Author compared achieved accuracy for base C4.5 and ADtree [23], as well as their boosted versions in a few experiments. The result of C4.5 was not satisfactory, but the result achieved by boosting of ADtree (83.30 %) was acceptable to the human experts. While Wozniak's approach has some similarity to the approach described in this chapter, the approach presented here deals with the success of hypertensive therapy, rather than diagnosis.

In another study by the same author [24] the development of a hybrid two-stage classifier for the diagnosis of the type of hypertension is proposed, once again focuse on essential hypertension and five types of secondary hypertension: fibroplastic renal artery stenosis, atheromatous renal artery stenosis, Conn's syndrome, renal cystic disease and pheochromocystoma, same as in previous described work. The first step is used to decide if the patient suffers from essential or secondary hypertension. This classification is done using the ADtree algorithm. The second step of classification specifies which type of secondary hypertension the patient is suffering from. The second stage of classification is done using human-expert-specified rules. The classification is once again based solely blood pressure, general information and basis biochemical data. The dataset contained 1425 patients with hypertension, 912 with essential and 513 with secondary, who had been treated in the Hôpital Broussais, Paris, France. Both WEKA and the author's own software were used to train and evaluate the proposed methodology. Once again, 10 fold cross-validation was used, as it is done in the study presented here. For the first stage of classification the best result was achieved by boosting ADTree (83.30 %), while for the second stage, the accuracy of 73.07 % was achieved, using human-expert-specified rules. The author's general conclusion is that boosting does not improve the performance of each classifier in each classification task.

Mevlut et al. [11] evaluated the performance of several classification techniques on the problem of predicting the risk of essential hypertension disease. A retrospective analysis was performed in 694 subjects and the performance of three decision trees, four statistical algorithms, and two neural networks has been compared. In this study, data were analyzed using Answer Tree 2.1, SPSS 10.5, S-plus 6.1 and NeuroSolutions 4.3. The study did not consider any freely available and/or open source software. Predictor variables (attributes) were age, sex, the family history of hypertension, smoking habits, lipoprotein (a), triglyceride, uric acid, total cholesterol and Body Mass Index (BMI). Furthermore, the performance of models was evaluated in terms of sensitivity, specificity, and the predictive rate. The same metrics are used in the study presented in this chapter. Mevlut et al. concluded that, although decision trees and statistical algorithms are capable of extracting patterns and relationships hidden deep in medical datasets, their results are useless when predicting the risk of essential hypertension disease. Neural networks produced the best results, both on the training set and the test set. They concluded RBF and Multi-Layer Perceptron (MLP) [25] neural networks were the techniques of choice to predict hypertension in control groups. They suggested that the use of several different methods should be explored in each specific future study, since the method with the best classification performance may differ from one data set to another. Taking the advice of Mevlut et al. we adopted the approach of evaluating a large number of different algorithms.

Methodology

Among several freely available data mining tools, WEKA is arguably the most popular and has therefore been selected to carry out the experiments conducted within our study.

WEKA is a collection of machine learning algorithms for data mining tasks. The algorithms can either be run using WEKA's graphical user interface or invoked within Java code. WEKA contains tools for data pre-processing, classification, regression, clustering, association rules mining, as well data visualization. It also facilitates the development of new machine learning schemes [26].

WEKA is open source software issued under the GNU General Public License. It allows its users to perform the necessary experiments efficiently and enables the subsequent realization of practical systems for prediction and classification [10].

Data Collection

The first step of any data mining study is to prepare the dataset, which will be used for model training and validation. Most clinical information systems still lack options to export data in a format compatible with data mining tools available. Data is dispersed across different databases and tables. Some of the data is confidential and confidential parameters need to be encrypted before they can be used. A major problem is that medical practitioners still mostly store data using Microsoft Excel or Word documents, making it hard to perform automatic extraction of relevant features. Even in clinical information systems, a lot of information pertinent to a patient, such as anamnesis and previous diseases, is stored in blob fields and there is no way to automatically retrieve features for the dataset. The medical information systems are still fragmented across institutions and some data is still stored on paper and has to be manually entered into datasets, especially in developing countries.

When creating the dataset used in this study the following procedure was used:

- Relevant database tables within the clinical information system were filtered to extract data of interest, e.g. for the specific period, type of disease etc. They were exported as Microsoft Excel files.
- The Excel files were imported into a new database to enable to facilitate further processing.
- Tables and fields were de-normalized in order to get one joint table with redundant data, which could later be converted to files compatible with WEKA. WEKA supports its native format 'arff' or Comma Separated Values (CSV) files.
- For multi-valued attributes the values were binarized. For each of the multiple values, a new binary attribute was created to indicate the presence of the value in an instance. The reason behind this is in the fact that some of the data could not

be de-normalized in a straight forward manner. Consider, for instance, the therapy information used in this study. Each patient can have more than one therapy prescribed. In the joint table this information could not be represented by a single field, without violating the requirement of having a single row per patient (instance). Therefore, the therapy information attribute had to be binarized, yielding 260 new attributes, each describing the use of a single type of therapy for a patient. The attributes' values were 'YES' or 'NO' and indicated whether the patient received that therapy or not.
- The final joint table was exported to a CSV file.
- ARFF header was subsequently added to the file, containing the specification of the names of all attributes and their types. As WEKA requires all possible values to be specified for categorical attributes, database queries were used to identify these.

Pre-Processing Data

Data pre-processing is an important step in the knowledge discovery process, since high-quality decisions must be based on high-quality data. Detecting data anomalies, rectifying them early, and reducing the amount of data to be analyzed can lead to huge payoffs for decision making.

Datasets often contain errors or missing values. Data-input methods are often loosely controlled, resulting in out-of-range values (e.g., blood sugar value of 123), impossible data combinations (e.g., gender: Male, pregnant: Yes), etc. Analysis of data that has not been carefully screened for such problems can produce misleading results. Thus, ensuring the quality of data is first and foremost requirement for quality knowledge discovery [27].

In medical studies, data pre-processing is usually done manually, as the datasets are commonly relatively small. In the study presented in this chapter, several actions were performed on the initial dataset. Incomplete rows with a lot of attributes missing were removed from the dataset. Noisy rows containing errors or outlier values that deviate significantly from the expected were removed. Consistency of data was improved by ensuring that the dataset does not contain attributes with different values having the same semantics. Some aggregate attributes were added to the dataset, such as the total number of patient's visits to the hospital.

After the pre-processing, the dataset contained data pertinent to 388 patients.

Machine Learning Algorithms

WEKA includes implementations of a large number of algorithms and machine learning approaches [28]. Several of these algorithms are of interest when it comes to the research presented in this chapter (listed by their WEKA denominations): ADTree, RandomTree, J48, J48graft, IB1, KStar, NaiveBayes, DecisionStump, AdaBoost and CostSensitiveClassifier.

Decision trees have widespread application, when it comes to classification in medicine. A decision tree is a non-linear discrimination method, which uses a set of independent variables to split a sample into progressively smaller subgroups. The procedure is iterative at each branch in the tree. It selects the independent variable that has the strongest association with the dependent variable according to a specific criterion. A large number of algorithms for decision tree construction exist.

Decision stump induction is an algorithm designed to build a simple one-level binary decision tree with an extra branch for missing values [28]. As it has limited capabilities, it is usually used in combination with boosting.

C4.5 [20] builds decision trees from a set of training data, using the concept of information entropy. The training data is a set of already classified samples. Each sample consists of a p-dimensional vector, where each element represents attributes or features of the sample, as well as the class in which sample falls. At each node of the tree, C4.5 chooses the attribute of the data that most effectively splits its set of samples into subsets enriched in one class or the other. The splitting criterion is the normalized information gain (difference in entropy). The attribute with the highest normalized information gain is chosen to make the decision. The C4.5 algorithm then iteratively continues on the subsets. J48 is an open source Java implementation of the C4.5 algorithm, available within the WEKA data mining tool.

Decision tree *grafting* adds nodes to an existing decision tree with the objective of reducing the error of prediction. The grafting algorithm considers a single set of training data for each leaf of the initial decision tree, consisting of a set of cases that fail at most one test on the path to the leaf. In this manner, new branches that can be added productively to the tree are identified. Then they are grafted to the existing tree to improve the decision making process. Grafting can be done by adding new branches in place of single leafs or by grafting them within leaves. *Pruning* and grafting are complementary methods to improve the decision tree.

Pruning is a technique in machine learning that reduces the size of decision trees by removing sections of the tree that provide little power to classify instances. The dual goal of pruning is reduced complexity of the final classifier as well as better predictive accuracy by the reduction of overfitting and removal of sections of a classifier that may be based on noisy or erroneous data.

Pruning allows cutting parts of decision trees to provide for better generalization, while grafting adds nodes to the decision trees to increase the predictive accuracy. J48graft is the WEKA implementation of a machine learning algorithm for generating a grafted (pruned or unpruned) C4.5 decision tree [29].

AdaBoost is an implementation of a meta-learning algorithm based on the approach of Freund and Schapire [30]. Boosting is a general method for improving the accuracy of any given learning algorithm. It is based on a well-known methodology for combining multiple models by explicitly seeking models that complement one another. AdaBoost is adaptive in the sense that subsequent classifiers built are tweaked in favor of those instances misclassified by previous classifiers. While it is sensitive to noisy data and outliers, it can be less susceptible to the overfitting problem than most learning algorithms, in some problems. The classifiers it uses can be weak (i.e., display a substantial error rate), but as long as their performance is not random (resulting in an error rate of less than 0.5 for binary classification), they will improve the final model. Even classifiers with an error rate higher than what would be expected from a random classifier will be useful, since they will have negative coefficients in the final linear combination of classifiers and hence behave like their inverses. AdaBoost generates and invokes a new weak classifier in each of a series of its iterations. After each classifier execution, a distribution of weights is updated that indicates the importance of examples in the data set for the classification. In each iteration, the weights of incorrectly classified examples are increased and the weights of correctly classified examples are decreased, so the new classifier focuses on the examples which have so far eluded correct classification.

Alternating Decision Tree (ADtree) [31] is a machine learning method for classification which generalizes decision trees and is associated to boosting. Boosting algorithms typically use either decision stumps or decision trees as weak hypotheses. As an example, boosting decision stumps creates a set of T weighted decision stumps (where T is the number of boosting iterations), which then vote on the final classification according to their weights. Individual decision stumps are weighted according to their ability to classify the data. Boosting a simple learner results in an unstructured set of T hypotheses, is making it difficult to infer correlations between attributes. Alternating decision trees introduce structure to the set of hypotheses by requiring that they build off a hypothesis that was produced in an earlier iteration. The resulting set of hypotheses can be visualized in a tree based on the relationship between a hypothesis and its "parent". As in boosting, the data is given a different distribution in each iteration. Once again, instances that are misclassified are given a larger weight while accurately classified instances are given reduced weight. An alternating decision tree consists of decision nodes and prediction nodes. Decision nodes specify a predicate condition. Prediction nodes contain a single numeric value. ADTrees always have prediction nodes as both root and leaves. An instance is classified by an ADTree by following all paths for which all decision nodes are true and summing any prediction nodes that are traversed. This is different from binary classification trees such as CART (Classification and regression tree) [32] or C4.5 in which an instance follows only one path through the tree.

RandomTree is used for constructing a tree that considers K randomly chosen attributes at each node. No pruning is performed in this case [28].

Random forest [33] is an ensemble classifier that consists of many random decision trees and outputs the class that is the mode (majority vote) of the classes output by individual trees. The algorithm for inducing a random forest was developed by

Breiman and Cutler. To classify a new object from an input vector, the input vector is propagated down each of the trees in the forest. Each tree gives a classification—the tree "votes" for that class. The forest chooses the classification having the most votes (over all the trees in the forest). It is one of the most accurate learning algorithms available. For many data sets, it produces a highly accurate classifier [34].

IB1 and KStar are instance-based, so-called "lazy learners", since they store the training instances and do no real work until classification time. IB1 is a basic instance-based learner [35]. It uses a simple distance measure to find the training instance closest to the given test instance, and predicts the same class as this training instance. If multiple instances are the same (smallest) distance to the test instance, the first one found is used.

KStar is a nearest-neighbour method with a generalized distance function based on transformations, proposed by Cleary and Trigg [36]. It is an instance-based classifier and the class of a test instance is determined based on the class of training instances similar to it, as determined by the distance function.

NaiveBayes algorithm implements the probabilistic Naive Bayes classifier [37]. It is widely used in medical data mining experiments. In simple terms, a Naive Bayes classifier assumes that the presence (or absence) of a particular feature of a class is unrelated to the presence (or absence) of any other feature, given the class variable. A Naive Bayes classifier considers all these features to contribute independently to the probability that an instance is a member of a certain class, whether or not they're in fact related to each other or to the existence of the other features.

For certain types of probability models, Naive Bayes classifiers can be trained very efficiently in a supervised learning setting. In many practical applications, parameter estimation for Naive Bayes models uses the method of maximum likelihood. In other words, one can work with the Naive Bayes model without believing in Bayesian probability or using any Bayesian methods.

When the input dataset is unbalanced, as it is the case in the study presented, *cost-sensitive* [38] classification is typically applied to achieve reliable prediction of the minority-class instances. By default, WEKA treats all types of classification errors equally. However, in many practical cases, this is not a good approach. Cost-sensitive classification allows one to assign different costs to different types of misclassification [39]. In WEKA this is done by creating a cost matrix [28].

Results and Performance

Different metrics can be used to evaluate the performance of data mining algorithms.

For classification tasks, the terms true positives, true negatives, false positives, and false negatives compare the results of classification on a test set with true data obtained

Table 9.1 Confusion matrix

	Actual class (observation)	
Predicted class (expectation)	tp (true positive)	fp (false positive)
	fn (false negative)	tn (true negative)

from external sources. The terms positive and negative refer to the classifier prediction, and the terms true and false refer to whether that prediction corresponds to the real classification (sometimes known as the observation). This is illustrated in Table 9.1:

In a classification task, the *precision* of classification for a class is the number of true positives (i.e., the number of items correctly labeled as belonging to the positive class) divided by the total number of elements labeled as belonging to the positive class (i.e., the sum of true positives and false positives, which are items incorrectly labeled as belonging to the class). *Recall* in this context is defined as the number of true positives divided by the total number of elements that actually belong to the positive class (i.e., the sum of true positives and false negatives, which are items which were not labeled as belonging to the positive class but should have been). Therefore, precision and recall equations are calculated as (9.1)

$$\begin{aligned} \mathrm{Pr}ecision &= \frac{tp}{tp+fp} \\ \mathrm{Re}call &= \frac{tp}{tp+fn} = Sensitivity \end{aligned} \tag{9.1}$$

Recall is sometimes referred to as the True Positive Rate or Sensitivity, and precision is also referred to as Positive predictive value (PPV). Other related measures used in classification include True Negative Rate and Accuracy. True Negative Rate is also called Specificity. The specificity and accuracy are calculated as (9.2):

$$\begin{aligned} Specificity &= \frac{tn}{tn+fp} \\ Accuracy &= \frac{tp+tn}{tp+tn+fp+fn} \end{aligned} \tag{9.2}$$

Accuracy is widely used for presenting and evaluation results.

The area under the ROC (Receiver Operating Characteristics) curve, or simply AUC, has been traditionally used in medical diagnosis since the 1970s. It has more recently been proposed as an alternative single-number measure for evaluating the predictive ability of learning algorithms [40].

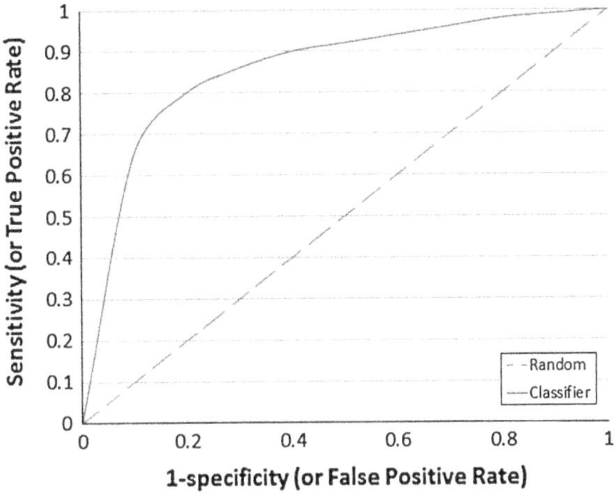

Fig. 9.1 Sample ROC *curve*

The area under the ROC curve reflects the relationship between sensitivity and specificity for a given test. High-quality tests will have an AUC-ROC approaching 1, and high-quality publications about clinical tests will provide information about the AUC-ROC. Cutoff values for positive and negative tests can influence specificity and sensitivity, but they do not affect AUC-ROC.

We used both accuracy and AUC to evaluate the performance of algorithms in the study presented here. Figure 9.1 shows a sample ROC curve.

Experiments and Results

The data used in the study was obtained for 388 patients who were hospitalized in the Clinic of Cardiology of the Institute of Cardiovascular Diseases of Vojvodina, situated in Sremska Kamenica, Serbia. The data was collected between 2004 and 2008 for patients diagnosed with arterial hypertension. Patients with previous diagnoses of ischemic heart disease were removed from the collected data, in order to create a dataset restricted to patients with hypertension as sole and primary cardiology disease.

The sample contains equal number of men and women, aged from 23 to 86 years, with the mean age of 60.34 and standard deviation of 10.23. The age distribution of patients is shown in Table 9.1. The clinical information system stores diverse information about the patients and their medical conditions, such as patient's medical history, previous therapies, risk factors, patient's social status etc.

In the study, each patient was described with 385 attributes. Each patient was initially described using 106 attributes which include: demographic and clinical

Table 9.2 Age distribution of patients in the sample

	Age of patient	Number of patients	% of dataset
1	23.000–27.846	2	0.515
2	27.846–32.692	2	0.515
3	32.692–37.538	4	1.030
4	37.538–42.385	7	1.804
5	42.385–47.231	23	5.928
6	47.231–52.077	49	12.629
7	52.077–56.923	45	11.598
8	56.923–61.769	77	19.845
9	61.769–66.615	69	17.783
10	66.615–71.462	55	14.175
11	71.462–76.308	38	9.793
12	76.308–81.154	14	3.608
13	81.154–86.000	3	0.773

characteristics, biochemical analysis of blood parameters and diagnosis codes. The first 13 attributes represent general information, such as patient personal data (age, sex, marital status, occupation, and social status) and anamnesis data (risk factors, systolic blood pressure on reception, and diastolic blood pressure on reception). Parameters from blood analysis on reception and on release of patient were represented by 53 attributes. Previous diagnoses of the patient were represented by 58 binary attributes, while certain therapies for regulating blood pressure were represented by further 260 of such attributes.

The dependent variable we are trying to predict is the class in terms of the success of antihypertensive therapy, represented with two labels: 'YES' for successful antihypertensive therapy, otherwise 'NO'.
On average, control examinations were performed about 6 months after the hospitalization by ambulatory 24 h blood pressure and ECG monitoring.

The sample contained 226 patients (58.24 %) who regulated blood pressure and 162 patients who did not (41.76 %). Figure 9.2 shows the distribution of the classes over age groups, where patients who regulated their blood pressure are indicated in black and those that did not in grey.

Machine Learning Algorithm Evaluation

We evaluated a number of algorithms available within WEKA as predictors of antihypertensive therapy: DecisionTable, RandomTree, J48 (C4.5), J48graft, Lazy IB1 and Lazy Kstar, NaiveBayes, and DecisionStump Boosting—(AdaBoostM1). Cost sensitive classification was explored as an additional methodology to enhance results.

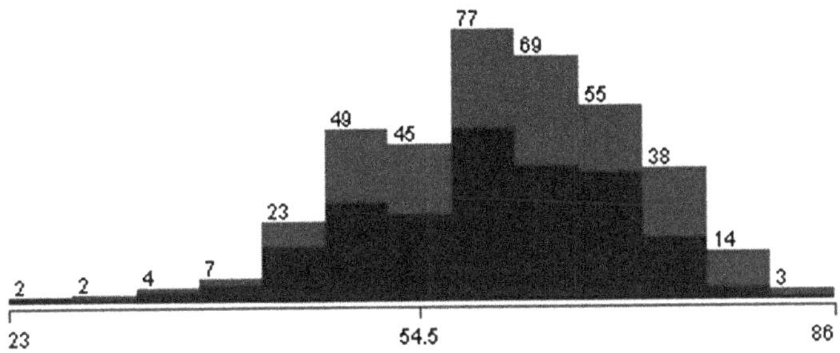

Fig. 9.2 Class distribution over different age groups

Table 9.3 Evaluation results

Algorithm	Accuracy (%)	AUC parameter
Decision stump boosting	71.65	0.692
Lazy.IB1	65.20	0.603
Lazy.KStar	56.70	0.523
Random tree	66.75	0.678
Random forest	72.93	0.783
Naive bayes	73.71	0.745
ADtree	70.10	0.700
J48	79.89	0.761
J48graft	80.92	0.767
J48graft tuned	81.70	0.794

Table 9.4 Cost matrix used

0	1.5
3	0

The performance of algorithms was assessed using cross-validation. The process consists of withholding a randomly-selected part of the data for testing and using the rest to train the algorithm. This is repeated n times with a different testing and training subset. Thus, multiple rounds of cross-validation are performed using different partitions and the validation results are averaged over the rounds [10]. When n iterations are performed, the process is referred to as n-fold cross-validation, as the dataset has been "folded" n times. The number of folds is usually kept between 3 and 10. We used 10-fold cross-validation, which is the default value in WEKA.

The results, in terms of accuracy and AUC, achieved by different algorithms are shown in Table 9.3. As the table shows, C4.5-based decision trees performed significantly better than other algorithms evaluated.
The predictive model based on J48graft is able to predict the success of antihypertensive therapy with more than 80 % accuracy (80.92 %). The AUC parameter achieved was 0.767.

Table 9.5 Confusion matrix for the best results experiment

A	B	
209	17	a = YES
54	108	b = NO

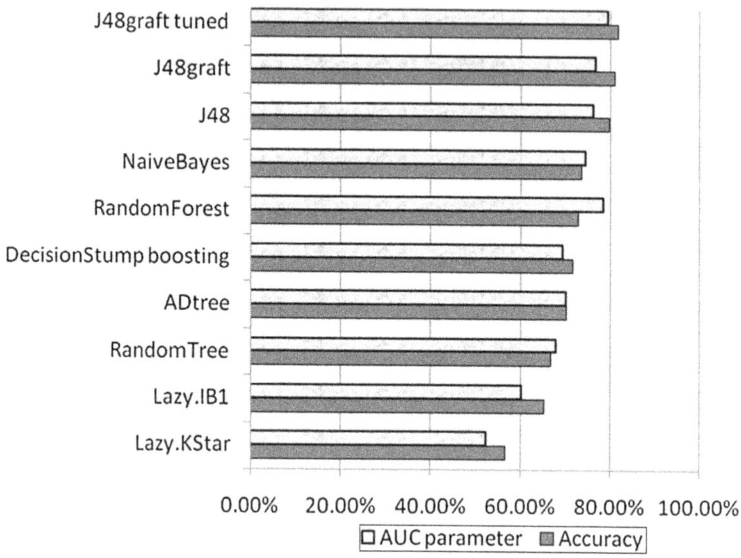

Fig. 9.3 AUC and accuracy of different classifiers

Since the dataset is slightly unbalanced it was reasonable to try to tweak the results by adjusting the cost matrix values. This yielded a small improvement over the base classifier. Applying cost matrix provided in Table 9.4 as input for WEKA CostSensitiveClassifier produced the classification result represented by a confusion matrix shown in Table 9.5.

As the table shows 317 (81.70 %) instances are classified correctly, while 71 (18.30 %) were classified incorrectly. The AUC obtained is 0.794.

Figure 9.3 provides a comparison between the AUC and the achieved accuracy for all the learning algorithms.

Figure 9.4 shows the ROC curve obtained for J48graft. The ROC is evaluated using the results obtained for each fold of cross-validation.

The resulting tree obtained from the J48graft algorithm is shown in Fig. 9.5. All attributes that have been selected as important predictors are listed in the figure. The child nodes of each node are indicated by indenting them.

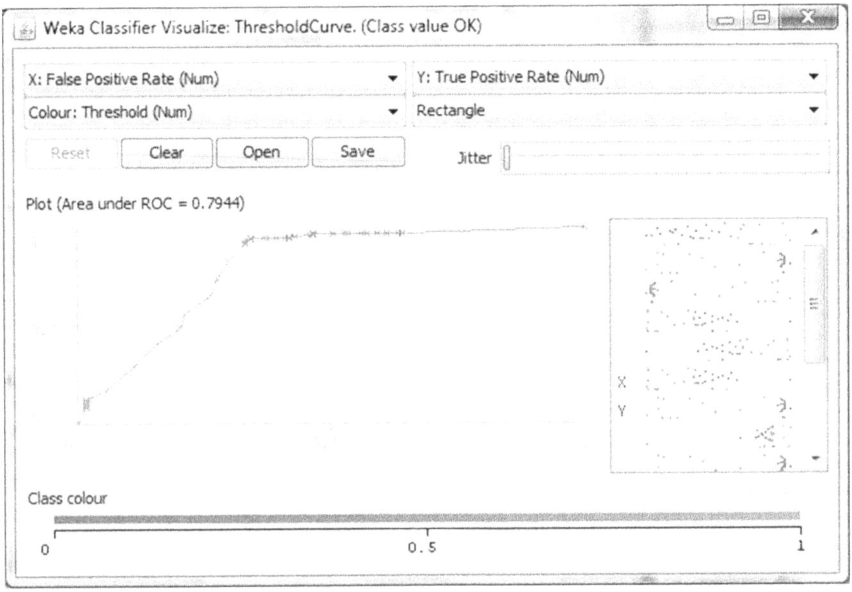

Fig. 9.4 AUC obtained for J48graft

Table 9.6 Laboratory parameters which affect prediction results

	Attribute	Attribute meaning
1	LABP70	Leukocytes (WBC)
2	LABP110	Total cholesterol
3	LABP170	Blood sugar
4	LABP270	AST

The predictive model developed relies on 32 attributes to reach its decision. These are the predictors that affect the outcome of antihypertensive therapy the most. They are to a large extent attributes related to those therapies, which were expected to have biggest impact on the outcome. However, some laboratory parameters and previous diagnoses have also been selected by the machine learning algorithms and deserve to be analyzed in more detail.

The decision tree included 4 attributes from the group of laboratory parameters, shown in Table 9.6.
It was expected that some of laboratory test values will affect the prediction results. The ties between them and hypertension are already known. WBC count is an important risk factor for hypertension, and the increased risk for hypertension associated with WBC count is more pronounced in non-smokers [41].

Since cardiovascular risk is high in hypertensive patients with the metabolic syndrome, it would appear advisable to pursue a rigorous blood pressure control in such cases, i.e., to lower blood pressure to values less than the high normal ones that are

```
LERCANIL10MG = NO
|   DIUNORM25MG = NO
|   |   AMLOPIN5MG = NO
|   |   |   INDAPRESSR1Z5MG = NO
|   |   |   |   MYCOSEB200MG = NO
|   |   |   |   |   METHYLDOPA250MG = NO
|   |   |   |   |   |   TRITACE5MG = NO
|   |   |   |   |   |   |   YURINEX1MG = NO
|   |   |   |   |   |   |   |   ZORKAPTIL12Z5MG = NO
|   |   |   |   |   |   |   |   |   NORVASC5MG = NO
|   |   |   |   |   |   |   |   |   |   GLUFORMIN500MG = NO
|   |   |   |   |   |   |   |   |   |   |   DAONIL5MG = NO
|   |   |   |   |   |   |   |   |   |   |   |   PRILAZIDPLUS5P125MG = NO
|   |   |   |   |   |   |   |   |   |   |   |   |   INDAPAMID2Z5MG = NO: OK (261.0/45.0)
|   |   |   |   |   |   |   |   |   |   |   |   |   INDAPAMID2Z5MG = YES
|   |   |   |   |   |   |   |   |   |   |   |   |   |   AMLOPIN10MG = NO: NO (4.0)
|   |   |   |   |   |   |   |   |   |   |   |   |   |   AMLOPIN10MG = YES: OK (2.0)
|   |   |   |   |   |   |   |   |   |   |   |   PRILAZIDPLUS5P125MG = YES
|   |   |   |   |   |   |   |   |   |   |   |   |   LABP270 <= 33.5
|   |   |   |   |   |   |   |   |   |   |   |   |   |   LABP170 <= 4.75: OK (0.0|14.0)
|   |   |   |   |   |   |   |   |   |   |   |   |   |   LABP170 > 4.75
|   |   |   |   |   |   |   |   |   |   |   |   |   |   |   AGE <= 43.5: OK (0.0|13.0)
|   |   |   |   |   |   |   |   |   |   |   |   |   |   |   AGE > 43.5
|   |   |   |   |   |   |   |   |   |   |   |   |   |   |   |   OCCUPATION =OtherCraftsmen: OK (0.0|19.0/1.0)
|   |   |   |   |   |   |   |   |   |   |   |   |   |   |   |   OCCUPATION !=OtherCraftsmen
|   |   |   |   |   |   |   |   |   |   |   |   |   |   |   |   |   LABP70 <= 11.05
|   |   |   |   |   |   |   |   |   |   |   |   |   |   |   |   |   |   LOMETAZID10P5MG = YES: OK (0.0|46.0/6.0)
|   |   |   |   |   |   |   |   |   |   |   |   |   |   |   |   |   |   LOMETAZID10P5MG != YES
|   |   |   |   |   |   |   |   |   |   |   |   |   |   |   |   |   |   |   MONOPRIL10MG = YES: OK (0.0|78.0/12.0)
|   |   |   |   |   |   |   |   |   |   |   |   |   |   |   |   |   |   |   MONOPRIL10MG != YES
|   |   |   |   |   |   |   |   |   |   |   |   |   |   |   |   |   |   |   |   GENDER = Z: OK (0.0|132.0/24.0)
|   |   |   |   |   |   |   |   |   |   |   |   |   |   |   |   |   |   |   |   GENDER != Z: NO (2.0)
|   |   |   |   |   |   |   |   |   |   |   |   |   |   |   |   |   LABP70 > 11.05: OK (0.0|24.0/2.0)
|   |   |   |   |   |   |   |   |   |   |   |   |   LABP270 > 33.5: OK (0.0|16.0)
|   |   |   |   |   |   |   |   |   |   |   DAONIL5MG = YES
|   |   |   |   |   |   |   |   |   |   |   |   I652121N = YES: OK (2.33/0.33)
|   |   |   |   |   |   |   |   |   |   |   |   I652121N = NO: NO (4.67)
|   |   |   |   |   |   |   |   |   |   GLUFORMIN500MG = YES
|   |   |   |   |   |   |   |   |   |   |   LABP70 <= 8.3: NO (6.43)
|   |   |   |   |   |   |   |   |   |   |   LABP70 > 8.3: OK (2.57/0.57)
|   |   |   |   |   |   |   |   |   NORVASC5MG = YES
|   |   |   |   |   |   |   |   |   |   LABP270 <= 33.5
|   |   |   |   |   |   |   |   |   |   |   LABP170 <= 4.75: OK (0.0|14.0)
|   |   |   |   |   |   |   |   |   |   |   LABP170 > 4.75
|   |   |   |   |   |   |   |   |   |   |   |   LABP110 <= 4.05: OK (0.0|14.0)
|   |   |   |   |   |   |   |   |   |   |   |   LABP110 > 4.05: NO (7.0/1.0)
|   |   |   |   |   |   |   |   |   |   LABP270 > 33.5: OK (0.0|16.0)
|   |   |   |   |   |   |   |   ZORKAPTIL12Z5MG = YES: NO (8.0/1.0)
|   |   |   |   |   |   |   YURINEX1MG = YES
|   |   |   |   |   |   |   |   AGE <= 43.5: OK (0.0|13.0)
|   |   |   |   |   |   |   |   AGE > 43.5
|   |   |   |   |   |   |   |   |   OCCUPATION =OtherCraftsmen: OK (0.0|19.0/1.0)
|   |   |   |   |   |   |   |   |   OCCUPATION !=OtherCraftsmen
|   |   |   |   |   |   |   |   |   |   E780 = YES: OK (0.0|43.0/5.0)
|   |   |   |   |   |   |   |   |   |   E780 != YES: NO (2.0)
|   |   |   |   |   |   TRITACE5MG = YES: NO (4.0)
|   |   |   |   |   METHYLDOPA250MG = YES: NO (14.0/1.0)
|   |   |   |   MYCOSEB200MG = YES: NO (4.0)
|   |   |   INDAPRESSR1Z5MG = YES: NO (7.0)
|   |   AMLOPIN5MG = YES: NO (7.0)
|   DIUNORM25MG = YES: NO (21.0/1.0)
LERCANIL10MG = YES: NO (29.0)
```

Fig. 9.5 J48graft decision tree

a common component of the syndrome [42]. One of the most important attributes, identified in this study, is the total plasma cholesterol. The recommended target levels are <5 mmol/L (less than ~190 mg/dL) for total plasma cholesterol and <3 mmol/L (less than ~115 mg/dL) for LDL cholesterol for subjects at low or moderate risk [43]. There are no differences in the beneficial effects of cholesterol lowering between men and women and between younger and older age groups, even individuals [44].

Individuals with hypertension commonly have other risk factors for cardiovascular diseases as such diabetes, insulin resistance, dyslipidaemia and target organ damage. Because risk factors may interact, the overall risk of hypertensive patients is increased, although the blood pressure elevation is only mild or moderate [9]. Based on the above, it is reasonable for the blood glucose to appear as one of the predictors in the presented study. The normal value for blood glucose is 5.5–6.9 mmol/L. Intensive glycogenic control significantly reduces the total number of major macrovascular events (death from cardiovascular causes, non-fatal myocardial infarction, nonfatal stroke) and major microvascular events (new or worsening nephropathy or retinopathy), but only the reduction in microvascular events is statistically significant [45].

Aspartate aminotransferase (AST) is an enzyme associated with liver parenchymal cells. AST is found in the liver, heart, skeletal muscle, kidneys, brain, and red blood cells. It is commonly measured clinically as a part of diagnostic liver function tests, to determine liver health, but may also be elevated due to diseases affecting other organs, such as myocardial infarction, acute pancreatitis, acute hemolytic anemia, severe burns, acute renal disease, musculoskeletal diseases, and trauma. It has been shown to be a marker for chronic alcoholism [46]. Jeanne and Clarc at al. in their work [47] showed that in both men and women, unexplained aminotransferase elevation was significantly associated with higher body mass index, waist circumference, triglycerides, fasting insulin, and lower HDL, as well as with type 2 diabetes and hypertension in women. Not surprisingly, the dataset used in our study contains more women with higher AST values.

When it comes to previous diagnoses, the identified important predictors are listed in Table 9.7.

Once again, it is not surprising that these diagnoses affect the outcome of therapies. Previous genetic and pathological studies, as well as observational and interventional studies, have established the crucial role of dyslipidaemia, especially hypercholesterolaemia, in the development of cardiovascular disease.

Regarding I652121, in the domain of medicine, the relationship between carotid IMT (Intima-Media Thickness) and cardiovascular events is a continuous one. There is evidence, derived from routine examination, showing that, in untreated hypertensive individuals without target organ damage such alterations are common, and thus

Table 9.7 Previous diagnoses which affect prediction results

	Attribute	Attribute meaning
1	E780	Pure hypercholesterolaemia
2	I652121	Occlusion and stenosis of left carotid artery

carotid ultrasound examination may often detect vascular damage and make risk stratification more precise [48].

The age of the patient affects outcome of the therapy. If a patient's age is below 43.5 years, the likelihood of a successful outcome is higher. The risk of hypertension increases with age. This result is confirmed by the work of Hermida et al. [49].

Conclusions and Future Directions

We presented a study in which a predictive model, able to predict the outcome of antihypertensive therapy of cardiology patients, has been developed. The model is able to make its predictions using patient's personal data, anamnesis, therapies and medical history collected from new patients. The applicability of different machine learning algorithms, available within the open-source data mining tool WEKA, as ways to learn such a model from empirical data, has been explored. The data set used in the study has been provided by the Clinic of Cardiology of Institute of Cardiovascular Diseases Vojvodina, Serbia.

Working with this unbalanced data set, cost sensitive classification was employed and the best prediction was achieved with the grafted C4.5 decision tree classifier.

The implementation of predictive models, such as that developed in this study, in medical practice could increase the success of therapy in patients with hypertension, especially when they help correct the antihypertensive therapy at an early stage.

In the future, acquisition of more data from the public health institutions in Vojvodina is planned, aimed at making a predictive model for hypertension occurrence in asymptomatic patients. In addition, the research will be widened to other problem in cardiology, with the final goal of developing a decision support system for the clinical practice in Serbia.

References

1. World Healt organization International Society of Hypertension Writing Group 2003World Healt Organisation stasment of hypertensionJ Hypertens 2003; 21: 1983–92.
2. MacMahon S, Peto R, Cutler J, Collins R, Sorlie P, Neaton J, Abbott R, Godwin J, Dyer A, Stamler J. Blood pressure, stroke, and coronary heart disease. Part 1, Prolonged differences in blood pressure: prospective observational studies corrected for the regression dilution bias. Lancet 1990; 335:765–774.
3. Wattigney WA, Mensah GA, Croft JB. Increasing trends in hospitalization for atrial fibrillation in the United States, 1985 through 1999: implications for primary prevention. Circulation 2003; 108:711–716.
4. Skoog I, Lernfelt B, Landahl S, Palmertz B, Andreasson LA, Nilsson L, Persson G, Oden A, Svanborg A. 15-year longitudinal study of blood pressure and demen-tia. Lancet 1996; 347:1141–1145.

5. Ong KL, Cheung BM, Man YB, *et al.*: Prevalence, awareness, treatment, and control of hypertension among United States adults 1999–2004. Hypertension. 2007, 49: (1): 69–75.
6. Lawes CM, Vander Hoorn S, A Rodgers. International Society of Hypertension: Global burden of blood-pressure-related disease, 2001. Lancet. 2008, 371: (9623): 1513–1518.
7. Chobanian AV, Bakris GL, Black HR, *et al.*: Joint National Committee on Prevention, Detection, Evaluation, and Treatment of High Blood Pressure; National Heart, Lung, and Blood Institute; National High Blood Pressure Education Program Coordinating Committee: Seventh report of the Joint National Committee on Prevention, Detection, Evaluation, and Treatment of High Blood Pressure. Hypertension. 2003, 42: (6): 1206–1252.
8. Giuseppe Mancia *et al.*, "2007 Guidelines for the management of arterial hypertension", European Heart Journal (2007) 28, 1462–1536 doi:10.1093/eurheartj/ehm236.
9. Joep Perk *et al.*, "European Guidelines on cardiovascular disease prevention in clinical practice (version 2012)", European Heart Journal (2012) 33, 1635–1701, doi:10.1093/eurheartj/ehs092.
10. Ian H. Witten, Eibe Frank, Len Trigg, Mark Hall, Geoffrey Holmes, and Sally Jo Cunningham, "WEKA: Practical Machine Learning Tools and Techniques with Java Implementations", Department of Computer Science, University of Waikato, New Zealand.
11. Ture, Mevlut, *et al.* "Comparing classification techniques for predicting essential hypertension." Expert Systems with Applications 29.3 (2005): 583–588.
12. Cios, Krzysztof J., and G. William Moore. "Uniqueness of medical data mining." Artificial intelligence in medicine 26.1 (2002): 1–24.
13. Bhatia, Sumit, Praveen Prakash, and G. N. Pillai. "SVM based decision support system for heart disease classification with integer-coded genetic algorithm to select critical features." In Proceedings of the World Congress on Engineering and Computer Science, pp. 34–38. 2008.
14. Saunders, Craig, *et al.* "Support vector machine-reference manual." (1998).
15. Goldberg, David E. "Genetic algorithms in search, optimization, and machine learning." (1989).
16. Park, Jooyoung, and Irwin W. Sandberg. "Universal approximation using radial-basis-function networks." Neural computation 3, no. 2 (1991): 246–257.
17. Li, Jinyan, Xiuzhen Zhang, Guozhu Dong, Kotagiri Ramamohanarao, and Qun Sun. "Efficient mining of high confidence association rules without support thresholds." Principles of, data mining and knowledge discovery (1999): 406–411.
18. Braunwald, Eugene. "Unstable angina: a classification". Springer Berlin Heidelberg, 1990.
19. Srdjan Sladojevic, Miroslava Sladojevic, Dubravko Culibrk, "Predicting the post-therapeutic ECG status of cardiology patients using data mining", 55th ETRAN conference, Banja Vrućica, BIH, June 2011.
20. Quinlan, J. R. "C4.5: Programs for Machine Learning", Morgan Kaufmann Publishers, 1993.
21. Vaithiyanathan V., Rajeswari K., P. Amirtharaj, "Application of Decision Tree Classifiers in Diagnosing Heart Disease using Demographic Data", American Journal of Scientific Research, ISSN 2301–2005 Issue 70 (2012), pp. 77–82, EuroJournals Publishing, Inc. 2012.
22. Wozniak, Michal. "Boosted decision trees for diagnosis type of hypertension." Biological and Medical Data, Analysis (2005): 223–230.
23. Moore, Andrew, and Mary S. Lee. "Cached sufficient statistics for efficient machine learning with large datasets." arXiv preprint cs/9803102 (1998).
24. Wozniak, Michal. "Two-stage classifier for diagnosis of hypertension type." Biological and Medical Data, Analysis (2006): 433–440.
25. Pal, Sankar K., and Sushmita Mitra. "Multilayer perceptron, fuzzy sets, and classification." IEEE Transactions on Neural Networks 3.5 (1992): 683–697.
26. Mark Hall, Eibe Frank, Geoffrey Holmes, Bernhard Pfahringer, Peter Reutemann, Ian H. Witten (2009); "The WEKA Data Mining Software: An Update", SIGKDD Explorations, Volume 11, Issue 1.
27. Pyle, D., "Data Preparation for Data Mining", Morgan Kaufmann Publishers, Los Altos, California, 1999.
28. Ian H. Witten & Eibe Frank, Data Mining -, Practical Machine Learning Tools", The Morgan Kaufmann, 2005.

29. Webb, Geoffrey I. "Decision tree grafting from the all-tests-but-one partition." International Joint Conference on Artificial Intelligence. Vol. 16. Lawrence Erlbaum Associates Ltd, 1999.
30. Yoav Freund, Robert E. Schapire: Experiments with a new boosting algorithm. In: Thirteenth International Conference on Machine Learning, San Francisco, 148–156, 1996.
31. Freund, Yoav, and Llew Mason. "The alternating decision tree learning algorithm." Machine learning - International workshop then conference - Morgan Kaufmann publishers, Inc., 1999.
32. Lewis, Roger J. "An Introduction to Classification and Regression Tree (CART) Analysis," presented at Annual Meeting of the Society for Academic Emergency Medicine." Annual Meeting of the Society of Academic Emergency Medicine in. 2000.
33. Breiman, Leo. "Random forests." Machine learning 45.1 (2001): 5–32.
34. Caruana, Rich; Karampatziakis, Nikos; Yessenalina, Ainur, "An empirical evaluation of supervised learning in high dimensions". Proceedings of the 25th International Conference on Machine Learning (ICML), 2008.
35. D. Aha, D. Kibler (1991). Instance-based learning algorithms. Machine Learning. 6:37–66.
36. John G. Cleary, Leonard E. Trigg: K*: An Instance-based Learner Using an Entropic Distance Measure. In: 12th International Conference on, Machine Learning, 108–114, 1995.
37. George H. John and Pat Langley (1995). Estimating Continuous Distributions in Bayesian Classifiers. Proceedings of the Eleventh Conference on Uncertainty in Artificial Intelligence. pp. 338–345. Morgan Kaufmann, San Mateo.
38. Bianca Zadrozny, John Langford, Naoki Abe, "Cost-Sensitive Learning by Cost-Proportionate Example Weighting", Mathematical Sciences Department IBM T. J. Watson Research Center, Yorktown Heights, NY 10598.
39. Kai Ming Ting, "Cost-Sensitive Classification using Decision Trees, Boosting and MetaCost", School of Computing and Information Technology, Monash University, Churchill, Victoria 3842, Australia.
40. Huang, Jin, and Charles X. Ling. "Using AUC and Accuracy in Evaluating Learning Algorithms." IEEE Transactions on Knowledge and Data Engineering 17.3 (2005): 299–310.
41. Nakanishi, Noriyuki at al. "White blood cell count as a risk factor for hypertension; a study of Japanese male office workers"; Journal of Hypertension: May 2002 - Volume 20 - Issue 5 - pp 851–857.
42. Mancia G. *et al.* "Metabolic syndrome in the daily life blood pressure, cardiac damage, and prognosis". Hypertension 2007; 49:40–47. OS.
43. Reiner Z. "How to improve cardiovascular diseases prevention in Europe?", Nutr Metab Cardiovasc Dis 2009; 19:451–454.
44. Preis SR *et al.*, "Trends in all-cause and cardiovascular disease mortality among women and men with and without diabetes mellitus in the Framingham Heart Study", 1950 to 2005. Circulation 2009; 119:1728–1735.
45. Patel A. *et al.*, "Intensive blood glucose control and vascular outcomes in patients with type 2 diabetes". N Engl J Med, 2008; 358:2560–2572.
46. Nalpas B, Vassault A, Charpin S, Lacour B, Berthelot P (1986). "Serum mitochondrial aspartate aminotransferase as a marker of chronic alcoholism: diagnostic value and interpretation in a liver unit". Hepatology 6 (4): 608–614. doi:10.1002/hep.1840060410.PMID3732996.
47. Clark, Jeanne M., Frederick L. Brancati, and Anna Mae Diehl. "The prevalence and etiology of elevated aminotransferase levels in the United States." The American journal of gastroenterology 98.5 (2003): 960–967.
48. Hunt SA, Haddad F. "The changing face of heart transplantation", J Am Coll Cardiol 2008; 52: 587–598.
49. Hermida, Ramón C., *et al.* "Influence of age and hypertension treatment-time on ambulatory blood pressure in hypertensive patients." Chronobiology International (2012): 1–16.

Chapter 10
Cloud Computing Approach to Novel Medical Interface Design

Maya Dimitrova, Lubomir Lahtchev, Siya Lozanova and Chavdar Roumenin

Introduction

Interface technologies and devices need to be developed with novel functionalities for pattern analysis and data transfer in order to receive helpful and reliable healthcare service "from the Cloud". The complexity of implementing Cloud computing for healthcare relates to a number of issues such as privacy, data protection, medical record access and update, high performance computation (HPC), etc. [1–4]. At the same time interoperability needs to be achieved at all levels of provision of Cloud services—from the novel interface, via Hardware as a Service (HaaS), Software as a Service (SaaS) and Infrastructure as a Service (IaaS).

New interface technologies for medical instrumentation, compatible with web platforms, have been recently developed like h'andy sana GSMs for mobile electrocardiogram (ECG) recording [5], improved portable defibrillators [6], digital stethoscopes [7], and other newly emerging medical peripheries based on multimodal data fusion [8, 9]. These have to be integrated in a novel framework for provision of medical Cloud services on subscription, adjusted to the individual user needs and health status.

A novel view of future information technologies for healthcare has been recently proposed [10, 11], based on the following *four pillars* of technological advancement. The first pillar is the transition from design of large-scale medical instrumentation to smart micro-system technologies—i.e. towards Hardware as a Service (HaaS) in the medical domain; the second is the transition from large telecommunication infrastructures, needed for health record transfer, towards mobile and secure data transmission via the appropriate middleware—i.e. towards Infrastructure as a Service (IaaS); the third is the transition from isolated islands of medical data towards integrated end-to-end healthcare solutions "in the Cloud" i.e. towards Software as

M. Dimitrova (✉) · L. Lahtchev · S. Lozanova · C. Roumenin
Bulgarian Academy of Sciences, Institute of Systems Engineering and Robotics, Sofia, Bulgaria
e-mail: dimitrova@iser.bas.bg

B. Furht and A. Agarwal (eds.), *Handbook of Medical and Healthcare Technologies*,
DOI: 10.1007/978-1-4614-8495-0_10, © Springer Science+Business Media New York 2013

a Service (SaaS) in the medical domain. The fourth pillar is the transition from intrusive and expensive health examinations towards harmless indirect health monitoring via novel devices—i.e. towards User Interface as a Service (UIaaS in the medical domain.

The main ideas behind the new concept of User Interface as a Service (UIaaS) for healthcare are the following:

- *Design of Cloud compatible new interfaces for harmless medical examination.* An h'andy sana GSM device [5] is just one of the possible Cloud compatible interfaces for medical examination in indirect and harmless way in the absence of a doctor. Data is transmitted via Bluetooth to the Cloud services the user has subscribed for—personalized search and retrieval of diagnostic information, GPS tracing, online medical consultation, etc. The subscription plan may change dynamically to conform best to the user health condition through time. Health records and new data can always be available, no matter where the user location is, via e-Health portals.
- *New principles guiding the design of Cloud compatible medical devices.* Artificial intelligence (AI) based solutions are essential for the UIaaS and therefore new principles of data registration need to be explored. The existing patents for electronic BP measurement are based on some mathematical ratio of the signal for the volume of the vessel and the pressure inside this volume (e.g. cardio-ankle vascular index CAVI [12]). It is proposed in our work to add to these a signal for the exerted vibration and the vessel wall response via high fidelity measurement [10].
- *New materials needed for the design of Cloud compatible medical interfaces.* In [11] a novel device intended to collect, analyze and transmit data obtained from registration of peripheral vibrations of the arteries of the human body is proposed. It is an attempt to overcome the electrical wiring of patients, including wearing smart fabrics for diagnostics and alerting on health issues. Instead, we propose the development of smart rubber implementing novel properties. *Smart rubber* has large future potential especially for implementing in novel devices to be used as Cloud compatible medical interfaces. A material of similar type is being developed at the Eindhoven University of technology and is called acyprop e.g. ([13], p. 16). The main idea is that its layered structure may help tune the vibration signal and provide useful and precise information.

Figure 10.1 illustrates two possible cases of health examination for consultation with medical Cloud services. The left case includes wired devices for recording health indicators. The right case involves taking measurements from body surface areas via wireless devices. Therefore the new framework includes both cases of examination via either lightweight health monitoring device (right) or via more substantial data-intensive wired instrumentation (left).

The overall aim of the present research is the development of a new integrated, smart, mobile and useful technology for doctors and patients to monitor and explore *cross-diagnosis conditions* and causal relationships among diseases in non-obtrusive, indirect and harmless way, which is designed for a Cloud computing framework. We

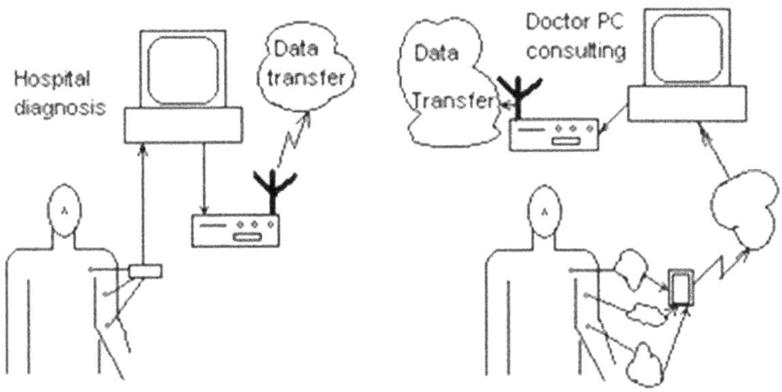

Fig. 10.1 Cloud compatible novel medical interfaces (*see text*)

focus on cardiology for the fact that the majority of the emergency cases are heart related conditions [14]. The design of novel health monitoring devices, based on indirect and harmless registration of functional heart indicators, is necessary for reliable Cloud services, explicitly aiming at supporting seamless and ubiquitous health monitoring and online access to medical help.

Complexity of Symptom Representation in Medical Diagnostic Systems for Cloud Services

Symptom representation and visualization in the existing medical diagnostic systems is a complex task, intended to aid the cognitive representations of the medical experts on the current condition, the history of illness and the prognosis of treatment outcome. Due to the ability of the natural cognitive systems to grab and process vast amounts of visual information, the most developed aiding systems deal with symptom visualization and 3D vessel reconstruction for medical diagnostic support [3, 8].

It has been proposed to approach the problem of designing a useful interface to health monitoring devices from a cognitive perspective and distinguish two levels of modalities in symptom representation—abstract level modality and physical level modalities [15, 16]. On the abstract level *knowledge discovery* takes place, which requires *abstract visualization* of the symptoms and health condition. On the physical level *fusion of data* takes place in order to obtain real visual image of a specific health condition (e.g. fusion of the ultrasound signal with ECG, angiography or magnetic tracking signal). Medical technology has achieved sophistication in data fusion and symptom representation in hospital instrumentation for medical interventions [17–19]. Novel technologies for medical peripheries needed to be developed in order to produce adequate symptom visualization in mobile devices for health monitoring. There is urgent societal need for such devices [20, 21].

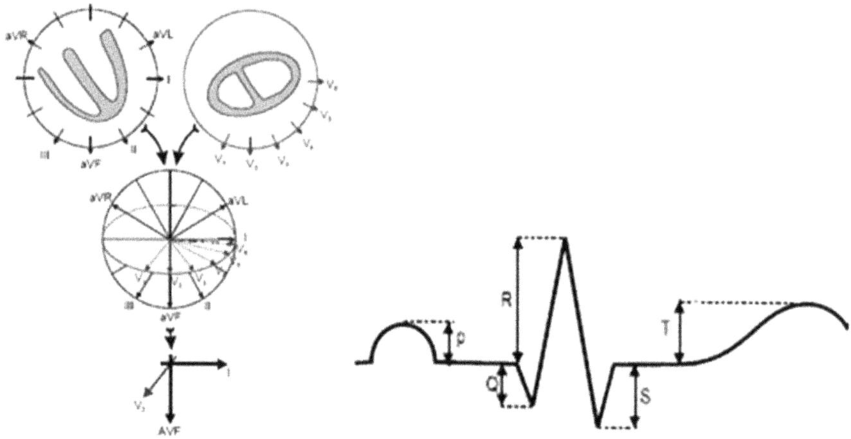

Fig. 10.2 Mental reconstruction of the heart geometry by a medical expert from reading a 12 channel ECG record. The picture is adapted from [14] with the permission of Dr. S. Marchev

Figure 10.2 illustrates how cardiologists read an electrocardiogram—in terms of the spatial position of the heart and its physical deformation. In abstract terms, they use the ECG record as a measuring instrument for geometric distance and infer the *actual geometry of a hidden object* (the heart) [14].

Despite modern advancement of diagnostic and interventional instrumentation—the 12 channel electrocardiograph remains one of the most reliable diagnostic tools in cardiology. Profiles of record patterns signify, first of all, deformations of heart tissue structure (spatial relations) and, based on this, causal relations between different organ malfunctions, and the respective heart deformation. We forwarded a hypothesis that patterns of the electrical activity of heart the can be obtained from peripheral areas of the body, which can be monitored by appropriate interfaces to medical diagnostic systems [16]. These we compare to patterns of artery wall vibrations and analyze them from a diagnostic perspective for novel medical interface design, compatible with Cloud infrastructures for healthcare.

From an electro-technical and an engineering perspective, current medical technology follows the miniaturization path, which is justified on the grounds of the strict reliability and safety regulations for design of large-scale medical instrumentation. With the increased awareness of the society of the *processual* nature of the *illness* a lot of concern is devoted to patient self-management via home monitoring of health indicators [20, 21]. Cardiology is being central in this concern for dealing often with the outcome of ill-managed consequences of other diseases. For example, recent studies have shown that home monitoring of blood pressure levels (nonintrusive method) can be more relevant for control and prevention of diabetes mellitus and subsequent heart problems than home monitoring of blood sugar levels (intrusive method) [22].

There is a level of construction of health monitoring devices where applying miniaturization did not produce devices that are displaying saliently the monitored symptoms. Patients find it difficult to manage the sphygmomanometers—either mercury or anaeroid—require assistance or are confused to understand the output of the electronic devices regarding their current condition. This situation is complicated by the imprecision of the electronic equipment for measuring blood pressure [23]. Therefore novel approaches are needed as the basis for design of home monitoring devices of the health condition.

Design of new sensor elements for smart devices can be sought both ways—from the particular to the general and from the general to the particular—by implementing modularity, well-adopted in electro-mechanical engineering, and less included in medical machinery. In technical sense this means that the high-fidelity sensors of unimodal nature of the useful signal usually carry efficient target information for a particular medico-biological symptom, but may be filtered out in large-scale instrumentation. Examples are thermo, photo, vibro sensors, electro- or magneto-sensor registration in devices such as electrocardiographs, functional magnetic resonance imaging (fMRI) machines, positron emission tomographs (PET) and ultrasound imaging devices such as intra-vascular ultra-sound (IVUS) equipment. On the other hand a multisensor device with several sensitive elements and areas can produce arrays of data of diagnostic relevance, characteristic for a symptom, illness or condition of the organism. The latter case relates and forwards artificial intelligence and cognitive systems accounts of medical symptom representation. New peripheries have to be designed and investigated where a multimodal sensor device with several sensitive elements and areas can produce arrays of data of diagnostic relevance (Fig. 10.3).

The patent search on blood pressure measurement devices has shown that most electronic devices employ some ratio of the signal for the volume of the blood vessel

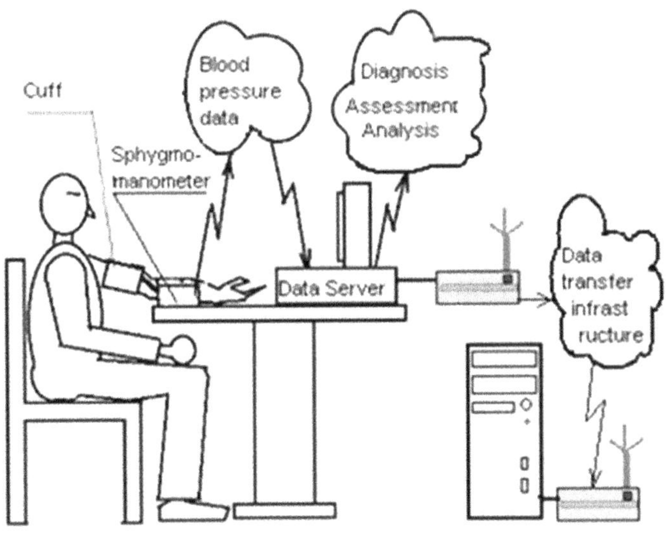

Fig. 10.3 Sensor configuration management for Cloud compatible medical interface design

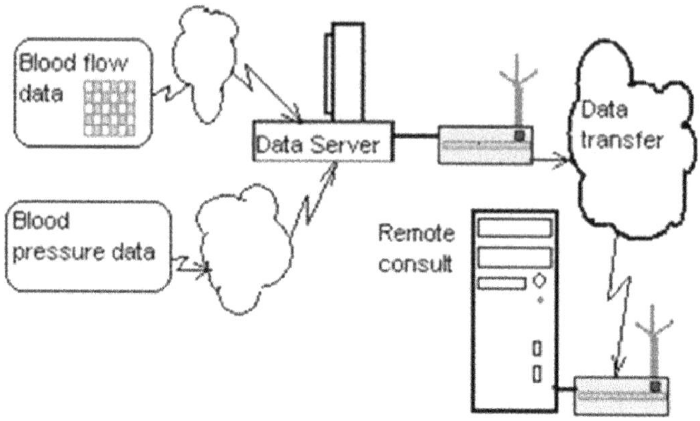

Fig. 10.4 Examples of periphery for symptom signal transmission (*see text*)

and the signal for the pressure inside this volume e.g. [12]. We propose to add two additional parameters—the velocity of the blood flow in the vessel, based on a principle similar to the patented cases and a control mechanism of registration the micro-vibration of the vessel wall at different points of the body. The idea is to add new means of non-invasive medical examinations of prognostic/predictive validity with cognitive abilities and smart technical solutions. The analysis of these combined measurements is the foundation of the current research.

We aim at finding a sensor or sensor combination, which are able to generate relevant and precise data for medico-biological parameters that can undergo different types of signal processing, including time/spectral analysis and artificial intelligence algorithms. For this purpose maximal discretization of the signals is sought.

The sensors are grouped in sensor segments, based on unified time discretization on a chessboard principle (see Fig. 10.4). This allows obtaining massive signal samples, which can be tested for correlational repetitiveness along segments and devices.

New Trends in Sensor Technology for Cloud Compatible Medical Interfaces

One aspect of the invention process of new principles of sensor design is hypothesizing complexity of sensor registration of influences and issuing useful signals. New sensors are being investigated with the advances of miniaturization and new silicon based technologies. Being of its own scope of research, the development of genuine (by origin) multi-sensors in parallel with combining specialized micro-sensors is a fruitful approach for translation of ideas from one research focus into another and bringing interdisciplinary focus on the sensor level between *physics*- and *biology*-inspired technical systems for medicine.

The aim of the future investigations in the domain of smart systems and devices, for example of the electromechanical and microelectronic mechanical units, supported by variety of sensors, like acoustic thermal and electromagnetic sensors, is to develop maintenance tools for complex time varying and time-frequency transform methods of medico-biological measurements. This sensor configuration set will bring high correlative data samples with a better filtration and amplification for adequate medical diagnosis and for deeper understanding of the human body as a biological system cognitively adapting and guided—in a manner, which is both interiorized (knowledge and self-awareness) and exteriorized (discussed with medical experts and economic establishments like health funds and insurance companies).

Description of the Sensor Configuration of the Novel Medical Interface

The information about blood pressure, heart rhythm, temperature and sound is contained in devices used in medicine such as manual and automated sphygmomanometers (including mercury and anaeroid devices), electrocardiographs, Holters, thermometers and echographs. The electrocardiographic (ECG) and the Holter devices operate over and analyze the electrical impulses of the heart [14]. Apart from the information about the form of the electrical impulse of the heart, the ECG registers the heart rhythm. These registrations can be made for longer durations via Holters, which store them in memory for 1, 2 or 3 days, and can be subsequently analyzed and evaluated in considering the patient case off-line and over time. Investigation on modules for *technical diagnosis of medical instrumentation* has been carried out during the recent years [24]. The level of noise in such devices can blur the symptoms and delay treatment if relied upon as the only health monitoring method.

The modern view on the illness extends to novel sensor modalities as well as to multisensor and multispectral analysis of disease symptoms within *a priory* defined modes of functioning of the organism. These modes of the organism can be addressed as cognitive systems (sympathetic, parasympathetic, adrenaline/noradrenaline, endorphine/placebo and others), subject to rationalized/engineering modeling based on functional and anatomical structures (according to the works of Torrent-Guasp [25]) and possessing certain autonomy, adaptation to novel situations via mode-switching and predictive abilities.

Non-invasive examinations can implement high-frequency (HF) and low-frequency (LF) vibration sensors as well as touch sensors providing useful information about the blood flow [12]. The sensor set for arterial pressure and cardiac pulsation can include sensor units, pre-processing units, intermediate memories, microprocessor, RAM and Flash memories, address controller, clock unit, outside periphery—programming and check units (Fig. 10.5).

Multi-purpose system configurations with powerful graphical systems, supporting a variety of models, communication and processing technologies, can be easily con-

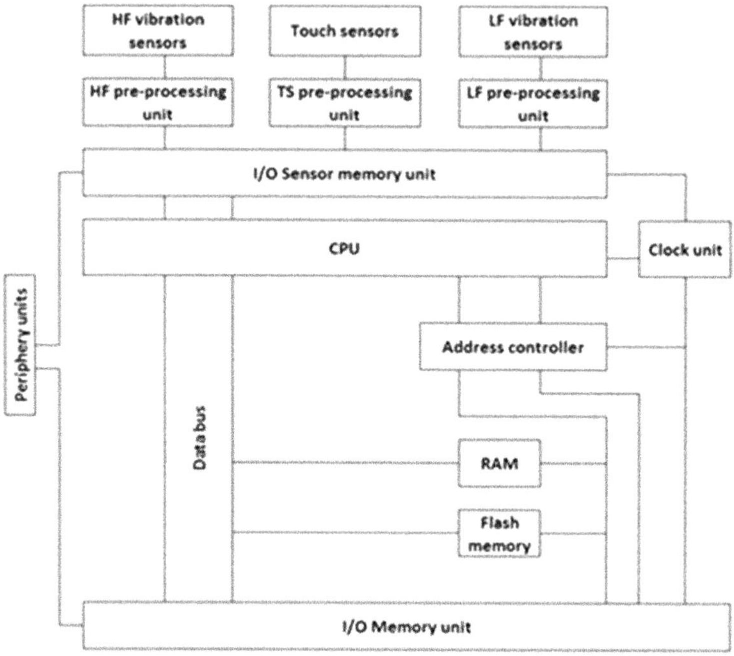

Fig. 10.5 Configuration of the sensor device

nected to many digitalized analogous and digital sensors of the sensor configuration for condition modeling and healthcare provision. The sensor configuration will remotely communicate with a central PC providing time, blood pressure and blood flow data. The new sensor device requires analogous-digital transformation on the input, digital pre-processing and basic calculations of the end data. A unit of I/O-memory supplies the communicative module with digital-sign and time data for communication to the central PC and from there—to the Cloud. In order to achieve desirable signal quality, a variety of signal processing algorithms need to be developed, fulfilled and tested.

For the design of the sensor configuration input keyboard, output digital display, PC, oscilloscope and function generator are the required equipment. The HF and LF vibration sensor groups consist of own power supply, transmitter and receiver sensor group and analogous digital conversion (ADC) unit. The touch sensor group uses ADC, too. The frequency and the touch sensors' pre-processing units convert data from the ADC to digital format and transform the input levels to the digital I/O levels of the microprocessor. The microprocessor controls the modes of the sensor groups and their pre-processing units. It also fulfils the low-level supporting and tracking algorithms, calculates the required work parameters and finishes with communication to the central PC and to the Cloud. The periphery units include database, display, indicators, supporting hardware diagnostic elements. All of them operate in dialog mode with the microprocessor.

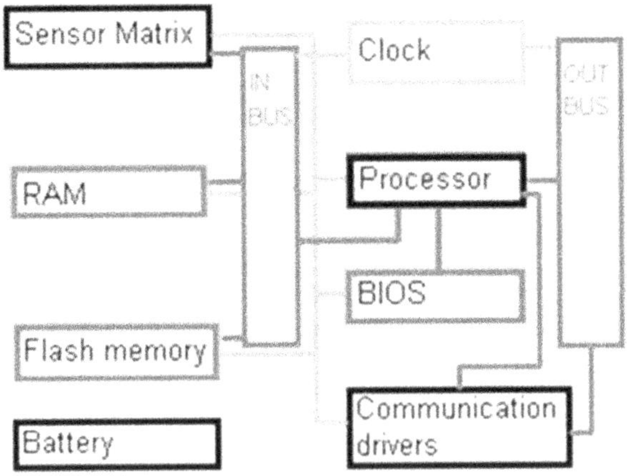

Fig. 10.6 Chart diagram of the sensor module with a micro-processing system

The diagram of the sensor module is based on analogy with a PC configuration (Fig. 10.6). It has to be equipped with operation system (OS) working in real time with automatic and semiautomatic mode of operation of the digital device. In semi automatic mode it is necessary that the device is able to receive commands from a central server, a keyboard or via the communication channel and perform on compatible platforms. The manufacturing of the module is possible with standard computer elements.

Engineering Principles of Design of the Novel Medical Interface

In the machine constructions the main sources of information for their mechanical state are located in the supportive elements—the bearings and the dynamic joints. In previous studies on turbo-generator sets a large amount of vibro-acoustic data was collected from the areas of the supporting sliding bearings and a classificatory array of system states was built [26]. The examination of the "Atlas of Human Anatomy" [27] has shown that the nervous, arterial and vein leads are placed closest to each other in the joint areas. The sensors for the non-invasive tests can receive reliable information if placed in these zones. Zones of the kind in the human body are the fingers, the wrists, the elbows, the neck, the shoulders, and the knees.

The blood artery stems are pervaded by neural leads. It is reasonable to consider each stem as a combined electro-hydraulic lead. We assume that in this *complex* the artery is a hydraulic tube and the nerves are the electrical conductor of its pulsations. Such engineering construct is well supported by other sources (textbooks and electrocardiographic manuals) as well as by the nature of the nervous cell with the axon and the dendrites being carriers/transmitters of electric impulses (Fig. 10.7).

Parallel to these theoretical assumptions it is reasonable to include in the engineering construct the pneumatic/gas component which is always present in any hydraulic

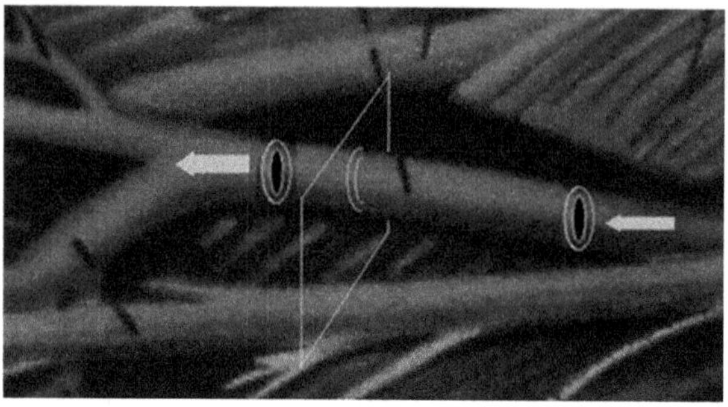

Fig. 10.7 Visualization of the tissue around the artery in the elbow area

system. This results in a reasonably complete scheme of the interaction of the joint, the blood vessel and the innervations and, in some sense, of the skeleton, vascular, endocrine and nervous systems, where the laws of mechanics, electrostatics, electrical chemistry, hydraulics and pneumatics co-act with probably different degree of intensity on different time scales during functioning.

If the trans-membrane potential at rest or activity is included, it will become evident that in general, at the present moment, the understanding of the cardio-vascular and the endovascular systems is fragmentary rather than integral from engineering sciences perspective.

Registration of Functional Heart Signals from Peripheral Areas of the Body: Preliminary Study

In a preliminary study of the feasibility of the proposed approach pairs of sensitive elements—electrodes Skintact F55 [28]—were placed around the blood artery stems in the areas of the heart, the neck, the wrists, the elbows, the finger joints of the indicator and middle fingers, the knees and the left and right anterior shoulder area. The aim of this preliminary experiment was to test a hypothesis that large blood vessels near the surface of the human body reflect the main pattern of the PQ RST complex in an ECG record [29]. This was reliably confirmed in signals taken either from the neck artery, the shoulder or the elbow artery by applying Holter microelectrodes to these areas (Fig. 10.8).

The Skintact electrodes were used in pairs placed around the arteries. Figures 10.9 and 10.10 display the recorded signals from the pairs of electrodes placed at the neck and the shoulder areas where the arteries reach the surface of the body. The information is unipolar and provides data for the energy spectrum of the signals with amplitude up to 2.49 V. The main outcome is that these parallel sensors register correlated electrical signals in the range of 0–6 Hz from the areas they were applied to. Strong correlation between the neck and the shoulder was obtained—which makes the shoulder the most appropriate place since the neck artery has to be protected from contact.

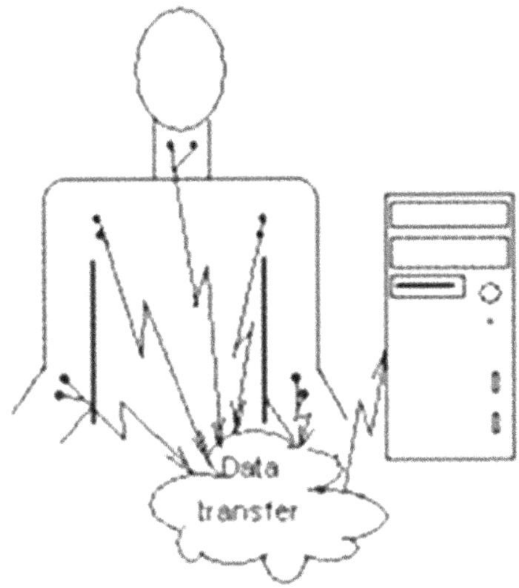

Fig. 10.8 Placement of the sensor matrix at the arterial locations on the neck, shoulders, and elbows

The PQ RST complexes are clearly visible in the senor data configuration. From the individual profile of the electric signal diagnostic conclusions can be made about the functioning of the heart. A very similar signal configuration was taken from the elbow zone, too.

The second aim was to test the Holter mini-electrodes used for response to ultrasound. Full insensitivity to sound was observed, which confirmed the assumption that the received signal is pure electrical (but not vibration) signal [29].

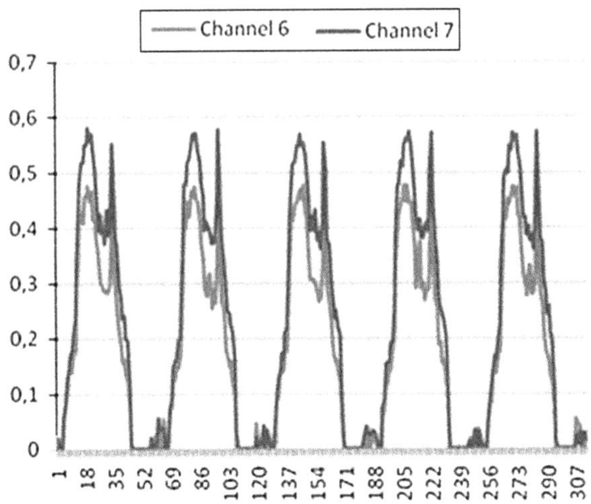

Fig. 10.9 The signal configuration (voltage), received from the *left* (Channel 6) and *right* (Channel 7) sides of the neck artery

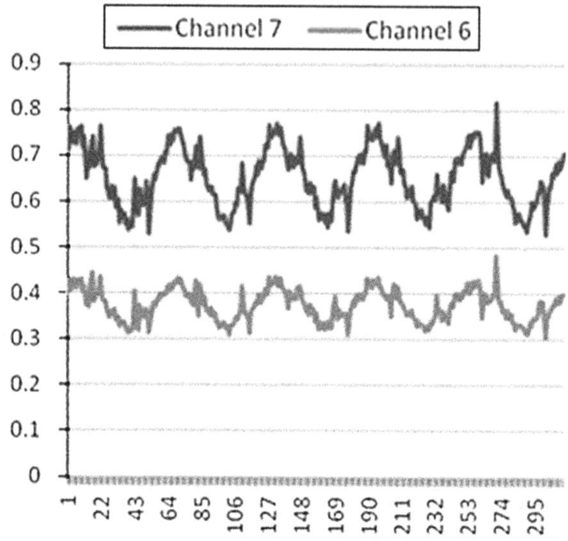

Fig. 10.10 The signal configuration (voltage), received from the *left* (Channel 6) and *right* (Channel 7) sides of the right shoulder area

Registration of Artery Vibration Data from Peripheral Areas of the Body

The next experiment focuses on investigating other sensor modalities (vibration of the artery wall) in order to receive correlates of the electrical signals for nonelectrical assessment of the heart condition. The configuration of the sensors measures blood flow data—systolic-diastolic blood pressure levels, rhythm and flow speed. The low frequency sensors measure speed of the blood flow. The high frequency vibration sensors measure the outside fluctuations of the medium. This device is currently under construction. The present experiments were taken with the help of an adapted commercial digital sphygmomanometer as described further in this section.

The sphygmomanometer contains sensors for BP signals: oscillometry, air pressure and osculate level. Every sensor produces analog voltage proportional to the measured parameter. The voltage signals are transferred to the computer with use of analog-digital converter. In the figures below the vertical axis represents a fraction of the pressure level in the cuff, which we denote as *P*. Tensoval® duo control blood pressure (BP) measuring device was adapted for taking vibration data from the artery wall above the elbow where usually blood pressure is measured (Fig. 10.11).The device was connected via wires welded to 8 points on the wafer surface of the Tensoval® electronic chip [30].

Materials and Procedure. The device for recording data was a USB Data Acquisition (DAQ) Module, DT9810, 10-bit, 25 kHz, 8 analog inputs (10-bit, 25 kS/s), analog input range: 0 to 2.44 V, 20 digital I/O lines, 32-bit counter/timer, software and drivers compatible with Windows XP/Vista/7 [31]. Twelve subjects took part

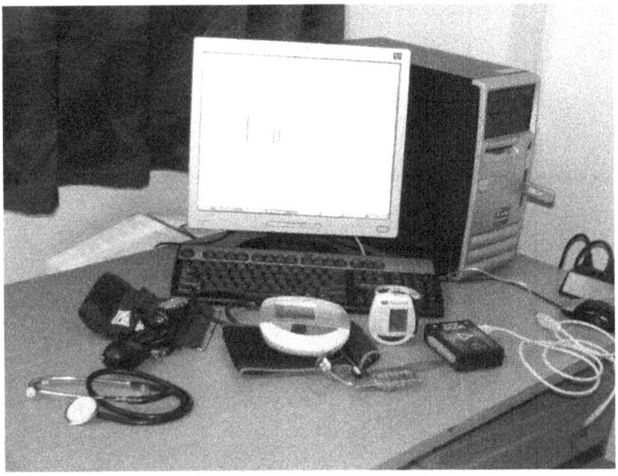

Fig. 10.11 The data recording set comprised of Tensoval® duo control with electronic chip welded to DT9810 USB data acquisition module

in the experiment—7 women and 5 men. They were invited in random order and signed informed consent, stating that the purpose of the experiment was testing the device Tensoval® duo control and did not assess health condition. Measurements were taken from both arms—first left, then right. The age range was from 25 to 65 years.

Results and Discussion. Data profiles were recorded in an Excel database and displayed via the DT9810 visualization interface. Patterns of artery vibrations are clearly distinguishable with the decrease of the cuff pressure during measurement. Profiles of arrhythmia (left and right hand) are evident in the data taken from the DT9810 visualization interface (Fig. 10.12). Table 10.1 presents the BP levels of the experimental data from measurement of artery wall vibration.

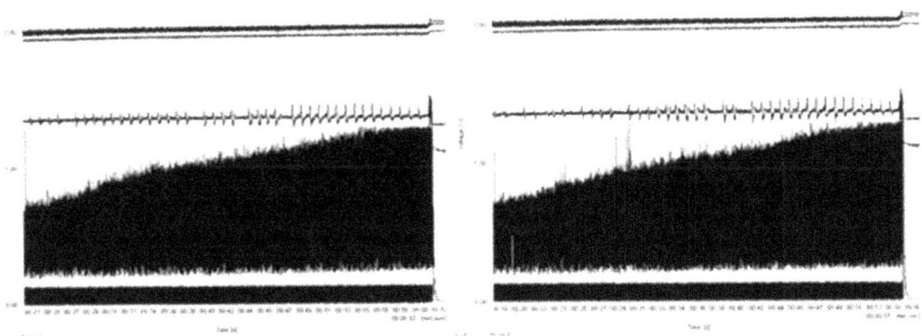

Fig. 10.12 Patterns of artery vibrations for arrhythmia (*left* and *right hand*) visualized by the DT9810 USB data acquisition module

Table 10.1 BP levels of the experimental data from measurement of artery wall vibration

Patient	Gender	Systolic BP left	Diastolic BP left	Pulse left	Systolic BP right	Diastolic BP right	Pulse right	Date of measurement	Interval min	Note
A	M	113	76	60	115	78	56	08.07.09	12	Normal BP
B	F	104	69	75	105	68	78	09.07.09	3	Low BP
C	M	155	84	72	157	76	70	09.07.09	7	High BP
D	M	117	87	98	124	90	104	09.07.09	4	Normal BP
E	F	137	96	85	124	88	87	09.07.09	3	High BP
F	F	98	66	72	101	74	75	09.07.09	3	Low BP
G	M	128	91	94	110	78	94	09.07.09	3	Normal BP
H	F	94	64	72	92	62	71	09.07.09	3	Low BP
I	F	122	82	89	108	71	80	09.07.09	21	Normal BP
J	F	117	78	70	108	74	65	09.07.09	2	Normal BP
K	F	118	73	67	127	67	69	09.07.09	3	Arrhythmia
L	M	116	80	77	107	97	77	09.07.09	3	Normal BP

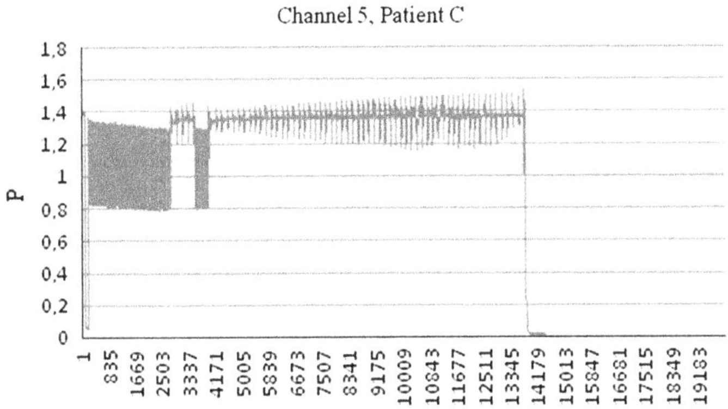

Fig. 10.13 Excel chart of high BP pattern (14,179 data points)

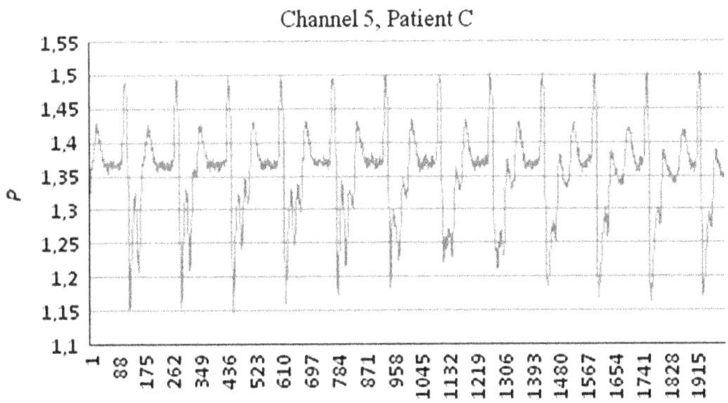

Fig. 10.14 Excel chart of high BP pattern (2,000 data points)

The high fidelity of the measurement procedure is the main result evident also from the inspection of Figs. 10.13, 10.14, 10.15, 10.16, 10.17, 10.18, 10.19 and 10.20. For a time window of approximately 60 s and approximately 70 heartbeats, the procedure is capable of recording between 13,000 and 31,000 data points. This makes 25–45 data points for every heartbeat—5 to 9 data points for every element of the PQ RST complex in an ECG. Therefore the device provides high fidelity of the measurement of vibration patterns, suitable for implementing in novel health monitoring interfaces with enhanced symptom visualization.

Figures 10.13, 10.14, 10.15, 10.16, 10.17, 10.18, 10.19 and 10.20 display different patterns of Excel data—one high BP pattern (Figs. 10.13 and 10.14) one low BP pattern (Figs. 10.15 and 10.16), one normal BP pattern (Figs. 10.17 and 10.18) and one arrhythmic BP pattern (Figs. 10.19 and 10.20) taken from the right arm.

Figures 10.13, 10.15, 10.17, and 10.19 visualize the entire patterns of vibration during automatic BP measuring. They represent the process of lowering the pressure in the cuff until the external and internal pressure values become equal. Figures 10.14,

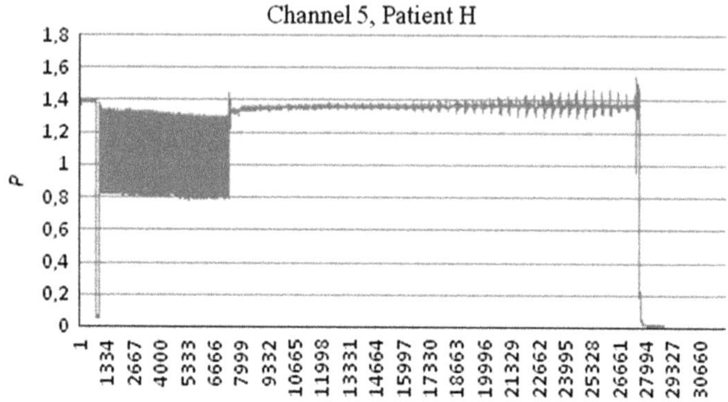

Fig. 10.15 Excel chart of low BP pattern (27,994 data points)

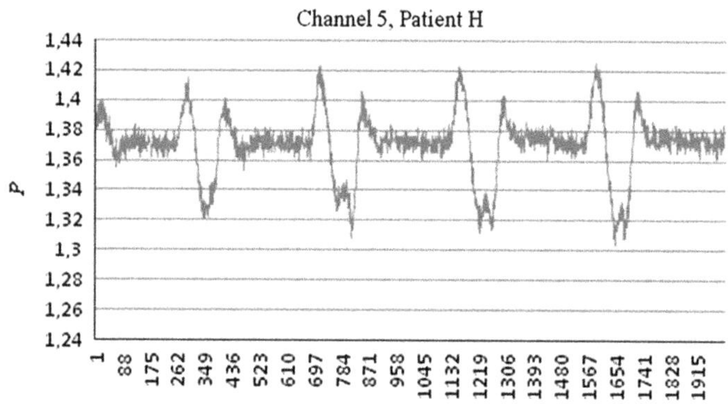

Fig. 10.16 Excel chart of low BP pattern (2,000 data points)

10.16, 10.18 and 10.20 visualize fractions of this process towards the end of the measurement. Figure 10.13 displays the data points from 10,000 to 12,000. Figures 10.16, 10.18 and 10.20 display data points from 20,000 to 22,000. Channel 5 is the point for data retrieval from the microprocessor of the Tensoval device, where the vibration pattern of the artery wall is most clearly visible.

High BP is characterized above all by short (10,000 data points) clear pattern of cuff pressure decrease (Fig. 10.13). The stiffness of the artery wall is clearly visible from Fig. 10.14 where the vibration pattern is very uniform and undistorted by noise.

The low BP pattern, visualized in Fig. 10.15, has a specific profile of mild vibrations at the start and clear resonance at the end of the measurement process. The wall of the artery is soft when BP is low so the vibration signal is distorted by noise from the surrounding tissue (Fig. 10.16).

The normal BP profile is smooth and very regular in comparison with the abormal profiles (Fig. 10.17). The normal BP reflects the flexibility of the artery wall and is

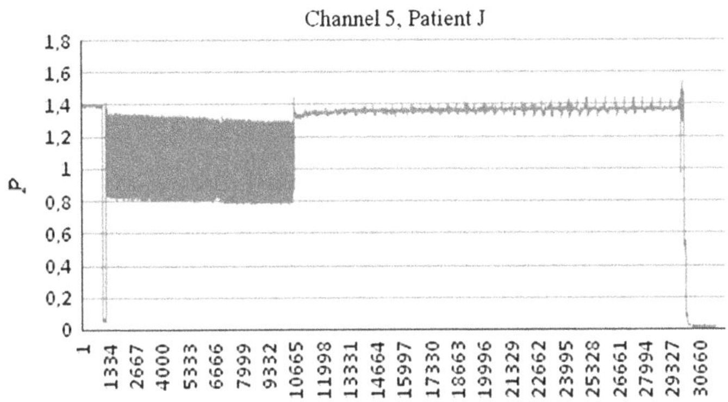

Fig. 10.17 Excel chart of a normal BP pattern (30,660 data points)

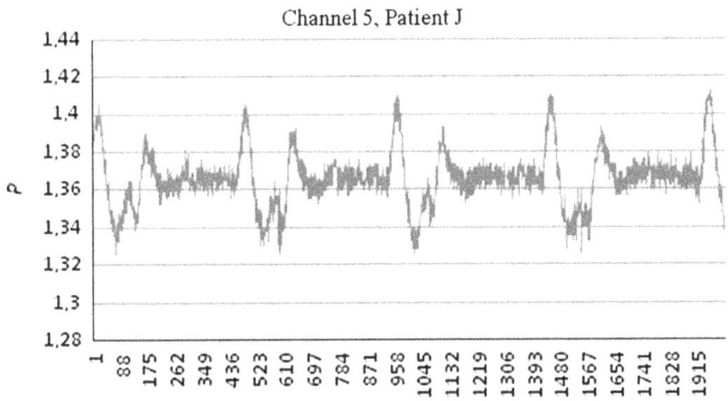

Fig. 10.18 Excel chart of normal BP pattern (2,000 data points)

similar to the low BP profile. The specific Q and T waves are more markedly expressed than in the case with low BP (Fig. 10.18).

The arrhythmic profile is clearly visible and unambiguous. It is accompanied with noisy and distorted profile of the PQ RST complex due to the deficient way the blood flows in the cardio-vascular system (Fig. 10.19). The inspection of the arrhythmic profile by magnifying the vibration signal can provide useful information for emergency intervention (Fig. 10.20).

The entire *complex* of monitoring artery wall vibrations in indirect and harmless way provides novel way for monitoring the health condition outside the clinic. Patterns are clearly visible and easily distinguishable and can be used for AI-based symptom analysis. Novel devices implementing the described principles in this chapter are especially appropriate for implementation in Cloud-based healthcare applications.

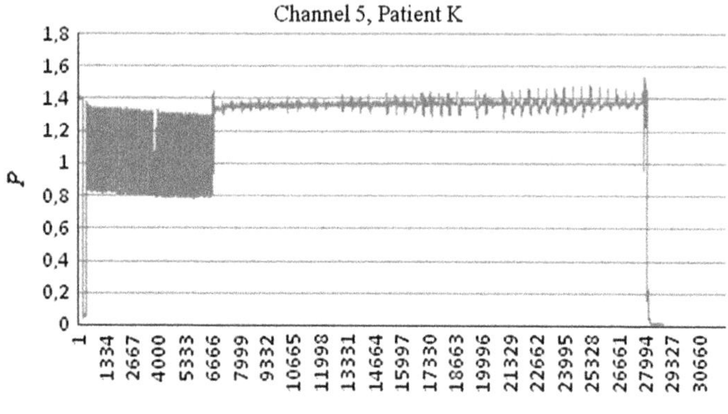

Fig. 10.19 Excel chart of arrhythmic BP pattern (27,994 data points)

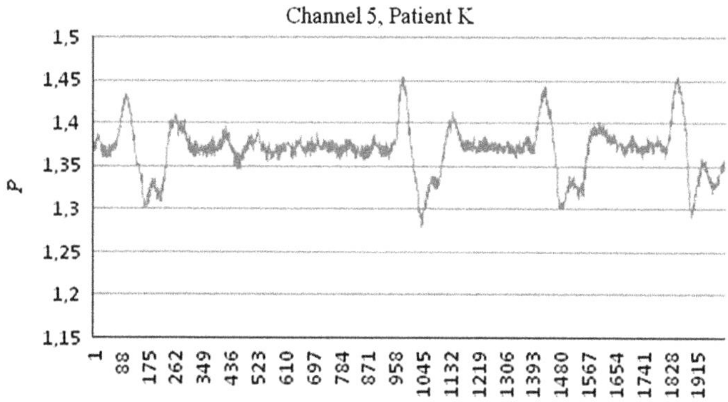

Fig. 10.20 Excel chart of arrhythmic BP pattern (2,000 data points)

3D Visualization of the Vessel: How Much about the Heart Can an Artery Reveal?

Cardiologists say that the sound of the 'healthy heart' has to be different from the sound of the 'ill heart'. This expert intuition has inspired one of the aspects of the current research—continuous and simultaneous listening of the heart beat and possibly reconstruction of the spatial position and actual geometry of the heart inside the chest based on the distortion of sound wave. This is an unexplored sufficiently topic because it was only recently the discovery of an important aspect of the anatomical and electrophysiological structure of the heart muscle—the spiral character of the single muscle that comprises the ventricles of the heart [25]. This anatomical structure has evolutionary meaning of efficient hold of the contracting container, which purpose is powerful blow of the liquid with minimal organ displacement.

Within the medical studies it has not been considered necessary for the fact that the ECG provides diagnosis of all aspects of the heart disease including 3D position and anatomical deformation, which can be supported by ultrasound, Xray and catheter intervention. On the other hand, medical experts intuitively diagnose based on sound (despite the imprecision of the stethoscope sensors, adapted to the average sensitivity of the human ear) and suggest that it is worth investigating how an intelligent system can analyze the vibrations of the heart and the artery to discover clinically relevant symptoms of early disease.

In summary, for building patient health records compatible with the Cloud-based healthcare applications new sensor technologies for representation of medical symptoms are needed as well as new health indicators for early and prospective diagnosis, implementing smart solutions for inclusion in relatively low-cost devices with higher fidelity than the existing ones.

Conclusions and Future Work

We are developing a device to collect, analyze and transmit data, obtained from registration of peripheral vibrations of the arteries of the human body. The gathered data profiles can be symptomatic for a number of diseases, which can be revealed by investigating heart problems. The current research is an attempt to overcome the electrical wiring of patients, including wearing smart fabrics, for diagnostics and alerting on health issues. Instead, we propose the development of *smart rubber* implementing novel health monitoring functionalities (or similar plastic material). Smart rubber has large future potential especially for implementing in novel devices to be used as User Interface as a Service (UIaaS) technologies for healthcare. By implementing the proposed approach the following technological transitions in Cloud computing for healthcare are expected:

- From lists of health indicators to AI based health condition assessment;
- From cable-wired health examination and medical-record management to wireless communication, secure transmission and translation of health data;
- From smart fabrics to smart rubber based health monitoring;
- From modality dependent and large-scale machinery-based imaging to compact and meaningful 3D organ/symptom visualization.

The proposed approach to development of new interface technologies provides the doctors and patients with useful tools to explore conditions and perform monitoring across diagnoses—in an indirect, safe, secure and harmless way—operating as new UIaaS. Future work includes design of the visualization module and tests of the compatibility with Cloud services as a step towards modern and ubiquitous healthcare based on Cloud computing.

References

1. B. Harris, "5 Ways Cloud Computing Will Transform Healthcare", http://www.healthcareitnews.com/news/5-ways-cloud-computing-will-transform-healthcare (accessed January 2013).
2. https://cloudsecurityalliance.org/research/him/ (accessed January 2013).
3. http://www.corp.att.com/healthcare/docs/medical_imaging_cloud.pdf (downloaded January 2013).
4. N. Hemsoth, "Opening Sequences for HPC on Demand", http://www.hpcinthecloud.com/hpccloud/2011-05-11/opening_sequences_for_hpc_on_demand.html.
5. http://www.independent.co.uk/life-style/health-and-families/health-news/smartphone-may-keep-the-cardiologist-away-1916652.html (accessed January 2013).
6. http://bblmedia.com/home_defibrillator.html (accessed January 2013).
7. C. Kaiser, "Cardio Notes: Docs Listen for Sound Arteries", http://www.medpagetoday.com/Cardiology/Atherosclerosis/36933 (accessed January 2013).
8. A. Freudenthal, T. Studeli, P. Lamata, and E. Samset, "Collaborative Co-design of Emerging Multi-technologies for Surgery", Journal of Biomedical Informatics, 44, 2011, pp. 198–215.
9. M. Dimitrova, Ch. Roumenin, D. Nikolov, D. Rotger, and P. Radeva, "Multimodal Data Fusion for Intelligent Cardiovascular Diagnosis and Treatment in ActiveVessel Medical Workstation", Journal of Intelligent Systems, Freund Publishing House Ltd., Vol. 18, No. 1–2, 2009, pp. 32–47.
10. M. Dimitrova, S. Lozanova, L. Lahtchev, and Ch. Roumenin, "New Interface Technologies for Cloud Healthcare Services", Comptes rendus de l'Académie bulgare des Sciences, Tome 65, No 1, 2012, pp. 83–88.
11. M. Dimitrova, S. Lozanova, L. Lahtchev, and Ch. Roumenin, "A Framework for Design of Cloud Compatible Medical Interfaces", In: B. Rachev and A. Smrikarov (Eds.), Proceedings if the International Conference on Computer Systems and Technologies (CompSysTech'12), Russe, Bulgaria, ACM New York, USA, ISBN 978-1-4503-1193-9, 2012, pp. 195–200.
12. A. Takaki, H. Ogawa, T. Wakeyama, T. Iwami, M. Kimura, Y., Hadano, S. Matsuda, Y. Miyazaki, T. Matsuda, A. Hiratsuka, and M. Matsuzak, "Cardio-ankle Vascular Index Is a New Noninvasive Parameter of Arterial Stiffness", Circulation Journal, 71, 2007, pp. 1710–1714.
13. G.J. van Beek, M.T. Boot, M. Claessens, O. Scheepstra, and Y. Zouhair, "Project DPK 10: Autarkic Living. Litter in Strijp", University of Technology Eindhoven, 08th January 2010, http://fritsvanbeek.com/evidens/B1.1.pdf (downloaded January 2013).
14. S. Marchev, "How to Read an Electrocardiogram", Sofia: TEVA, 2007 (In Bulgarian), http://sotirmarchev.tripod.com/EKG_Marchev.pdf (downloaded January 2013).
15. E. I. Barakova and T. Lourens, "Event Based Self-Supervised Temporal Integration for Multimodal Sensor Data", Journal of Integrative Neuroscience, Vol. 4, No. 2, 2005, pp. 265–282.
16. M. Dimitrova, L. Lahtchev, S. Losanova, and Ch. Roumenin, "Interface for Representation of Multimodal Information in Medical Applications", In: R. Romansky (Ed.) Proceedings of the International Conference on Information Technologies (InfoTech-2009), Varna, Bulgaria, ISBN: 978-954-438-771-6, 2009, pp. 157–164.
17. C. Nafis, V. Jensen, and R. von Jako, "Method for Evaluating Compatibility of Commercial Electromagnetic (EM) Micro Sensor Tracking Systems with Surgical and Imaging Tables", 2008, www.ascension-tech.com (accessed January 2013).
18. W. Wein, A. Khamene, D. A. Clevert, O. Kutter, and N. Navab, "Simulation and Fully Automatic Multimodal Registration of Medical Ultrasound", In: N. Ayache, S. Ourselin and A. Maeder (Eds.), Proceedings of MICCAI 2007, Part I, LNCS 4791, 2007, pp. 136–143.
19. Ch. Roumenin, " Microsensors for Magnetic Field". In: J. Korvink and O. Paul (Eds.), "MEMS Handbook", Chapter 11, William Andrew Publishing, USA, 2003.
20. W. H. Curioso and P. N. Mechael, "Enhancing 'M-Health' With South-To-South Collaborations", Health Affairs, Vol. 29, No 2, 2010, pp. 264–267.

21. J. Symonds, D. Parry, and J. Briggs, "An RFID-based System for Assisted Living: Challenges and Solutions," The Journal on Information Technology in Healthcare, Vol. 5, 2007, pp. 387–398.
22. M. Heisler, "Actively Engaging Patients in Treatment Decision Making and Monitoring as a Strategy to Improve Hypertension Outcomes in Diabetes Mellitus", Circulation, Journal of the American Ilcart Association, 117, 2008, pp. 1355–1357.
23. E. O'Brian, B. Waeber, G. Parati, J. Staessen, and M. G. Myers, "Blood Pressure Measuring Devices: Recommendations of the European Society for Hypertension", British Medical Journal, 322, 2001, pp. 531–536.
24. L. Lahchev, M. Dimitrova, and D. Rotger, "A Classifier of Technical Diagnostic States of Electrocardiograph", In: B. Rachev and A. Smrikarov (Eds.) Proceedings of the International Conference on Computer Systems and Technologies (CompSysTech'06), 2006, pp. III.A.15.1-III.A.15.6.
25. F. Torrent-Guasp, M. Ballester, G.D. Buckberg, F. Carreras, A. Flotats, I. Carrió, A. Ferreira, L. E. Samuels, and J. Narula, "Spatial Orientation of the Ventricular Muscle Band. Physiologic Contribution and Surgical Implications", Journal of Thorac and Cardiovascular Surgery, 2001, pp. 389–392.
26. L. H. Lahchev, J. D. Zaprianov, and I. B. Jonov, "Acoustic Interface to an Expert System for Turbo-Generator Shaft System Diagnosis", Proceedings of the IFAC Symposium on Control of Power Plants and Power Systems, Munich, March 9–11, 1992, pp. 195–200.
27. R. D. Sinelnikov, "Atlas of Human Anatomy, "Vol. III, Moscow: Medicine, 1981 (in Russian).
28. www.skintact.org (accessed January 2013).
29. L. Lahtchev and M. Dimitrova, "Systematics and Analysis of Computer-based Biomedical Research," In: R. Romansky (Ed.) Proceedings of the International Conference on Information Technologies (InfoTech-2008) vol. 2, Varna, Bulgaria, ISBN: 978-9549518-56-6, 2008, pp. 243–250.
30. http://www.datatranslation.com/products/dataacquisition/usb/DT9810/ (accessed January 2013).
31. http://www.tensoval.com/tensoval_duo_control.php (accessed January 2013).

Chapter 11
Tissue Engineering Triangle and its Development

Mirjana Pavlovic, John Mayfield and Bela Balint

Introduction

This chapter analyses the basic triangle in TE: cells, scaffolds, molecules in terms of their discovery, production and upgrading procedures within last decade. The most important researchers and their discoveries and breakthrough achievements are emphasized and elaborated.

Tissue engineering: definition and impact

There are two definitions of TE quoted in this chapter: NIH and Pittsburgh TE Initiative definitions.

NIH Definition of Tissue Engineering

Tissue engineering is an emerging multidisciplinary field involving biology, medicine, and engineering that is likely to revolutionize the ways we improve the health and quality of life for millions of people worldwide by restoring, maintaining, or enhancing tissue and organ function. In addition to having a therapeutic application, where the tissue is either grown in a patient or outside the patient and transplanted, tissue engineering can have diagnostic applications where the tissue is made in vitro and used for testing drug metabolism and uptake, toxicity, and pathogenicity. The foundation of tissue engineering for either therapeutic or diagnostic applications is the ability to exploit living cells in a variety of ways. Tissue engineering research includes biomaterials, cells, biomolecules, engineering design aspects, biomechanics, informatics to support tissue engineering and stem cell research.

M. Pavlovic (✉) · J. Mayfield
Department of Computer and Electrical Engineering and Computer Science,
Florida Atlantic University, Boca Raton, FL, USA
e-mail: mpavlovi@fau.edu

B. Balint
Military Medical Academy Belgrade, Belgrade, Serbia

B. Furht and A. Agarwal (eds.), *Handbook of Medical and Healthcare Technologies*,
DOI: 10.1007/978-1-4614-8495-0_11,

The Pittsburgh Tissue Engineering Initiative Definition

Tissue engineering is the development and manipulation of laboratory-grown molecules, cells, tissues, or organs to replace or support the function of defective or injured body parts. Although cells have been cultured, or grown, outside the body for many years, the possibility of growing complex, three-dimensional tissues—literally replicating the design and function of human tissue—is a recent development. The intricacies of this process require input from many types of scientists, including the problem solving expertise of engineers, hence the name tissue engineering. Tissue engineering crosses numerous medical and technical specialties: cell biologists, molecular biologists, biomaterial engineers, computer-assisted designers, microscopic imaging specialists, robotics engineers, and developers of equipment such as bioreactors, where tissues are grown and nurtured.

Although definitions of TE involve a lot of descriptions, this field is still evolving and once will be better defined. The perspective of this subject is greatly due to dramatic breakthroughs in different sections of TE such as: nanotechnology, scaffolds, robotics, artificial organs, etc. Quite distinctive field is stem cell technology the development of which is more convincingly conquering the regenerative and replacement issues in human pathology. The most important category within the concept of TE is an integral thinking, the process which requires not only broad individual education, but broad professional orientation of each individual within the team. The integration of the ideas is necessary for good foundation of the knowledge of the basic principles of science in general, functioning first in normal and then in pathologically changed tissues. Rational approach that involves mathematical, physical, chemical, biological and engineering principles is possible only if each particular problem solver has intention to act in synchrony with others. In that way the productive outcome can be achieved and novel approach to the old concept designed and executed.

Background and Significance

What is the difference between bioengineering and biomedical engineering?

Bioengineering: **biological engineering**, **biotechnological engineering** or **bioengineering** (including **biological systems engineering**) is the application of concepts and methods of physics, chemistry, mathematics, and computer science to solve problems in life sciences, using engineering's own analytical and synthetic methodologies and also its traditional sensitivity to the cost and practicality of the solution(s) arrived at [1, 2]. In this context, while traditional engineering applies physical and mathematical sciences to analyze, design and manufacture inanimate tools, structures and processes, biological engineering uses the same sciences, as well as the rapidly-developing body of knowledge known as molecular biology, to study many aspects of living organisms.

Thus, biological engineering **is a science-based discipline founded upon the biological sciences in the same way that chemical engineering, electrical engineering, and mechanical engineering are based upon chemistry, electricity and magnetism, and classical mechanics, respectively** [3].

Biological engineering can be differentiated from its roots of pure biology or classical engineering in the following way. Biological studies often follow a **reductionist approach** in viewing a system on its smallest possible scale which naturally leads toward tools such as **functional genomics**. Engineering approaches, using classical design perspectives, are constructionist, building new devices, approaches, and technologies from component concepts. Biological engineering utilizes both kinds of methods in concert, relying on reductionist approaches to identify, understand, and organize the fundamental units which are then integrated to generate something new. In addition,**because it is an engineering discipline, biological engineering is fundamentally concerned with not just the basic science, but the practical application of the scientific knowledge to solve real-world problems in a cost-effective way**.

Although engineered biological systems have been used to manipulate information, construct materials, process chemicals, produce energy, provide food, and help maintain or enhance human health and our environment, our ability to quickly and reliably engineer biological systems that behave as expected is at present less well developed than our mastery over mechanical and electrical systems [1].

The differentiation between biological engineering and **overlap with Biomedical Engineering can** be unclear, as many universities now use the terms "bioengineering" and "biomedical engineering" interchangeably. However, according to Prof. *Doug Laufenberg* of **MIT**, Biological Engineering (like biotechnology) has a **broader base** which applies engineering principles to an enormous range of size and complexities of systems ranging from the molecular level—molecular biology, biochemistry, microbiology, pharmacology, protein chemistry, cytology, immunology, neurobiology and neuroscience (often but not always using biological substances)—to cellular and tissue-based methods (including devices and sensors), whole macroscopic organisms (plants, animals), and up increasing length scales to whole ecosystems. Neither biological engineering nor biomedical engineering is wholly contained within the other, as there are **non-biological products for medical needs and biological products for non-medical needs** [2].

ABET the U.S.-based accreditation board for engineering B.S. programs, makes a distinction between Biomedical Engineering and Biological Engineering; however, **the differences are quite small**. Biomedical engineers must have life science courses that include **human physiology** and have experience in performing measurements on living systems while biological engineers must have **life science courses (which may or may not include physiology**) and experience in making measurements not specifically on living systems.

Foundational engineering courses are often the same, and include: thermodynamics, fluid and mechanical dynamics, kinetics, electronics, and materials properties.

How bioengineering relates to areas such as stem cell research?

They are fundamentally inter-related, since stem cells are known to be the building blocks of entire organism, the "blank chips" with great potential to Trans-differentiate into different tissues, and so regenerate, repopulate and recruit new cells in order to heal the process caused by the initial tissue damage [3]. Here we are in the Tissue Engineering area, the sub-area of Biomedical engineering, where stem-cell application is still debatable in some respect, but the results of which are also encouraging. The great breakthrough is the discovery and use of adult stem cells, which can be found and taken out of the human body and used either for classical transplantation or tissue reparation when necessary. There is a considerable advance in computer aided tissue engineering (CATE), where the dimensions of tissue damage can be determined, and tissue samples designed by the use of stem-cells and scaffolds, (the supportive structures made from biocompatible biomaterial), which are enabling stem cells to differentiate and grow in accordance with original tissue architecture, leading toward complete and perfect reparation. It is also strengthen by *ink-jet printing system,* where the stem cell patterns are layered by dispensing them through notorious ink-jet cartridge [3]. Stem cells have the capability of self-renewal, expansion under hypoxic conditions, and multipotency-capacity to differentiate into many directions dependent on the conditions. There are even trials with cells of an old organ which behave like stem cells when introduced into damaged one. Stem-cell researchers explain that those cells already know their environment and are well instructed; in fact they memorize how to arrange and to what extant to grow. This approach is developed by Dr. Anthony Atala and known as "*transplantation without a donor*". A great success of stem-cell application is especially noticed in the disease known as *osteogenesis imperfecta*, where the bones in children are extremely fragile, and when applied in early stage of child development they can dramatically improve their future life. I am personally collaborating with two groups from Europe, and they have very good results with application of autologous adult stem cells in acute myocardial infarction and other ischemic diseases.

What are the discipline's main sub-areas? Is it OK to specialize in only one of these areas?

They are really numerous, and I think that each is equally important since either bioengineering or biomedical engineering have so many sub-disciplines which are interrelated that it is difficult to make strict distinctions. In fact, the heart of these two disciplines is INTEGRATIVE THINKING and as such, involves the ideas for the solutions that are coming from life scientists and engineers at the same time. The first such "crossing over" happened between Alexander Fleming who has discovered Penicillin but did not have the possibility to expand its production, and Howard Florey who was a pharmacologist (chemical engineer) and who invented technology for Penicillin production using Fleming's frozen samples [2]. Today, for example, for a good Rational Vaccine Design (RVD) you need the interaction of Bioinformatician and Immunologist in order to do it well. The first one will do the data mining and necessary mathematical transformations in order to find the best possible candidate for the vaccine, while another will lead the bioinformatician through the field of immunology known as vaccination and finally check it experimentally in the wet-lab. So, the hypothesis is tested and either confirmed or rejected. Yes, it is OK to specialize in only one of these areas if you understand that the team work is the ESSENTIAL request for successful bioengineering solution.

What are the typical jobs that engineers perform in industry?

Biological Engineers or *bioengineers* are engineers who use the principles of biology and the tools of engineering to create usable, tangible, economically viable products. Biological Engineering employs knowledge and expertise from a number of pure and applied sciences, such as mass and heat transfer, kinetics, biocatalysts, biomechanics, bioinformatics, separation and purification processes, bioreactor design, surface science, fluid mechanics, thermodynamics, and polymer science. It is used in the design of medical devices, diagnostic equipment, biocompatible materials, renewable bioenergy, ecological engineering, and other areas that improve the living standards of societies.

In general, biological engineers attempt to either mimic biological systems to create products or modify and control biological systems so that they can replace, augment, or sustain chemical and mechanical processes. Bioengineers can apply their expertise to other applications of engineering and biotechnology, including genetic modification of plants and microorganisms, bioprocess engineering, and biocatalysis.

Because other engineering disciplines also address living organisms (e.g., prosthetics in mechanical engineering), the term biological engineering can be applied more broadly to include agricultural engineering and biotechnology. In fact, many old agricultural engineering departments in universities over the world have rebranded themselves as **agricultural and biological engineering** or **agricultural and biosystems engineering**. Biological engineering is also called bioengineering by some colleges and Biomedical engineering is called Bioengineering by others, and is a rapidly developing field with fluid categorization. The Main Fields of Bioengineering, and therefore, the typical jobs that they can find may be categorized as:

- **Bioprocess Engineering**: Bioprocess Design, Biocatalysis, Bioseparation, Bioinformatics, Bioenergy.
- **Genetic Engineering**: Synthetic Biology, Horizontal gene transfer.
- **Cellular Engineering**: Cell Engineering, Tissue Culture Engineering, Metabolic engineering.
- **Biomedical Engineering**: Biomedical technology, Biomedical Diagnostics, Biomedical Therapy, Biomechanics, Biomaterials.
- **Biomimetics**: The use of knowledge gained from evolved living systems to solve difficult design problems in artificial systems.

How is the market for fresh graduates? What are the typical salaries?

This is developing field in a rapid expansion, so the market is open to fresh graduates, either at Universities, Hospitals, or Industry. The typical salaries are: \$45,000–\$55,000 and within a year can reach even \$60,000.

What are the hot research and development topics?

One of the greatest is growing organs from patient's own tissue. A very good example of that is the bladder. Clinical trial is going on to collect the data. Great "hit" is drug delivery through particular vectors, the surface of which has the molecules that bind to specific receptors on damaged tissues. In that way, drug delivery is targeted toward only damaged tissue (cancer, inflammation, etc.) and the medication affects only sick cells without touching normal ones. This enables precise dosage and individual targeted therapy. The Bioinstrumentation has brought up also incredible solutions such as eradication of cancer cells by using golden nanoparticles in combination with laser technique. Gene therapy has raised the hope in treatment of hemophilia. Almost unbelievable, but true, the mouse eye is developed to the certain point in one experimental trial.

What are the long term challenges and future directions?

Since the very first use of stem cells in bioengineering they have been used with hope that they can have anti-ageing and life-improvement effect. Is the longevity the ultimate goal? For those who really live in that hope I think that, as a human race with defined life we cannot live much longer then we do. But as long as we leave, we should have a good quality of life. And that for sure, will be better. So, let us say that it is the ultimate goal and in my vision that is on its way to be achieved.

What are the academic prerequisites (science and math, software tools etc.) and what is the key academic bottlenecks en-route to graduation?

In my experience, at least here, at FAU I have found that students with good understanding of basic sciences (math, chemistry and physics) even without any biological experience can "conquer" biological knowledge to that extent that they feel very comfortable in becoming independent in their work. Especially if they are scientifically oriented and therefore, very resourceful, they can surprise you pleasantly with problem solving and creativity skills. Both are important for bioengineering and their own growth. My students were amazingly interested in what they were doing and therefore their knowledge was/is exceptionally solid.

What are typical topics for senior design projects?

I would say: nanotechnology, rational vaccine design, gene therapy, stem-cell application, bioinstrumentation, etc.

How much of the engineer's work is done at the "systems level" and how much at the "individual device level"?

It is really hard to say. I do believe that it goes in parallel, since both directions are challenging and necessary to be developed, and as long as we as humans are different, so there will be those who are interested in one and those who have an interest in another direction. In that sense, both directions will be and I think they are, developed with great enthusiasm and intellectual investment. An especially important application is the analysis and cost-effective solution of problems related to human health, but the field is much more general than that. For example, biomimetics is a branch of biological engineering which strives to understand how living organisms, as a result of the prolonged trial-and-error processes known as evolution, have solved difficult problems in the past, and to find ways to use this knowledge to solve similar

Table 11.1 Diagram of TE triangle

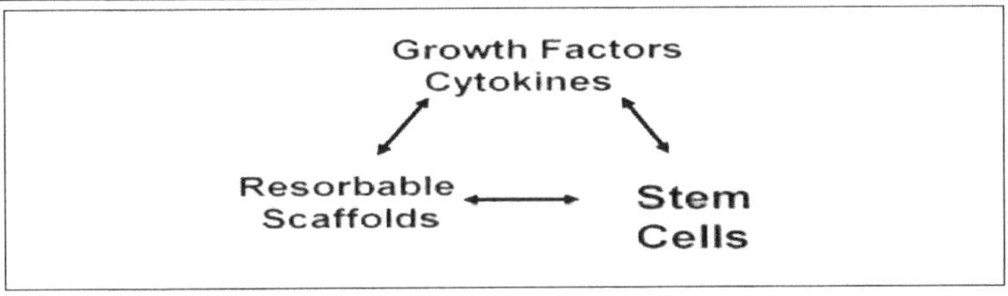

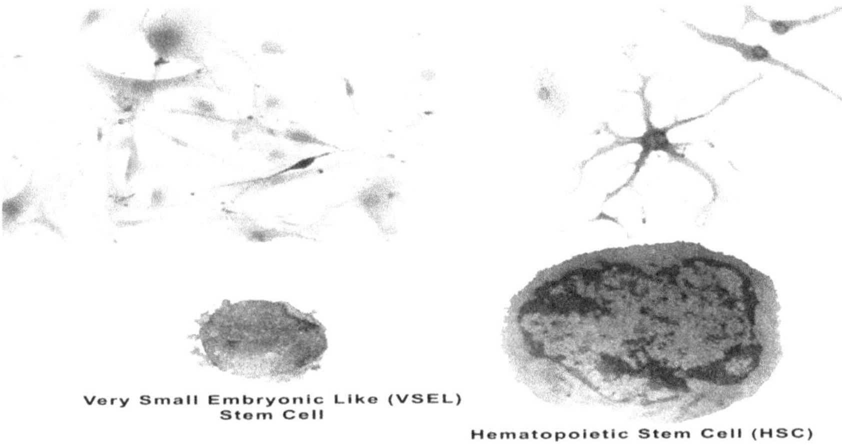

Fig. 11.1 Hematopoietic stem cells and Very Small Embryonic-like cells as patterns for TE

problems in artificial systems. Systems biology, on the other hand, seeks to utilize the engineer's familiarity with complex artificial systems, and perhaps the concepts used in "reverse engineering", to facilitate the difficult process of recognition of the structure, function, and precise method of operation of complex biological systems (Fig. 11.1).

Tissue engineering as a Substantial Advance in Medicine

- The triangle of TE

One of the fundamental features of TE is its "triangle", the participation of three fundamental components such as: cells, scaffolds and active molecules. Together, they contribute to the significant breakthrough in TE: 3-D (three-dimensional growth of tissue, which was before that only planar and limited to relatively simple cell culture technique)(Table 11.1).

Cells: Cell is either one (unicellular) organism or the physiological unit of multicellular organisms (animal and/or plant). It is open but limited-border-lined system involving very functional cell membrane. It communicates with external environment through plasma membrane (open pores and active transport); while at the same time makes a borderline toward it. The cellular components of different tissues are different assuming that we have about 200 different types of cells and about 10–100 trillion of cells within human body (according to different sources) which is just an estimate, since there is no method so far developed for determination of the exact total body cell count.

Talking about the cells on scaffolds, there are mainly two types of cells today: either those are chosen patterns of stem cells [4–6], or old cells taken from biopsy sample and seeded through ink-jet printer into the biodegradable and bioresorbable scaffold molds that are helping shaping of the organ [7]. This latter approach is known as "transplantation without a donor" and is used in connection with diseases of bladder so far. While clinical trials are going on, researchers are trying to

Understand how the cells of differentiated tissue have the memory for the environment that they have left and where is that memory stored and if so, is that different than in stem cells? Many questions are open with this breakthrough of Dr Athala, but two important facts are achieved: the body does not engage immunological mechanisms to destroy the cells since they belong to the same organism, and the patient does not have to wait for organ donor to be found and then transplanted since he has his own, made by this TE technique.

Scaffolds

The essential idea of 3-D growth is to get the cells to grow in three dimensions, while in tissue culture (growing in the flasks, on their surface) they had quite planar growth. The 3-D growth is facilitated by introduction of scaffolds, supportive structures for cell growth made from different materials, but unique in that that they are stimulating stem cells for movement-mobilization in all directions and interaction with the molecules of extra cellular matrix that facilitate the 3-D growth (Table 11.2).

Thus, scaffolds are probably one of the most prominent breakthroughs in TE enabling tissue architecture to grow in three dimensions and layers, if necessary. Scaffolds have been initially made from the hard material or at least solid, however, the last news are the liquid scaffolds that can be ink-jet printed into the specific environment where the replacement of defected tissue is expected to happen ( ).

Growth Factors

When talking about growth factors, we have to emphasize the role of extracellular matrix in the tissues, especially solid tissues. While blood as the liquid tissue has HS

Table 11.2 Characteristics of different scaffolding approaches in tissue engineering

Characteristics of different scaffolding approaches in tissue engineering

Scaffolding approach	(1) Pre-made porous scaffolds for cell seeding	(2) Decellularized extracellular matrix for cell seeding	(3) Con cells with secreted extracell matrix
Raw materials	Synthetic or natural biomaterials	Allogenic or xenogenic tissues	Cells
Processing or fabricating technology	Incorporation of porogens in solid materials; solid free-form fabrication technologies; techniques using woven or non-woven fibers	Decellularization technologies	Secretion extracellu matrix by confluent
to	Seeding	Seeding	Cells pres

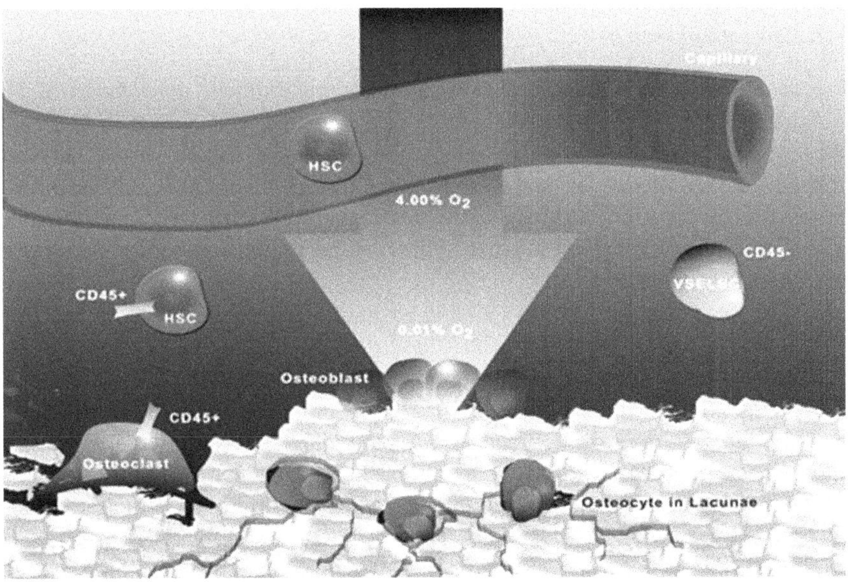

Fig. 11.2 Adult stem cell (HSC) and VSEL in the niche of Bone Marrow, exposed to hypoxia and impact of other environmental molecules, including growth factors

and VSEL cells in the niches with a specific environment (Fig. 11.2), solid tissues have the extracellular matrix (ECM), the interconnected complex substances between the cells, (laminins, integrins, etc) filled with different growth factors which may alter proliferation and differentiation of the given stem cells in different manners. Dependent on the sort of cell and the level of cellular evolution and maturation, different active molecules with the role of growth factors will attach to the cell surfaces producing signals that could convey crucial messages resulting in movement, proliferation and/or differentiation of these cells.

Table 11.2 is showing the functions of ECM in native tissues and on scaffolds. And really, the best scaffold should be the ECM of the target tissue in its native state. However, due to complexity of ECM it is difficult to be mimicked exactly. It is replaced therefore with the most appropriate biomaterials in the form of scaffolds, analogous to the functions of ECM in native tissues and associated with their architectural, biological and mechanical features.

Technical Breakthroughs

- Microscopy (light, compound, phase contrast, electron : transmission and freeze fracture, atomic force)

Probably one of the greatest discoveries and breakthroughs in evolution of TE is construction of the compound microscope greatly facilitated even in sixteenth and seventeenth centuries by J. Jenssen, A. Loevenhook and R. Hook, who all have realized the role of magnifying glass in visualization of invisible structures and entities, and by upgrading and solving the resolution problems to the highest possible extent, open the door for formulation of the cell theory. Schwan and Schliden will later on introduce the term cell in the biology as the unicellular organism or smallest functional part of the organism or building block of organ and tissue structures. This will inspire the researchers to look into the shape, size and behavior of the cells and with the introduction of vital dyes, for specific organelle, they will show that the cell, like the atom, is particulated. This will trigger the curiosity of scientists in order to look into the growth of the cell and in order to be able to see the cells trough the culture medium, it was necessary to use physical phenomenon known as the phase contrast and incorporate it into microscope. The first microscope with phase contrast has been constructed in 1934 by Dutch physicist Frits Zernike who will later on get the Nobel Prize for that discovery. The addition of phase contrast optical accessories to a standard bright-field microscope, can be employed as a technique to render a contrast-enhancing effects in transparent specimens that is reminiscent of optical staining. Light waves that are diffracted and shifted in phase by the specimen (termed a *phase object*) can be transformed by phase contrast into amplitude differences that are observable in the eyepieces (Fig. 11.3).

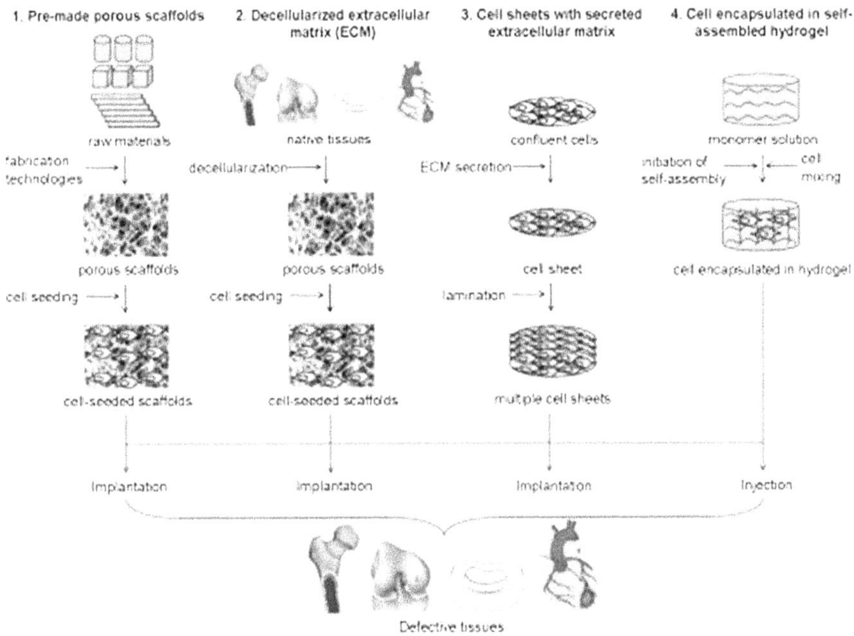

Fig. 11.3 Schematic diagram showing different scaffolding approaches in tissue engineering

Table 11.3 Functions of extracellular matrix (ECM) in native tissues and of scaffolds in engineer

Functions of extracellular matrix (ECM) in native tissues and of scaffolds in enginee

	Functions of ECM in native tissues	Analogous functions of scaffolds in engineered tissues	Architectural, biolo features of scaffolc
1.	Provides structural support for cells to reside	Provides structural support for exogenously applied cells to attach, grow, migrate and differentiate in vitro and in vivo	Biomaterials with bi porous structure wit migration and for nu temporary resistanc implantation
2.	Contributes to the mechanical properties of tissues	Provides the shape and mechanical stability to the tissue defect and gives the rigidity and stiffness to	Biomaterials with su properties filling up t defect and simulatin

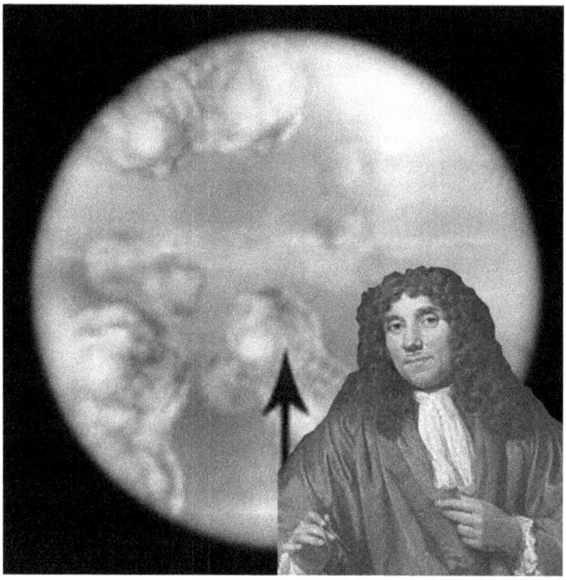

Fig. 11.4 Antoine de Leuwenhoek and his microscope

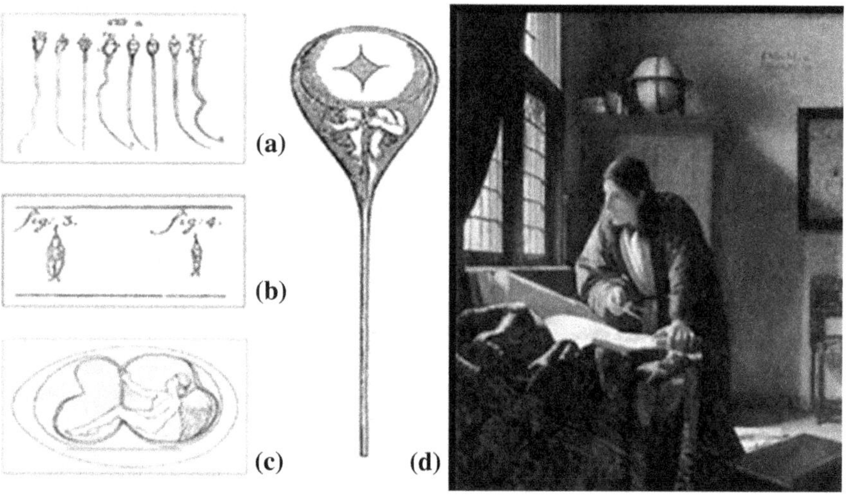

Fig. 11.5 Not only a great innovator but a great thinker as well

Zernike's development of phase contrast optical theory is an excellent example of how research results from a highly specialized field (in this case, theoretical physics) can yield innovative new developments in seemingly unrelated disciplines, such as biology and medicine. During the Second World War, the Zeiss Optical Works in Jena, Germany, was the first manufacturer to incorporate practical phase contrast optics into their microscopes. The immediate impact on biological research was significant, and widespread application of the technique continues to the present day. Modern phase contrast objectives, designed and produced by Nikon and other optical manufacturers, are capable of operating in combination with auxiliary contrast-enhancing techniques, such as differential interference contrast, fluorescence, and polarized light. Thcsc objectives are available with internal phase plates that have varying levels of absorption and phase displacement of the surround (undiffracted) illumination to produce a wide spectrum of specimen contrast and background intensity choices for phase contrast microscopy (Fig. 11.4).

- Patch clamp technique

One of the most prominent biological technologies that has found its application very quickly in vital medical situations is a Patch clump technique invented by Bert Sackman who has got a Nobel Prize for that in 1991. Everything is based on a microelectrode. The electrode is sealed to the patch of membrane, and the cell remains intact [8]. This allows for the recording of currents through single ion channels in that patch of membrane, without disrupting the interior of the cell. Our nerve cells convey the electric signal through ion channels of different kinds, and it is possible to be measured by this device. The microelectrodes will later on be used even on alive humans and gather a lot of information necessary for understanding of the work of nervous system (Fig. 11.5).

For ligand-gated ion channels or channels that are modulated by metabotropic receptors, the neurotransmitter or drug being studied is usually included in the pipette solution, where it can contact what had been the external surface of the membrane. While the resulting channel activity can be attributed to the drug being used, it is usually not possible to then change the drug concentration. The technique is thus limited to one point in a dose response curve per patch [8, 9]. This technology is with different modifications elevated to much higher level than it was 20 years ago and used in animal models for better characterization of different neurological phenomena including diseases and defects (Fig. 11.6).

- Neural Growth Factor (NGF)

On molecular level, probably the biggest discovery was that of Rita Levi Moltanzini and Stanley Cohen who have isolated and shown that this molecule has neural cell growth effect (1934) t. It took them 20 years to convince the humanity that it really works. They have got the Nobel Prize for their work, which has become the basis for differentiation procedures in stem cell cultures and tissue engineering where the growth of neural cells is necessary. This is the molecule without the influence of which, the growth of neural tissue is impossible, vital for that and many other tissues and fundamental for neuroscience development [10].

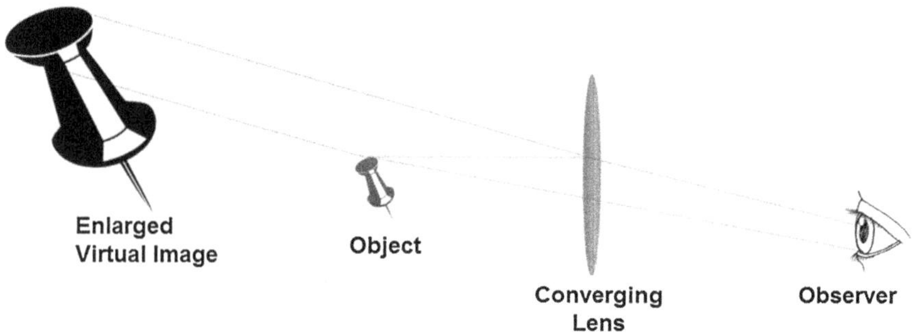

Fig. 11.6 The principle of work of magnifying glass

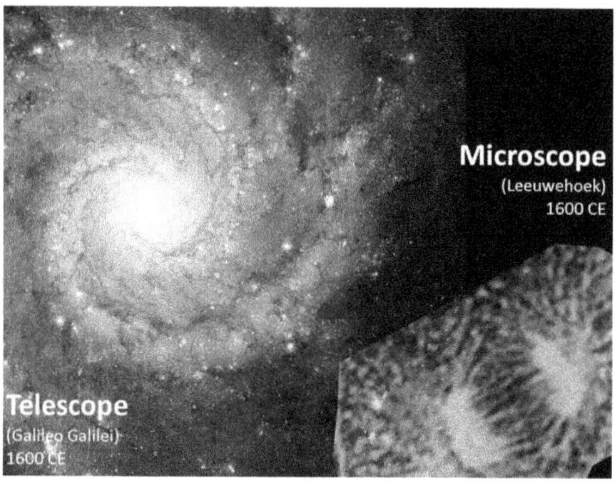

Fig. 11.7 The humans have looked into the Universe and into the cell at almost the same time

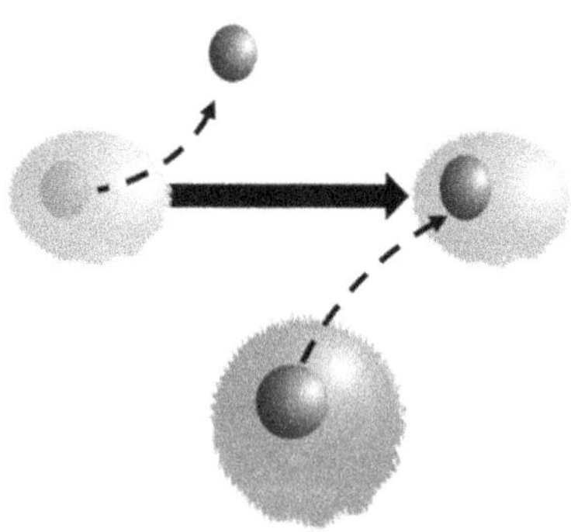

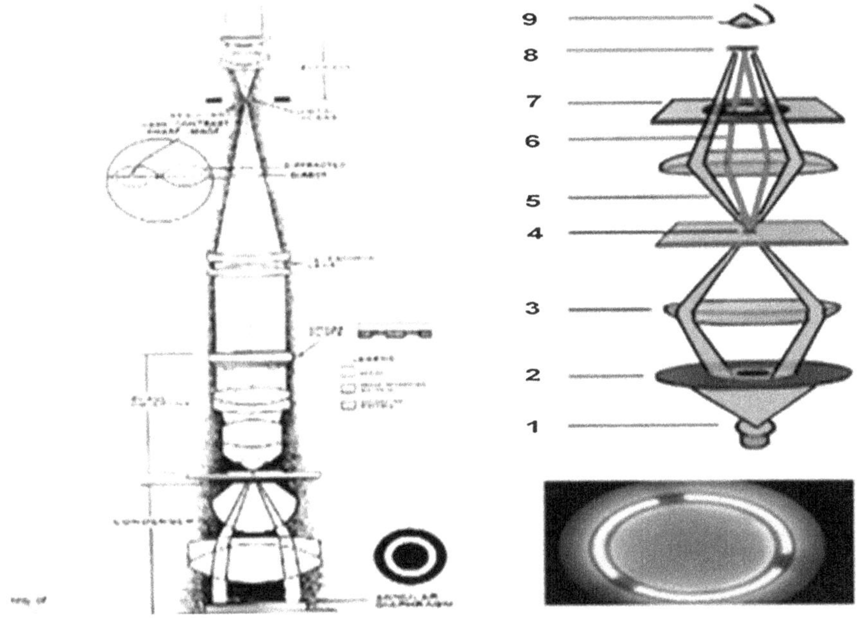

Fig. 11.8 Phase contrast microscope

Fluorphore	Excitation (nm)	Emission (nm)
Hoechst 33342	343	483
DAPI	345	[illegible]
R-Phycoerythrin (PE)	480;565	578
EGFP	488	507
Fluorescein	495	519
Cy3	(512);550	570;(615)
TRITC	547	572
Texas Red	589	615
Cy5	(625);650	670
Allophycocyanin (APC)	650	660
Cy7	743	767

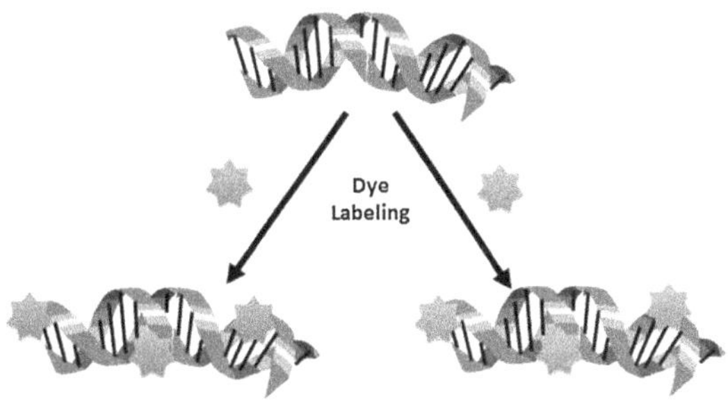

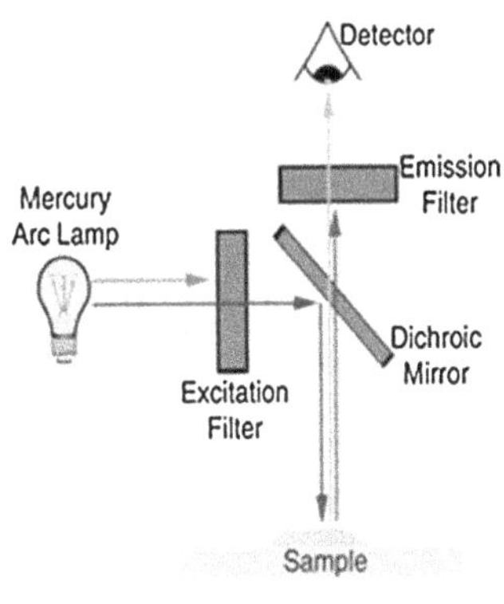

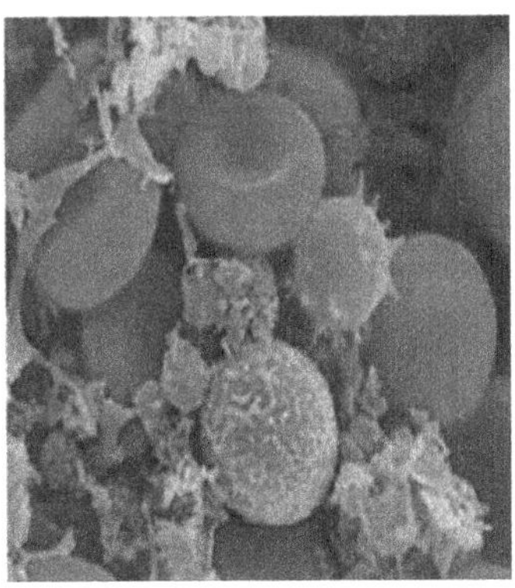

• FC and FACS

Understanding of the fluorescence and fluorescent dyes has supported further development of knowledge on stem cells and cells in general since it was possible to label monoclonal antibodies for specific protein markers with characteristic dye and then detect it in the cell or on it by using fluorescent microscope or Flow cytometry. The classification of the cells in categories and their separation was facilitated by introduction of cell sorter (fluorescence acquisition cell sorter (FACS)) (Fig. 11.7).

• What else?

Probably the development of fluorescent dyes and staining with use of labeled monoclonal antibodies was fundamental breakthrough for establishment of criteria at molecular level on and within the cells, the Flow Cytometry and Cell Sorter were also of strong impact upon the understanding of the molecular basis of stem cells and different techniques in scaffolding have characterized the new era of TE. However, transplantation without a donor, the great innovation of Dr Anthony Atala is looking into the future with a bright smile [8–10]. Gene therapy trials, nanorobotics and entire nanotechnology will change the quality of life of future civilizations tremendously (Fig. 11.8).

References

1. S.A.Berger, W.Goldsmith, and E.R.Lewis (eds):Introduction to bioengineering 1996, Oxford University Press, Oxford New York.
2. W.Matk Saltzman:Biomedical Engineering. 2009, Cambridge Univerosty Press, New York.
3. M.Pavlovic (Ed) and B.Balint: Stem cells and Tissue engineering, Springer Brief, 2013.
4. Kucia M, Reca R, Campbell FR, Surma-Zuba E, Majka M, Ratajczak M, and Ratajczak MZ A population of very small embryonic - like (VSEL) CXR4+SSEA-1+Oct4+ stem cells identified in adult bone marrow. Leukemia 2006, 20: 857–69.
5. Balint B, Ljubenov M, Stamatović D, Todorović M, Pavlović M, Ostojić G, et al. Stem cell harvesting protocol research in autologous transplantation setting: large volume vs. conventional cytapheresis Vojnosanit Preg 2008; 65(7): 545–51.
6. Todorović V, Marković D, Milošević-Jovčić N, Petakov M, Balint B, Čolić M et al. Dental pulp stem cells - potential significance in regenerative medicine. Stom Glas S 2008; 55: 170–9.
7. A.Atala, Bauer S, Soker S, Yoo JJ, Retik Ab: Tissue-engineered bladders for patients needing cytoplasty. The lancet, 367, 9518,:1241–1246, 2006.
8. Hamill OP, Marty A, Neher E, Sakmann B, Sigworth FJ. (1981). "Improved patch-clamp techniques for high-resolution current recording from cells and cell-free membrane patches". Pflügers Archiv European Journal of Physiology 391 (2): 85–100. doi:10.1007/BF00656997. PMID 6270629.
9. J. I. Lee, M. Sato, H. W. Kim, and J. Mochida, "Transplantatation of scaffold-free spheroids composed of synovium-derived cells and chondrocytes for the treatment of cartilage defects of the knee",European Cells and Materials Journal, vol. 22, pp. 275–290, 2011.
10. Hamburger V. The history of discovery of nerve growth factor. J Neurobiol 1993, 24(7):893–7.

Part II
Healthcare Technologies

Chapter 12
Brief Overview of Various Healthcare Tools, Methods, Framework and Standards

Timothy Cyr, Ankur Agarwal and Borko Furht

Abstract There exists a multitude of standards with regards to health information systems (HIS) and the electronic exchange of commercial transactions containing private data that must be used amongst various service providers to adequately perform their duties to patients. The evolution of health information systems has been guided by business interests as well as from government legislation creating a somewhat fragmented system with many marginally compatible components exchanging patient sensitive information electronically. The many standards in use today include: HIPAA, EDI, HL-7, DICOM, IEEE 11073, ICD-9, and CPT. In this chapter, we discuss various healthcare standards listed above and their history briefly.

Introduction

A key to gaining knowledge in a system such as the healthcare industry is the ability to correctly interpret information that is received through processing of precise and accurate data collected within a standardized guideline for conformity amongst multiple coordinating agencies to develop the most comprehensive information system with effective and efficient outcomes for the state of a patients' well-being. The knowledge of standards allows the healthcare industry to deliver its services in an effective and efficient manner. The core of a Health Information System (HIS) is the flow/exchange of complete, timely, and accurate data within a healthcare delivery organization as well as among various healthcare delivery systems. This allows

T. Cyr · A. Agarwal (✉) · B. Furht
Department of Computer & Electrical Engineering and Computer Science, Florida Atlantic University, Boca Raton, FL 33431, USA
e-mail: ankur@cse.fau.edu

B. Furht
e-mail: bfurht@fau.edu

B. Furht and A. Agarwal (eds.), *Handbook of Medical and Healthcare Technologies*,
DOI: 10.1007/978-1-4614-8495-0_12, © Springer Science+Business Media New York 2013

the creation of a fully integrated information infrastructure to service patients and maximizes the outcome of delivered healthcare [1].

The healthcare system is much dispersed in nature. There are public and private entities in existence for delivery of complete healthcare. These entities exchange information among themselves (between public to public, private to private, private to public or public to private) in order to render healthcare services to the individual and society at large. Such coexistence has led to fragmentation. The result of this fragmentation has caused severe challenges for evolving standards for healthcare industry. For instance, the private hospital may interact with a private lab for getting medical condition testing while they seek the reimbursement for their services from government organizations such as Medicaid or a Medicare or from a private health insurance companies such as Humana healthcare.

All of these interactions such as patient medical data, billing information among others, must be kept private and secured at all time in order to respect the patient privacy. All these requirements have posed challenges for adoption and integration of technology in healthcare domain. The exponential growth of information and information exchange capabilities creates an increasingly arduous task of providing interoperability and integration between heterogeneous healthcare information systems while maintaining data security.

There is a legislative push in the healthcare industry to move towards interoperability of health and medical information [2]. Better health outcomes and reduced healthcare cost are the driving factors for this push to adopt interoperability. Such interoperability is impossible to achieve until all health information systems adopt electronic standards (moving away from paper) for data generation. This effort has led to vast amount of health and medical data generation. As a result of this various organization and workgroups had been formed which are aimed to conduct research and provide solutions to help alleviate the information overload of the healthcare system. These organizations are seen as the leaders and advisory group for leading the path for healthcare industry. Institute of Medicine (IOM) and the Workgroup for Electronic Data Interchange are two examples for such organizations.

IOM was established in 1970 servers as a branch of the National Academy of Sciences. A report released by IOM in 1991 stated the need for a computer-based patient record defining it as an electronic patient record. As per the report the electronic patient record was to be used within a healthcare specific framework for allowing patients, physicians, insurance companies, healthcare facilities, and any other necessary institutions or agencies with timely access to complete unaltered data accurately through a secure network [3]. WEDI was established in November of 1991 comprising of volunteer representatives from the public and private healthcare industries [4]. The main objective of WEDI was to gain insight and perspective into the issue of Electronic Data Interchange (EDI), reduce administrative costs, and streamline healthcare administration. The 1993 WEDI report presented a vision for the future healthcare industry which is equipped with a system that is fully interoperable, providing a secure electronic health information technology infrastructure and operating under a universal standard used for all business transactions. In the report WEDI defined a strict federal role in EDI where, federal government is solely responsible for the definition of the mechanisms to be used in EDI. These reports helped to fuel the formation of legislation to guide implementation of electronic information in healthcare standards [5].

In 1994 the Health Security Act was debated on the senate floor for the first time and that law developed into the Health Insurance Portability and Accountability Act of 1996 (HIPAA) signed into law August 1996 [4]. This was a milestone for the healthcare industry as it was the first major legislation on healthcare information standards in the United States.

Standards

HIPAA created a baseline for conformity standards amongst the healthcare industry providers applying holistically to all agencies from the federal level on to the state level and further down to the individual Physician. HIPAA states its purpose is "to improve…the efficiency and effectiveness of the healthcare system, by encouraging the development of a health information system through the establishment of standards and requirements for the electronic transmission of certain health information" [6]. HIPAA legislation outlined general requirements, definitions, and security standards for the healthcare industry.

HIPAA created many laws governing the adoption of standards and regulations concerning the technical capabilities of EDI systems especially concerning the security and privacy of an individual patient's record. HIPAA was the basic legislation defining Individual Identifiable Health Information (IHII). This definition gives rise to Protected Health Information (PHI). PHI is an important part of an Electronic Medical Record (EMR) or an Electronic Health Record (EHR) that is available to various healthcare organizations for facilitating the effective and efficient delivery of healthcare services to patients [6].

HIPAA helped to push the healthcare industry towards implementing holistic HIS standards. However the lack of further legislation to enforce these standards left the industry fragmented and incomplete. In 2009 the American Recovery and Reinvestment Act (ARRA) and the Health Information Technology for Economic and Clinical Health Act (HITECH) were passed [7]. HIPAA and ARRA HITECH provide legislation to regulate the privacy and security of personal health information with great emphasis on protecting the rights of patients [6, 8]. These laws help to further define the regulations concerning Electronic Protected Health Information (e-PHI), and IIHI and their implications to the implementation of EHR systems conforming to specified security requirements [8]. These laws do not specify the exact implementations of HIS standard protocols. As a result many electronic communication protocols have been developed. The most widely accepted international electronic communication standard issuing protocols is Health Level Seven International (HL-7).

HL-7 has standards adopted by several organizations such as the U.S. Department of Health and Human Services. The American National Standards Institute (ANSI) has adopted standards under their clinical and administrative domain standards [9].

The International Organization for Standardization (ISO) has several standards such as data exchange standards, EHR standards, health informatics standards, and electronic business extensible markup language (ebXML) standards using HL-7 [10].

HL-7 provides a broad set of standards creating domain specific protocols to achieve interoperability among healthcare service providers. Two specific standards are the clinical document architecture (CDA), and the Continuity of Care Document (CCD). These systems target healthcare providers, healthcare information technology vendors, EHR and PHR systems. One other major HL-7 standard is the Clinical Context Object Workgroup (CCOW). CCOW is a system developed to allow hospital and healthcare facilities utilizing more than one information system to streamline data interchange providing a foundation for meeting HIPAA and ARRA HITECH requirements [9].

HL-7 Reference Information Model (RIM) is the basis for deriving working ebXML message documents to be used in standardized information exchange protocols such as Transmission Control Protocol/Internet protocol (TCP/IP). RIM is a pictorial object model representing data domains and the life-cycle of a message or a group of messages [9, 11, 12]. HL-7 provides some specific codified language protocols that are widely accepted and used globally by many health care organizations. Further a highly specified standard for medical imaging has been developed.

The National Electrical Manufacturers Association (NEMA) and the American College of Radiology teamed up to form a committee to develop standards for capturing, storing, and viewing radiological images. The result is the digital imaging and communication in medicine (DICOM) non-proprietary data exchange protocol [13, 14]. This standard has been accepted and put into use as an international interchange for digitized medical imaging.

Medical imaging involves tremendously complex computer based processing techniques to obtain high resolution 3-dimensional images. These digital images are large data files that need to be stored, retrieved and processed rapidly. This has led to the evolution of a standard Picture Archiving and Communication System (PACS). Almost all PACS utilize the DICOM standard [15]. DICOM and PACS are well designed to allow the interoperability of all medical imaging. Other medical equipment and devices have such defined information protocols as outlined in the Institute of Electrical and Electronic Engineers (IEEE) standards.

IEEE has provided the standards of Medical Device Communication ISO/IEEE 11073 [10]. One standard is IEEE 11073-20601 which defines precise secure information transfer protocols for a manager/agent communication system. In this context ISO/IEEE, 11073 defines the implementation of communication standards to be used between agents such as a blood pressure monitors and other medical data collection equipment and managers such as smart phones or personal computers responsible for collecting, displaying, and re-transmitting the collected data [16].

As discussed there are numerous standards regarding privacy, security, electronic use of data, and electronic communication in healthcare. There are also standards that healthcare providers must follow when billing and insurance providers. This is a major part of the medical information infrastructure as this is how a healthcare provider will ultimately be able to receive compensation for rendered services.

The American Medical Association (AMA) provides the official Current Procedural Terminology codes for medical billing [17]. CPT codes are set for specific procedures and diagnostics with a reimbursement value assigned to them declaring how much compensation will be received by the healthcare provider thereby creating a schedule of fees. CPT codes are contained in an EMR which must get transmitted to an insurance provider in a secured and efficient manner. Determining which CPT code to use is a critical decision that must be made by the healthcare provider requiring the provider to have timely, accurate, and complete data when making a diagnosis and codifying procedures. Errors in this process can result in future misdiagnosis by healthcare providers and cause a negative economic impact [18]. Correct diagnosis of a condition or disease is the first step in identifying the proper CPT code so disease classification becomes a key factor in making a diagnosis. A worldwide standard exists for the classification of diseases.

Standards encompassing worldwide disease classification are set by the World Health Organization (WHO) and known as the International Classification of Diseases, Ninth Revision (ICD-9) [19]. This classification is used to collect, process, classify, and house mortality statistics. A related classification the International Classification of Diseases, Clinical Modification (ICD-9-CM) exists. ICD-9-CM is the official classification system of codifying diagnosis and procedures associated with the utilization of hospitals in the US [20].

All of the standards and regulations reviewed in this paper are for the content of health information. Implementations of systems that operate using the content of healthcare information exist as tools and frameworks for data processing. The frameworks developed must conform to the healthcare standards and regulations, utilizing tools that provide interoperability and timely access to accurate and complete data.

Tools, Methodologies, and Frameworks

Developing a healthcare product that is robust and provides effective and efficient processing of information is a complex process. It requires implementing healthcare standards and regulations and knowledge of many heterogeneous subsystems. An EMR is a primary information source for patient records and data providing the initial contact information for patients in a healthcare environment. There are several EMR solutions present today. The new generation of EMR solutions provide interface with mobile device such as a tablet for easy access to a patient data. Further the EMR solutions of current generation have becomes more specialized in providing disease specific solutions. For instance an EMR can be designed to provide the data management for a specific speciality such as Cardiology or Dermatology. While the other EMR are also designed to provide a template based solutions. These templates are customizable in nature for providing a better layout of information exposure which is customized for a specific speciality. All the EMRs are required to be certified by National Institution of Standards and Technology (NIST) for Meaningful User

One (MU-1) certification. The MU-1 certification dictates on the minimum interfaces and information capture for an EMR system.

On the other hand there are simple EMR solutions. One such open source EMR solution is OpenEMR [21]. OpenEMR is a small open source software tool for mainly research and development efforts. The software provides its usage in medical practice management. OpenEMR allows the integration of patient health records with electronic billing data, insurance data, and scheduling. The software also incorporates administrative functions for the EMR such as a backend billing function to insurance companies and clearinghouses. Report generation is also incorporated into OpenEMR as well placing orders for laboratory tests and procedures [22]. In the end the software is well developed to provide a good model for understanding the EMR system functionality and allowing new research method to be developed based on the existing solution. One concern for the development of frameworks and tools is conformity to legislation based regulations on healthcare information.

Implementing cloud computing architecture into healthcare information systems is one methodology being adopted at a fast pace. This requires special concern for data security as information is traveling to and from a data storage facility over a data network. The Implementation of cloud computing brings forth the possibility for patients to have access to and control over their Personal Health Record (PHR) as long as the information is kept secure through privacy protection mechanisms [23].

The PHR mainly contain the patient specific information such as learning resource specific to a disease or medicine, results of lab, medication lists, patient past medical history, and appointment schedule among others. Now PHR have advanced to provide a web-based interface where the data may reside on a cloud which is either accessible through a computer connected through internet or even a mobile device [24]. PHRs have been mandated by HIPAA and HITECH to ensure the data availability for patient usage and learning resources [6, 8]. One methodology in providing accountability requires authentication of a digital signature for any access to a PHR through a data repository. This ensures that data repositories are maintained and monitored [24]. Ensuring data security is paramount in PHR requiring strict transmission protocol.

The National Health Information Network (NHIN) is being developed to provide a robust health information infrastructure needed to support cloud computing technologies and user control of their PHR [25]. The NHIN framework addresses the connectivity issue between healthcare providers and health information exchange (HIE). The NHIN is essentially a "Network of Networks" [25].

Core capabilities of these HIE networks include the ability to access and exchange health information in a secure manner giving users control over information exchange preferences. In accomplishing this goal, NHIN has developed two sub components: (1) NHIN CONNECT which services large organizations and (2) NHIN Direct which targets at smaller physician practices. These two systems are tailored to the specific health information network architectures of large organizations such as HIE systems versus smaller information networks in a practicing physician's office [24]. NHIN Direct poses a specific challenge for providing data security knowledge to users of PHR systems. Techniques and methods for enhancing data security exist in encryption methods and protocols.

Having a robust health information infrastructure in today's personal communication market includes the ability of users to be able to securely access a PHR system from mobile devices outside of trusted domains of healthcare facility networks. Preventing unauthorized access to data is a major concern with cloud computing. Another major issue is exposing the data to other network during the data transmission such as over the wireless network. One method used to address the issue of data privacy and security in cloud computing is attribute-based encryption (ABE) [26].

ABE has provided a proof-of-concept for secure mobile encryption of health data [27]. Within the framework patient-centric EHR systems and cloud computing, ABE allows for the encrypted storage of personal health data in the cloud with access to that information being directly controlled by the patient. The key to this system is the ability of a patient to encrypt data under healthcare provider attributes so that deciphering the information can only be accomplished by a healthcare provider with those attributes such as (provider attribute: Dr. Jones and identification attribute: 12345). In this method metadata associated with patients files is also hidden so that repositories cannot identify any particular file thereby, a user insuring the privacy of data is protected [26].

HL-7 encoding also allows the information encryption and therefore data security. HL-7 encoding is complex ebXML code format used to transmit health information messages between health care facilities [9]. One framework for DICOM and HL-7 implementation is Mirth Connect. Mirth Connect addresses the interoperability problem with disparate healthcare information systems providing integration in information exchange. Mirth Connect is a standards-based integration engine for healthcare information systems making use of communication messaging interfaces or channels to send and receive data [28]. These channels carry data in many formats including standardized medical information formats such as HL-7. Mirth Connect is open source platform coded using the JAVA programming language [29].

DICOM is the specialized coding format for radiological images [13]. Mirth Connect helps to solve the interoperability problem translating messages to and from coded formats for display and manipulation. The open source environment of Mirth Connect allows for individual tailoring of data acquisition, data storage, and data presentation to the needs of an individual health care facility. This ability to select plug-ins and modules for a specific interest gives Mirth Connect the power to create efficient and effective solutions to HIE for healthcare organizations. One module focusing on HIE security and individual entity identification is Mirth Match [29].

Mirth Match is a solution cross referencing patient data files between providers that creates a master patient index used by providers. This is especially important when implementing HIE's. Using a cross referencing index for matching patient records is vital in providing interoperability in a HIS. Mirth Connect is powerful framework for using DICOM objects.

Mobile diagnostic devices are becoming available as technology goes into the mobile domain. With the strict privacy guidelines needed for data security this is a challenging process. A diagnostic mobile ultrasound system research framework

Table 12.1 List of acronyms used in the chapter

Health Care Standards and Information			
Legislation/Organizations		*Definitions*	
AMA	American Medical Association	ABE	Attribute Based Encryption
ANSI	American National Standards Institute	CIED	Cardiovascular Implantable Electronic Devices
ARRA	American Recovery and Reinvestment	CPT	Current Procedural Terminology Act
HIPAA	Health Insurance Portability and Accountability Act	EDI	Electronic Data Interchange
HITECH	Health Information Technology for Economic and Clinical Health Act	EMR	Electronic Medical Record
		e-PHI	Electronic Protected Health Information
ICD-9	International Classification of Diseases, Ninth Revision	EHR	Electronic Health Record
IEEE	Institute of Electrical and Electronics Engineers	HIS	Health Information Systems
IOM	Institute of Medicine	IHII	Individual Identifiable Health Information
ISO	International Organization for Standardization	PHI	Protected Health Information
NEMA	National Electrical Manufacturers Association	PHR	Personal Health Record
WEDI	Workgroup for Electronic Data Interchange	SDK	Software Development Kit
WHO	World Health Organization		
Data Exchange		*Networks*	
CCD	Continuity of Care Document	ebXML	Electronic Business Extensible Markup Language
CCOW	Clinical Context Object Workgroup	HIE	Health Information Exchange
CDA	Clinical Document Architecture	NHIN	National Health Information Network
DICOM	Digital Imaging and Communication in Medicine	TCP/IP	Transmission Control Protocol/Internet Protocol
HL-7	Health Level Seven International		
PACS	Picture Archiving and Communication System		
RIM	Reference Information Model		

has been developed that includes DICOM capabilities accessed with cloud connectivity. Implementing DICOM compliant encryption in the cloud is accomplished by the development of the DICOM Mobile software development kit (SDK) [30]. The

SDK includes a DICOM conversion module and a DICOM communication module to further divide the task of converting raw image files to DICOM standards and transmitting DICOM images to the cloud storage facility or to a PACS. This SDK interacts with m-Health applications and provides an intermediate transport protocol for data transfer to a cloud DICOM server or to a PACS. The application is Windows based utilizing Azure server software for the cloud connectivity portion and utilizing mobileUS open source software for the data acquisition from the mobile ultrasound equipment [31]. This application for mobile imaging diagnostics gives the implementation of a working prototype for such a system. Another domain for timely research requiring adherence to healthcare standards is cardiac monitoring.

Telemonitoring of Cardiovascular Implantable Electronic Devices (CIED) can be an extremely powerful tool indicating the onset of cardiac arrest or other heart conditions. With the timely monitoring of data received from such devices, the quality of life for patients can be improved. The iCARDEA project delivers CIED data form CIED vendors to adaptive care planners to make informed decisions concerning the well-being of patients. The iCADREA project uses protocols outlined in IEEE 11073 (Health Informatics, Point-of-care Medical Device Communication) and HL-7v2 in the implementation of telemonitoring. Even with communication standards this research cites a problem with development in that there are many CIED vendors with a variety of operational protocols.

Conclusion

Healthcare standards have evolved slowly along with the development of technology to provide medical knowledge through electronic medical systems. These standards have been regulated through legislation that does not fully address the interoperability and security issues associated with electronically collecting, storing, and transmitting personal health information. Disparate business interests developing medical equipment devices and technologies have further compounded the problem of interoperability. Implementing the standards that are in place is a challenging process, but with improved interoperability comes the benefit of greater efficiency and effectiveness in providing healthcare services leading to maximization of positive results in patient driven healthcare.

References

1. R.S. Dick, E.B. Steen, D.E. Detmer, "The Computer-Based Patient Record: An Essential Technology for Health Care" Revised Edition, Washington, D.C.: National Academy Press, 1997. pp. i-xii.
2. K.A. Wager, F.W. Lee, J.P. Glaser, "Healthcare Information Systems: A Practical Approach for Healthcare Management", San Francisco, CA., John Wiley & Sons, 2009, pp. 65–107.

3. Institute of Medicine (IOM). (2012, Sept. 14). [Online]. Available: http://www.iom.edu/About-IOM.aspx
4. W.R. Braithwaite, "The federal role in setting standards for the exchange of health information", Proceedings of the Symposium on Pacific Medical Technology (PACMEDTEK '98). IEEE Computer Society, Washington, D.D., USA, 2012, pp. 340–347.
5. Workgroup for Electronic Data Interchange (WEDI). (2012, Sept. 15). [Online]. Available: http://www.wedi.org/public/articles/details.shtml
6. Heath Insurance Portability and Accountability Act of 1996 (HIPAA). (2012 Sept. 12). [Online]. Available: http://www.gpo.gov/fdsys/pkg/PLAW-104publ191/pdf/PLAW-104publ191.pdf
7. T. Piliouras, et al., "Impacts of legislation on electronic health records systems and security implementation", Systems, Applications and Technology Conference (LISAT) IEEE Long Island, 2012, pp. 1–7.
8. HITECH Act, The Health Information Technology for Economic and Clinical Health Act (HITECH) Act, ARRA Components–January 6, 2009 HITECH. (2012 Sept. 12). [Online]. Available: http://www.hipaasurvivalguide.com/hitech-act-text.php
9. Health Level 7 (HL7). (2012 Sept. 16). [Online]. Available: http://www.hl7.org/
10. International Organization for Standardization (ISO). (2012 Sept. 17). [Online]. Available: http://www.iso.org
11. M. Vida, O. Lupse, L. Stoicu-Tivadar, "Improving the interoperability of healthcare information systems through HL& CDA and CCD standards", 7th IEEE International Symposium on Applied Computational Intelligence and Informatics. Timisoara, Romania 2012. pp. 157–161.
12. T. Namli, G. Aluc, A. Dogac, "An interoperability test framework for HL7-based systems", IEEE Transactions on Information Technology In Biomedicine, vol. 13, no. 3, May 2009. pp. 389–399.
13. Digital Imaging and Communications in Medicine (DICOM). (2012 Sept. 15). [Online]. Available: medical.nema.org.
14. M. Mustra, K. Delac, M. Grgic, "Overview of the DICOM standard", IEEE 50th International Symposium ELMAR, Zadar, Croatia, 2008. pp. 39–44.
15. L. Yang, Y. Gu, "Design and realization of DICOM/HL7 gateway in PACS", IEEE 2011 International Conference on Electronic & Medical Engineering and Information Technology, Shanghai, China, 2011. pp. 2164–2167.
16. N. Goga, S. Costache, F. Moldoveanu, "A formal analysis of ISO/IEEE P11073–20601 standard of medical device communication", 3rd Annual IEEE International Systems Conference, Vancouver, Canada, 2009. pp. 163–166.
17. Current Procedural Terminology (CPT). (2012 Sept. 14). [Online]. Available: http://www.ama-assn.org/ama/pub/physician-resources/solutions-managing-your-practice/coding-billing-insurance/cpt.page
18. M.S. King, M.S. Lipsky, L. Sharp, "Expert agreement in current procedural terminology evaluation and management coding", Archives of Internal Medicine, vol. 162, no. 3. 2002, pp. 316–320.
19. International Classification of Diseases, Ninth Revision (ICD-9). (2012 Sept. 14). [Online]. Available: http://www.cdc.gov/nchs/icd/icd9.htm
20. International Classification of Diseases Ninth Revision, Clinical Modification (ICD-9-CM). (2012 Sept. 14). [Online]. Available: http://www.cdc.gov/nchs/icd/icd9cm.htm
21. OpenEMR. (2012 Sept. 14). [Online]. Available: http://www.oemr.org/
22. J. Noll, S. Beecham, D. Seichter, " A qualitative study of open source software development: the OpenEMR project", 2011 IEEE 5th International Symposium on Empirical Software Engineering Measurement, Banff, Canada, 2011. pp. 30–39.
23. Z. Li, et al. "A secure electronic medical record sharing mechanism in the cloud computing platform", IEEE 15th International Symposium on Consumer Electronics, Singapore, 2011, pp. 98–103.
24. D. Mashima, M. Ahamad, "Enhancing accountability of electronic health record usage via patient-centric monitoring", The 2nd ACM SIGHIT International Health Informatics Symposium (IHI 2012), Miami, Florida, 2012, pp. 409–418.

25. National Health Information Network. (2012 Sept. 14). [Online]. Available: http://www.hhs.gov/healthit/healthnetwork/background/
26. S. Narayan, M. Gagne, R. Safavi-Naini, "Privacy preserving HER system using attribute-based infrastructure", Proceedings of the 2010 ACM Workshop on Cloud Computing Security, Chicago, IL., 2010, pp. 47–52.
27. J.A. Akinyele, et al., "Securing electronic medical records using attribute-based encryption on mobile devices", 18th ACM Conference on Computer and Communications Security (CCS), Chicago, Il., 2011, pp. 75–86.
28. Mirth Corp., Mirth Connect. (2012 Sept. 16). [Online]. Available: http://www.mirthcorp.com/products/mirth-connect
29. Mirth Corp., Mirth Match. (2012 Sept. 16). [Online]. Available: http://www.mirthcorp.com/products/mirth-match
30. C. Teng, et al. "Mobile ultrasound with DICOM and cloud connectivity", Proceedings of the IEEE-EMBS International Conference on Biomedical and Health Informatics", 2012, Hong Kong, China, pp. 667–670.
31. M. Yang, et al., "Guideline-driven telemonitoring and follow-up of cardiovascular implantable electronic devices using IEEE 11073, HL7 & IHE profiles", 33rd Annual International Conference of the IEEE EMBS", Boston, Massechusets, 2011, pp. 3192–3196.

Chapter 13
Predicting Hospital Readmission Risk for COPD Using EHR Information

Ravi Behara, Ankur Agarwal, Faiz Fatteh and Borko Furht

Abstract Hospital readmission is an important quality of care indicator. It reflects challenges in quality of in-patient care and the difficulty of coordination of care after the transition back into the community. It is also a significant financial burden, especially as it relates to Medicare and Medicaid costs now and into the future. Chronic Obstructive Pulmonary Disease (COPD) is also one of the leading causes of disability and mortality worldwide. So it is a quality, cost and demographic imperative to design and develop predictive clinical support systems to better manage patients with this condition so as to simultaneously improve the quality of care while controlling costs through avoiding preventable hospital readmissions for patients with COPD.

Introduction

The Office of the National Coordinator for Health Information Technology (ONC), in the U.S. Department of Health and Human Services, was formed in 2004. It is the key federal government entity responsible for the coordination of efforts to implement and use advanced health IT and electronic exchange of health information in the U.S. As part of its mandate, the ONC has initiated a $60 million advanced research project in 2010 called Strategic Health IT Advanced Research Projects (SHARP) to focus on developing products and services based on breakthrough advances that overcome barriers to adoption and meaningful use of health IT. The five areas of work being pursued are [1]:

R. Behara · A. Agarwal · B. Furht (✉)
Florida Atlantic University, Boca Raton, FL, USA
e-mail: bfurht@fau.edu

F. Fatteh
SorenTechnology Inc., Plantation, FL, USA

B. Furht and A. Agarwal (eds.), *Handbook of Medical and Healthcare Technologies*,
DOI: 10.1007/978-1-4614-8495-0_13,

1. Security and Health Information Technology: Development of technologies and policy recommendations that reduce privacy and security risks and increase public trust (led by The University of Illinois at Urbana-Champaign).
2. Patient-Centered Cognitive Support: Use of health IT to integrate and support physician reasoning and decision-making in patient care (led by the University of Texas, Houston).
3. Health Care Application and Network Design: Creation of new and improved system designs that facilitate information exchange while ensuring the accuracy, privacy, and security of electronic health information (led by Harvard University).
4. Secondary Use of EHR Information: Development of strategies to improve the overall quality of healthcare by leveraging existing EHR data to generate new, environmentally appropriate, best practice suggestions (led by Mayo Clinic of Medicine).
5. Prototype Healthcare Intranet: Development of technology, software, standards, and tools to provide higher quality patient data by enabling medical device manufacturers to create products that will allow interoperability with other manufacturers' devices, EHRs, and health IT systems (at Massachusetts General Hospital).

The research described in this chapter relates to the secondary use of EHR information. The specific focus is to address avoidable hospital readmissions, as it relates to patients with Chronic Obstructive Pulmonary Disease (COPD).

Hospital readmission rates are considered to be an important indicator of quality of care because they may be a consequence of actions of commission or omission made during the initial hospitalization of the patient, or as a consequence of poorly managed transition of the patient back into the community [2–5]. There is also an economic cost to readmission. A study reported in 2009 that 19.6 % of Medicare fee-for-service beneficiaries who had been discharged from a hospital were readmitted to the hospital within 30 days, 34.0 % within 90 days, and more than half (56.1 %) within one year of discharge [6]. Also, the Medicare Payment Advisory Commission (MedPAC) found that 17.6 % of hospital admissions resulted in readmissions within 30 days of discharge, 11.3 % within 15 days, and 6.2 % within 7 days. MedPAC also reported that readmissions within 30 days accounted for $15 billion of Medicare spending [7]. More recently, according to the Institute for Healthcare Improvement, of the 5 million U.S. hospital readmissions, approximately 76 % are preventable, at an annual cost of about $25 billion. Medicare is the payer for about half of these readmissions.

To address this, the Affordable Care Act established the Hospital Readmissions Reduction Program that requires the Center for Medicare and Medicaid Services (CMS) to reduce payments to IPPS (Inpatient Prospective Payment Systems) hospitals with excess readmissions, effective for discharges beginning on October 1, 2012. Hospitals receiving inpatient prospective payment by Medicare are penalized 1 percent for high rates of avoidable readmissions with the three highest diagnosis-related groups (DRG) of cardiac and pulmonary conditions. The focus of our study is on Chronic Obstructive Pulmonary Disease (COPD) which is one of the leading causes of disability and mortality worldwide, and is expected to become the third cause of death and fifth cause of disability adjusted life years in 2020 [8]. In 2003–2004, 22.6 % of fee-for-service Medicare beneficiaries admitted to the hospital for COPD were readmitted within 30 days [9]. The COPD related readmission rate was 21.4 %, with an 18 % to over 50 % increase in cost for readmission (compared to the initial admission), in a more recent 2008 study based on data of 15 states [10].

The negative impact on patient quality of life and huge burden on healthcare system have made reducing hospital readmissions a central goal of healthcare delivery and payment reform efforts. So it is both a clinical and financial imperative to address the patient readmission problem. At the same time, there are growing technical capabilities to develop predictive analytic solutions in a variety of domains including healthcare. Outside healthcare, companies have begun utilizing both structured and unstructured data to gain a better understanding of the underlying business processes as well as to predict customer outcomes. It is these concepts and technologies that make it feasible to address the readmission problem.

This chapter presents the framework, design and development of a predictive COPD clinical decision-support system to help reduce the number of readmissions by identifying those patients who need preventive interventions to reduce the probability of being readmitted. Based primarily on patient's clinical discharge summary, the system would be able to determine the readmission risk profile of patients treated for COPD. Suitable transitional care interventions could then be initiated with the objective of providing quality and timely care that helps prevent avoidable readmission.

Readmission Risk Modeling

The extant literature indicates that predictive modeling in hospital readmission is generally being developed for two uses, to provide a basis for transition of care interventions aimed at reducing readmissions based on clinically-based readmission risk metrics, and to develop risk-standardized readmission rates as a quality metric for reporting and reimbursement. The focus of this chapter is the former, to categorize patients hospitalized with COPD into groups based on clinically-based readmission risk, with an aim to reducing avoidable readmissions.

Readmission models have been developed for specific conditions such as congestive heart failure, acute myocardial infraction, and pneumonia. Such readmission studies also used administrative data such as utilization or primary data such as chart review or patient survey based data. Such data that is based on patient chart or discharge reports related to the index hospitalization is referred to as retrospective data. Predictive models are evaluated based on the proportion of times the model correctly discriminates a pair of high and low risk patients.

For instance, in one study predicting 30-day heart failure related readmissions for an urban socioeconomically disadvantaged population [11], variables from electronic medical records (EMR) including social factors such as number of address changes, drug use, and marital status, resulted in a model with moderate discriminant ability.

Another study [12] also found that models that included functional status of the patient (from surveys) performed better than using administrative data such as utilization and comorbidity data. Yet a different study [13] found that a simple non-clinical Charlson comorbidity-based model was only slightly different in its discrimination than a complex model based only on diagnosis and procedures. So it appears that non-clinical data need to certainly be considered in the development of readmission prediction models.

But very few readmission risk models have been developed for COPD [14]. Amongst those, one study [15] used the BODE index. This comprises Body mass index, Obstruction of the airway, Dyspnoea (difficulty in catching breath or in breathing) score based on the modified Medical Research Council questionnaire, and Exercise capacity based on a 6 minute walk test. This study found that their clinical and survey based model had a better predictive capability than one that was based only clinical data. In another study [16], prospective data was collected on patients recruited into the study. Clinical and sociodemographic data on potential risk factors such as clinical and functional status, medical care and prescriptions, medication adherence, lifestyle, health status, and social support, was collected from patients at the recruitment admission. Prediction models showed that physical activity and certain clinical indicators were good predictors of readmission.

So we find a variety of information being used in developing readmission risk predictive models. These models also generally tend to be different type regression models. But [17] highlights the complex nature of readmission risk prediction and its inherently limited predictive ability, and calls for developing better approaches. The remainder of this discussion presents the methodology developed in this study and presents its development.

Methodology

The predictive COPD clinical support system is based on predictive analytics using structured and unstructured patient data to develop a readmission risk profile for a patient being discharged after an initial COPD related hospital admission. The framework for this system is shown in Fig. 13.1. This was developed in response to the limitations in research on risk prediction for hospital readmissions that is highlighted in the literature [17]. A thorough review of patient medical records or patient reports is suggested as on approach to address the many factors that may contribute to readmission. Since this is primarily in unstructured text form, the proposed framework includes text analysis of such data from patient records. Also, given the limited predictive ability of many models, it is suggested that the value of clinician gestalt be considered. Our framework addresses this by including specific structured and unstructured patient demographic data that is also related to patient social history that is recorded by physicians in their assessment. Finally, the framework considers specific COPD related laboratory test results as part of the structured patient data. These data types are used in the development of appropriate regression models to

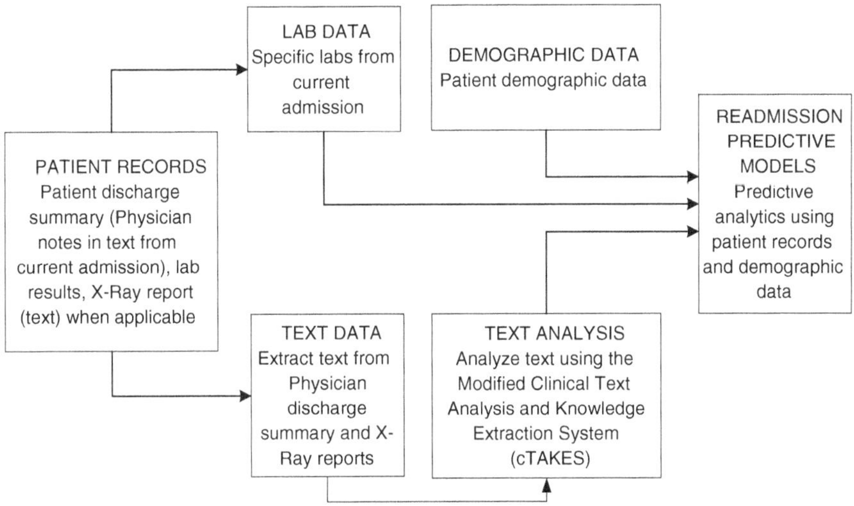

Fig. 13.1 Framework for predictive COPD readmissions clinical support system

predict readmission. The models developed will be designed to predict risk categories rather than specific readmission probabilities alone. This "banding" of readmission risk would also help in informing hospitals in development of discharge strategies based on readmission risk. The details of the implementation of the unstructured and structured analysis in this framework are further discussed in the following sections.

Unstructured Data Analysis

Since free text is an important part of patient records reflecting the thought process of the physician and other care givers, including it in predictive analysis is important. But a manual review of free text records is time-consuming, despite the inherent value in the clinical information it contains. So there is interest in developing a natural language processing based approach to extract such information from patient records. But this is not a simple task due to the ambiguity and variety of language used in the description and evaluation of any specific patient condition. There is also context and user specific use of terminology, abbreviations, and acronyms.

There are ongoing efforts at natural language process in the biomedical sciences. For instance, the U.S. National Library of Medicine's MetaMap program is used for data mining and indexing of biomedical text [18]. Other specific clinical applications have also been attempted, including smoking status [19–21], diagnosis of angina or heart failure [22, 23], family history [24], quality of life scores [25], and cause of death [26].

In this study, Mayo Clinic's Clinical Text Analysis and Knowledge Extraction System [27] (cTAKES) open source clinical natural language processing system is being adopted. It can be used to create one or more pipelines to process clinical notes and to identify mentions of clinical named entities such as diseases and disorders, signs and symptoms, anatomical sites/ and procedures, and drugs in patient records. cTAKES, which was primarily developed for is built on the UIMA framework, and is being adapted to address COPD in this study. This is initially being done by utilizing the NLM bio-ontology [28].

Most of the data in enterprise systems is in unstructured form like in handwritten notes etc. It is information that was not specifically encoded for machines to process but rather authored by humans for humans to understand. There is a need of a framework which can convert these unstructured data into a structured view to extract concepts of interest, relation between them or facts. The Unstructured Information Management Architecture (UIMA) is a component-based architecture and software framework for creating, discovering, composing and deploying a broad range of multi-modal analysis capabilities and integrating them with search technologies [29]. The UIMA architecture is divided into three parts: type systems, Annotators and Analysis Engines. A type system defines the various types of objects that may be discovered in documents by Analysis Engine's that subscribe to that type system. An Analysis engine (AE) is a program that analyzes documents/texts and extracts information from them. An analysis engine may contain a single annotator (Primitive AE) or it may contain a composition of multiple annotators (Aggregate AE). Analysis engines are constructed from building blocks called Annotators. The meta-data information associated with a particular location or span in the original unstructured data is implemented in the form of an annotator. An annotator is a component that contains analysis logic. Examples of annotations that may be applied to text documents include annotations that identify sequences of characters as a numeral, fraction or word. The Common Analysis System (CAS) is the data structure in which all the information is logically bundled. The UIMA plug-in system allows users to deploy their own analyzing components or assemble components in a convenient way [30].

The data in most hospital systems are of unstructured, such as in physician's notes, patient discharge summaries, and x-ray radiology reports. IE (Information Extraction) in natural language process aims to help humans extract useful information automatically from such corpus of data [31]. The component architecture of UIMA can be used efficiently to extract such information at an enterprise level. UIMA provide the platform for unstructured information process and allows developers to reuse building analysis components thereby reducing development time [32]. The Clinical Text Analysis and Knowledge Extraction System (cTAKES) is Mayo Clinic's information extraction system for the clinical domain which was developed using IBM's Unstructured Information Management Architecture (UIMA). The system was developed to process and extract information from free-text clinical notes for PAD (Peripheral Artery disease). Annotators are strung together to build a pipeline for the discovery of clinical named entities such as diseases, signs/symptoms, anatomical sites and procedures, drug mentions, side-effects etc. Attributes related to these named entities such as the context, status and relatedness to patient, are also extracted from the text. The pipeline consists of a elements including context free tokenizer, abbreviation disambiguation annotator, lexical normalizer annotator, sentence detector, context dependent tokenizer, part of speech tagger, shallow parser, dictionary look-up annotator, a machine learning component, and a negation annotator.

The predictive COPD clinical support system is being developed on the cTAKES platform, and it adopts several basic Analysis Engines from UIMA such as for creating tokens, a phrase builder, and a POS tagger. It also adds a new Analysis Engines to extract information including Drug Named Entity Recognition and Disease conditions, and uses the cTAKES smoking status extractor.

A layered architecture with output from one layer serving as an input to another is utilized as shown in Fig. 13.2. There are 5 layers in this system: Document preprocessor Layer, Lexical Analyzer Layer, Assertion Layer, COPD Layer (with term spotter, drug name recognition, and smoking status recognition) and the Readmission Predictive Model. The input to this system will be a text document or CDA (Clinical Document Architecture) documents. The Document Preprocessor Layer converts all the CDA documents into plain text and creates sections and tokens. It also extracts information such as all date mentions, fraction mentions, and numeral notations which can later be used to assess details such as medication dosage and frequency. The Lexical Analyzer Layer parses all word tokens and tags each word with their corresponding part-of-speeches and generating their lexical variant to build phrases which later becomes key factor in predicting readmission. The next layer, the Assertion Layer, determines if the text being discussed is related to the 'patient' or a 'family member'.

The COPD Layer, is the most important layer for this text analysis system. It extracts all the COPD related terms such as disease terms and location/disorder terms based on prebuilt dictionaries. The unique part that is being developed in this project is that COPD which is condition-centric is unlike PAD which is anatomically-based in its presentation. Descriptive text of disease specific terms are paired descriptors

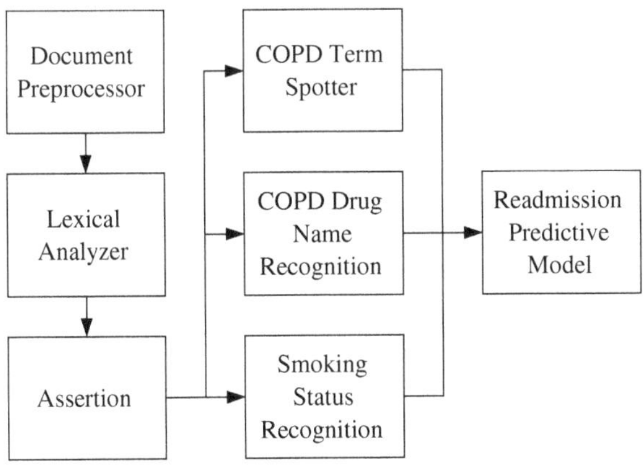

Fig. 13.2 Layered architecture of the cTAKES-based text analyser for COPD

Table 13.1 Sample COPD Bio-Ontology and Medication Terms

Primary standalone terms	Primary associated terms	Secondary terms	Drug terms
COPD	Wheezing	Severe	Ipratropium
Chronic obstructive pulmonary disease	Cough	Productive	Atrovent
Pulmonary embolism	Infiltrate	Lung	Tiotropium
Shortness of breath	Respiratory infection	Upper	Spiriva
Hypoxemia	Hypertension	Pulmonary	Salmeterol

Table 13.2 Sample COPD text extractions

Annotations extracted:

Medication Annotations:

- COMBIVENT

COPD Term Annotations:

- COPD=EXACERBATION
- LUNG INFILTERATE
- INFILTERATE
- LEFT LUNG INFILTERATE
- SHORTNESS OF BREATH
- COPD

of the condition or location to build a relational tie, indicating a *hit*. There are two main dictionaries involved: COPD_Primary_Terms and COPD_Secondary_Terms. Primary terms can be Primary Standalone terms which fully represent the clinical condition positively, or Primary Associated terms which together with appropriate Secondary terms positively identify COPD. The dictionaries involved were initially built using different medical ontologies provided by NLM. They were further refined based on physician feedback, COPD clinical diagnosis literature, and tested against a sample data set. The COPD layer also extracts drug mentions with all related information such as dosage frequency, unit, start date and end date, and extracts side that may occur later on due to medications and disorder combination. Examples of these disease and drug terms are shown in Table 13.1.

The COPD Term Spotter processes clinical notes textual extractions specifically pertaining to the diagnosis and treatment of Chronic Obstructive Pulmonary Disease (COPD). The main feature is classifying each document for terms positively identifying the presence of COPD and its related assessment and treatment. Descriptive text of diagnosis and illness terms are paired with the site designated terms to build a relational tie, indicating a 'hit'. The pipeline assesses presence of phrases indicative of COPD in one or more sentences contained in discharge summaries from doctors. A sample of text extractions in a sample data set is shown in Table 13.2.

The Smoking Status part of the COPD layer that is from the original cTAKES system, processes patient records into five pre-determined categories: past smoker (P), current smoker (C), smoker (S), non-smoker (N), and unknown (U). The definition of smoking status is adapted from I2B2 Natural Language Processing Challenges for Clinical Records. These are defined as, Past Smoker (P): A patient whose record asserts either that they are a past smoker or that they were a smoker a year or more ago but who have not smoked for at least one year, Current Smoker (C): A patient whose record asserts that they are a current smoker (or that they smoked without indicating that they stopped more than a year ago) or that they were a smoker within the past year, Smoker (S): A patient who is either a CURRENT or a PAST smoker but, whose medical record does not provide enough information to classify the patient as either a CURRENT or a PAST smoker, Non-Smoker (N): A patient whose record indicates that they have never smoked, and Unknown (U): The patient's record does not mention anything about smoking.

Finally, the Readmission Predictive Model would predict the patient's probability of being readmitted and flags a patient according to different categories of readmission risk on a scale from very high risk to very low risk of readmission. But, as shown in the framework in Fig. 13.1, this analysis also requires structured data inputs that relate to patient clinical laboratory test results and patient demographics. These are discussed in the following section.

Structured Data Analysis

This study will develop appropriate predictive statistical models to predict patient readmission that also uses structured data, in addition to the unstructured text data discussed in the previous section. Specifically the structured data will include relevant laboratory test results including Spirometry and Arterial Blood Gas (ABG) tests, and non-clinical patient demographic data.

For instance, normal and abnormal ABG test result values are shown in Table 13.3. Normal respiratory function is indicated by a partial pressure of oxygen (PaO_2) that is between 75 and 100 millimeters of mercury (mmHg), a partial pressure of carbon dioxide ($PaCO_2$) between 35 and 50 mmHg, and a pH between 7.35 and 7.45.

A person with COPD may have an increased pH and rising partial pressure of carbon dioxide because not enough carbon dioxide is being exchanged in the

Table 13.3 Arterial blood gas (ABG) analysis (COPD vs normal)

	pH	PaCO2	Pa02	O2 Sat (%)
Normal ABG	7.4	40	60–90	>95
Compensated	7.39	50	60–90	>92
Decompensated	<7.35	Rising	Falling	<92

lungs. People with COPD may also display low levels of dissolved oxygen and oxygen saturation. Oxygen saturation is a measurement of how much oxygen is bound to hemoglobin and is expressed as a percentage. Oxygen saturation less than 94 % indicates a decrease in respiratory function. Respiratory failure is defined as a PaO_2 <60 mmHg or $PaCO_2$ >50 mmHg. Other clinical tests that will be investigated for being relevant input variables of interest include sputum analysis, spirometry results that test the capacity of the lungs, and chest x-ray results. Appropriate patient demographic data will also be included in the structured data component of the readmission analysis.

Conclusion

The clinical support system described here is designed to predict hospital readmission risk for COPD using EHR information such as disease specific conditions extracted from the free text of physician notes in patient discharge summaries. It leverages recent advances in text analysis of unstructured clinical records to do so. It would also utilize specific laboratory test results and appropriate patient sociodemographic information in the analysis.

As discussed earlier, predictive modeling of readmission is a complex effort with varying degrees of accuracy. It has been suggested in the literature that many different models be investigated with an aim to achieve increased prediction reliability. This study is a part of that ongoing effort in addressing the important challenge of reducing avoidable readmission for patients with COPD. Since readmission rates have remained approximately constant for the past few years, such efforts are not just timely, they are also critical in helping improve quality of service while reducing associated healthcare costs.

References

1. ONC, Strategic Health IT Advanced Research Projects (SHARP) http://www.healthit.gov/policy-researchers-implementers/strategic-health-it-advanced-research-projects-sharp accessed on 4/10/2013
2. Friedman, B. and Basu, J., "The rate and cost of hospital readmissions for preventable conditions," Medical Care Research and Review 61(2):225240, June 2004.
3. Miller, M.E., "Statement of executive director of the Medicare Payment Advisory Commission, before the Subcommittee on Health, Committee on Energy and Commerce," U.S. House of Representatives. April 18, 2007.
4. Halfon, P., Eggli, Y., PretreRohrbach, I., et al., "Validation of the potentially avoidable hospital readmission rate as a routine indicator of the quality of hospital care," Medical Care 44(11):972981, November 2006.
5. Kripalani, S., LeFevre, F., Phillips, C.O., et al., "Deficits in communication and information transfer between hospital based and primary care physicians," JAMA 297(8):831841, February 28, 2007.

6. Stephen F. Jencks, M.D., Mark V. Williams, M.D., and Eric A. Coleman, M.D., M.P.H., "Rehospitalizations among patients in the Medicare Fee-for-Service Program," New England Journal of Medicine, vol. 360 (April 2, 2009), pp. 1418–1428. These data refer to years 2003–2004.
7. Medicare Payment Advisory Commission (MedPAC), "Report to Congress: Promoting Greater Efficiency in Medicare," June 2007, Chapter 5. See http://www.medpac.gov/documents/Jun07_EntireReport.pdf. These data refer to 2005.
8. Murray CJL, Lopez AD., "Alternative projections of mortality and disability by cause 1990–2020: global burden of disease study," Lancet, 349:1498–504, 1997.
9. Jenecks S. F., Williams M. V., Coleman E. A., "Rehospitalizations among patients in the Medicare fee-for-service program," NEJM, 360:1418–1428, 2009.
10. Elixhauser A., Au D.H., Podulka J., "Readmissions for Chronic Obstructive Pulmonary Disease," Statistical Brief #121, Healthcare Cost and Utilization Project, Agency for Healthcare Quality and Research, Sept. 2011.
11. Amarasingham R, Moore BJ, Tabak YP, et al., "An automated model to identify heart failure patients at risk for 30-day readmission or death using electronic medical record data", Med Care., 2010, 48(11), 981–988.
12. Coleman EA, Min SJ, Chomiak A, Kramer AM, "Post-hospital care transitions: patterns, complications, and risk identification", Health Serv Res., 2004, 39(5), 1449–1465.
13. Halfon P, Eggli Y, Prêtre-Rohrbach I, Meylan D, Marazzi A, Burnand B, "Validation of the potentially avoidable hospital readmission rate as a routine indicator of the quality of hospital care", Med Care., 2006, 44(11), 972–981.
14. Bahadori K, FitzGerald JM, "Risk factors of hospitalization and readmission of patients with COPD exacerbation—systematic review", Int J Chron Obstruct Pulmon Dis., 2007, 2(3), 241–251.
15. Ko, F.W.S., W. Tam, A.H.M. Tung, J. Ngai, S.S.S. Ng, K. Lai, K. Au, D.S.C. Hui, "A longitudinal study of serial BODE indices in predicting mortality and readmissions for COPD", Respiratory Medicine, 2011,105,266–273.
16. Garcia-Aymerich J, E Farrero, M A Félez, J Izquierdo, R M Marrades, J M Antó, "Risk factors of readmission to hospital for a COPD exacerbation: a prospective study", Thorax, 2003, 58, 100–105.
17. Kansagara D, H Englander, A Salanitro, D Kagen, C Theobald, and S Kripalani, "Risk Prediction Models for Hospital Readmission: A Systematic Review", Evidence-based Synthesis Program (ESP) Center, Portland VA Medical Center, Portland, OR (prepared for the Department of Veterans Affairs), October 2011.
18. Alan R Aronson AR, Lang FM., "An overview of MetaMap: historical perspective and recent advances," J Am Med Inform Assoc, 17:229–236, 2010.
19. Savova GK, Ogren PV, Duffy PH, Buntrock JD, Chute CG, "Mayo clinic NLP system for patient smoking status identification," J Am Med Inform Assoc, 15:25–28, 2008.
20. Uzuner O, Goldstein I, Luo Y, Kohane I, "Identifying Patient Smoking Status from Medical Discharge Records," J Am Med Inform Assoc, 15:14–24, 2008.
21. Clark C, Good K, Jeziernyb L, Macpherson M, Wilsonb B, Chajewska U: Identifying Smokers with a Medical Extraction System. J Am Med Inform Assoc, 15:36–39, 2008.
22. Pakhomov S, Hemingway H, Weston S, Jacobsen S, Rodeheffer R, Roger V, "Epidemiology of Angina Pectoris: Role of Natural Language Processing of the Medical Record," Am Heart J, 153(4):666–673, 2007.
23. Pakhomov S, Weston SA, Jacobsen SJ, Chute CG, Meverden R, Roger VL, "Electronic medical records for clinical research: application to the identification of heart failure," Am J Manag Care, 13 (6 Part 1):281–288, 2007.
24. Melton GB, Raman N, Chen ES, Sarkar IN, Pakhomov S, Madoff RD, "Evaluation of family history information within clinical documents and adequacy of HL7 clinical statement and clinical genomics family history models for its representation: a case report," J Am Med Inform Assoc, 17(3):337–340, 2010.

25. Pakhomov S, Shah N, Hanson P, Balasubramaniam S, Smith SA, "Automatic quality of life prediction using electronic medical records", AMIA Annu Symp Proc, 2008:545–549, 2008.
26. Shah AD, Martinez C, Hemingway H., "The Freetext Matching Algorithm: a computer program to extract diagnoses and causes of death from unstructured text in electronic health records," BMC Medical Informatics and Decision Making, 12:88, 2012.
27. Savova1 GK, Masanz JJ, Ogren PV, Zheng J, Sohn S, Kipper-Schuler KC, Chute CG, "Mayo clinical Text Analysis and Knowledge Extraction System (cTAKES): architecture, component evaluation and applications," J Am Med Inform Assoc, 17:507–513, 2010.
28. Bodenreider O, Stevens R., "Bio-ontologies: current trends and future directions", Brief Bioinform, 7(3):256–74, Sept 2006. Epub Aug 9, 2006. http://www.ncbi.nlm.nih.gov/pmc/articles/PMC1847325/
29. Egner MT, Lorch M, Biddle E., "UIMA GRID: Distributed Large-scale Text Analysis," IEEE, 2007.
30. Cao Q, Guo W, Cui Y., "The semantic search based on UIMA," IEEE, 2009.
31. Han X, Rao R., "The Method of Medical Named Entity Recognition Based on Semantic Model and Improved SVM-KNN Algorithm," IEEE, 2011.
32. Zhipeng Z., "Knowledge Acquisition Framework for Unstructured Information," Microcomputer Applications, 26, 2010.

Chapter 14
Modeling Personalized and Context-Aware Multimedia e-Health Framework

Md. Abdur Rahman and Abdulmotaleb El Saddik

Introduction

The term context-aware e-Health system is coined with the vision that each person is surrounded by a smart space, which will be able to identify him/her in home or outdoor, recognize his/her actions, emotions, intentions, physiological activities, and health conditions and assist the person according to his/her individual preferences and needs, anytime and anywhere. Hence, e-Health related research has been a center point of many entities such as government, research institution, medical hardware and software industry, and healthcare institutions. This is because context-aware e-Health research domain offers high quality of healthcare by leveraging recent advancements in multidisciplinary research domains such as wireless sensors, smartphones, high speed body area networking and mobile communication (3.5/4G). For example, various wired or wireless sensors can capture different vital phenomena such as heart beat rate, blood pressure, glucose level, and sweat condition; activities such as walking, sleeping, driving, falling, running, talking, and in a conversation; environmental parameters such as humidity, temperature, location, altitude etc.

To add to this advancement, rapid growth in smart phones has made them a ubiquitous personal computing device for e-Health applications where a smart phone can create an ad-hoc network (also called body sensor network) with the sensors, store the sensory data, analyze the raw sensory data and generate a high level sensory data to take further actions. Several technologies at the personal area network level such as zigbee or Bluetooth and local/wide area network level such as Wi-Fi or mobile data communication technologies such as 3.5/4G have made it possible to disseminate the sensory data from a body sensor network to remote e-Health service

Md. A. Rahman (✉)
Department of Computer Science, Umm Al-Qura University, Makkah, Kingdom of Saudi Arabia
e-mail: marahman@uqu.edu.sa

A. El Saddik
School of Information Technology and Engineering University of Ottawa, Ottawa, ON, Canada

B. Furht and A. Agarwal (eds.), *Handbook of Medical and Healthcare Technologies*,
DOI: 10.1007/978-1-4614-8495-0_14, © Springer Science+Business Media New York 2013

providers or concerned community of interest. This requires a context-aware e-Health framework, which is aware of the events and context of each person, and is sensitive, flexible, and responsive to the needs, practices, gestures and emotions of a person. Using smart user interfaces, it can then seamlessly provide health services when or where ever it is needed.

Although capturing user context by analyzing sensory data is a popular trend, Rahman [1] have shown that user context is also embedded in the information available through online sources, for example, SMS message containing the change of appointment date of a patient, email containing date of refilling medicine, checking online prescription, alert message sent to the caregiver family member of a patient, and push message regarding severe weather information, to name a few. Recently, consuming such heterogeneous Internet-based services has become commonplace. Several multi-disciplinary breakthrough technologies in the areas of Web2.0 and modern smartphones have further fueled the usage of these services. Instead of creating, managing, sharing and accessing information on a specific place and time, a person can now provide as well as consume many diversified Internet-based services that are somehow related to e-Health such as weather, calendar, medical, serious games, sports, educational etc. any-time and anywhere. This propels the sharing and consumption of e-Health services ubiquitously. To add to these advancements, we envision the incorporation of user context in the e-Health domain by leveraging sensory data as well as Internet-based services, which offer personalized and context specific interaction and consumption of different e-Health services.

Context-awareness has been in center position of many e-Health researches. Context-awareness deals with the adaptation of computing systems to the user's current e-Health context. An e-Health framework can be called Context-Aware if: "it uses context to provide relevant e-Health information and/or services to the user, where relevancy depends on the user's task [2]." By analyzing information such as "I am in a shopping mall now" or "I am in a doctor's office" gives us an indication about a user's location, "I am driving a car" tells us about a user's current activity and "I have high blood pressure" provides the physiological condition of a user [3–7]. Previous researches show that user context can be captured using both multimedia information stored in different Internet-based services and using sensory media [8–12].

The main focus of this article is to design and model a context-aware framework that can dynamically determine a subset of e-Health services, a particular user needs at a particular context. The contributions of this article are as follows:

1. Design and development of mathematical and conceptual models to express e-Health services consumed from one's body sensor network (BSN) and the Internet.
2. Design and development of mathematical and conceptual models to express user context in terms of sensory data and different heterogeneous Internet-based services.
3. Show mapping methodology to find a subset of relevant e-Health services depending on user context.

4. Present a proof of concept open source framework that leverages the modeling technique shown in this article. The implemented framework can dynamically extract context information from BSN and diversified Internet-based services and depending on the inferred user context, the framework is capable of providing a subset of e-Health services to a user.

The rest of the chapter is organized as follows: section "Literature Review" outlines some closely related works. In Section "Framework Modeling", we illustrate the modeling of the proposed context-aware framework. In Section "Prototype Implementation" we describe the implementation details while in Section "Test Results" we present the test results followed by conclusive remarks and our future research plan in Section "Conclusions and Future Directions".

Literature Review

In this section we cite some interesting frameworks that either provide context-awareness, e-Health services or have potential to be used as context-aware e-Health services. Capturing user context is an attractive area of research in the e-Health domain and numerous techniques have been studied in the past [4–6]. Previous research show that user context can be captured using multimedia information stored in Internet-based services [7, 13–15]. Joly et al. [16] built a prototype called "Meeting Room Assistant," where different Internet-based services are triggered by sharing contextual artifacts such as content or personal information. Gartrell [15] presents a framework for building context-aware Internet-based services that reflect the preferences of one or more users engaged in collaborative works together. Koolwaaij et al. [7] presented a context management framework called Context Watcher that enables mobile phone users to easily and unobtrusively share personal context data such as their location, heart rate, speed or view with members of social networks. In addition to sharing data, the context framework can adapt applications to the contexts such as "meeting with a doctor" or "is a regular visitor". The application integrates a context management framework for context discovery, exchange and reasoning. The functionalities provided by the framework are: the ability of knowing where people are located, easy access to services (input parameters automatically provide context parameters like local weather, public transport information, etc.), remote logging of activities and preferences, and the sharing of such information across different applications. Although the above works in [7, 13, 15, 16] provide user context from data coming from a limited subset of social network sites, they did not include sensors in their context-aware system. They work only inside an indoor environment and hence, do not support user mobility.

A context-aware middleware, called the Socially Aware and Mobile Architecture (SAMOA), has been proposed in [14], which supports anytime, anywhere semantic and context-aware social networks. SAMOA takes into account two types of a mobile user's context: location-based context and user profile-based context. SAMOA tries to decouple social network management functionalities from application requirements by integrating a set of common management facilities for personalizing location-dependent social networks and for propagating social networks' visibility up to the application level. SAMOA can dynamically update services based on location and profile context. However, SOMOA does not provide context from sensory media, does not support existing heterogeneous Internet-based services.

Numerous sensor network platforms have been introduced in the literature, proving that sensors are suitable for capturing user context. Beutel et al. [17] have proposed a context sensing platform for wearable and ubiquitous computing. A medical sensor network that acts as a human Brain Computer Interface has been used to understand user context [18] while an online context tracking system has been used in [19]. iBadge [20] is a lightweight context-aware sensor badge wearable by a human being which can capture human interactions and send the captured data wirelessly to a base station. The Wireless Body Sensor Network proposed in [21] comprises of tiny wireless sensor nodes that can be comfortably carried by any human, such as an older patient and provide diversified context information.

A wireless sensor node has been presented in [22], which can monitor several activities of elderly people such as detection of arrhythmia disease, norm calculation, orientation calculation and fall detection using multiple sensors such as ECG and accelerometer. The sensor node is capable of sending the live sensory data to a server where it is analyzed for possible health risks. If needed, the server can send the data to the doctor's PDA. A Medical Embedded Device for Individualized Care (MEDIC) [12] is a wearable sensor platform, intended for capturing and diagnosing remote patients' live physiological and contextual information. In [23], a prototype of a mobile sensor network has been developed called cartel, which facilitates collecting and processing sensory data locally from a human body and then delivering and visualizing it in remote locations in real time or with a delay, based on the availability of the delivery networks. The prototype shown in [23] facilitates collecting and processing sensory data locally from a human body and then delivering and visualizing it in remote locations in real time or with a delay, based on the availability of the delivery networks. Another interesting context extraction framework is BeTelGeuse [24], which gathers data from a BSN and forwards it to a remote server. Although the above works i.e. [12, 22–24] provide contextual information from sensory media, they do not support context extraction from diversified Internet-based services and dynamic adaptation of different services based on the current user context.

BSN has been employed to develop different e-Health applications as well. The context sensing system captures the sensory data from a patient's body and then sends the information to the nearest monitoring server. The server in turn transforms the data to the end user standard and sends it to a remote patient database. Several applications of home health monitoring systems have been implemented that use wearable sensor nodes [25, 26]. The framework designed by [27] incorporates different types of sensors that communicate with a PDA using Bluetooth. The framework enables remote users to access the sensor network and query the sensory data via GPRS. The

PDA acts as a control node which coordinates and stores data from various sensors, and transmits to remote health providers using an XML based protocol.

Another health monitoring model is designed by [28] where a ring sensor is used for healthcare automation. The ring can be worn by a patient for monitoring pulse waves and blood oxygen saturation. The data collected by the ring sensor is transmitted to a home computer where the actual processing takes place. The ring is capable of detecting emergency situations since it is enriched with location estimation and activity recognition algorithms. The work presented by [9] tends to improve patient monitoring and response tracking. The system coordinates the communication among different entities of a health center, including medical professionals in a hospital, and other specialists available online through the system. A central web portal is used to enlist a patient's health records augmented with location information, and remote users can access patient information in real-time. The system also provides historical sensory information once the patient is taken to the emergency. However, they do not consider providing heterogeneous services support.

An interesting research conducted by [29] facilitates monitoring a patient's stress level using a distributed wireless intelligent sensor system. The system consists of a body area network which uses different sensors attached to a patient's body and a PDA as a gateway between sensors and end-point terminals on the Internet. However, the work does not include any Internet-based services for deducing user context. Other related research has shown the potential of involving context-aware social network services in e-Health applications. For example, Smith and Christakis [30] have studied the impact of interconnection between health specialists and patients' social networks. Results show the trends of Web 2.0 developments and provide recommendations to leverage context-aware social network services.

In light of the works presented above, although sensors provide rich sources of user context and have been used extensively by researchers in the past, there is lack in literature about user context extraction from multimedia content in Internet-based services. In this article we have combined both of context sources to extract a rich set of user context and modeled them such that it can be adapted to any system requiring user context based services. As a proof of concept, we apply the model in designing an e-Health system in which user-context plays an important role. Also, both Internet-based services and sensors are widely used nowadays in e-Health domain. In our case, we consider context as sampled information about people's environment and actions in time, and information contained in the multimedia information within the social network space. We propose to leverage this context information to give more opportunities for a user to consume e-Health services.

Framework Modeling

Before we go into the framework modeling, let us assume a scenario where a person named Alice interacts with different e-Health services throughout a day. According to Alice, e-Health services comprise of services she uses that are related to the sensory data as well as services she uses from Internet. Alice wears several sensors that keep track of her physiological phenomena, activities and ambient condition. The sensors are paired with her smartphone that has ubiquitous access to the Internet. Alice uses several Internet-based services to communicate, consume and share information with the members of her e-Health community. On a typical day after getting up from bed, Alice was informed by Google calendar service that she had an online meeting from 10 a.m. to 11 a.m. with a group of three research teams from three different hospitals. She also needs to take her child to the family physician's office for a medical appointment from 12:30 p.m. to 1:30 p.m., and then must join another project meeting from 2:30 p.m. to 4:00 p.m. with a group of industrial collaborators. At 5:00 p.m., she has to teach a course at the university. While coming from the afternoon meeting, due to severe weather and traffic conditions, she predicts she will be about 2 min late arriving to class, which is to start at 5:00 p.m. sharp. She needs to relay this delay to the students immediately.

After finishing teaching, Alice feels severe pain in her heart while driving home which is noted by the wearable ECG sensor. This alarming event needs to be instantaneously relayed to her concerned community of interest, such as the family physician, caregiver family members, nearby friends, living partner and emergency services. The family physician receives the alert message but needs to verify the severity level and sends an SMS message to Alice's smartphone requesting last five minutes of raw ECG sensory data in order to analyze the context. After receiving the SMS message, Alice's smartphone begins sending the requested sensory data directly to the family physician. In case of emergency, the family physician recommends that emergency services bring Alice to the hospital, and notifies her caregiver family members. The family physician also checks Alice's medical history from the Electronic Health Records, which is regularly updated.

In the above scenario, the types of people Alice interacts with and the types of services she uses at different occasion may be completely different and require her to manually invoke these services and maintain the appropriate community of interest. Technically, the above scenario requires a framework that has the knowledge of the global set of social ties and the services Alice is attached with. Then, depending on Alice's context, the framework can map necessary services depending on her context. For example, in case Alice has severe heart pain, she only needs to notify the caregiver family member who is in close vicinity, the family physician, the health care institution and emergency services. The framework should be able to track user context using the information coming from BSN and different services throughout the day ubiquitously, irrespective of time and location [1, 31]. Similar to Alice, every person's context is different and everyone maintains different associations with people and services.

In this section at first we focus on context-aware framework modeling steps without making any assumptions on the underlying domains of context. The purpose of context modeling is to try to capture different states of user context and represent them using mathematical expressions. User context can be expressed as a collection of user information which is obtained from diversified Internet and ad-hoc sources such as a body sensor network that can be used to characterize a user's ambient,

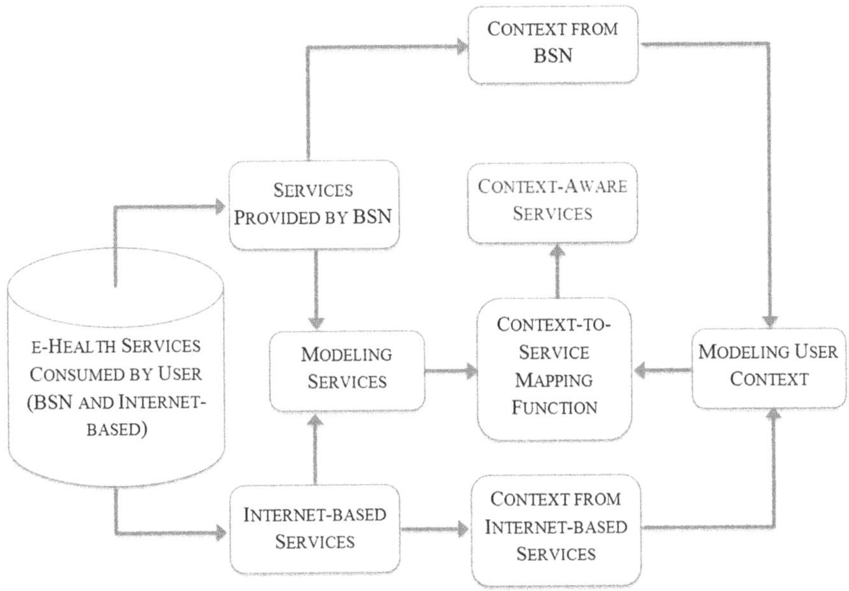

Fig. 14.1 Different entities involved in modeling context-aware internet-based services

personal, physiological and consumed service state. In our approach, user context is captured from two different sources: body sensor network and Internet-based services [12]. Our proposed modeling scheme is portrayed in Fig. 14.1. As shown in Fig. 14.1, the framework follows two steps of modeling. One is modeling services while the other is context modeling. Finally, a mapping is done between each user context with a set of services. Now we describe the modeling steps in details.

Modeling User Context

We first define necessary variables of user context needed during different stages of context modeling. This serves as a context vocabulary or schema that can be used to verify the completeness of a unique context. In order to model user context, we take into consideration the following types of contexts:

- Personal context data including user profile, user location (home, school, gym, shopping mall, airport, hospital, doctor office, etc.), time of day or week (week day, week-end, vacation, etc.), user activities (walking, sleeping, lying, talking, running, driving, etc.), user physiological information (heartbeat, blood pressure, etc.), to-do lists, and types of end-device used, to name a few.
- Social context data including contact lists, social ties through social networks and interactions and types of information shared.

- Event-based context such as appointments and meetings.
- Application-based context data such as types of web services used, bandwidth and reliability requirements of each service, types of protocols and access mechanism needed for each service, and URI of each service.
- Historic context such as a subject's past context information stored in a database similar to user profile or resource profile.
- Intra-user context difference, which is a result of change in one particular user's context throughout a day. For example, every user needs to access different e-Health services or communicate with different categories of people related to his/her health during different periods of a day.

Modeling user context is an attractive area of research and numerous techniques have been studied in the past [22, 23]. In order to simplify the context modeling, similar to the recommendations found in [13, 14], we use the context topology shown in Fig. 14.2. The tree-based context topology shown in Fig. 14.2 helps in expressing different combinations of context expressions using four context categories. These four categories of contexts are spatial, temporal, task-based and personal. The next level, like the children of each category, helps in defining fine-grained and low-level user context. For example, the spatial context might fall into one of the three sub-categories namely the location, direction and orientation. The third level of user context actually deals with a primitive class of user context. For example, in the case of location-based context, user location can be expressed in high level notation such as room number 2016 of School of Information Technology and Engineering of the University of Ottawa, ON, Canada or it might be low level such as in terms of latitude, longitude pair. Each path through one of the leaves of the topology tree leads to one unique expression of user context.

Now we formally express the user context modeling technique. We express the set of context primitives as following:

$$C = \{c_1, c_2, c_3, \ldots, c_l\} \tag{14.1}$$

where C is the set of all atomic context primitives in terms of vocabulary from one of the four categories i.e., spatial, task, temporal and personal. Each granular context expression from set C is formed using the tree shown in Fig. 14.2. For example, let us consider a physiological context of a user such as a "user is stressed". Using the topology tree, we can break down this high level context into smaller chunks of atomic context primitives as shown below. Note that the following breakdown of primitives might vary from user to user, the sensors available to the user, e-Health services that a user has subscribed, and how the user wants to express his/her health condition in that particular context. Assume that a user has sensors to measure heart rate, body temperature and sweat level, time of the day, current location, and surrounding temperature. Using each sensory data reading, a user can model several atomic context primitives. For example, using HeartRate data, a number of different contexts can be inferred such as USER HeartRate HIGH, USER HeartRate Low, USER HeartRate NORMAL, USER HeartRate ALARMING…Assuming the existence of such sets

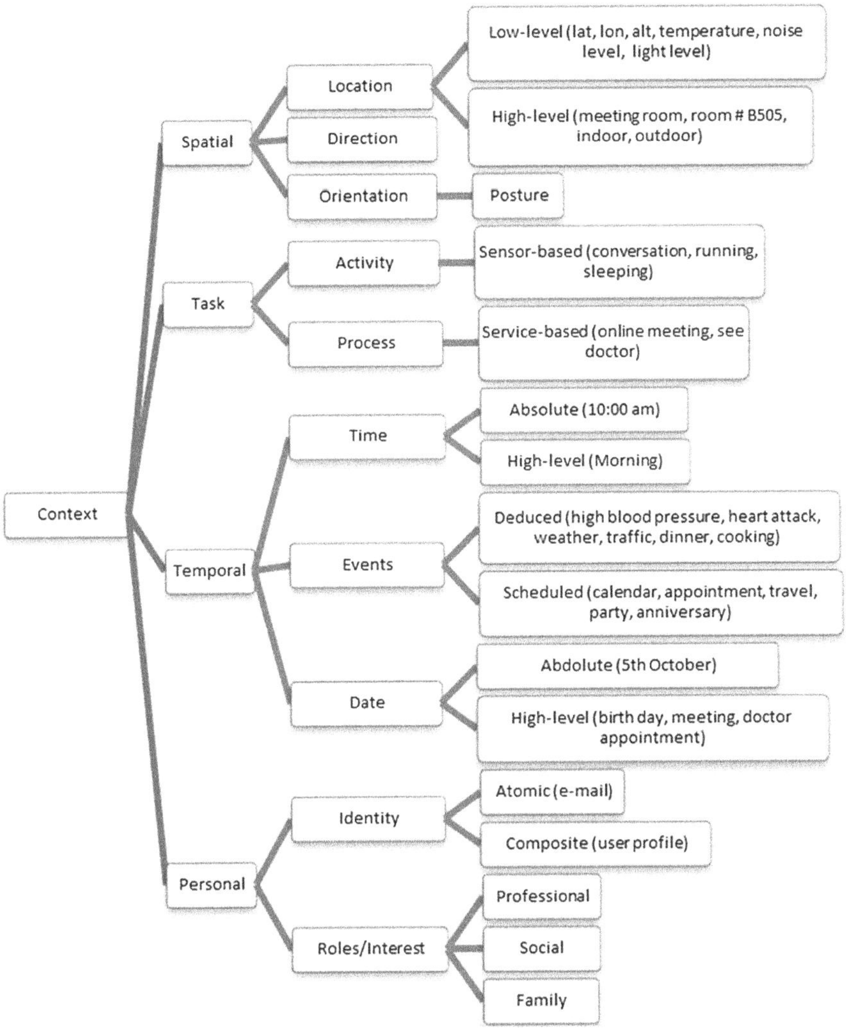

Fig. 14.2 Context topology for modeling different levels of context primitives

of atomic context primitives, we can infer a high level user context "user is stressed" as follows.

c_1 = USER HeartRate HIGH [Events Context]
c_2 = USER BodyTemperature HIGH [Events Context]
c_3 = USER SweatLevel HIGH [Events Context]
c_4 = TIME is MIDNIGHT [Temporal Context]
c_5 = LOCATION is HOME [Spatial Context]
c_6 = AMBIENT Temperature NORMAL [Events Context]
c_7 = USER not MOVING [Events Context]

If (c_1) and (c_2) and (c_3) and (c_4) and (c_5) and (c_6) and (c_7) Then
Context = *User is stressed*

To illustrate the context primitives pertaining to some other dimensions of life, let us consider the following additional contexts of a user such as *sleeping at night, taking a shower, cooking at kitchen,* and*engaged in meeting.* Using the topology tree, we can break down each of the four high-level contexts into smaller chunks of primitive contexts as shown below. Again, the following breakdown of primitives is just an instance from many possibilities, which might vary from subject to subject.

c_1 = SUBJECT LocatedIn BEDROOM [Spatial Context]
c_2 = BEDROOM LightLevel LOW [Spatial Context]
c_3 = TIME is MIDNIGHT [Temporal Context]
If (c_1) and (c_2) and (c_3) Then
Context = *sleeping at night*

c_4 = SUBJECT LocatedIn WASHROOM [Spatial Context]
c_5 = WATERHEATER LocatedIn WASHROOM [Spatial Context]
c_6 = WASHROOM DoorStatus CLOSED [Task Context]
c_7 = WATERHEATER Status ON [Task Context]
If (c_4) and (c_5) and (c_6) and (c_7) Then
Context = *taking a shower*

c_8 = SUBJECT LocatedIn KITCHEN [Spatial Context]
c_9 = ELECTRICOVEN LocatedIn KITCHEN [Spatial Context]
c_{10} = ELECTRICOVEN Status ON [Task Context]
If (c_8) and (c_9) and (c_{10}) Then
Context = *cooking at kitchen*

c_{11} = SUBJECT LocatedIn MEETINGROOM [Spatial Context]
c_{12} = SMARTPHONE LocatedIn MEETINGROOM [Spatial Context]
c_{13} = SMARTPHONE Status ON [Task Context]
c_{14} = CALENDAR AlertMessage ACTIVE [Temporal Context]
If (c_{11}) and (c_{12}) and (c_{13}) and (c_{14}) Then
Context = *engaged in meeting*

For example, Table 14.1 shows some examples of deducing context primitives. The rule how to formulate a high level user context is completely flexible and an e-Health domain expert can help in deducing all such user contexts using the above model. Raw context data gathered from heterogeneous sources including Internet-based sources such as calendar, email, SMS, social portals, etc. and ad-hoc sources such as BSN tend to preserve diversified proprietary formats which should be transformed into a unified form. To this end, we adopt the Actor, Activity and Asset (3A) interaction model [32] to serve the goal of context data alignment. We employ the 3A model to map every service and sensor in a BSN to one of the entities of the 3A model. An Actor is the owner of an Asset (in our case a user), which is connected to

Table 14.1 Deducing context primitives from sensory data and internet-based Services

(*User : Alice*)→ Registered user
(*Temperature* : 31 °C) → Hot region
(*Light Intensity : 10,100 lx*) → Less light condition
(*Latitude* : 45° 19′N, *Longitude*: 75° 40′W)→Ottawa, Canada
(Blood pressure : 160) →Unusual blood pressure
(Pulse : 145) →Higher than regular
(*Email-Attachment : CalendarEvent*)→Meeting between Tom and Alice
(*Facebook-StatusMessage-Sender : Tom*)→Doctor's office till 2:30 p.m.
(*Twitter-Message-Sender : Pharmacist*)→Prescription refill ready to be picked up at 5:30 p.m. from Pharmacy
(*Weather-Message : WeatherService*) →Heavy rainfall this morning
(*Calendar : CalendarService*)→ Doctor's appointment at 9:30 a.m.

an e-Health service through an Activity. An Asset represents the sharable information source such as sensory data, a Twitter message containing current location and event, etc. Thus, context information can be modeled as system Assets. An Activity is the formalization of a common objective to be achieved by the user. Activity can be, among others, information related to acceleration or ECG sensor or user location/activity tracking from his/her twitter profile page. Finally, the mapping produces a unified context format that can be easily converted to a context primitive shown in Table 14.1.

Similarly, each element of the set C is called specific user context because it represents one single and unique aspect of the context definition. The context primitives are bounded by a universe of discourse, for example defined by a vocabulary of context. More than one specific context can be happening at the same time such as time related context units: time::afternoon, time::meeting etc. and location related context units: location::doctor-office, location::emergency-unit, location::(latitude, longitude) etc. Please note that the parameters of Eq. (14.1) do not indicate which categories of context they belong to.

In order to express categorized contexts, Eq. (14.2) can be re-written as follows:

$$C' = \{C'_1, C'_2, C'_3, C'_4\} \tag{14.2}$$

where C' is the set of context sets classified according to each category; C'_1 is a set of spatial context primitives, C'_2 is a set of task-related context primitives, C'_3 is a set of temporal context primitives and C'_4 is set of personal context primitives. The following expressions define the relation between different variables of Eqs. (14.1) and (14.2):

$$C'_i \subseteq C \tag{14.3}$$

$$\bigcup_{i=1}^{4} C'_i = C \tag{14.4}$$

Once the atomic context primitives have been defined for a user, the next task in modeling is to define a unique and complete context expression, which is performed as follows:

$$C^* = \{c_1^*, c_2^*, .., c_n^*\} \tag{14.5}$$

where c_i^* is formed using a combination of primitive contexts chosen from one or more elements from C_1', C_2', C_3' and C_4' (see Eq. (14.4)). However, it is not a necessary condition that at least one context primitive has to be present from each context category. Sometimes one or more context categories might be absent within the expression of c_i^*, depending on the type of context. Sometimes, one or more context primitives might be chosen from a single category. A particular element of C^* i.e. c_i^* is a complete and unique context definition such as *user is having a heart pain at the mall in the afternoon*. Because the actual sources of events that will trigger an existing high level context-primitive are obtained from sensors or Internet-based services, we express the user context in terms of low level context primitives as follows:

$$C'' = \{C_s, C_{sc}\} \tag{14.6}$$

where C'' is the set of contexts classified according to their source, i.e. C_s is the set of context primitives that are triggered by the sensory data and C_{sc} is the set of context primitives that are triggered by the multimedia information contained in diversified internet-based services. The relationship between C'' and C can be expressed as $C_s \cup C_{sc} = C$. We can expand Eq. (14.6) using context primitives based on the source of each context using the following expressions:

$$C_s = \{c_{s1}, c_{s2}, c_{s3}, \ldots c_{sk}\} \tag{14.7}$$

$$\text{where } c_{si} \in C \text{ and } C_s \subset C.$$

$$C_{sc} = \{c_{sc1}, c_{sc2}, c_{sc3}, \ldots c_{scj}\} \tag{14.8}$$

$$C'' = C_s \bigcup C_{sc}$$

$$\text{where } c_{scj} \in C \text{ and } C_{sc} \subset C \text{ and.}$$

Services Modeling

We assume that a user has subscribed to m numbers of diversified types of e-Health services, whose total set can be defined as S. The set of services S can be expressed as follows:

$$S = \{S_1, S_2, S_3, S_4, ..., S_m\} \tag{14.9}$$

where $s_i | \{1 \leq i \leq m\}$ is an instance of service interaction that takes place between a subject and a particular e-Health service. For example, sensor-assisted services provided by BSN, Internet-based services such as a subject checks his electronic health record, online drug availability, email from pharmacist, current weather for jogging outside, bus schedule, driving direction in a map, etc.

We assume that a user uses d number of sensors (wearable on the human body and/or deployed to surrounding environment) to observe a particular phenomenon. We express the set of sensors as the following:

$$SEN = \{sen_1, sen_2, sen_3, \ldots sen_d\} \tag{14.10}$$

Each sensor can be a source of several context primitives. For example, the sensor can be used to define locations such as home, doctor's office, shopping mall, healthcare center, etc. If a person has d number of wearable sensors, then the problem would be to map each sensory data type with a context primitive of set C_s as following:

For any instance of context $c \in C_s$ and $sen \in SEN$ (derived from Eqs. (14.7) and (14.10) respectively), we define some one-to-one function f on sen into $cf : sen \rightarrow c$, so the following relation holds:

$$C_s(\mathrm{c_{si}}) = \{(\mathrm{c_{si}}) | \exists \mathrm{sen_i} \in \mathrm{SEN}, \mathrm{f}(\mathrm{sen_i}) = \mathrm{c_{si}}\} \tag{14.11}$$

For any Internet-based service $s \in S$ and any instance of context $c \in C_{sc}$ (derived from Eq. (14.8) and (14.9) respectively) we define some one-to-one function f' on s into $cf' : s \rightarrow c$,. With respect to a particular context $c_{scj} \in C^*$, a set of services is defined as:

$$C_{sc}\left(c_{scj}\right) = \left\{(c_{scj}) \exists s_i \in S, f'(s_i) = c_{scj}\right\} \tag{14.12}$$

It should be noted that a sensor such as ECG might be used to produce several user contexts such as "stressed", "normal", "doing exercise", "panicked", "heart attack". However, all the different variations has to be first modeled as primitive contexts according to our proposed modeling methodology and then these primitives can be used in different compound context expressions to produce higher level context scenarios. Hence, we use the term "one-to-one function" such as f and f' to refer to the unique context primitives. These unique context primitives form the context vocabulary of our framework model.

Context-Aware Services

Now that we have formally defined the context primitives, complete context expressions and services based on their source, we can proceed in mapping a set of services with a particular complete context expression. For any service $s \in S$ and any instance of context $c \in C^*$, we define some one-to-one function g on s into c, $g : s \rightarrow c$.

With respect to a particular context $c_i^* \in C^*$, a context-aware service can be mapped as follows:

$$CS(c_i^*) = \{(s_i)|s_i \in S,\ \forall s_i : g\,(s_i) = c_i^*\} \tag{14.13}$$

Equation (14.13) maps each complete context from the set of C^* with a subset of services from S. Therefore, the set of context-aware services (*CS*) can be thought as a set mapping each instance of context with a set of services:

$$CS = \{CS(c_i^*)|c_i^* \in C^*\} \tag{14.14}$$

Equations (14.13) and (14.14) do not specifically mention the source of context. Hence, we express the context-aware services based on the source of the context. Context-aware services based on sensory data can be expressed as follows:

$$CS(c_{si}^*) = \{(s_i)|s_i \in S, \forall s_i : g\,(s_i) = c_{si}^*\} \tag{14.15}$$

Similar expressions of set of context-aware Internet-based services can be deduced as the following:

$$CS(c_{scj}^*) = \{(s_i)|s_i \in S', \forall s_i : g\,(s_i) = c_{scj}^*\} \tag{14.16}$$

Equation (14.14) can then be rewritten based on source of context as follows:

$$CS = \{(CS(c_{scj}^*)|c_{scj}^* \in C^*)U(CS(c_{si}^*)|c_{si}^* \in C^*)\} \tag{14.17}$$

Equation (14.17) can be used to deduce a complete user context by combining a subset of context primitives from both sensors and Internet-based services. Table 14.2 shows two sample expressions of complete definition of user context that uniquely defines two distinct states of a user. Please note that the complete context definition is domain specific and can be designed by subject matter expert (SME) during the modeling and design time. For example, an SME can provide the threshold of each category of heart beat sensor data such as normal, abnormal, critical, during-exercise, alarming, etc.

In order to map each context with a set of services, we use fuzzy ontology using the Mamdani inference engine through the following four steps, details of which can be found in [11]:

(1) fuzzification, where we map each crisp input data type into a fuzzy set;
(2) determining the individual context rule to semantically map the input and the output in the fuzzy domain;
(3) determining the aggregate context output of all the fuzzy rules;
(4) defuzzification, which means finally mapping each fuzzy output to a crisp set of outputs, i.e., a vector containing the context-aware e-Health service.

Prototype Implementation

The high level implementation view is portrayed in Fig. 14.3. The framework collects contents from both sensors and diversified Internet-based services and then infers user context by analyzing the content. The BSN comprises of a smartphone with several internal and external sensors. The smartphone chosen was HTC G1 Dream running Android 2.2 OS. We leverage the internal sensors of HTC G1 such as orientation, accelerometer, light, magnetic field, proximity, temperature, audio and camera. As external sensors, we have used a Garmin Forerunner 50 attached with a heart rate monitor that provides the smartphone instantaneous, maximum and average heart rate in beats per minute. Android 2.2 comes with some built-in communication facilities including SMS, telephony, email and HTTP POST method. We have ported the i-jetty[1] personal web server within the HTC G1 phone to communicate with the external server i.e. the *User-Context Manager*.

In order to collect content from heterogeneous Internet-based services, we have ported some popular e-Health services written in PHP and Python programming language that help us in extracting and analyzing contents [33] from their respective service providers within the *User-Context Manager* module (see Fig. 14.3). For proof of concept, we have tested with the following types of services: (a) IM and audio/video conferencing (Skype, MSN/Yahoo messenger), (b) Social portals (Facebook, Twitter, YouTube), (c) E-mail (Yahoo, Gmail, Hotmail), (d) Location (Google street view), (e) Communication (SMS, Fax, MMS, Voice mail, RSS and APRS), (f) Event-oriented (Google/Yahoo Calendar, Yahoo Weather). Since the framework is open source, we can add as many web services as needed with the framework. For a comprehensive list of our implemented services, readers are requested to refer to [1, 8, 33].

Both content as well as context extraction modules have been deployed into an XAMPP[2] server which stores the context primitive in a MySQL database. Web portal has been implemented using open source iMoogle, which uses PHP and JSON[3] to

Table 14.2 Deducing context primitives from sensory data and multimedia information of diversified internet-based services

Values received from sensors/services	Complete context
(*Agenda received from online meeting client*) **and** (*people nearby are co-authors*) **and** (*location is university*) **and** (*cell phone status off*)	The subject is in a meeting with researchers at the university
(*Blood pressure* $\geq$ 160) **and** (*pulse* $\geq$ 140) **and** (*sweat flag is on*) **and** (*Latitude*—45° 19′*N*, *Longitude*—75°40′*W*) **and** (*GPS signal is absent*)	The subject is doing exercise

[1] http://code.google.com/p/i-jetty/

[2] http://www.apachefriends.org/en/xampp.html

[3] http://www.json.org/

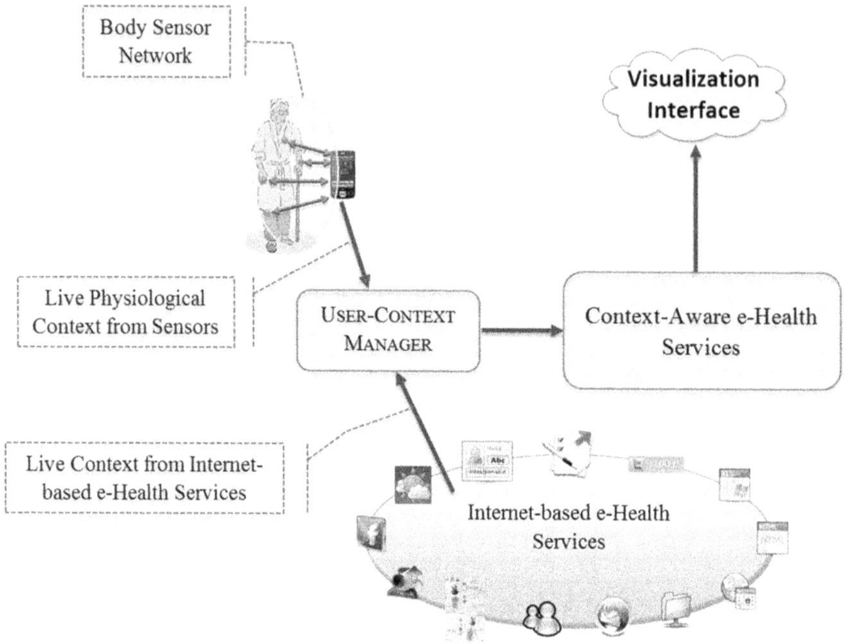

Fig. 14.3 High level implementation scenario of the proposed system

dynamically control the layout and content of each portlet. iMoogle portal is based on Javascript and the number of portlets, their layout, spatial location and the size of each of them can be dynamically changed by server side PHP script. We have deployed a demo framework environment for public access. We have configured PHP modules as a XAMPP service cron that can be configured to automatically run at a specific interval to discover any update to a user's e-Health service list. In order to implement the context-aware services and load balancing, we have configured three proxy servers with two of them having open IP that are not bound to any corporate firewall. The following are the configuration of the proxy servers:

- *Proxy server 1*: OS-Windows XP professional, RAM-2GByte, Processor-32 bit, 3.6 GHz Intel Pentium 4, IP address-137.122.89.108, Java Version - jdk1.6.0.
- *Proxy server 2*: OS-Windows Server 2003, RAM-4GByte, Processor-32 bit, 3.1 GHz Intel Xeon with 4 processors, IP address-137.122.89.112, Java Version - jdk1.6.0.
- *Proxy server 3*: OS-Virtual Machine running Ubuntu 9.10 using vmware-server.2.0.2-203138, RAM-2GByte, Processor-3.1 GHz Intel Pentium 4, Java Version - jdk1.6.0, Database-Postgresql 8.4.1.

Using AJAX, the smartphone web server can push sensory data to the *User-Context Manager*, while using reverse AJAX the BSN receives remote server pushed data over the web, which allows a server to push events to the smartphone web server.

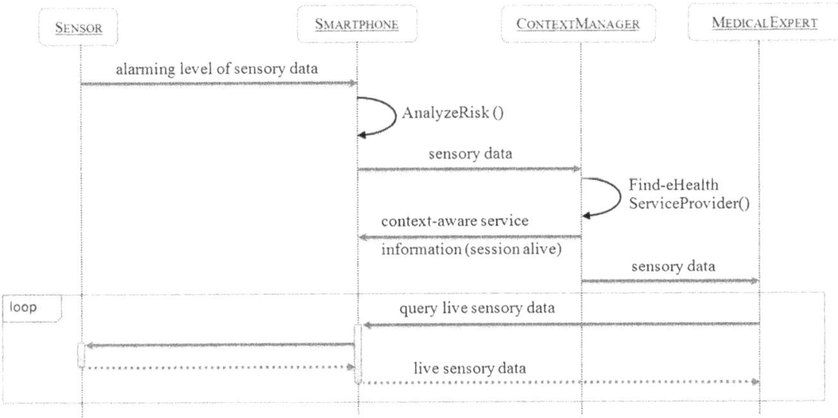

Fig. 14.4 A scenario describing live sensory data communication between a BSN and an e-Health service provider at a given physiological context

An implementation scenario has been illustrated in Fig. 14.4 where a BSN establishes two-way communication with a medical expert of an e-Health service provider via *User-Context Manager*. The medical expert can act as subject matter expert and check for erroneous sensory data coming from the BSN. The BSN context extraction service module has been implemented using an XAMPP server which stores the sensory data primitive in a MySQL database. Finally, the context extraction logic has been developed using different third party applications written in Perl, Python, Java and PHP programming language. In order to store user context, we have defined the context schema as shown in Table 14.3. This serves as a context vocabulary that can be used to verify the completeness of a unique context. Table 14.3 provides context parameters that together express a complete definition of user context.

Figure 14.5 shows an instance of scenario when a user logs in to the portal and visualizes dynamically calculated context-aware services. We assume a user uses Google email as single sign-on. After Google email server authenticates the user, the portal renders the context-aware services with spatial layout and size of each portlet. Figure 14.5 shows how a relative change in a user's context is reflected within the portal.

Test Results

In this section, we provide the subjective evaluation of the proposed framework, i.e. users' feedback collected from questionnaires. These measures are obtained by the combination of logging data as a result of user interaction with the framework and subsequent fill up of online questionnaires. The subjective evaluation is based on a sample of 45 test persons with 25 % females, which was conducted between May 15,

Table 14.3 Context schema definition

Context definition	Description
context-ID	Unique ID of the context
context-Name	Name of the context
context-CreationDate	Date of creation of the context
context-LastModified	Date of last modification of the context
context-URI	Location where the context schema is stored
context-Creator	Human or non-human subject who created the context
context-Events	Event(s) that should trigger the context. In this modeling, sensors and live event information coming from diversified sources of Internet are the event sources
context-Location	Physical location(s) related to the context
context-Objective	Purpose of the context
context-Services	Services/applications/resources necessary or related to realize the context. For example, communication devices (smartphone) and sensors, applications, software agents, and network resources (bandwidth, data rate)
context-AccessControl	Information or parameters needed to access different services and events information from the Internet, BSN or other private sources defined at the current context. Privacy or security issues are also part of this parameter
context-Quality	Precision, probability of correctness, trustworthiness, resolution and up-to-date

2010 and August 30, 2010. The majority of the users belong to an age group older than 25 while 10 % under 25 years. All the test users used various Internet-based services in different scale since the past 4–6 years. Twenty percent of the test users are non-technical and they use Internet sparingly only at their home desktops or laptops.

Before the test begins, the subjects were first given a brief introduction of each of the functionalities they have to test, as outlined in the questionnaires and give their feedback about. Users were guided to define their complete context expressions using a wizard that facilitates choosing different primitives in pursuant to the context topology (see Fig. 14.2). Then, each user was requested to test the framework at different locations and time for duration of their choice. Some took several days to test different contexts while some were in hurry to finish the test with one or two distinct contexts within a day. Finally, each subject was requested to fill up an online web-based feedback form. Each question had five possible answers ("Strongly Agree", "Agree", "Not Sure", "Disagree", and "Strongly Disagree"). The questionnaires are shown in Table 14.4.

As the questionnaires were online, the users had the option to provide their feedback regarding their test experience at any moment of a day from their home or any other location over the Internet. Because user privacy is out of scope of this research, providing login information about services was kept optional for the users. To facilitate the testing process, we created demo accounts for each of the services and kept

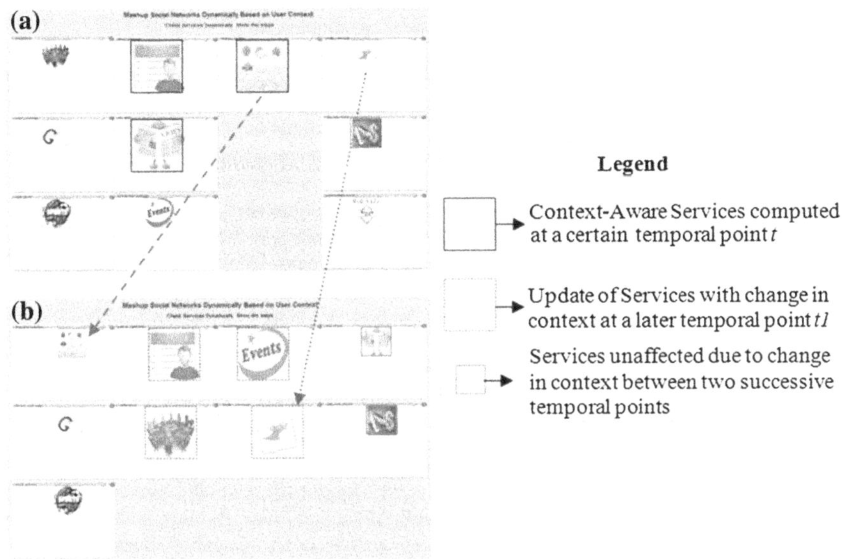

Fig. 14.5 Web portal showing the effect of context-awareness (**a**) services with large rectangular icon are services that have fresh content with context value, (**b**) updated user context dynamically updates the portal content as well as layout

operational for about a year prior to this usability test so that users can see the content of each service. However, some users were kind enough to provide their login information, with the assurance that current testing infrastructure would not store any personal or login information in the server. Some users needed special assistance due to their age and inability to either see properly or read some fonts or understand some user interfaces. Proper onsite help was arranged for those accessibility issues.

The portal presents not only those services that a user defined for a particular context a priori but also those services (from the pool of one's all registered services) that have new content are also brought within the service dashboard. The services having new or unread content or having context value were shown with some noticeable size and graphical annotations. The variants that we considered capturing through this usability test are following:

Variant-1: User view regarding context modeling from primitives

Users were presented with interfaces that showed some basic context primitives selected from the login information such as location of the user, semantic time (e.g. time showed according to hourly time slice, portion of the day, day of the week and so on). The context primitives were categorized to reflect the context topology shown in Fig. 14.2. A subject had the flexibility to add as many distinct context expressions into his/her profile. A user can visualize or edit the context expressions that he/she has already defined in the past to facilitate the formation of new context expressions. The resulting user feedbacks related to this idea is shown in Fig. 14.6. Fifty-five percent

Table 14.4 Usability and user satisfaction questionnaire (adapted from ISO 9241-11)

Questionnaires	
Q1	*I appreciate the concept of context-aware services and community of interest. If my privacy is protected, I might consider using the framework*
Q2	*I communicate with my social ties through emails, instant messages, and mobile phones and so on*
Q3	*I consume different categories of e-Health services such as through emails (Hotmail, Gmail, Yahoo...), instant messaging (MSN, Skype...), social networks (Facebook, Twitter...), audio/video conferencing (Skype, Google Talk...), checking weather, checking bus schedule and so on*
Q4	*I appreciate that I do not have to login at each service individually to check its current content*
Q5	*The framework collects user context from different categories of services (e.g. email, calendar...) in real time. Do you agree with that?*
Q6	*The delay/waiting time in showing the services within the portal/home-page is within your tolerable limit*
Q7	*The orientation/presentation of the dynamically available services based on the context value is quite interesting and I liked the idea*
Q8	*I like the concept that the framework checks the content of all my registered services and extracts the context value*
Q9	*Incorporating sensors to extract important context information (e.g. high heart rate, room and body temperature) looks appropriate to me*
Q10	*I am happy with the idea of categorizing the services according to the type of services (e.g. email, video conferencing, calendar, and sensory data)*
Q11	*You are at your work and engaged in a meeting. You only allow certain services until your meeting is over or you manually permit a particular service or certain members of your COI. These kinds of scenarios portray the benefit of adding context-awareness to my services*
Q12	*It is useful to see the list of all my social ties organized according to my social categories (e.g. family, kin, friends, colleague...)*
Q13	*I like the idea of organizing my social ties based on the services (e.g. Gmail, Yahoo, Skype, Facebook) through which I communicate with them*
Q14	*It is interesting to show a subset of my social ties (community of interest) at any given context (e.g. location: home and/or event: meeting with Doctor and/or time: evening)*

http://zing.ncsl.nist.gov/iusr/documents/cifv1.1b.htm

of the users strongly accepted the proposition while 40 % showed their support and the rest 5 % did not have either positive or negative view.

Variant-2: User view about collecting context from sensors

The test environment was bundled with four sensor based services and users had the option to test a subset or all of them. The first two services were to check user stress level using both heart rate and body temperature sensors. The rest two services are based on accelerometer and GPS sensors, which tells the framework whether a user was doing some physical activities for a certain amount of duration. Figure 14.7 shows that 65 % of the subjects strongly supported the idea of incorporating sensors to monitor different vital parameters and advise them some suggested services they

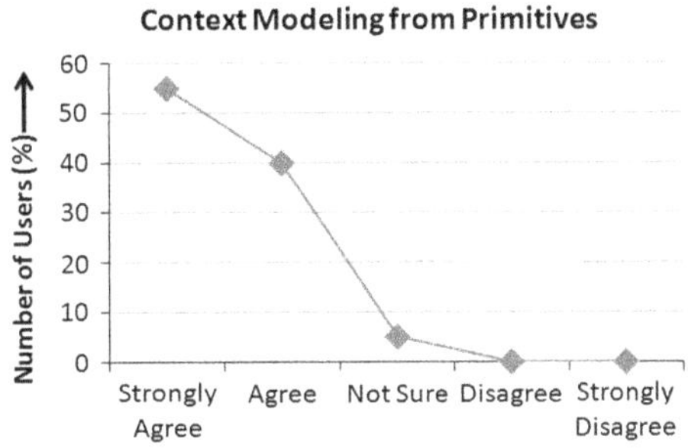

Fig. 14.6 User comments about creating fine grained user context from context primitives

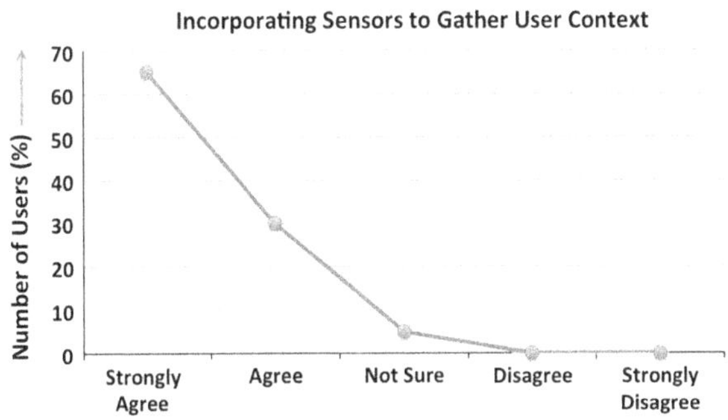

Fig. 14.7 User view of collecting a user and his/her ambient context information from a body sensor network

prefer in those contexts. Thirty percent subjects showed approval and 5 % did not have any clear opinion. Moreover, some users raised voice regarding privacy issues while others were concerned about the prices of those sensors. Some showed pessimism to carry them always to get those services. The overall recommendations were very encouraging and optimistic.

Variant-3: User view about collecting context from Internet-based services

Users were presented with several services mentioned in section "Framework Modeling" to demonstrate the concept of extracting live content that might carry important context information such as weather data, location and addresses in maps, and events from calendar, to name a few. As shown in Fig. 14.8, 75 % users showed their strong support of this variant while the rest of them approved the concept. User feedbacks show encouraging prospect of collecting context from Internet-based e-Health services.

Variant-4: Overall user feedback regarding the framework

Figure 14.9 shows the overall test results collected through the questionnaire initiative. This variant reflects the user feedbacks regarding the overall framework and the demonstrated features. The figure also portrays the integrated view of user satisfaction and experience. Question numbers four and eight scored the highest approval rating

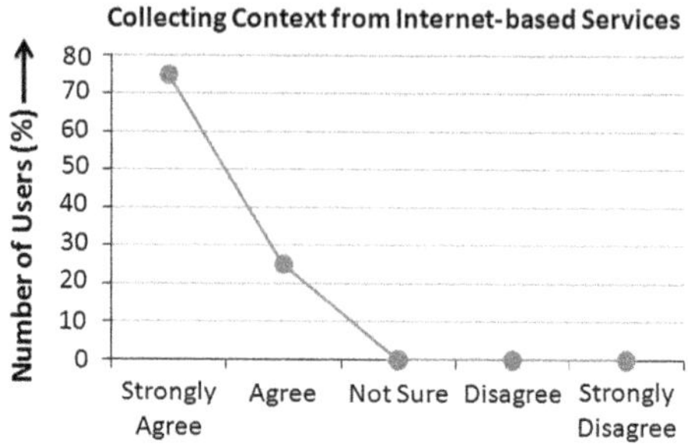

Fig. 14.8 User view of collecting online context information from heterogeneous services

(90 %) under the category "Strongly Agree," both of which showed the potential of the research value presented through the proposed framework. On the other hand, question numbers five and six of the same category earned the lowest score (50 %). In the case of question number five, we analyzed the subjects who did not approve strongly and found that they either belonged to non-technical user group or were those who only tested the framework once then provided their feedback. In the case of question number six, user-tolerable delay is found to be vague and follows no pattern.

The mean value of subjective approval of "Agree" is approximately 30 %. The highest approval in the category "Not Sure" was given to question number five, which shows that users were skeptical about the idea of collecting user context from the analysis of content coming from heterogeneous services. One reason we unearthed was that many of the users do not use many Internet-based services on a regular basis, and so some could not pick up the concept of context extraction from service content. On the other hand, context extraction from sensors showed a better approval rating than its service counterpart, while both did the same job (providing context

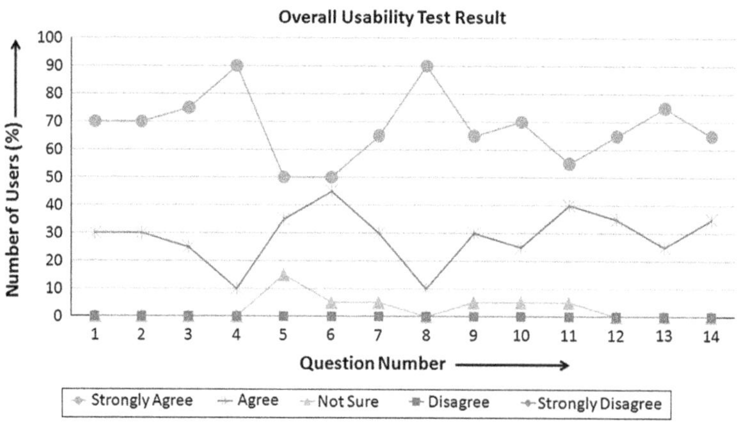

Fig. 14.9 Integrated feedback results from all the test subjects regarding the framework

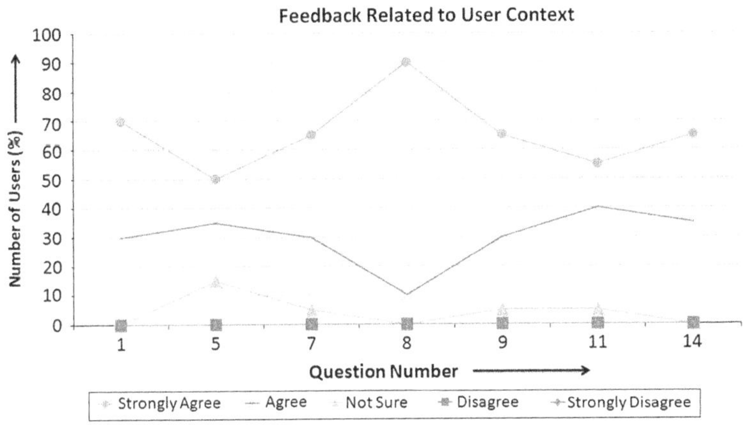

Fig. 14.10 User feedbacks regarding global view of context-awareness

value to the framework). The average value of user ratings in "Not Sure" category is about 5 %. The most interesting information is that no user chose the categories "Disagree" and "Strongly Disagree".

Variant-5: Overall user view about context-awareness in e-Healthdomain

Although different aspects of user context are evaluated through this subjective evaluation test, this variant provides the set of questionnaires that are fully or somewhat related to users' view of context. As shown in Fig. 14.10, question numbers one, five, seven, eight, nine, eleven and fourteen were meant to collect context related user feedbacks. Around 70 % of users on average strongly accepted the notion about importance of user context in the area of e-Health, 25 % of users showed their positive view and the rest were undecided, leaving their answers empty for the category "Disagree" and "Strongly Disagree".

Variant-6: Overall user view about the context-aware e-Healthservices

This variant helps us in collecting user feedback regarding the central idea and one of the most important contributions of this research—how interesting the idea of "context-aware services" is to users. Question numbers one to eleven either directly or indirectly brings forth user views regarding this important phenomenon. From the obtained test data, as shown in Fig. 14.11, we observe that about 70 % of the users strongly agreed the concept of providing services based on user context while around 25 % of users agreed upon the concept and the rest were unsure what to respond. No user completely disapproved of the idea.

Variant-7: Non-technical users' view

Figure 14.12 shows non-technical users' (businessman, construction worker, housewife, elderly person, etc.) views regarding all the aspects of the e-Health framework. This variant is intended to capture how the people outside the university and research domain feel about the necessity of the concept proposed in this research.

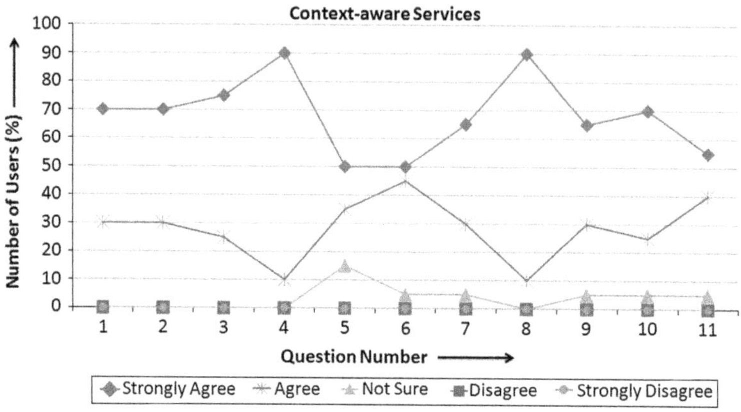

Fig. 14.11 Users' view about providing e-Health services based on a given user context

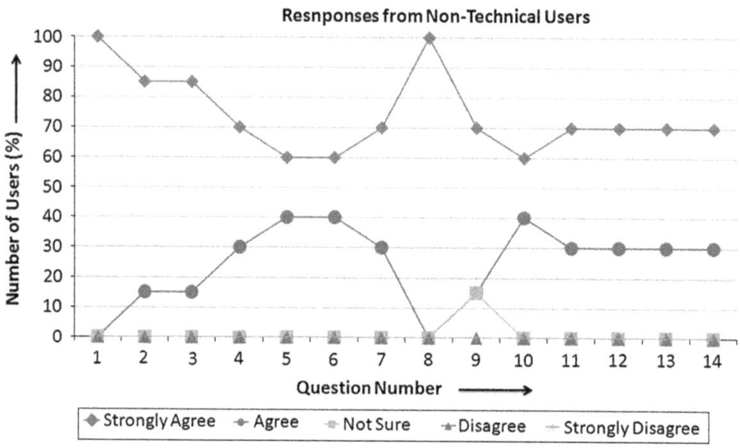

Fig. 14.12 Non-technical users' feedback about different aspect of the framework

Non-technical users were first introduced to different key words and concepts through real life examples that were introduced through all 14 questions. Many users were not familiar or did not use some aspects of the framework in the past, which led to the "Not Sure" option. From the captured feedback, we were enlightened by their feedback and their urge in seeing the concepts serve their daily life. For example, services such as location, weather, maintaining doctor appointment and local bus schedule based on user context such as location and time were very appealing to this group.

As seen in Fig. 14.12, all the subjects in this category strongly supported the framework and its ability to check the content of each registered services (question numbers one and eight). On the average 75 % strongly supported the features provided by the framework while a mean value of 20 % showed their support. A mean value of about 5 % was undecided. We are in the process of doing a second round of usability tests in a large scale which will occur once we enhance both interfaces and functionalities as suggested by the test subjects.

Conclusions and Future Directions

Due to the recent popularity of diversified Internet-based services and usage of sensory media, we have recognized the need for a context-aware framework that is capable of identifying user context at any given moment and provide relevant services. The framework facilitates a user in defining simple or complex context expressions from context primitives. We have argued that user context can be collected from two sources: sensors attached to a person's body sensor network and/or surrounding environment and multimedia content from Internet-based services. We have presented details about modeling of such framework. The framework has been validated by conducting a usability test where users were presented with a demo environment. The usability test gives us encouragement and boosts our confidence in carrying out research to its next stage.

We have compiled a list of user recommendations that were gathered while conducting the usability test. Based on the user recommendations, we have targeted the following aspects that we are also planning to incorporate in our framework. First of all, we will be investigating existing and state of the art privacy models that would fit the framework and will adopt a suitable privacy model so that users have full control over how the framework uses the sensitive and personalized e-Health data originating from sensors and Internet-based services. Secondly, we are contemplating adding new media with the framework in addition to sensory and Internet-based multimedia. We have already added second life virtual work and Microsoft Kinect-based serious game environment to add more modality. Moreover, two media candidates that we are planning to incorporate are haptics and emotion. Adding the emotional state with each e-Health service will enable users to semantically understand the importance of each service. Then, through haptic devices, a user could feel the emotions tagged with each service. Thirdly, we will investigate and incorporate appropriate models to deal with incorrect measurements while analyzing content and context values. Finally, we are interested to model the following metrics that are related to user context in near future: accuracy of service prediction, user satisfaction in terms of Mean Absolute Error (MAE), compound context error rate, quality of context and confidence on context information.

References

1. Md. A. Rahman, A. El Saddik, and W. Gueaieb, "Augmenting Context-Awareness by Combining Body Sensor Networks and Social Networks", IEEE Transaction on Instrumentation and Measurement, Vol. 60, No. 2, February 2011, pp. 345–353.

2. P. Killworth et al., “Estimating the Size of Personal Networks”, Social Networks, Vol. 12, 1990, pp. 289–312.
3. A. K. Dey, “Understanding and Using Context”, Personal Ubiquitous Computing, Springer-Verlag, Vol. 5, No. 1, 2001, pp. 4–7.
4. D. Phung, B. Adams, K. Tran, S. Venkatesh, M. Kumar, “High accuracy context recovery using clustering mechanisms”, Proc. IEEE Int. Conf. Pervasive Computing and, Communications, pp. 1–9, Mar. 9–13, 2009.
5. J. An, S. Pack, S. An, M. Kim, and Y. Jeon, “A novel service architecture for personalized context aware services”, Proc. 11th Int. Conf. Advanced Communication Technology, 15–18 February, Vol. 1, pp. 554–559, 2009.
6. Y. Kawahara, H. Kurasawa, and H. Morikawa, “Recognizing User Context Using Mobile Handsets with Acceleration Sensors”, Proc. IEEE Int. Conf. Portable Information Devices, pp. 1–5, May 25–29, 2007.
7. J. Koolwaaij, M. Wibbels, S. Böhm, and M. Luther, “ContextKing: Virtual Kingdoms in Real Life”, Proc. 1st IEEE Int. Conf. Games and Virtual Worlds, pp. 61–67, Mar. 23–24, 2009.
8. Md. A. Rahman, Sadek Hamdan, A. El. Saddik, and W. Gueaieb, “Context-Aware Social Networks Mashup: A Personalized Web Perspective”, Proc. IEEE Int. Instrumentation and Measurement Technology Conference (I2MTC 2010), Austin, Tx, USA, pp. 1228–1233, May 3–6, 2010.
9. T. Gao, D. Greenspan, and M. Welsh, “Improving patient monitoring and tracking in emergency response”, Proc. Int. Conf. Information Communication Technologies in Health, July 2005.
10. D. Wyatt et al”., Towards Automated Social Analysis of Situated Speech Data”, Proc. Ubicomp, Vol. 344, 2008, pp. 168–171.
11. R. K. Ganti, T. Yu-En, T. F. Abdelzaher, “SenseWorld: Towards Cyber-Physical Social Networks”, Proc. Int. Conf. Information Processing in Sensor, Networks, pp. 563–564, 2008.
12. W. H. Wu, “MEDIC: Medical embedded device for individualized care”, Journal of Artificial Intelligence in Medicine, Elsevier, Vol. 42, No. 2, 2008, pp. 137–152.
13. S. Gaonkar, J. Li, R. R. Choudhury, L. Cox, and A. Schmidt, “Micro-Blog: sharing and querying content through mobile phones and social participation”, Proc. 6th Int. Conf. Mobile systems, applications, and services, pp. 174–186, 2008.
14. D. Bottazzi, A. Corradi, and R. Montanari, “Context-Aware Middleware Solutions for Anytime and Anywhere Emergency Assistance to Elderly People”, IEEE Communications Magazine, 2006, pp. 82–90.
15. C. M. Gartrell, “SocialAware: Context-Aware Multimedia Presentation via Mobile Social Networks”, University of Colorado. Masters Thesis. [Online] Available: http://www.cs.colorado.edu/rhan/Papers/Mike_Gartrell_CU_MS_thesis-final.pdf
16. A. Joly, P. Maret and J. Daigremont, “Context-Awareness, the Missing Block of Social Networking”, International Journal of Computer Science and Applications, Technomathematics Research Foundation, Vol. 6, No. 2, 2009, pp. 50–65.
17. J. Beutel, O. Kasten, and M. Ringwald, “Btnodes a distributed platform for sensor nodes”, ACM SenSys, Los Angeles, California, USA, pp. 292–293, 2003.
18. S. Sarikaya, M. A. Alim, and S. Rezaei, “Integrating wireless EEGs into medical sensor networks”, ACM IWCMC, Vancouver, British Columbia, Canada, pp. 1369–1373, 2006.
19. X. An, and J. Wang, “Opt: online person tracking system for context awareness in wireless personal network”, in ACM REALMAN, Florence, Italy, pp. 47–54, 2006.
20. S. Park et al., “Design of a wearable sensor badge for smart kindergarten”, Proc. of the 6th International Symposium on Wearable Computers, pp. 231–238, 2002.
21. O. Aziz et al., “A pervasive body sensor network for measuring postoperative recovery at home”, ACM IPSN, Journal of Surgical Innovation, Vol. 14, No. 2, 2007, pp. 83–90.
22. S. Bhardwaj, D-S. Lee, S. C. Mukhopadhyay and Wan-Y. Chung, “Ubiquitous Healthcare Data Analysis and Monitoring Using Multiple Wireless Sensors for Elderly Person”, Sensors & Transducers Journal, Vol. 90, 2008, pp. 87–99.
23. S. B. Eisenman, ”The bikenet mobile sensing system for cyclist experience mapping”, ACM SenSys, pp. 87–101, 2007.

24. P. Nurmi, J. Kukkonen, E. Lagerspetz, J. Suomela, P. Floreen, "Betelgeuse a tool for bluetooth data gathering", Helsinki Institute for Information Technology (HIIT). [Online]. Available: http://www.cs.helsinki.fi/group/acs/betelgeuse/articles/betelgeusebodynets07.pdf
25. J. Yao, and S. Warren, "Applying the ISO/IEEE 11073 standards to wearable home health monitoring systems", Journal of Clinical Monitoring and Computing, Springer, Vol. 19, 2005, pp. 427–436.
26. L. Schmitt, T. Falck, F. Wartena, and D. Simons, "Novel ISO/IEEE 11073 standards for personal telehealth systems interoperability", Joint Workshop on High Confidence Medical Devices, Software, and Systems and Medical Device Plug-and-Play Interoperability, pp. 146–148, 2007.
27. S. Krco, "Health care sensor networks-architecture and protocols", Ad Hoc and Sensor Wireless Networks, Vol. 1, August 2004, pp. 1–25.
28. B. H. Yang, and S. Rhee, "Development of the ring sensor for healthcare automation", Robotics and Autonomous System, Vol. 30, 2000, pp. 273–281.
29. E. Jovanov, et al. "Stress monitoring using a distributed wireless intelligent sensor system", IEEE Engineering in Medicine and Biology Magazine, Vol. 22, No. 3, 2003, pp. 49–55.
30. K. P. Smith, and N. A. Christakis, "Social networks and health", Annual Review of Sociology, Vol. 34, August 2008, pp. 405–429.
31. R. Upendra, and O. Max, "Predicting network availability using user context", Proc. of the 5th Annual International Conference on Mobile and Ubiquitous Systems, pp. 1–8, 2008.
32. S. El Helou, C. Salzmann, S. Sire, and D. Gillet, "The 3A Contextual Ranking System: Simultaneously Recommending Actors, Assets, and Group Activities", Proc. 3rd ACM Conference on Recommender Systems, New York, USA, pp. 373–376, Oct. 22–25, 2009.
33. Md. A. Rahman, A. El Saddik, and W. Gueaieb, "Building Dynamic Social Network From Sensory Data Feed", IEEE Transaction on Instrumentation and Measurement, Vol. 59, No. 5, 2010, pp. 1327–1341.

Chapter 15
Personal Web in Healthcare

Aniket Bochare, Kristen Brady, Kristianne Oristian, Omar El-Ghazawi, Yelena Yesha and Yaacov Yesha

Abstract In this chapter we discuss the innovation and perspective of the Personal Web and its wide impact in the healthcare domain. We approach the Personal Web from a Web 2.0 perspective and how it can benefit both practitioners and consumers in the medical field. The demand for personal web in healthcare is analyzed, as well as how it can be beneficial for key players involved in its development and maturity. The current role of personal web in the health industry and technologies is identified along with its advantages over conventional practices of diagnosis and treatment. Coupled with this, we isolate factors that may contribute to the success or failure of such a platform. Highlighted are the key aspects of Web 2.0 elements and features that are intrinsic to such innovation in the medical field. The relationship between personal web and personalized medicine is also discussed. Additionally, the

A. Bochare · Y. Yesha (✉) · Y. Yesha
Department of Computer Science and Electrical Engineering,
University of Maryland, Baltimore County,
1000 Hilltop Circle, Baltimore, MD 21250, USA
e-mail: yeyesha@cs.umbc.edu

A. Bochare
e-mail: aniketb1@umbc.edu

Y. Yesha
e-mail: yayesha@cs.umbc.edu

K. Brady
University of Maryland, College Park, MD 20742, USA
e-mail: kristenbrady80@gmail.com

K. Oristian
Elon University, Elon, NC 27244, USA
e-mail: koristian@elon.edu

O. El-Ghazawi
George Mason University, 4400 University Drive, Fairfax, VA 22030, USA
e-mail: omarghazawi@yahoo.com

B. Furht and A. Agarwal (eds.), *Handbook of Medical and Healthcare Technologies*,
DOI: 10.1007/978-1-4614-8495-0_15, © Springer Science+Business Media New York 2013

current nature of personal web within the industry is analyzed in the context of these proposed ideas.

Introduction

The following chapter introduces the reader to the basic concept of personal web and its application in the medical domain. It identifies the current technology in the medical industry and advantages of the personal web model and Web 2.0. The chapter walks you through the role of personal web in the health domain. We have also highlighted in detail the users who will benefit most from the proposed technological innovation, as well as the capacity in which they would use it. The factors that may potentially enhance or stymy the forward momentum of personal web use in this field are identified. The following sections will acquaint the reader with, and provide an accurate picture of the ideas discussed above.

Personal Web

The following is an overview of the concepts of Web 2.0 that are essential to the understanding of Personal Web. Personal web and Web 2.0 are related in the following section and the emergence of these technologies simultaneously in Healthcare is discussed. According to TechPluto [1], Web 2.0 is a combination of various characteristics of web technology including the user-centric model, platform independence, collaborative contributions, self service systems free from administration, software as service and an engaging user interface. In essence, this means that most of the web components can work independently by providing rich user interface to end users on any platform. The capacity for web users to collaborate information and share dynamic content is essential to the Web 2.0 model [1]. In December 2006 Tim O'Reilly defined the next generation of software and Web 2.0, "*Web 2.0 is the business revolution in the computer industry caused by the move to the internet as platform, and an attempt to understand the rules for success on that new platform. Chief among those rules is this: Build applications that harness network effects to get better the more people to use them*" [2]. According to O'Reilly, software should not be treated as a static entity, but rather, involve dynamic users. He makes the concept of reusability of data and services an important conversation in the web development community [2]. Joanna Ng et al. notes that the web is currently viewed as "Smart Internet" which provides the end user with relevant information aggregated from online resources. The importance of providing the user with an appealing user experience to navigate throughout the web is demonstrated. There is a transformation from the conventional server-driven model of web development to a more user-driven model. Essential to this model is the understanding that a non-technical user should be easily able to navigate across websites [3].

Ng proposes that substantial technical expertise should not be required for using the Personal Web. The Personal Web should enable the combination of information from various sources on the web in order to address a specific issue that is of particular relevance to the user. That said, the architecture should be both autonomous and user-driven [4]. According to Kinley and Tjondronegoro [5] the idea of personal web focuses on a general user or individual who lacks technical knowledge of programming. As such, we cannot ignore the importance of human/computer interaction while designing systems used for the personal web. Rather, there is a need to analyze how a web user accumulates information and to delve into those patterns of its usage. Study of the literature reveals that holistic users employ disparate approaches to searching and processing information as compared to analytical ones [5]. We can expect the personal web platform, then, to help such users gather necessary and reliable information from a variety of authentic sources and to present them in a standardized and readable form. This provides the capability to integrate various sources to those who might otherwise not employ the skill set required for such a task. The consumer of the web service should be able to integrate the various web components through a personal account. In essence, the internet era necessitates a dynamic integration of web elements and information to be navigated by any user without the need for extraordinary skills.

In her work, Joanna Ng identifies the following components as essential to the design of personal web:

- The user is the most important element of web integration.
- The aggregation of web elements over the web should consider semantics relevant to the user.
- The user should have absolute control over integration of web elements and the proposed social interaction [4].

The following section identifies the current direction of modern healthcare and its relationship to personal web.

Identifying the Need for Personal Web in Healthcare

The drawbacks of the current web model serve as the impetus for the emergence of personal web. Shortcomings are identified in the literature as follows:

- Lack of control for the end users when collecting information from multiple relevant sources
- Lack of customizable features or personalization at run time for user's context
- Lack of support for carrying out complex tasks at user's end.
- Restricted functionality for collaboration and combined features for information across the web [3].

The healthcare industry is extensive, and is a large consumer of funding both for the treatment and care of patients and for infrastructure improvement. In the last few years, the information technology movement has gained substantial momentum in the United States, making drastic transformations possible. According to the President's Council of Advisors on Science and Technology, Health IT has the potential to:

- Eliminate the onerous task of data entry by integrating information technology in the clinical setting.
- Assist physicians in decision-making processes by providing access to the clinical/genomic data of the patient at the point of care.
- Facilitate both patients and caretakers to be involved in self-health management and health care of dear ones.
- Facilitate research and monitoring at the general population level.
- Induce an upturn in personalized treatment in Healthcare via personalized medicine.
- Provide a more transparent process as well as policies within the health domain with reduced overhead as a result of current paperwork and bureaucracy procedures.
- Make high end jobs available in the market.
- Help tackle nation's economic challenges and reforms in the healthcare industry [6].

Healthcare in the US is at a turning point and the right steps in health IT can aid in improving and solving critical problems. Due to the expansive and variant nature of the health industry in this country, managing health records across institutions is not an easy task. To understand the need for the personal web in healthcare, one has to understand Electronic Health Records (EHRs). EHR refers to records generated and maintained by healthcare software in order to archive medically relevant information about patients undergoing care in a particular institution. They contain the complete medical history of an individual to be assessed for diagnosis, treatment and long-term care.

According to Berges, Bermudez, Go, and Illarramendi in the First International Workshop on Model-Driven Interoperability, EHRs boast long-term benefits in the healthcare industry, but an obstacle lies in the operation of various proprietary information systems and standards followed across institutions. This generates a need for better interoperation between systems [7]. Wilijer points out that the data set generated by physicians, clinicians, hospitals, and research institutions to monitor the health of an individual is both enormous and dynamic [8]. Additionally, the existence of EHRs in many health care institutions and organizations allow for patient access in order to facilitate self-health monitoring. Although this results in improved health planning on the part of patients, it also raises concerns regarding standards for implementation and maintenance of privacy and security [8]. Integration of data across the medical domain will not only benefit medical practitioners, patients, and insurance companies, but also students and researchers for whom medical data analysis at the academic level offers significant benefit.

Users and Uses of Personal Web

The personal web should benefit a majority of society. The key players involved in the healthcare industry need to be targeted as consumers and features of Web 2.0 and personal web should be catered to maximally benefit these groups. Ng indicates that the proposed technology can be beneficial to healthcare providers if we take into consideration the following conceptual principles of personal web:

- The consumer controls integration of web elements effortlessly
- Web integration is contingent upon a particular frame of reference and relevance to user.
- Personal web control and customization by user should be treated with utmost seriousness.
- The personal web has to be social, allowing data to be shared across the web platform with ease [4].

The following is a discussion as to how the above parameters, once applied in the healthcare domain, directly benefit patients, physicians, researchers, insurance companies, and other proprietors of the medical industry.

For Patients

As articulated by Deloitte Center for Health Solutions, the consumers of technology can benefit through self-management and monitoring of their own health on wireless devices. The display of one's personal health status and alerts (through electronic mail or another form of wireless communication) allow for the direct and real-time monitoring of his or her own health [9]. A simple user-centric model of web can be applied to control web elements in order to allow for the definition of specific alerts and real-time monitoring of health status. The health status alerts can theoretically be set personally by patients depending on individual priorities and needs. This demonstrates the possibility of complete personalization of self-health over the web.

A pilot study was conducted by the University Health Network in Toronto, Canada to understand how the internet could enhance the patient-physician relationship [10]. The result was a strong indication that the internet can potentially aid the patient when communicating his or her symptoms and laboratory results via electronic messages and updates. Specifically, this study helped heart failure patients utilize a tool designed to manage their disease by facilitating the sharing of data between patient and physician and allowing patients to effectively communicate health-related concerns to their caretakers. Their results indicated a reduction of communication over time between doctors and patients as evidence of overall improvement of patients' health [10]. It is important to clarify that the proposed web tool is not limited to certain groups of patients and specific symptoms or syndromes. Rather, the tool will incorporate personal web aspects in order to share large amounts of information from recent appointments, prescriptions, and cancellations to laboratory results, allergies, and other pertinent medical data.

Similarly, the user can personalize his or her account in order to share health records or information with *specific* clinicians, healthcare providers or insurance companies. For instance, "Google Health" allows users to share key information or keep certain information confidential, demonstrating effective privacy handling. Here, the user has absolute control over web elements they share with family members and care providers [11]. The patients can share personal medical records with anyone across the globe through their personalized account with ease. This is the feature of personal web called "sharing context-specific information with other users", which will be beneficial for patients if incorporated effectively.

We can infer, then, that the utmost importance is given to the "social" aspect of personal web and to efficient communication to and from end users of the service. The non-technical user will be able control his or her web information with other members easily. With personal web, dynamic content aggregation is possible, allowing users to gather information about healthcare providers in the network and other information personally relevant to the individual user [4].

Even though Google Health had positive influence, it was discontinued because of lack of sufficient user base [12]. Google Health was retired on January 1, 2013 [12, 13].

To Physicians

The personal web scenario explained in this section facilitates accurate diagnosis and treatment by physicians by analyzing the medical information made accessible to them by their patients over the web. This type of sharing has already been implemented in some sectors. For example, personal health records from Aetna health insurance can be securely shared with family members and physicians [14]. In this manner, physicians have access to their patient's health records at the point of care in order to diagnose and provide treatment with the most complete knowledge of the patient's health status.

Alex Jadad notes that in the age of internet, the majority of individuals turn to the internet to their first and often primary source of information [15]. As such, the deluge of information available to physicians is vast, but varied, and credible information is often indistinguishable from non-credible information. As a result, decision making can be both positively and negatively impacted. Combining the positive potential of the internet with expert knowledge and credible information can lead to improved treatment techniques. This necessitates efficient and up-to-date information in an accessible format to decision makers [15]. Since physicians are generally considered non-technical users, they must be provided with simple, user-friendly controls to access papers, journals, reports, and the most recent medical literature at the point of care.

The standardized PHR (personal health record) systems like Google Health can help accumulate information from different users for physicians. The user-centric experience of personal web can allow physicians to subscribe to patients' specific health updates or feeds. Depending on the availability of clinical and genomic data for patients, this data can also be made available for research and analysis at the patient's discretion. The additional function of managing customizable alerts, risks and reminders can be optimized for better treatment of patients under clinicians care.

Research Institutions and Healthcare Institutions

Anderson and Edwards at the Association for Computing Machinery indicate that healthcare is not limited to those who provide care to patients, but also involves researchers within the biomedical field investigating better practices in healthcare environments and detecting disease patterns across large populations. Large organizations such as the National Center for Biomedical Computing, National Cancer Institute, and other such institutions often act as forerunners in biomedical research. These organizations motivate the sharing, discovering and analyzing of clinical and genetic data. However, there is a long and arduous process that researchers must go through in order to gain access to relevant data to analyze. The medical data to be collected by any research institute passes through an Institutional Review Board (IRB) or other governing body before use in research [16]. While a personal web platform facilitates research and better healthcare, it also raises concerns with respect to privacy and confidentiality of patients' data. In addition to academic institutions, organizations in the commercial sector, such as pharmaceutical companies, seek access to current medical data in order to evaluate their products before going on the market. A study by the United States General Accounting Office shows that pharmaceutical companies actively participate in research to evaluate drug and treatment efficacy based on clinical data and seek to understand additional factors such as patient's subsequent susceptibility to disease and expenses associated with the use of their product [17].

Hian Chye Koh and Gerald Tan highlight the fact that data mining is a widely used practice and is very popular in healthcare research. Many academic institutions are actively involved in data mining and the arena of machine learning research would benefit greatly from managed data sharing over the web. Proper standardization and distribution of medical data across institutions can drastically improve efficient data mining for healthcare purposes. Insurance companies also benefit by mining healthcare data. The practice allows for the monitoring of insurance fraudulence, as well as understanding customer relations in order to provide decision support and affordable healthcare to patients [18]. The KDD (knowledge discovery in databases) process, that involves data mining, is very helpful for automated analysis of health care data [19]. The complex tasks of authorization and integration can be minimized by embracing web 2.0 technologies along with personal web. By automating routine tasks of authorization to specified institutions, crippling overheads that often stymy progressive research within institutions can be minimized.

Driving Forces for Personal Web in Health Care

The success or failure of any new technology or concept for end users depends on numerous factors. The architect of new technology must take into consideration both positive and negative components that may potentially impact its progress. In the following section, the driving forces and barriers for personal web in healthcare are underlined.

Medical Information on the Web

According to Margaret A. Winker et al. many users who seek information on the internet are not aware of the plethora of inaccurate information made available to them. Therefore, web users who seek information are made susceptible to inaccurate and incomplete information which can be misleading when trying to make educated decisions about their healthcare [20]. Houston and Allison explored the usage of health information found by patients online. According to their study, the subjects learn from and assign credibility to new health information that becomes accessible on the web. As a result, there is also a tendency for many patients to debate information with their physicians. This tool must aid patients in consuming accurate information related to their health [21]. The understanding of information as credible or non-credible is one of the largest obstacles to modern healthcare's use of the web.

According to Eysenbach and Jadad, one of the primary hurdles preventing consumers (or end users) from obtaining accurate information is an accessible standard format online. Health care decision-making is a bipartisan process, where both patients and physicians use knowledge from medical literature and health information on the web to make informed health care decisions. An inferior quality of health information available online is injurious not only to patients, but also to their healthcare providers [22]. As suggested above, a web tool should be designed that employs all of the features of personal web that empower users to gather information from sources that are validated and verified.

WebMD is one tool that has contributed much to the standards of personal web today by providing users with the ability to customize their needs and gain access to accurate disease information, physician information, and other care providers [23]. WebMD has developed a mobile app for Android and iPhone users so that they are connected to that health information wherever they go [24]. This tool provides a symptom checker, first aid information, drug information and information pertaining to counter interactions with other medicines, as well as referrals to local physicians, clinics, or hospitals based on the patient's current location.

WebMD is now prompting patients to maximize the opportunity to become active members of their healthcare teams. Websites such as these help to provide basic health information, but lack personal web features that can truly optimize the healthcare experience for patients. Medical information as provided on the web cannot replace a physician's knowledge, but a personal web tool in conjunction with a team of medical professionals and governing members can actively facilitate the exchange of important and real-time information online. Personal web along with simple web 2.0 features for users can help to aggregate data from various authentic sources and present to it the end user in a useable format.

Personal Health Records (PHRs)

According to Tang et al. a personal health record can be defined as a record which allows the individual patient to actively maintain and share their own health information in a protected and confidential setting with family and healthcare providers [25]. Unlike EHRs, which are maintained by physicians, PHRs are managed by the patients themselves [25]. Solutions like Microsoft Health Vault [26] and Google Health [27] help web users maintain medical portfolios online in the form of PHRs.

The following section uses the example of Google Health to demonstrate the features available on such PHRs. Personal web features that are currently employed and specific areas of improvement are identified. The use case of Google Health analyzes various features provided by this website for their users.

Use Case: Google Health

A typical user of a Google Health PHR can create a profile for his or her self and for family members. The interface allows the members to maintain a summary of parameters related to their body such as blood glucose, height, weight, blood pressure, etc. The system provides an outline of important patient details and also provides the functionality to list ailments, symptoms and conditions in detail on the user's profile. One can include prescription medications and over-the-counter medicines they are taking presently and those taken in the past. It also allows tracking of laboratory diagnostics, results and reports from various healthcare providers. Outpatient, inpatient and surgical procedure information is also maintained by the Google health user as part of his or her personal health record. The system features the capability of storing immunization and vaccination records along with the ability to upload important documents or images. Detailed entry of insurance plans and dates can be maintained for later reference. This is an example of how standards of Personal web can be used to provide an attractive and user-friendly interface with sharing options with family members and care providers. Additionally, the site offers the capability to link a user's profile with third party health solutions. One can import medical records from pharmacies such CVS or Walgreens pharmacy by linking their profile to that of the pharmacy. One can explore various medical treatments or obtain second opinions of diagnosis by sharing his or her PHR with different healthcare providers. The user can also track his or her own activity easily with Google Health [26].

An important component of this program is that users are given complete control of their profile. It is an excellent example of the concept of user-centered design and simple sharing features, fostering the integration of various web elements involved in healthcare. This provides evidence that extensive and efficient use of personal web features and web 2.0 characteristics in the medical domain can provide easy navigation to the users. A personal account to manage medical information is attractive to a market of users and helps to maintain data in a standard format, which helps to overcome the disadvantages of conventional heterogeneous medical databases that are currently available. There is potential for better interoperability as well as development of national standards to be followed. An architect of personal web can develop an even better user-centric model with improved usability and attractiveness for patients and healthcare professionals.

Personalized Medicine

The honorable Mr. Michael Leavitt, secretary of Health and Human Services (HHS), has indicated that, "Personalized Medicine means knowing what works, knowing why it works, knowing who it works for and applying the knowledge for patients" [28]. In other words personalized medicine is a form of treatment targeted at individuals that is unique and works precisely for the patient under care. Many researchers and institutions are studying the underlying mechanisms of individual human genes in an attempt to identify what components of the genetic code might be targeted to improve the quality of life of individual patients. One example of this type of research would be the *23andMe* program that aims to collect genetic data of individuals along with online surveys to find links between their genetic profile and their health [29].

At Duke Medicine, in the forefront of the modern medical community, experts believe in 5 principles of personalized medicine, known as the "5Ps":

Predictive: Predict precise risk to patient's health and final outcomes with the help of high end diagnostic tools and molecular signatures.

Personalized: Is defined by every patient's distinct information pertaining to DNA, environment, and medical symptoms and history of diagnosis and treatment.

Preventive: Put emphasis on preventing diseases before it reaches a more advanced stage.

Preemptive: Include planning that is tailored specifically for each patient and is based on action.

Participatory: This requires the patient to be proactive and participate in self-care by managing disease and also treatment from health care support team [30].

Utilizing the personal web platform judiciously to aggregate authorized clinical data from PHRs and genetic data from individuals to researcher or healthcare providers can assist physicians better to provide effective personalized treatment.

Social Network in Healthcare

The introduction of social networking in healthcare has the potential to be a great evolution for the next generation. The social network Facebook [31] is used to connect to friends and family, share personal information, photos, and other social information. It is the quintessential example of user-centered personal web where a user with minimal technical expertise can connect to the world at large and share data with ease. On the heels of this phenomenon, it becomes reasonable to imagine a similar network within the medical community. One can imagine a "social network" just for healthcare involving all of the various entities belonging to the healthcare industry.

A Study by Pew Internet finds that about 65% of adults use social networking sites. This data suggests that a social network utilizing all tenants of personal web design in healthcare can be a successful tool for users and perhaps even improve the general health of the country [32].

Eysenbach discusses the impact of both social networking and participation. Social network is a kernel of many Web 2.0 and Medicine 2.0 applications where there are complex relationships among its members and how they collaborate or eliminate impertinent information. They can explicitly control the information from peers (family, friends, etc) and follow specific health topics. It gives them control over their personal accounts and quality of information. It also helps to build trust and reputation across the network and enables "viral marketing" which allures health practitioners towards particular web applications. They show active engagement of teenagers with the social network, which provides the complete personalized experience. Absolute control over a personal account to modify, edit and share information attracts many web users. The study demonstrates the analogy between Facebook and a term coined by its authors as "Healthbook". Similarly, participation is also one of the core components of Medicine 2.0, which affects both healthcare professionals and patients. The integration of PHRs with the social networking concept leads to a unique innovation in personal web for healthcare. Patients actively participate by connecting formally or informally with caregivers, healthcare professionals or researchers [33].

User Centric Approach

The ideal personal web tool uses Web 2.0 technologies created for a user. The healthcare industry is comprised of technical and non-technical users among patients, healthcare professionals, insurance companies, and research groups. The Personal

Web system, which considers the user to be the integral part of its model and provides dynamic applications with rich consumer experience, illustrates the user-centric model.

While designing a user interface for end users, one has to know the target audience, its size and level of technical know-how with modern tools already on the market. Joseph Kramer et al. highlight the fact that while designing user systems one has to understand the linguistics, mental perspective, and beliefs of the users [34]. The paper "User-managed access to web resources" by Machulak at al. demonstrates the flexibility for the user to manage and control the information accessible to various third party hosts. It also indentifies the user interactions and abilities to share and access information across the web [35]. Finally, a notably conspicuous aspect of user centeredness is privacy, allowing for absolute control over who has access to every individual element of the profile of the end user.

After exploring Google Health as an example of a product on the market, it was clear that personalization for patients efficiently conforms to patient's needs. Similarly, a web technology which can be designed to cohesively include all consumers in healthcare (including, but not limited to the patients) is essential. User-centered design must guarantee that the transfer of information between patients and their caretakers is well coordinated and efficient while being managed by the user, as well as streamlined and accessible to both parties. The user should have all the rights to modify his or her information and change privacy settings for the medical records that they choose to share with a given institution.

Use Case: PatientsLikeMe

Another example of personal web within the medical community is PatientsLikeMe (PLM). It provides a complete social experience to the patients who connect to other users with similar medical problems, in order to share ideas and treatment options with each other and other members of the health community. The system uses secure forums and private messages to facilitate contact between users. Sharing specific information with other members provides a personalized experience to users with similar goals over the web. The integrated system makes use of the location of the user and allows them to search patients with similar conditions based on treatment, symptoms, age and profile characteristics. The website also provides suggestions about local clinicians, services, fundraising and support groups. The website offers a personal experience and relevant information based on user inquiry. It also provides the flexibility to share, track and comment on the health profiles of other patients with whom users have become connected. The autonomous nature and total control of one's profile to edit, delete, and update diseases, symptoms and treatment are features of the personal web well exhibited by PLM. The patients can subscribe to updates from other members in the form of incoming feeds and track others' progress as compared to their own. PLM demonstrates the potential for self-health management by allowing members to input information about prescriptions, dosage, drug efficacy and side effects as they experience them. Additionally, PLM encourages patients to participate in treatment and drug surveys monitored by the US Food and drug Administration to aid in the improvement of drug research and safety. Currently, doctors and physicians cannot access the profile of patients directly, but are granted access to profiles as authorized by patients after joining PLM in order to assist with diagnosis and treatment planning. PLM has utilized most of the conceptual elements of social networking, the user centric web model, participation and personal web in its design. This marks strong progress in the direction of improved personalization within the medical industry [36].

Barriers for Personal Web in Health Care

Security Concerns

Ting mentions the issue of confidentiality and privacy concerns as inhibiting people from sharing sensitive information such as healthcare records over the internet [37]. The general sentiment of the public is that personal information related to health, finances, or personal identity should be kept exclusively private, and individuals are rarely encouraged to seek contact with strangers. In spite of the existence of published privacy policies, laws and data security protection steps, the true nature of protection on the internet is often confusing and misunderstood by consumers [37]. The personal web interface should be an example of the utmost care in the security of information, with clear guidelines and protection against malicious activity on the web. The system would need to be in complete compliance with the Health Insurance Portability and Accountability Act (HIPAA) as well. According to the Department of Health and Human Services HIPAA helps to safeguard the rights of an individual and to protect health records that are transmitted electronically. The act clearly explains privacy, confidentiality and security rules and regulations. Every health organization must abide HIPAA policy while handling patient health records over the web, and this interface would be no exception to these regulations [38]. Proper legal and ethical standards must be followed to safeguard classified health information in a Personal web environment.

The Disorganization of Health Information Management and Characteristics of Internet

Shortliffe identifies numerous pitfalls in the new technology. It will be difficult for any health organization to keep pace with the rapid growth of the web including improved quality control, new software or high end computing tools, social and ethical concerns [39]. The information would be intrinsically dynamic, as would the platform with which that data is shared. According to Mittman and Cane, databases scattered across institutions and in heterogeneous formats could also limit usage of web technologies in healthcare [40]. In order to work successfully, there is a need for the combination of the personal web system with the heterogeneous medical data already in existence. The proprietary information systems that handle electronic medical records for various insurers, hospitals and physicians prevent users from integrating as well as trusting any new technology that enters the market. The above concerns suggest that substantial restructuring is needed before such systems can be integrated into the lives of the consumers. We can conclude that even though web and its many useful characteristics can provide momentum in healthcare, problems such as security concerns, inappropriate policies and ethical issues will potentially hinder its growth. In the future, these hurdles might be better accounted for as systems move toward a more standardized model [40].

The Mixed Quality of Information on the Internet

The study "Review of Internet Health Information Quality Initiatives" by Risk and Dzenowagis illustrates that poor quality of health information can misguide or harm the readers. Misinterpretation of medical information on the web can be due to disparities in language and culture between individuals, as well as a lack of medical education for the patients. The information might be directed toward a particular audience and therefore be misinterpreted by an unintentional consumer of the information. This becomes exceptionally relevant in the medical field as the medical literature is written with the assumption that the readers are educated medical professionals. Additionally, services and products may not be available in all the parts of world that have access to the information, creating unnecessary concern and misdirection. The credibility and accuracy of the medical information can also be questionable, as the information that is readily available may be biased or directed to a particular community with particular beliefs. The incorrect information not only potentially impairs the emotional, mental and physical health of a patient, but also affects the health care providers that are treating them by undermining their credibility and expertise [41]. The personal web should aim to provide the maximum amount of control over the source of information received by users. A well-designed architecture can help overcome some of the aforementioned hurdles in information quality.

Conclusions

The aspects of the personal web as applied in the healthcare industry have been discussed, along with the benefits that might be acquired after its implementation. Characteristics of personal web that should be considered when designing an interface for the healthcare industry have been identified and analyzed. Personalization of web elements will affect various aspects of the medical industry and the end users, as previously articulated. A variety of factors can help the personal web to prosper or decline, as evidenced by presented examples such as ‘Google Health’ and ‘Patients-LikeMe’. These examples illustrate various important factors that may contribute to the successful personalization of the web in healthcare. The issues and concerns regarding such technological advancement in healthcare have been duly noted and explored while providing feedback on the current personal web market and how it can be improved. By embracing this innovative technology, drastic and powerful improvements can be made in today’s world of healthcare.

References

1. Core Characteristics of Personal Web, http://www.techpluto.com/web-20-services/
2. Tim O’Reilly. “Web 2.0 Compact Definition: Trying Again” (2006).
3. Joanna W. Ng, Mark Chignell, and James R. Cordy. 2009. The smart internet: transforming the web for the user. In Proceedings of the 2009 Conference of the Center for Advanced Studies on Collaborative Research (CASCON ’09), Patrick Martin, Anatol W. Kark, and Darlene Stewart (Eds.). ACM, New York, NY, USA, 285–296. doi:10.1145/1723028.1723062http://doi.acm.org/10.1145/1723028.1723062
4. Joanna Ng. 2010. The Personal Web: smart internet for me. In Proceedings of the 2010 Conference of the Center for Advanced Studies on Collaborative Research (CASCON ’10). ACM, New York, NY, USA, 330–344. DOI=10.1145/1923947.1923981 http://doi.acm.org/10.1145/1923947.1923981
5. Khamsum Kinley and Dian Tjondronegoro. 2010. User-web interactions: How wholistic/analytic web users search the web? In Proceedings of the 22nd Conference of the Computer-Human Interaction Special Interest Group of Australia on Computer-Human Interaction (OZCHI ’10). ACM, New York, NY, USA, 344–347. DOI=10.1145/1952222.1952297 http://doi.acm.org/10.1145/1952222.1952297
6. President’s Council of Advisors on Science and Technology (PCAST). Realizing the Full Potential of Health Information Technology to Improve Healthcare for Americans: The Path Forward. Executive Office of the President. 2010.
7. Idoia Berges, Jesus Bermudez, Alfredo Go, and Arantza Illarramendi. 2010. Semantic interoperability of clinical data. In Proceedings of the First International Workshop on Model-Driven Interoperability (MDI ’10), Jean Bzivin, Richard Mark Soley, and Antonio Vallecillo (Eds.). ACM, New York, NY, USA, 10–14. DOI=10.1145/1866272.1866275 http://doi.acm.org/10.1145/1866272.1866275
8. Wiljer D, Urowitz S, Apatu E, DeLenardo C, Eysenbach G, Harth T, Pai H, Leonard KJ, Canadian Committee for Patient Accessible Health Records (CCPAEHR) Patient Accessible Electronic Health Records: Exploring Recommendations for Successful Implementation Strategies J Med Internet Res 2008; 10(4):e34 URL: http://www.jmir.org/2008/4/e34/ doi: 10.2196/jmir.1061
9. Deloitte Center for Health Solutions - “The Mobile Personal Health Record: Technology-enabled self-care” (2010).
10. Wu RC, Delgado D, Costigan J, MacIver J, Ross H Pilot Study of an Internet Patient-Physician Communication Tool for Heart Failure Disease Management. J Med Internet Res 2005;7(1):e8 URL: http://www.jmir.org/2005/1/e8/ doi: 10.2196/jmir.7.1.e8 PMID: 15829480
11. Google Health Privacy- http://www.google.com/intl/en_us/health/privacy.html
12. An update on Google Health and Google PowerMeter http://googleblog.blogspot.com/2011/06/update-on-google-health-and-google.html

13. Google Health has been discontinued http://www.google.com/intl/en_us/health/about/
14. Aetna's Personal Health Record* makes it easy to organize and store your health information online (share online) - http://www.aetna.com/showcase/phr/
15. Alex Jadad -"The Internet and evidence-based decision-making: a needed synergy for efficient knowledge management in health care" (J Med Internet Res 2000; 2(suppl2):e2) doi:10.2196/jmir.2.suppl2.e2.
16. Nick Anderson and Kelly Edwards. 2010. Building a chain of trust: using policy and practice to enhance trustworthy clinical data discovery and sharing. In Proceedings of the 2010 Workshop on Governance of Technology, Information and Policies (GTIP '10). ACM, New York, NY, USA, 15–20. DOI=10.1145/1920320.1920323 http://doi.acm.org/10.1145/1920320.1920323
17. United States General Accounting Office - "Medical Records Privacy, Access Needed for Health Research But Oversight Of Privacy protection Is Limited" (Feb 1999).
18. Hian Chye Koh and Gerald Tan - "Data Mining Applications in Healthcare", Journal of Healthcare Information Vol. 19 No 2.
19. Margaret A. Winker, Annette Flanagin, Bonnie Chi-Lum, John White, Karen Andrews, Robert L. Kennett, Catherine D. DeAngelis, Robert A. Musacchio, Special Communication Guidelines for Medical and Health Information Sites on the Internet: Principles Governing AMA Web Sites, JAMA. 2000;283(12):1600–1606.
20. Houston TK, Allison JJ,"Users of Internet Health Information: Differences by Health Status" J Med Internet Res 2002;4(2):e7 URL: http://www.jmir.org/2002/2/e7/ doi: 10.2196/jmir.4.2.e7 PMID: 12554554
21. Gunther Eysenbach and Alejandro R Jadad, Evidence-based Patient Choice and Consumer health informatics in the Internet age. J Med Internet Res 2001;3(2):e19 URL: http://www.jmir.org/2001/2/e19/ doi: 10.2196/jmir.3.2.e19 PMID: 11720961
22. WebMD: Better Information, Better Health http://www.webmd.com/
23. WebMD for Android, iPhone and iPad http://www.webmd.com/mobile
24. Tang Paul C, Ash Joan S, Bates David W, Overhage J Marc, Sands Daniel Z. Personal health records: definitions, benefits, and strategies for overcoming barriers to adoption. J Am Med Inform Assoc. 2006, 13(2), pp. 121–6. doi: 10.1197/jamia.M2025. http://www.pubmedcentral.nih.gov/articlerender.fcgi?tool=pubmed&pubmedid=16357345
25. Google Health - http://www.google.com/intl/en-US/health/about/
26. Microsoft Health Vault - http://www.microsoft.com/en-us/healthvault/
27. A statement by honorable Mr. Michael Leavitt, secretary of Health and Human Services. http://atavas.com/personalized-medicine-myth-pipe-dream-or-realizable-promise/
28. 23andMe - Genetics just got personal URL - https://www.23andme.com/you/faqwin/whatis23andmeresearch/
29. Duke Medicine's five principles denoted by 5Ps. http://www.dukepersonalizedmedicine.org/what_is_personalized_medicine
30. Facebook https://www.facebook.com/
31. Pew Internet: Pew Internet and American Life Project, 65% of online adults use social Networking sites. http://pewinternet.org/~/media/Files/Reports/2011/PIP-SNS-Update-2011.pdf
32. Gunther Eysenbach, Medicine 2.0: Social Networking, Collaboration, Participation, Apomediation, and Openness J Med Internet Res 2008;10(3):e22 URL: http://www.jmir.org/2008/3/e22/ doi: 10.2196/jmir.1030
33. Joseph Kramer, Sunil Noronha, and John Vergo. 2000. A user-centered design approach to personalization. Commun. ACM 43(8), August 2000, pp. 44–48. DOI=10.1145/345124.345139 http://doi.acm.org/10.1145/345124.345139
34. Maciej P. Machulak, Eve L. Maler, Domenico Catalano, and Aad van Moorsel. 2010. User-managed access to web resources. In Proceedings of the 6th ACM workshop on Digital identity management (DIM '10). ACM, New York, NY, USA, 35–44. DOI=10.1145/1866855.1866865 http://doi.acm.org/10.1145/1866855.1866865
35. T.C. Ting, "Privacy and Confidentiality in Healthcare Delivery Information System," Computer-Based Medical Systems, IEEE Symposium on, p. 2, 12th IEEE Symposium on Computer-Based Medical Systems (CBMS'99), 1999.

36. Health Insurance portability and Accountability Act of 1996 (HIPAA) Privacy and Security Rules - http://www.hhs.gov/ocr/privacy/
37. Shortliffe EH. The Next Generation Internet and health care: a civics lesson for the informatics community. Proc AMIA Fall, Symposium 1998: 8–14.
38. Robert Mittman and Mary Cain "The Future of Healthcare, Five Year Forecast, California Healthcare Foundation", Jan 1999.
39. Ahmad Risk, Joan Dzenowagis J. "Review of Internet Health Information Quality Initiatives" Med Internet Res. 2001 Oct-Dec; 3(4): e28. Published online 2001 December 26. doi: 10.2196/jmir.3.4.e28 PMCID: PMC1761913.
40. PatientsLikeMe - http://www.patientslikeme.com/
41. Usama Fayyad, Gregory Piatetsky - Shapiro, and Padhraic Smyth, The KDD Process for Extracting Useful Knowledge from Volumes of Data, Communications of the ACM, November 1996/Vol. 39, No. 11, pages 27–34.

Chapter 16
Secure Mobile Framework for Monitoring Medical Sensor Data

Ankur Agarwal, Borko Furht, Mark Conatser and Chris Baechle

Abstract Increasing elderly populations, medical facility under-staffing, and increased governmental spending on healthcare have created a shaky climate which could ultimately lead to bankrupting government healthcare programs and generally lower qualities of healthcare for all individuals. This chapter proposes a secure and reliable web-based architecture for a mobile platform based system for monitoring a wireless sensor network of medical devices which could effectively be used as a solution in mitigating costs on individual patient care while maintaining a high quality level of care. First we discuss related work in the area of wireless medical sensor networks. Then we describe our proposed solution and detail our experimental implementation and results.

Introduction

The healthcare domain is currently reaching unprecedented levels of duress and concerns are growing over the quality of patient care and government expenditures on healthcare. As technology and medical science proficiencies have grown elderly populations and individuals that need extensive assistance with one or more activities of daily living have increased. Another factor in this notable rise is that the "Baby Boomers" of post-World War II are entering their senior years generating an influx in elderly populations in the United States. In 2007 approximately 16 % of the gross domestic product of the U.S. was spent on medical related expenses with a large majority of this being apportioned to Medicare benefits for those aged 65 and

A. Agarwal (✉) · B. Furht · M. Conatser · C. Baechle
Department of Computer and Electrical Engineering and Computer Science, Florida Atlantic University, 777 Glades Rd, Boca Raton, FL 33431, USA
e-mail: agarwa2@fau.edu

Furht
e-mail: bfurht@fau.edu

B. Furht and A. Agarwal (eds.), *Handbook of Medical and Healthcare Technologies*, DOI: 10.1007/978-1-4614-8495-0_16, older [1, 2]. These figures are predicted to increase over the next several decades. Another issue facing the medical field is the gross under-staffing of medical facilities. Studies have shown that high patient to doctor or nurse ratios result in lower quality of health for the patient with some studies showing an increase in potential mortality rates in direct correlation to increase in nursing patient workloads [3, 4]. Although some states such as California have mandated minimum nurse to patient ratios there is no official federal legislation regarding this issue.

Another trend in today's society is the growing reliance upon smart devices as a gateway for communication and information. These smart-phones and personal digital assistant (PDA) devices have become ubiquitous in our world and as high speed data connections availability is on the rise it seems this technology will only further change the ways in which we interact with our environment. In consideration and recognition of this we believe that the problems mentioned formerly can be alleviated through the use of medical informatics systems based around these smart devices for monitoring and treating patients in a remote setting. These systems can allow a doctor or caregiver to maintain an acceptable quality level of patient care while at the same time maximizing the number of patients he or she can reliably attend to. These systems can also provide patients who would otherwise be forced to relocate to assisted living or nursing home facilities with the opportunity to remain at home as long as possible by utilizing medical sensors in place in their local environment which can monitor and report the patient's vital statistics and provide assistance with simple activities of daily living (such as activity reminders or item locating) which would otherwise force them to move. This extension of time, even if for only a month, can significantly reduce both individual and government spending on quality nursing home and assisted living care. This represents only one possible implementation of this technology however as the possibilities are really limitless. Figure 16.1 illustrates potential areas where this technology can be effectively utilized in the medical domain.

In an effort to provide a viable solution to these escalating problems we have developed an architecture for the monitoring of patient vital statistics in a local environment using wireless medical sensor devices and a smart-phone as a local hub. The goal of our design is to provide an architecture that is available, reliable, secure, and dependable. In the remainder of this chapter we will first briefly discuss related research in this area and then we will describe our proposed architecture as well as our experimental implementation results.

Background

As the needs for a solution to these ever growing healthcare problems increase much research has been invested in the area of remote medical healthcare informatics and tele-presence based systems. This section first discusses the unique requirements that a medical informatics system such as this should meet and then briefly discusses

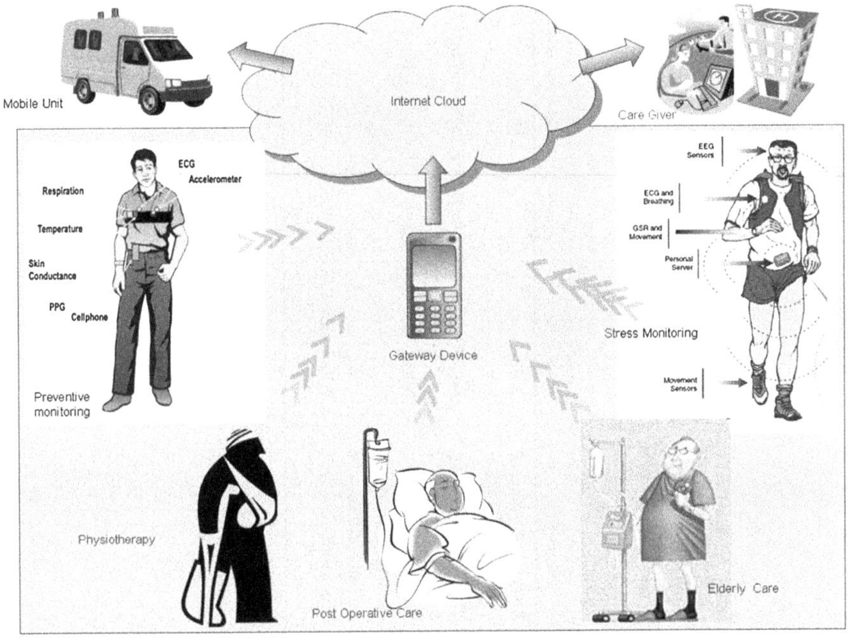

Fig. 16.1 Potential applications of sensor based medical monitoring system

several related research projects and concludes with a table which provides a general overview of the salient points relative to our research.

A. Medical Informatics System Requirements

With medical informatics systems there are certain requirements and standards that must be upheld for it to meet the strict demands necessary in dealing with a patient's vital statistics. First of all it is critical that a patient's safety is ensured. The system must never place the patient in a situation of danger. Secondly the system must be accurate in its data and provide a strict level of availability and accessibility to authorized users. Lastly the system must comply with both government standards as well as existing integrations. The most well-known standard for systems interchanging patient information electronically is the Health Insurance Portability and Accountability Act (HIPAA) regulations are designed to protect health information integrity and security by essentially ensuring that a security management process is in place in the health informatics system.

B. Research Related Projects

In this section we will discuss various implementations of homehealthcare systems. Table 16.1 summarizes these research projects focusing on points of interest in relationship to our efforts.

B1. Personal Assistant System: At the University of Illinois at Urbana-Champaign researchers have developed a system to provide an in-home alternative to assisted-

Table 16.1 Overview of wireless sensor network medical projects

	PAS	ITALH	Carenet	Mobihealth	MiLAN	Alarmnet
Video-monitoring	None	Only through user-granted access	Used in conjunction with fall detection algorithm	Attached to patient through BAN	None	None
Hub device	Standalone PC	Standalone PC + Mobile	Standalone PC	Mobile	Geared towards standalone but nonspecific	Standalone PC
Web services	RESTful + SOAP	Unspecified	XML based	Jini + Remote method invocation	XML + DAML based	Unspecified
Wireless protocols	Bluetooth + 802.11	Bluetooth + 802.15.4	802.11 + 802.15.4	Bluetooth + 802.15.4	Bluetooth + 802.11	802.15.4

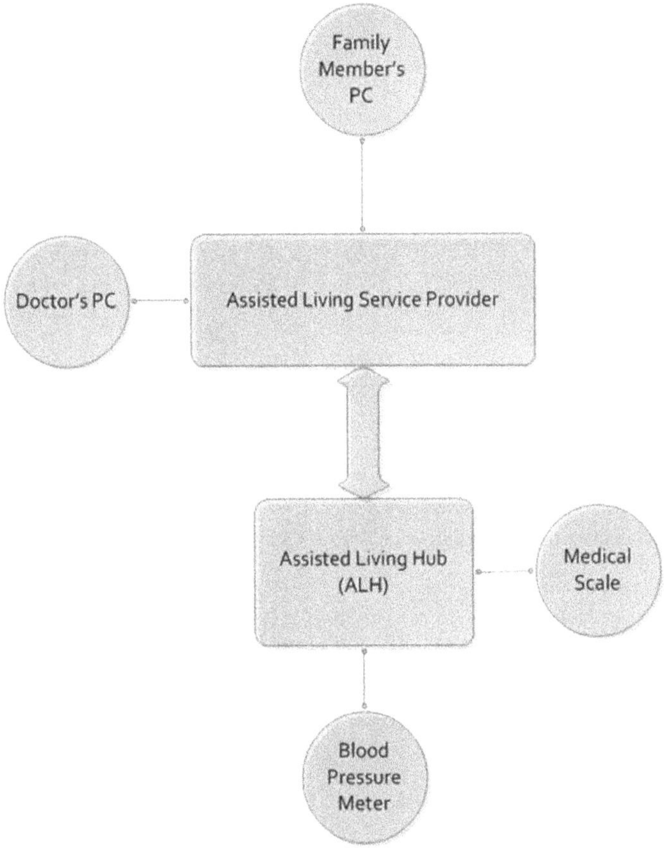

Fig. 16.2 Architecture of personal assistant system

living care using wireless sensor motes based primarily on RFID and Bluetooth technology.

This system, known as the Personal Assistant System (PAS), is designed with the goal in mind of providing an open environment that preserves patient privacy while maintaining security and dependability [5, 6]. The main services of their system are activity reminders, personal belonging localization, medical data monitoring, and emergency notification. Their design uses a drop-box style server in-home as the main hub for communications in their system.

B2. Information Technology for Assisted Living at Home: (ITALH) is a research project conducted at the University of California Berkeley aimed at providing a healthcare service for the elderly [7].

ITALH is a sensor based monitoring system that is designed to be an emergency intervention system. A large part of the focus of their efforts was in the engineering of a fall-detection sensor developed using several three-axis accelerometers

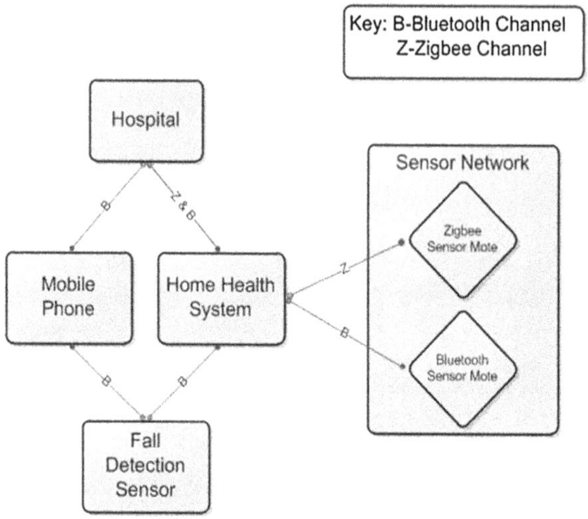

Fig. 16.3 Architecture of information technology for assisted living system

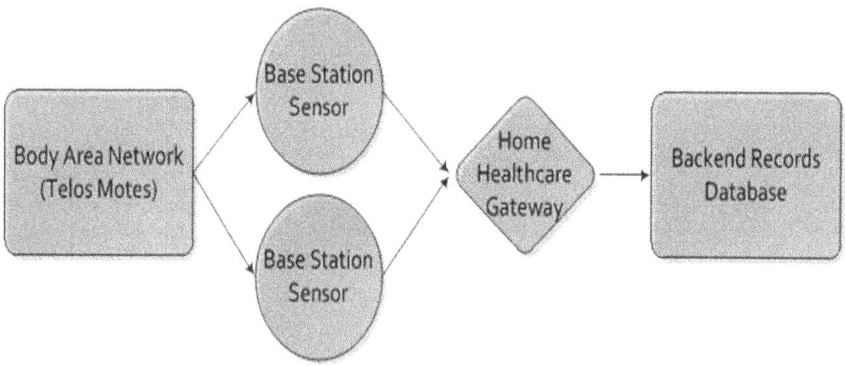

Fig. 16.4 Architecture of carenet system

in conjunction with heuristic fall-detection and analysis algorithms to determine and quantify fall characteristics and upon identification alert appropriate emergency response channels.

B3. CareNet: is a collaborative effort of several notable universities including Vanderbilt University with an emphasis on providing a scalable and reliable networking infrastructure for wireless medical sensor networks [8, 9].

Their system uses a multi-hop wireless sensor network design based around the ZigBee wireless standard as a middle-ware layer between monitoring sensors and a local desktop server. This design improves both availability and system robustness by taking away a possible single point of failure at this layer.

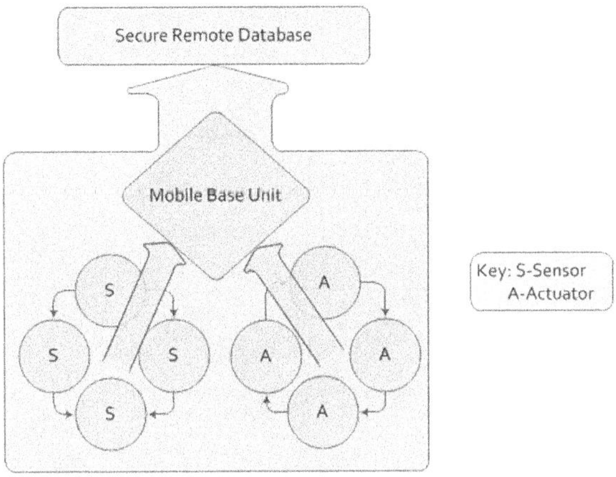

Fig. 16.5 Overview of mobihealth system

B4. MobiHealth: is a research project conceived at the University of Twente in Netherlands with large backing from the European Commission [10, 11].

Their research is focused upon the design of a body area network (BAN) of sensor and actuator nodes which monitor and interact with a patient through the use of an iPAQ H3870 PDA acting as a base unit hub. The primary goal of this project is aimed at providing a system that can monitor an individual anywhere and at any time without the limitations of the patient being constrained in a confined environment.

B5. Middleware Linking Applications and Networks: (MiLAN) is a research effort from a team at the University of Rochester with a goal of designing a system which can support a network of energy constrained resources with management and QoS parameters defined by the application using graphs of requirements [12, 13]. Their efforts allow an application to proactively interact with a network as opposed to traditionally reacting to constraints inherently imposed by the network itself.

B6. AlarmNet: is a development from the University of Virginia designed for continuous remote monitoring of assisted living patients at home [14, 15]. Their research is unique in that it allows for interconnection of heterogeneous devices in an ad-hoc style of wireless networking. They have developed services to monitor and be more responsive to a patient in a heuristic fashion by analyzing circadian activity rhythms. They have also provided applications to manage wireless sensor power requirements and configure security policies at the user level.

Proposed System Architecture

Figure 16.6 shows the architecture we have proposed for monitoring patient medical data in a mobile remote setting. This architecture is primarily composed of six different layers: the Medical Sensor Device Layer, the Mobile Device Application

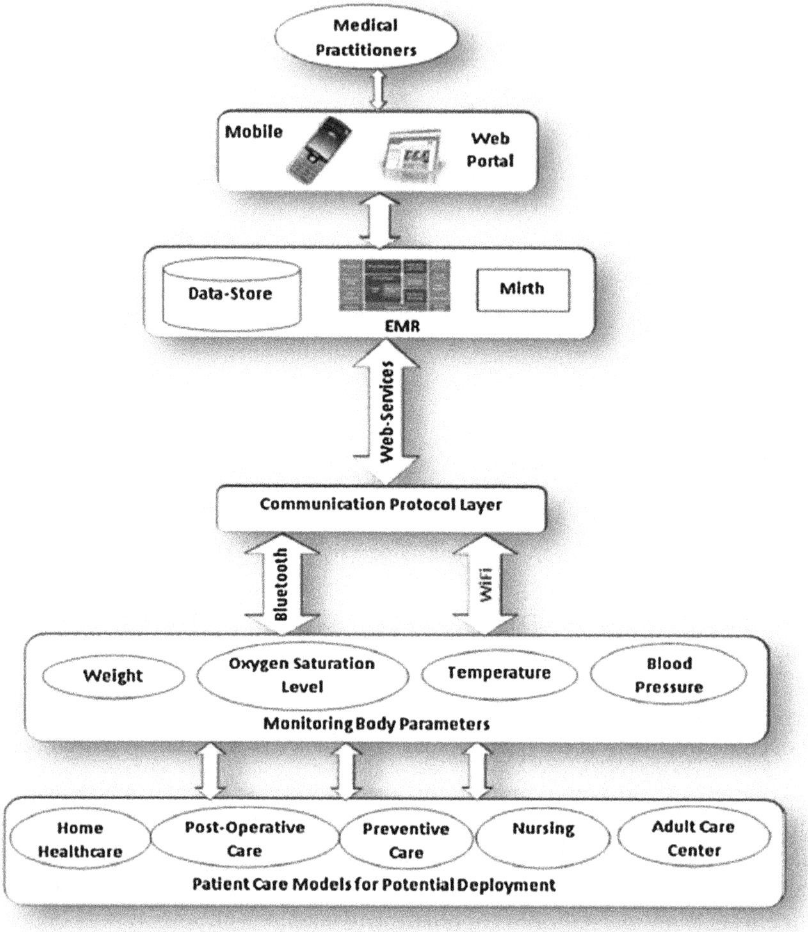

Fig. 16.6 System architecture of monitoring physiological data from mobile device for remote patients

Layer, the Web Services Cloud Middleware Layer, the Database Layer, the Web Server Layer, and the Electronic Medical Record (EMR) Layer. The remainder of this section discusses these layers in detail.

A. Medical Sensor Device Layer

This layer consists of the physical sensor devices and wireless motes we have created to provide these sensors with the capability to talk with the upper layers of our architecture. The most important facet of this layer is our wireless platform agnostic protocol which applies at the Application Layer of the well-known Open Systems Interconnection (OSI) networking model. The reasoning for the development of our own protocol is that there are no firm existing standards which meet our needs independent of any specific wireless interface. Our protocol consists of six command

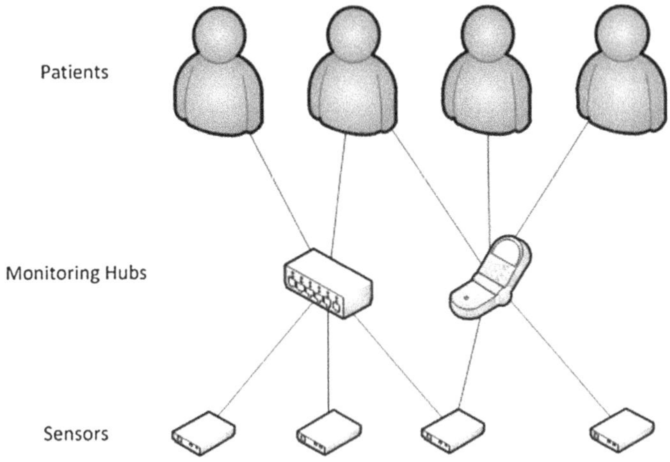

Fig. 16.7 Patient monitoring environment relationship

sets: Get Device Information, Get Device String Name, Get Reading Precision, Set Reading Precision, Get Reading, and Get Stream Readings. This protocol allows any valid hub device to communicate with any medical sensor device irrespective of the specific nature of the sensor device and the underlying technology it uses. It is important to notice in the command set that there are actually two commands to get a reading (Get Reading and Get Stream Readings). By having two commands such as this we allow for the introduction of both devices which only produce a single reading at a time (such as a thermometer or medical scale) and those which produce a constant stream of data over a certain period of time (such as an EKG or heart rate monitor). Figure 16.7 shows the patient monitoring environment relationship and Fig. 16.8 shows medical device communication protocol layer.

B. Mobile Device Application Layer

The Mobile Device Application Layer represents the monitoring hub with which all communications of data between the medical devices and the remote server are processed and transmitted. This layer is designed around the Android Mobile Operating System Platform which provides suitable Application Programming Interfaces (APIs) for performing wireless data communications using Bluetooth and 802.11 wireless communications standards as well as for networking, security, and web service communications parsing. Specifically we communicate with the server through messages passed using JavaScript Object Notation (JSON) which is a lightweight and human readable standard for data exchange between platforms. This layer also provides the Graphical User Interface (GUI) with which the patient or caregiver interacts with the system, registering devices and obtaining readings. Security is introduced into this layer through the use of Secure Sockets Layer (SSL) encryption of the JSON messages interchanged between the hub and the remote server and user authentication requirements at the User Interface component.

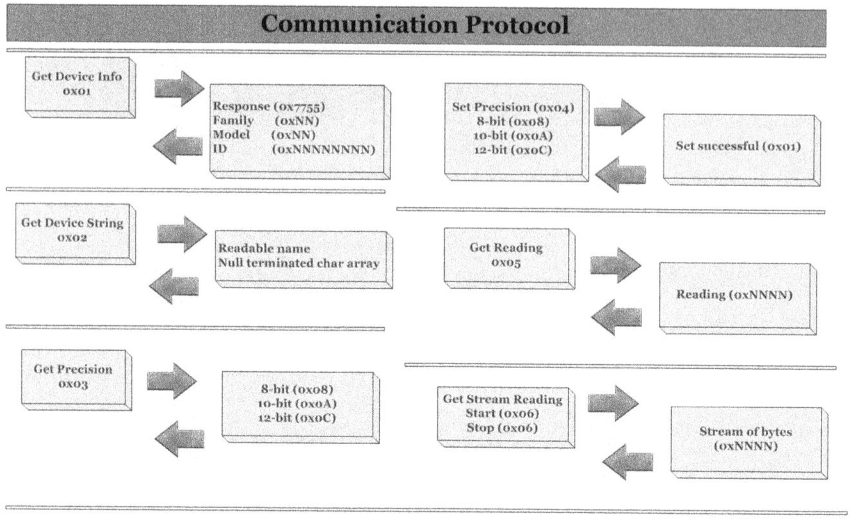

Fig. 16.8 Medical device communication protocol layer

C. Web Service Cloud Middleware Layer

Our desires for a server side component which could communicate easily with disparate hub devices and platforms to support an indeterminable number of separate patient monitoring systems necessitated an open standards server component which could provide services independent of the actual technologies in place. These requirements influenced our decision to design our middle-ware in the pattern of a service oriented architecture. We have developed our architecture to support Representational State Transfer (REST) based web services which are styled in such a way to treat data as a resource defined by a unique Uniform Resource Locator (URL). RESTful web services are lightweight and fast and have a large support base in the mobile development field making them most suitable for our architectural goals. These services are developed in Java EE using the Java API for RESTful Web Services (JAXRS) standards and deployed to a Tomcat Servlet Container.

D. Database Layer

The Database Layer manages patient/doctor/caregiver accounting and relationship information, device registration information, and keeps a log of all recorded device readings. This layer is used internally however should not be relied on for complete knowledge because the majority of patient information is to be maintained in an external EMR system which linked to at the EMR Layer. We use the MySQL RDBMS to persist all relevant medical data.

E. Web Server Layer

At the Web Server Layer we have designed a user portal which allows for doctors and patients to view medical devices and readings. Another feature at this layer allows a doctor to institute an alert level for a device. If the alert level is exceeded in

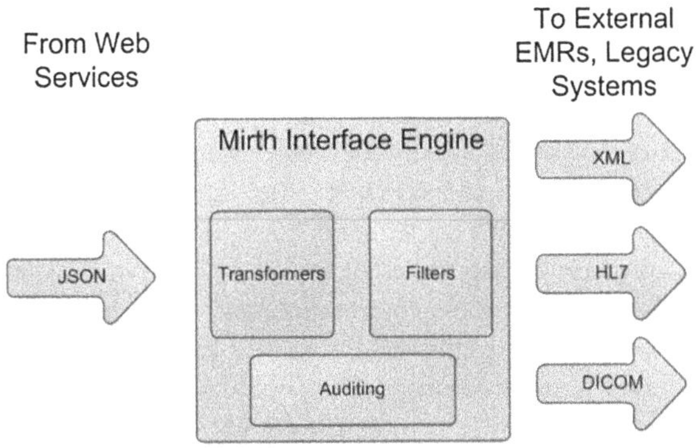

Fig. 16.9 EMR integration layer

any reading from that individual device the doctor is notified through e-mail. These pages are designed using HyperText Markup Language (HTML), Cascading Style Sheets (CSS), and the Yahoo User Interface (YUI) JavaScript libraries which provide progressive enhancement features for cross browser compatibility and custom components for rapid user interface development and web service communications.

F. Electronic Medical Records Integration Layer
To allow the integration with existing and future medical infrastructures we have used a Health Level Seven (HL7) interface engine to provide an interconnection point between our system and these external entities. HL7 represents a language of standards for the interchange of electronic health information between disparate new and legacy systems. For this integration we have implemented the Mirth Connect Interface Engine which is an open source platform that provides brokering channels between endpoints. Through this powerful engine we can interconnect with any number of external entities using several supported data interchange messaging formats including Extensible Markup Language (XML), HL7, Digital Imaging and Communications in Medicine (DICOM), and JSON. For our design we have developed a channel to request new readings from our service architecture and transform these into valid HL7 messages to be inserted into an EMR system. Figure 16.9 shows the EMR integration with our solution architecture.

Experimental Work

For the implementation of our proposed architecture we have developed an end-to-end deployment using two individual medical sensor devices for testing and evaluation. The following section discusses the details of this implementation.

A. Sensor Devices
For our sensor devices we are using a TMP102 Digital Temperature Sensor and a Polar T31 Coded Transmitter for Heart Rate Monitoring. The temperature sen-

sor allows for high accuracy measurements to within 0.5 °C. To utilize the coded heart rate monitoring transmitter we have deployed it in conjunction with a Polar Heart Rate Monitoring Interface. The need for this is predicated upon the proprietary communications protocol used by the transmitter. This interface converts these 5KHz frequency transmissions into a usable serial interface. To provide an wireless communications interface which implements our open protocol we have developed two motes one to provide an experimental test of 802.11 wireless communications and the other for Bluetooth wireless communications. These motes connect directly to the serial interfaces of our medical sensors and have at their core Atmel AVR ATmega8 RISC based microprocessors. The Bluetooth mote uses a RN-41 Class 1 Bluetooth Module while the 802.11 mote uses a WiFly GSX module that communicates specifically using both 802.11b and 802.11g. These chips have low power states and can easily be run for a long period (depending on usage an average of two years) on a set of AAA batteries.

B. Android Monitoring Application and Hub Device

To test our architecture we have developed a simple application for the Android platform that allows us to register both 802.11 and Bluetooth based medical devices and take readings from these registered devices. We are using a Motorola Droid X smart-phone running the Android operating system version 2.2. This device has a 1.0 GHz processor, 512 MB RAM, and 8 GB internal Flash ROM. It provides remote networking capabilities through a 3G cellular network.

Figure 16.10 shows the flow of the Android device monitoring application which begins with a user authentication step.

C. Server Side Platform

To provide a redundant and cloud-based server-side implementation we are using a solution provided by the hosting company Rackspace. This allows us to minimize our efforts in server administration by utilizing a virtual solution on their servers. On

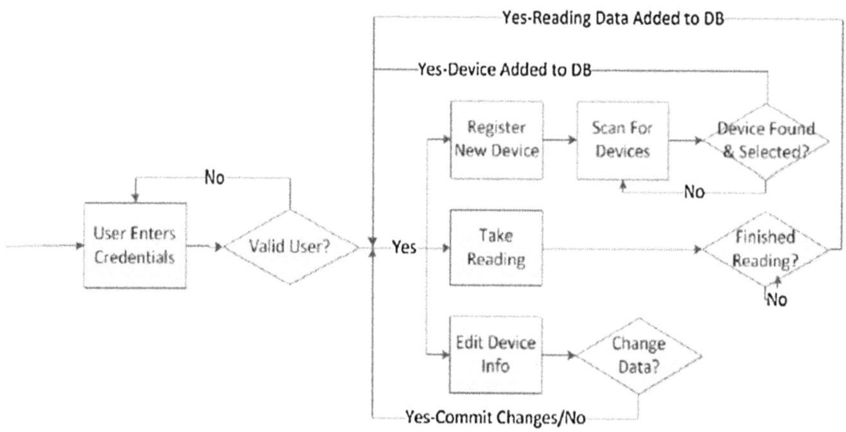

Fig. 16.10 Android application flow diagram

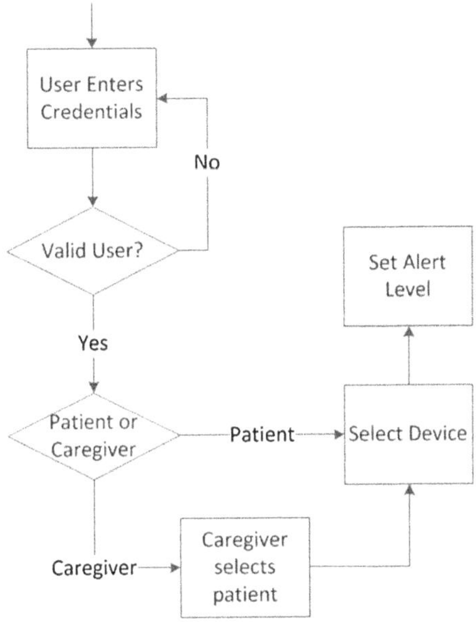

Fig. 16.11 Single sign-on behavior and flow of Android application

this server we have deployed a Tomcat instance for exposing our RESTful services, a MySQL instance for managing our persistent data, and an Apache HTTP server to host our web portal pages. The cloud server instance has 256 MB RAM and a 10 GB hard disk space with CPU capabilities variable at run-time. To secure external communications we expose only web port 80 where our Apache server is running and forward web service requests to the Tomcat Container. This allows us to blanket our exposed pages and services with SSL encryption.

D. EMR Platform and Web Portal

To provide a test external EMR implementation for our Mirth Engine to communicate with we have used the open source EMR system FreeMED which is an HL7 compliant EMR system that runs on a Linux platform and provides a web interface for interaction.

To test our architectural proposals for a web portal we have implemented a basic flow of pages that allows a doctor to view a patient's devices and device data in a visual graph and tabular format. Our web application also provides the capabilities for a patient to view his/her own personal device readings data. We have also implemented the discussed alert based system at this level. Figure 16.11 shows the flow of the web portal application which uses the same single-sign-on behavior as the Android application.

Conclusions

With difficulties in the medical field arising from under-staffing as well as governmental overspending compounded with a burgeoning population in need of quality medical care the need for a technology assisted solution proves apparent. Using a network of medical sensor devices to monitor a patient in a relaxed environment proves to be a possible and feasible solution to alleviating these issues. In this article we have introduced our proposed vital statistic monitoring solutions architecture and provided details of our developed system implementation. Our solution contributes to the efforts of solving these problems by using an Android based mobile platform to monitor disparate wireless devices independent of device types and wireless protocols. In addition we have developed our server side system to collaborate with the Mirth Connect Integration Engine which allows us to hook into existing EMR and legacy healthcare backbones further enticing healthcare providers to implement our system without loss of their own identity and without worry of future healthcare storage requirements. Our implementation has also provided an example web portal allowing a doctor or patient to easily view device readings from any web browser.

As technology continues to rapidly evolve along with research advancements in the area of wireless sensor based networks there is much work that can be done in the future to enhance our architecture and implementation. Along with the obvious inclusions of a larger feature set at the application levels, work can be done to utilize the growing number of sensors included in the hardware designs of many smart-phones available today. Possible applications of this lead themselves naturally towards localization based applications. Another area for future work is in the design of more patient-friendly user interfaces, possibly configurable according to disease types.

References

1. OECD, "OECD Health Data 2008", *OECD Publishing*, 2008.
2. Laurence Kotlikoff, and Christian Hagist, "Who's Going Broke? Comparing Healthcare Costs in Ten OECD Countries," *NBER Working Paper* 11833, 2005.
3. Jack Needleman, Peter Buerhaus, Soeren Mattke, Maureen Stewart, and Katya Zelevinsky, "Nurse-Staffing Levels and the Quality of Care in Hospitals," *New England Journal of Medicine*, vol. 346, pp. 1715–1722, 2002
4. Linda Aiken, Sean Clarke, Douglas Sloane, Julie Sochalski, and Jeffrey Silber. "Hospital Nurse Staffing and Patient Mortality, Nurse Burnout, and Job Dissatisfaction," *JAMA*, vol. 288, pp. 1987–1993, 2002
5. Qixin Wang, Wook Shin, Xue Liu, "I-Living: An Open System Architecture for Assisted Living," *Proceedings of the IEEE International Conference on Systems, Man and Cybernetics*, pp. 4268–4275, 2006
6. Jennifer Hou, Qixin Wang, Bedoor AlShebli, "PAS: A Wireless-Enabled, Sensor-Integrated Personal Assistance System for Independent and Assisted Living," *Proc. of Joint Workshop on High Confidence Medical Devices, Software, and Systems (HCMDSS) and Medical Device Plug and Play (MD PnP) Interoperability (HCMDSS/MD PnP'07)*, 2007

7. J. Mikael Eklund, Thomas Riisgaard Hansen, Jonathan Sprinkle and Shankar Sastry, "Information Technology for Assisted Living at Home: Building a Wireless Infrastructure for Assisted Living", *EMBC*, 2005
8. Shanshan Jiang, Yuan Xue, Annarita Giani, and Ruzena Bajcsy, "Robust Medical Data Delivery for Wireless Pervasive Healthcare," *IEEE Transactions on Information Technology in Biomedicine*, 2008
9. Shanshan Jiang, Yanchuan Cao, Sameer Iyengar, "CareNet: An Integrated Wireless Sensor Networking Environment for Remote Healthcare," *Third International Conference on Body Area Networks*, 2008
10. Val Jones, Aart van Halteren, Ing Widya, "MobiHealth: Mobile Health Services Based on Body Area Networks," *M-Health Emerging Mobile Health Systems, Springer-Verlag, Berlin, pp. 219–236*, 2006
11. Dimitri Konstantas, Val Jones, and Rainer Herzog, "Mobihealth–Innovative 2.5/3G Mobile Services and Applications for Healthcare," *Proc. Eleventh IST Mobile and Wireless Telecommunications Summit, Thessaloniki, Greece*, 2002
12. Amy Murphy and Wendi Heinzelman, "MiLan: Middleware Linking Applications and Networks," *University of Rochester, Technical Report TR-795*, 2002.
13. Salem Hadim and Nader Mohamed, "Middleware: Middleware Challenges and Approaches for Wireless Sensor Networks," *IEEE Distributed Systems Online*, vol. 7, no. 3, 2006
14. A. Wood, G. Virone, T. Doan, "ALARM-NET: Wireless Sensor Networks for Assisted-Living and Residential Monitoring," *University of Virginia Technical Report CS-2006-11*, 2006
15. Anthony Wood, John Stankovic, Gilles Virone, "Context-Aware Wireless Sensor Networks for Assisted Living and Residential Monitoring," *IEEE Network*, 2008

Chapter 17
Virtual Doctor: A WBAN Based Architecture for Healthcare Service

Deena M. Barakah and Muhammad Ammad-uddin

According to the United States Census Bureau (USCB) [1] the world's population became more than doubled in 50 years; it was six billion in late 1999 and up to March 2012 it reached more than seven billion [2, 3]. According to An Aging World (commissioned by the U.S. National Institute on Aging) the number of people older than 65 will double (14 % from 7 % of the world population). In next 30 years, it will be 1.4 billion by 2040 [4].

Due to this rapid growth of world population especially increasing trend of elder people, the current healthcare systems are estimated probable to face new challenges like providing ample health care facilities, provision of quality health care, the escalating cost of healthcare, and the emerging technological innovations for patient care outside medical institutions. A future healthcare system is expected to help people maintain their health profile by examining a wide range of vital signals, providing early-warning systems for people with some medical problems. Early warnings prevent patients critical health conditions, which cost more to healthcare providers. It is envisaged that remote patient monitoring/testing may save many lives and millions of dollars every year.

Continual advances in sensing technology, systems-on-a-chip (SoCs), wireless communication, better battery life, reduced sensor weight, increased processing power, and higher communication bandwidth all these make it possible to design cost-effective, robust, and unobtrusive WBAN networks for personal health monitoring. Using WBANs patients can continue their daily life while their medical data is examined continuously at their hospital and/or doctor's clinic.

D. M. Barakah (✉)
Dental Clinic Department, King Saud Medical City, Ministry of Health, Riyadh, Kingdom of Saudi Arabia
e-mail: drdeena@gmail.com

M. Ammad-uddin
Research Center for Sensor Network and Cellular Systems, University of Tabuk, Tabuk, Kingdom of Saudi Arabia
e-mail: mohammad.ammad@gmail.com

B. Furht and A. Agarwal (eds.), *Handbook of Medical and Healthcare Technologies*,
DOI: 10.1007/978-1-4614-8495-0_17, © Springer Science+Business Media New York 2013

The main contribution of this chapter is to present the role of sensors-based Virtual Doctor for improving quality of health facilities. The contents of this chapter are organized as follow: First, an introduction of Wireless Body area Network (WBAN) is presented. Its daily life use at various sectors is discussed. A whole picture of WBAN follows: including how to develop WBAN, which components are required, what are the available standards. The detail study for the role of WBAN in detecting and curing different diseases is also reviewed. Finally, we cover the concept of sensors network-based virtual doctor.

Introduction To Wireless Body Area Network (WBAN)

WBAN is an abbreviation of Wireless Body Area Network, also called Wireless Personal Area Network (WPAN). It is a network of interconnected nodes that are installed on/in/around the human body to take direct measurements of body vital parameters. Normally 10–20 nodes are deployed to measure different vital signals of the person under treatment/test and transmitted this data to the gateway node. The gateway node sends the aggregated data to remote location by using any of available networks in the surroundings (GSM, WiFi, satellite etc.) [5].

The most important challenge for this emerging technology is to keep the power consumption and side effect radiation as low as possible to guarantee long time continuous operation of the network and to restrain the radiation to which the person is subjected. This is very critical as the use of WBAN is prolonged process and the individual under test is a hospital patient, where radiation over longer period of time could affect his/her health condition. In addition, many medical testing devices can be erroneous if exposed to strong radiation. By using WBAN state of art technology, people will be connected to the grid gathering information about their health conditions, their location and mood. The benefits are endless, and at present state of this technology it is extremely appealing for building many interesting applications such as:

Medical Usage

Hospitals/health care is the domain where WBAN is invented. It represents the launching ground for this technology and has a potential to grow rapidly in future. From the medical point of view, a WBAN is a special purpose sensor network designed to operate autonomously to connect medical application with various sensors and actuators, deployed in or around the human body. WBANs can add flexibility, facilitate patient monitoring/diagnostic/treatment/rehabilitation and save cost in the medical facilities. WBAN achieves all these benefits while maintaining patient mobility. Patients wearing portable devices (sensors, actuators and cellular device) can move anywhere and enjoy their routine life. In the same time physician can get

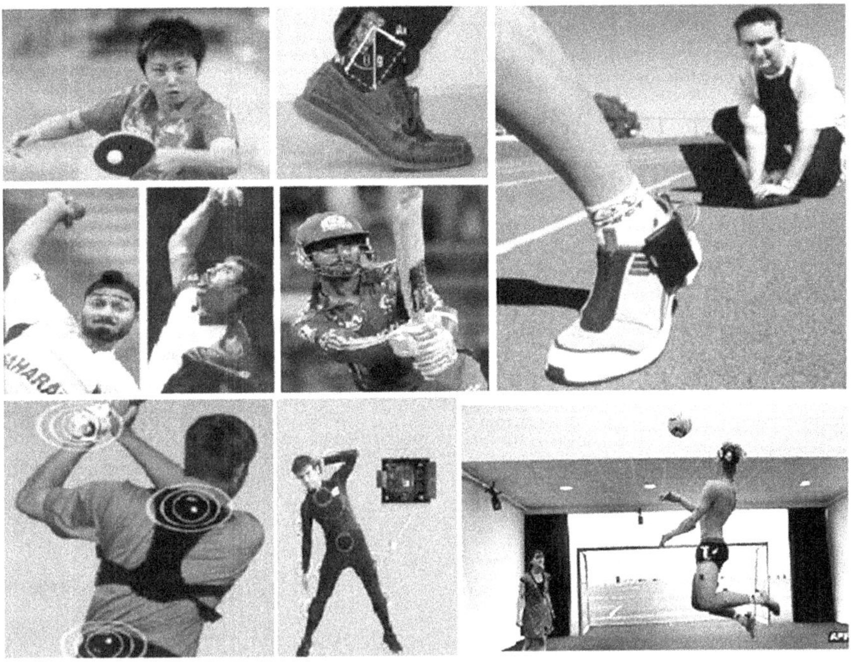

Fig. 17.1 Use of WBAN in sports activities

update information periodically, and it can help them in monitoring and diagnosing their patient without admitting them in hospital which will further reduce the cost of treatment. WBAN emerging technology can also help in monitoring elderly people at home, who are unable to fully manage their physical life. WBAN allows continuous monitoring of their needs and allows required assistance to be provided whenever it is critically needed.

Sport Applications

WBAN has wide range of utilities in this field of life (fitness and sport) [6–9]. Almost all sports like Bodybuilding, Weightlifting [10], Table tennis, Badminton, Cricket, and Football etc. can get benefit of this technology as shown in Fig. 17.1. Young players, who exercise a lot and want to keep track of their training progress, may use WBANtechnology to view their body conditions and to get future exercise plans.

Sensors can be deployed on players body, playing instruments and/or around playing ground. Analysis of measured parameters helps player to improve their game skills and techniques and gives them better chance to win. For example in table tennis angle of hand force can be measured and improved with practice. In cricket games, angle of wrist and arm is very critical for successful bating and bowling. In football angle of knee and ankle and positions of other players are very impartment to win a game. WBAN sensors can also provide useful information in other sport related fields such as: integrated bike sensors (speed, cadence), pedometer, GPS sensor, heart beat sensor, temperature sensor, etc. All these examples show that WBAN may have a vital role in supporting and performing many sports.

WBAN Application for Medical Safety

Human errors are one of the major factors of medical accidents and physician errors. It takes approximately, 98,000 lives very year [11]. WBAN technology can cope with this alarming situation by maintain a log of previous medical accidents, and can alarm the health care providers for occurrence of such errors. This technology is also being used in other public health safety related areas like monitoring diseases span and for fire safety and rescue system [12–14].

WBAN for Safeguarding of Uniformed Personnel

WBAN can help uniformed personals—e.g. Firefighters, policemen, civil defense or military personals—in carrying their tasks. In military, WBAN technology is being applied for several years [15–17]. WBAN monitors the level of toxics in the air and warns the firefighters or soldiers if a life-threatening level is detected. As uniformed personnel are often exposed to great risks and stressful situations, WBAN can be used to read physiological signals that indicate stress levels [18] of an individual. As a result, timely correction measures can be taken to mitigate stress. To develop the commercial standard for such application and to get maximum benefit of WBAN in this field is still an area for active research.

Application of WBAN in Health Electronics

Next to purely medical applications, a WBAN can include appliances that support health care such as an MP3-announcement player, head-mounted (computer) displays, control cameras, Advanced human-computer interfaces such as a neural interface, and Virtual Reality [19]. This technology is also being used in modern health clothing, infant monitoring and in many more applications for enjoying healthy daily life.

WBAN Architecture

WBAN consists of several heterogeneous devices. These may be categorized into three main components.

1. WBAN Hardware
2. WBAN Software/WBAN Operating system
3. WBAN Communication System.

WBAN Hardware

Special consideration is required for development and selection of hardware of WBN due to its power constraint, affordability, adoptability and portability from user point of view. WBAN hardware should have trivial radiation effect on BAN users. Battery life is an important factor, because WBAN nods needs to work continuously for continuous observing of parameters fatal to human life. Most WBAN nods are very low power devices. It's hardware mainly consists of:

(a) **Sensor Node (SN):** Several tiny Sensors Nodes are used in WBAN to build a network around body to monitor different activities. It can be placed close to human body (on every day clothing) or can be installed on the body as portable wearable devices or can be installed inside the human body. The SN are health monitoring sensors (such as ECG, EMG, biomedical sensors, eyeglass mounted displays, sensor equipped shoes) and mainly used to collect and transmit different parameters of person under test; details are given in Table 17.2.

(b) **Actuator Node (AC):** It operates as a drug-delivery system having a reservoir to hold the medicine and hardware to control the medicine. The medicine can be ejected on predetermined moments, triggered by an external source (i.e. a doctor who analyzes the data) or immediately when sensors notice a problem.

(c) **Central Unit (CU):** This unit is wired/wirelessly connected device to all sensors and actuators and have processing power and communication channels to external gateway for connecting WBAN to the outer world (internet, hospital etc). CU may be designed as an intelligent hub like PDA-class device or a cellular phone or Intel Personal Server [20–22].

WBAN Software/Operating System

WBAN requires more consideration for operating system and software development because of limited storage, limited processing, security constraints and battery conservation. The embedded sensor software is used for sampling and acquisition, event queuing, real-time processing, and WBAN communication. Some of the available software resources are discussed below.

- Tinyos [23]: TinyOS is a component-based open source operating system developed for wireless sensor networks (WSNs). It is an embedded operating system composed of cooperating tasks and processes written in the nes C programming language. It is developed with strong consideration for battery and memory limits of sensor networks.
- WinCE [24]: Microsoft Windows CE is an operating system developed by Microsoft for embedded systems. Windows CE is optimized for devices that have minimal storage. Its kernel may run in few megabytes of memory and can be configured without disk storage as a "closed system" (kernel is burned into ROM). Windows CE is classified as a real-time operating system, having deterministic interrupt latency. The fundamental unit of execution is the thread which leads to simplified interface and better execution time.
- nesC [25]: nesC (network embedded systems C is an event-driven, component-based programming language used to develop applications for the TinyOS platform. nesC is built as an extension to the C programming language where different threads are "wired" together to run applications on TinyOS at minimum execution time.
- MICA2 [26]: Data is transmitted wirelessly from the patient to the base station by using Crossbow's Mica2 motes. Mica2 mote is simply a processor/Thread designed to establish wireless connections for sensor network for Tinyos platform. The implementation has the following three main phases: (i) collecting data from the sensors (ii) sending the collected data to the base station and (iii) displaying the data in a user friendly interface on the PDA.

WBAN Communication System

The communication system could be a standard telephone network, mobile phone network, a dedicated link to medical center, hospital network, WLAN, Wi-Fi, Bluetooth, ZigBee or combination of any of these.

We can divide WBAN communication into two categories.

- Short-distance communication and
- Long-distance communication.

The short-distance communication means communication between various sensors and actuators to CU and CU to the personal device like mobile/PDA/Laptop. Short distance communication is used to collect all vital signals on a central location, and then these collected vital signals are transmitted to hospital and nursing station or emergency server unit by using long-distance communication.

Both long-distance and short-distance communication has its own radio spectrum, standers and technologies [27, 28]. WBAN mostly used ZigBee/IEEE 802.15.4 (915 and 2,450 MHz) [29], Bluetooth 802.15.1(2,450 MHz) [30] or Wi-Fi (2,450 and 5,800 MHz bands) for short-distance communication. WLAN, GSM, wired telephone cable, DSL are the standards mostly used for long-distance communication.

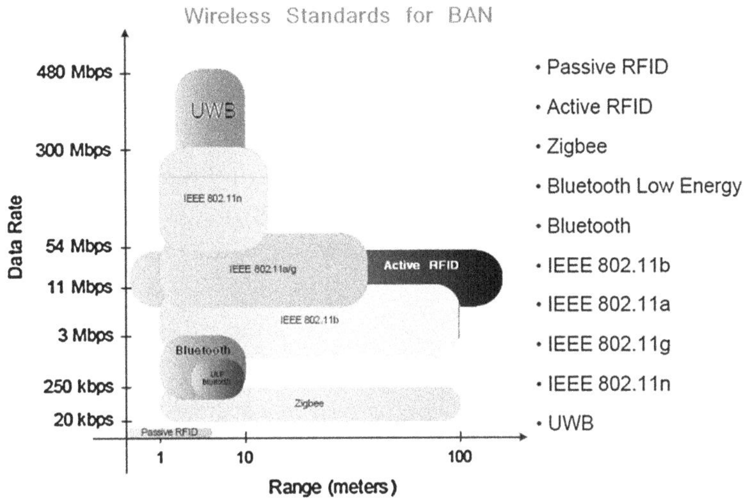

Fig. 17.2 Comparision of wireless standars for BAN

Short-distance communication is very important and critical for correct operation of WBAN due to many factors like energy/battery limitations, security issues, and reliability and availability constraints.

In-door wireless devices are mostly using unlicensed ISM (Industrial, Scientific and Medical) band for communication. In addition to ISM bands there are other medical bands such as MICS (Medical Implant Communication Service), WMTS (Wireless Medical Telemetry Service) and UWB (Ultra Wide Band) [31] that can be used for the WBAN implementation.

The Federal Communications Commission (FCC) [32] has approved and allocated 40 MHz spectrum (2,360–2,400 MHz) for medical communication. This will make WBAN communication liberated from already saturated standard Wi-Fi spectrum and move to a new standard band. FCC existing Medical Device Radio communication (MedRadio) Service will available on a secondary basis. WBAN devices using this band will operate under a "license-by-rule" basis which eliminates the need to apply for individual transmitter licenses. The 2,360–2,390 MHz frequencies band is restricted for usage of indoor communication at health-care facilities and it required registration and site approval of coordinators to prevent aerospace telemetry primary usage. Different potential wireless standards are shown and compared in Fig. 17.2.

WBAN Standards

The most essential part of WBAN standardization is the physical medium of communication. It is very critical to choose the wireless medium technology for WBAN.

The nature of communication channel determines the overall WBAN performance and may produce interference and life-threatening malfunctions. 802.15.4 Standard used three different specifications for radio communication: Narrow band, Ultra wide band (UWB) and Human Body Communication. Last two are most important from WBAN prospective. UWB transmits data with very minute power but on a very broader frequency band. Main advantage of UWB is preventing interference with other adjacent devices. It's extremely important for use in medical applications, where any interference with life support systems can have a catastrophic effect.

IEEE 802.15.4

IEEE 802.15.4 [33] defines communication in layers 1 and 2 (Physical and Data Link Layer) in the OSI reference model as shown in Figs. 17.3 and 17.4. Its main objective is to establish communication between two devices. At first layer (physical layer) basic units bits are organized and managed to become electromagnetic impulses. The basic functionality of this layer is similar to others known standards such as the common Ethernet-802.3 and WiFi-802.11 but 802.15.4 is developed with simple connectivity, lower data rate and battery constraints in mind. This standard operates in 27 different frequency channels and can be divided in three main bands:

868.0–868.6 MHz → 1 channel (Europe)
902.0–928.0 MHz → 10 channels (EEUU)
2.40–2.48 GHz → 16 channels (Worldwide)

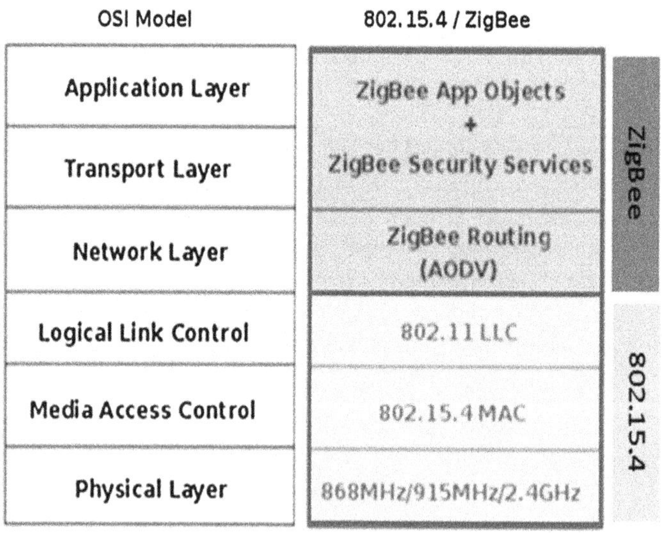

Fig. 17.3 Comparison of OSI model and 802.15.4/ZigBee

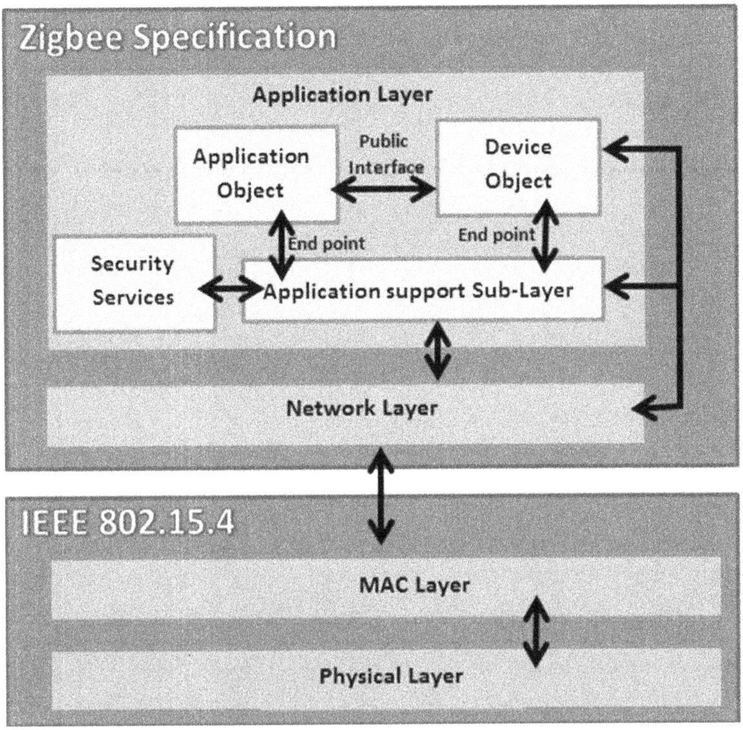

Fig. 17.4 IEEE 802.15.4 vs. ZigBee

The bandwidth associated with each frequency band is:

868.0–868.6 MHz → 20/100/250 Kb/s
902.0–928.0 MHz → 40/250 Kb/s
2.40–2.48 GHz → 250 Kb/s

The 802.15.4 standard allows point-to-point or a point-to-multipoint communication configuration. A typical application is to have a central coordinator node connected with multiple remote nodes.

ZigBee

ZigBee standard defines layer 3 and upper layers at in the OSI model as shown in Figs. 17.3 and 17.4. Its main purpose is to create a network topology to allow different devices to communicate wirelessly and to add additional communication features such as routing, encryption, authentication and association in the upper layers (Network, Transport, Application). It is created by a set of companies called ZigBee Alliance [34].

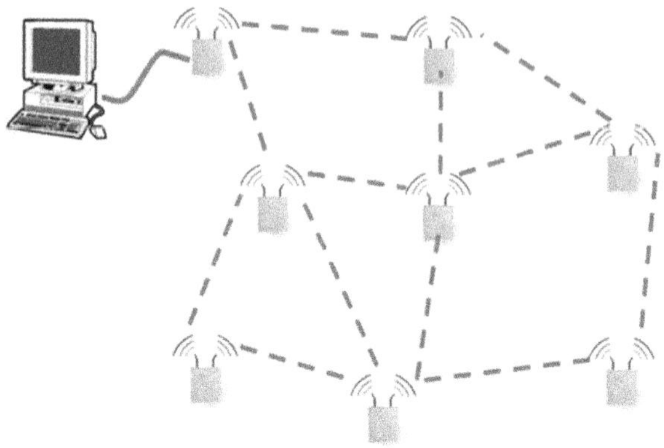

Fig. 17.5 ZigBee mesh network

ZigBee protocol is developed based on IEEE 802.15.4 standard and supplements some extra routing and networking features on upper layers. It adds mesh topology to the underlying 802.15.4 radios as shown in Fig. 17.5. Mesh networking is used in applications where the source and destination nodes are far away and directed communication is not possible, but intermediate nodes could forward this message to reach desired destination.

To illustrate the Fig. 17.5 shows how data to be transmitted from point A to point B, when the distance is too far to communicate directly. The message will be transmitted using a number of intermediate nodes including C to reach the destination. The ZigBee protocol is designed to build a whole network, consisting of many small radios devices and takes care of routing, acknowledgements, retries and self-heal etc within the whole network radios. If the point C radio is not available, a new path will be adapted to route messages from A to B. ZigBee protocol allows 802.15.4 to define the PHY and MAC layers, the signal bandwidth, frequency and modulation.

ZigBee is designed for low power applications, thus it is very suitable for WBAN where reliability is most important rather than high bandwidth RFID.

Table 17.1 shows a comparison of different features of ZigBee with other communication technologies.

ZigBee devices do not interfere with WiFi or Bluetooth devices, although both operate under IEEE Standard. Devices in the ZigBee specification can either be used as Coordinators, Routers or End devices these are described as follows:

- **Coordinator:** is the "master" device, it governs the entire network. It is always awake.
- **Routers:** They route the information received by the end devices. The routers can connect to each other and with the coordinator. It is also always awake.
- **End device:** The motes or sensor nodes, which take the information from the surroundings/environment. The end devices connect to a router or a coordinator. The end devices can be set to sleep.

Table 17.1 WBAN available standards and comparison

	ZigBee	802.11 (Wi-Fi)	Bluetooth	UWB (Ultra Wide Band)	Wireless USB	P-RFID	A-RFID	802.15.6
Data rate	20, 40, and 250 Kbits/s	11 & 54 Mbits/s	1 Mbits/s	100–500 Mbits/s	62.5 Kbits/s	900 kbps	10's of Mbps	10 Mbps up-to 1 Gpbs
Range	10–100 m	50–100 m	10 m	<10 m	10 m	3 m	100 m	10 m
Networking topology	Ad-hoc, peer to peer, star, or mesh	Point to hub	Ad-hoc, very small networks	Point to point	Point to point	Multipoint to point 1-Way	Multipoint to point 2-Way	Star, Star mesh hybrid, Ad-hoc, bi-directional link
Operating frequency	868 MHz (Europe) 900–928 MHz (NA), 2.4 GHz (worldwide)	2.4 and 5 GHz	2.4 GHz	3.1–10.6 GHz	2.4 GHz	900 MHz	860–960 MHz 13.5 MHz	400 MHz, 2.4 GHz, 3.1G~11.2 GHz
Complexity (device and application impact)	Low	High	High	Medium	Low	Low	Low	Low
Power consumption (battery option and life)	Very low (low power is a design goal)	High	Medium	Low	Low	Nil	Low	Ultra Low
Security	128 AES plus application layer security	Privacy, confidentiality, authentication and access control	64 and 128 bit encryption			No	Authentication mechanisms, public key encryption, embedded computation, Tame Transformation Signatures	3 level security mechanism

(continued)

Table 17.1 (continued)

	ZigBee	802.11 (Wi-Fi)	Bluetooth	UWB (Ultra Wide Band)	Wireless USB	P-RFID	A-RFID	802.15.6
Typical applications	Industrial control and monitoring, sensor networks, building automation, home control and automation, toys, games	Wireless LAN connectivity, broadband Internet access	Wireless connectivity between devices such as phones, PDA, laptops, headsets	Streaming video, home entertainment applications	PC peripheral connections	Healthcare supply chain High volume manufacturing Libraries / book stores Pharmaceuticals Passports Electronic tolls Item level tracking	Healthcare Auto dealerships Auto manufacturing Construction Mining Laboratories Remote monitoring IT asset management	WBAN
Setup time	30 ms	~10 s	~3 s Bluetooth Low energy <100 ms			~0.1 s per read	<1 ms per read	Insertion/De-insertion <3 s
Nodes	Unlimited	255	7+1	127+1		Only one tag read at once	1000+ tag cans read at once	256
Peak current /power	20 mA	150–200 mA	40 mA Bluetooth Low energy 10–20 mA	~400 mW		Nil	~1 mW	5 mA
Battery life	1,000 + days	2 days	5–10 days Bluetooth Low energy 1 year	1 day		Nil	~100 days	500 mAh battery for 1 year 50 mAh battery for 9 years

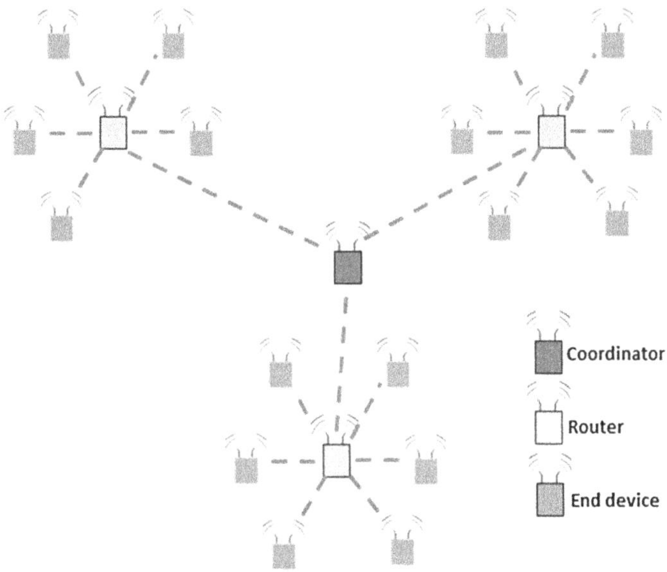

Fig. 17.6 ZigBee star topology

Ad-hoc "Mesh" communications is sometimes called peer to peer (P2P) network where all the devices in a network can directly communicate with each other. They can discover each other and can send broadcast messages to all the neighbors (**"hello! Is there anybody out there**?"). ZigBee may have a star topology not mesh as shown in Fig. 17.6. To create a completely mesh network all the nodes have to have the both roles as "end devices" as well as "routers" so that they can route their neighbors information and goes to sleep mode when no action is required (energy saving). Completely distributed network is possible in **DigiMesh** protocol over 802.15.4 where all the nodes can talk with each other using P2P (equal to equal) datagrams.

IEEE 802.11 - WLAN/Wi-Fi

WLAN or Wireless LAN (also called Wi-Fi) is a set of low tier, terrestrial network technologies for data communication. ISM frequency band of 5 GHz and 2.4 GHz ISM is reserved for the WLAN standards. It is a specification of IEEE 802.11 [35] standard and it has many variations like IEEE 802.11a/b/g/n. It is very famous wireless technology. In today world, almost all wireless devices use these standards to communicate freely over the available ISM frequency band. Wi-Fi is not suitable for WBAN communication because of the high energy requirement and interferences of many devices over the free frequency band, which is not acceptable in WBAN.

IEEE 802.15.1: Bluetooth

Bluetooth wireless communication technology is based on IEEE 802.15.1 standard [30]. It is an ad-hoc, low tier, terrestrial, wireless standard for short range communication. It is designed for low cost small end devices with small power consumption. The technology can have three different classes of devices: class 3, class 2 and class 1. The maximum range for each class is about 1,10 and 100 m respectively. Wireless LAN and Bluetooth both operate in 2.4 GHz frequency band but using different signaling method for communication which prevents interference. Bluetooth can be used for WBAN setup but ZigBee and IEEE 802.15.6 are better choices. IEEE 802.15.6 is however the best so far.

IEEE 802.15.6

IEEE 802.15.6 is a short range wirelesses communications standard specified transmission around, or inside the human body [36, 37]. It uses existing ISM frequency bands as well as other frequency bands approved by regulatory authorities. Provision of quality of service (QoS), 10 Mbps transmission rate, extremely low power consumption and use of secure frequency band make is best choice for WBAN technology. This standard is well immune to WBAN obstructions like the impact on transmission rate due to the user movement and effect of transition due to personal characteristics (e.g. being a male and female, skinny and heavy, etc.) and it has also the minimum absorption rate into the body. The comparison of all available communication standards for WBAN is shown in Radio-frequency identification (RFID).

Radio-Frequency Identification (RFID)

RFID technology has great potential in healthcare as it significantly reduces cost, and improves medical services and provides patient safety [38]. RFID works in two modes passive (read only) and active (read/write). Passive mode has no directly associated power source, while active mode does. The approved radio frequency range for RFID applications is 900 MHz for passive mode and either 13.56 MHz ISM Band or 860–930 MHz for active mode. More details of these modes follow:

Passive Mode: This kind of receiver collects power from incoming signals. The collected energy is then rectified and is used to power the receiver itself. Thus, when no signal is sent to the receiver, the receiver stays in the sleep mode. Although the RFID tag has quite low power consumption less than 1uW but its main challenge to be widely used in WBAN is its poor sensitivity. For some WBAN applications the transmitter power should not be limited. For example, if the sensor node only needs to communicate with the gateway node, a passive receiver can be used because the battery for the gateway node can be easily replaced. However, passive mode cannot be used. In other cases, whenever the node needs to communicate with other sensor nodes.

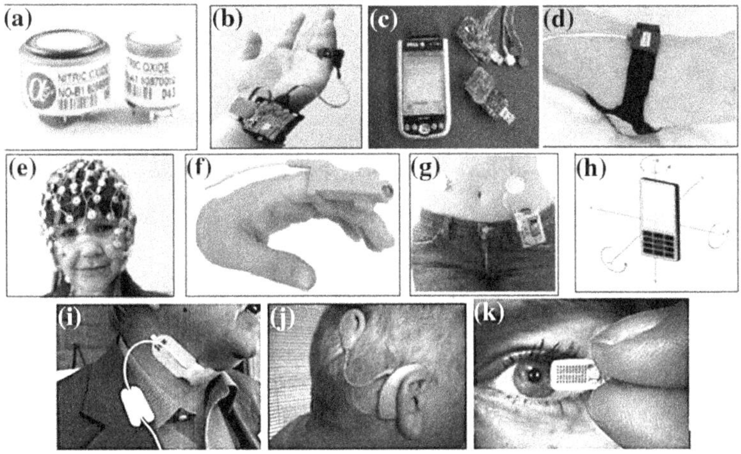

Fig. 17.7 WBAN sensor nodes

Active Mode: Sensitivity is guaranteed by using active devices but this mode has its own limitation like high power consumption.

WBAN Sensors

WBAN may consist of different kinds of sensors and actuators deployed around human body. Some of the well-known sensors specification used in WBAN are given in Table 17.2.

WBAN Application in Medical Fields

The biggest stake of WBAN is medical applications, it has unlimited applications in this filed. Almost every sector of health care fields can get benefit of this technology. In this section we will discuss various medical sectors where WBAN can play a vital role and we will show how QoS of each field can be improved dramatically if supported by this state of art technology. In a letter section we will show how QoS will be further enhanced by adding Virtual Doctor (VD) server in existing WBAN. We will discuss how WBAN equipped with VD will give a paradigm shift to existing medical facilities.

The medical applications of BAN may consist of:

- Gathering continuous waveform samples of biomedical data by each sensor
- Remote monitoring of different vital signal information of a patient

Table 17.2 WBAN sensors

Sensor	Purpose	Data rate	Bandwidth	Accuracy
Nitric oxide sensor Fig. 17.7a	Sensors which are able to detect nitric emitted by cancer cells	9600 bps	0–3 Hz	18 bit
Blood pressure Fig. 17.7b	Blood pressure monitoring	115.2 kbps		16 bit
ECG (12 leads) Fig. 17.7c	Monitoring heart activities	288 kbps	100–1000 Hz	12 bits
ECG (6 leads)	Monitoring heart activities	71 kbps	100–500 Hz	12 bits
EMG Fig. 17.7d	Monitoring muscle activity	320 kbps	0–10,000 Hz	16 bits
EEG (12 leads) Fig. 17.7e	Electroencephalography (EEG) is the recording of electrical activity along the scalp.	43.2 kbps	0–150 Hz	12 bits
Blood saturation Spo2 Sensor Fig. 17.7f	Monitoring the saturation of blood and oxygen	16 bps	0–1 Hz	8 bits
Glucose monitoring Fig. 17.7g	Monitoring the sugar level in blood	1600 bps	0–50 Hz	16 bits
Temperature	Monitoring the body temperature	120 bps	0–1 Hz	8 bits
Gyroscope Fig. 17.7h	An accelerometer is a sensor that measures acceleration with respect to gravity, and can be used to determine the orientation of a body part in the absence of movement.	35 kbps	0–500 Hz	12 bits
Accelerometer Fig. 17.7h	A gyroscope is a sensor that measures angular velocity and can be used to determine the orientation of a moving body part as a function of time	35 kbps	0–500 Hz	12 bits
Respiration Fig. 17.7i	Monitoring the respiration rate	640 bps	1–10Hz	
Cochlear implant Fig. 17.7j	The Clarion cochlear implant. Sound is received by a microphone, processed by a minicomputer (not shown), and the electric signals are transmitted to the implant by radio-frequency communication	100 kbps		
Artificial retina Fig. 17.7k		50–700 kbps		
Audio		1 Mbps		
Voice		5–10 Mbps		

- Remote control of medical devices (sensors and actuators).

WBAN can be broadly classified into two categories depending on its operating environments.

1. **Wearable BAN**: It is mainly operated around or on the surface of body, such as blood pressure monitoring and control.

2. **Implantable BAN**: It is operated inside the human body, e.g. capsule endoscope and pacemaker.

WBAN can improve health care services in many ways including:

- **Chronic Disease Monitoring**: it is the most important application, as the cost of treating diseases represents 75 % of total health care cost. Chronic diseases include a wide range of illnesses: diabetes, heart diseases, asthma and many more. Most of the diseases need constant long term monitoring to get accurate diagnosis and proper treatment.
- **Episodic Patient Monitoring**: in this category wide range of data is collected and further analyzed by taking periodical medical tests of a patient. It helps doctors to determine trends in patient's medical history. For example trends in blood pressure or sugar level disorder can help the doctor to diagnose the reason and to give a proper treatment.
- **Patients Alarm Monitoring**: in this category patients are monitored continuously to prevent health threatening response in case of emergency condition. For example a vital signals for a cardiac patient can be monitored and if some threshold level is exceeded, The patient case should be taken as emergency and an alarm is then generated or some health hazards prevention response need to be announced.
- **Elderly people monitoring**: This type of WBAN system is used for maintaining well being of old persons. It can help the senior citizens to get medical assistance at their homes/elderly nursing homes. It can also provide extra assistance in case of old age disability.

Role of WBAN for Diagnosis and Treatment

WBANs consisting of wearable devices, can provide unremitting remote health monitoring and proactive and affordable healthcare. With the help of sensors it's become easy to monitor a patient remotely and actuators can be used to control certain disease. In what follow we will discuss how WBAN controls different syndromes by using most modern way.

WBAN Applications for Chronic Disease

Cancer: Nowadays the second leading and alarming cause of human death is cancer. It is observed that nitric oxide is emitted by cancer cells and this disease can be diagnosed in early stage by observing the presence of this substance (nitric oxide). To prevent and detect this disease, tiny sensors which are able to detect nitric oxide are placed on human body. These sensors can differentiate between cancer causing cells and other cells.

Diabetes: Diabetes is the disease caused by disordered of blood glucose level. Diabetes further may cause high blood pressure, heart and kidney diseases. In order to closely and continuously monitor the glucose level, a bio-sensor is implanted in the patient to monitor the glucose level and to transmit the results to a fixed gateway. This type of WBAN can also automatically inject insulin in human body if a threshold level of glucose is reached.

Asthma: The patients suffering from asthma can also be saved from its attacks by using sensing nodes that detects allergic components in the environment and can alert the patient or doctor accordingly.

Epileptic Seizures: Any kind of abnormal brain activity can be detected by a portable unit "Mobi" which is designed to produce an alarm in case of seizure occurrence. When the signs of electrical trouble are picked and detected by the device it will transmit a warning to the patient or physician or any relative.

Pain treatment: An Actuator can be attached in spinal cord, having some pain killer which can be ejected in the body for long-term pain relief.

High Blood pressure: High blood pressure (HBP) is a serious problem that can lead to kidney failure, stroke, coronary heart disease, heart failure and other health problems, all these risks can be mitigated by continuously monitor and manage the blood pressure. A sensor and actuator can be installed on the patient body to measure and control high blood pressure [39].

Parkinson's disease: WBAN can help in rehabilitation of Parkinson's stroke patients as described in [40].

Eye Diseases Treatment: WBANs can also help the blind people by implanting retina prosthesis chips within a human eye. The people with limited vision or blind people can able to see at a reasonable level by using this technology.

In summary, there are many more chronic disease (Renal failure, Respiratory problem, blood sugar, Alzheimer, depression, Hypertension) in which WBAN can also play its role to monitor/manage/diagnose the problem during the routine life of the patient.

Cardiology

Cardiovascular Disease (CVD): Sudden deaths caused by cardiovascular diseases can be reduced significantly by installing some tiny sensor nodes on human body which are used to monitor vital parameters. The medical staff can prevent heart attack by continuously monitoring any kind of irregularities in heart function. Some actuators can also be installed to give lifesaving drug remotely or to produce an electric shock to re-activate normal heart functions.

Orthopedic/Rehabilitation/Physiotherapy

WBAN can help in monitoring the alignment and healing process of broken bones. WBAN can also play a vital rote to assist patient recovery. For example using hip guard system, the exact position of hip and leg (and their rotation movement) for a patient recovering from hip surgery can be continuously monitored with the help of embedded wireless sensors. Alarming signal is transmitted if the position or rotation of patient's leg or hip is not in proper position. Several medical studies proved that WBAN are useful in providing timely information for the rehabilitation process.

Dentistry

WBAN has wide range of applications in Dentistry like broken teeth replacement, building crowns and bridges and defective tooth positions treatments. It is also used to measure the growth of the jaw and the tooth status, by accurately supervising the duration of retainer use on the patient [41].

Emergency

WBAN can help in providing quality of emergency services like pre operation and post-operative monitoring etc.

Gynecology

WBAN can play a vital role to reduce the casualties during births, WBAN can be used for Fatal Heart Beat monitoring, fatal Position monitoring and Mother uterus/pelvis position monitoring [30–32].

Sleep Disordered

WBAN is very beneficial for people having sleep disorder. It can also help the doctor to fix the problem by remotely monitoring the patient vital signals during his sleep time [42].

WBAN Prototype

Architecture and prototype of WBAN are described in many studies [43–46]. We are classifying WBAN architecture into two categories as shown in Fig. 17.8, 17.9 with three tiers or four tiers architecture. The main objective of layered architecture is that any newly needed or invented module can easily be incorporated into existing architecture. New sensor type can be added in WBAN layer, new source of communication can be supplemented in communication layer and similarly new services can be integrated in services layer. A discussion for WBAN three tier architecture (TTA) and four tier architecture (FTA) follows.

WBAN Three Tier Architecture (TTA)

TTA [47] is shown in Fig. 17.8 and mainly consists of following layers.

WBAN Layer

This layer can consist of different sensor nodes and actuator nodes installed on human body. Samples of these include: Sensors, actuators, Central unit and personal device collectively form a WBAN around the human body connected with ZigBee, Blue tooth or Wi-Fi.

Connectivity Layer

This layer is used to connect WBAN Layer with Services Layer by wireless media using cellular network or wired media using home servers. A WBAN could allow a user to store this collected data on his PDA, iPad, Laptop or any other portable device and then transfer that information to remote hospital or physician computer for diagnostic or prescription purpose.

Services Layer

The facilities and services need to provide quality of health care and monitoring is collected in this layer and can be expanded as per needed or invented by modern technology. Some of the services are:

(a) Emergency and Ambulance services
(b) Weather forecast services
(c) Medical server and global storage services
(d) Paramedic services.

WBAN Four Tier Architecture (FTA)

As shown in Fig. 17.9 FTA consists of four layers with first three layers are same as TTA. The extra fourth layer includes following components but not limited to it.

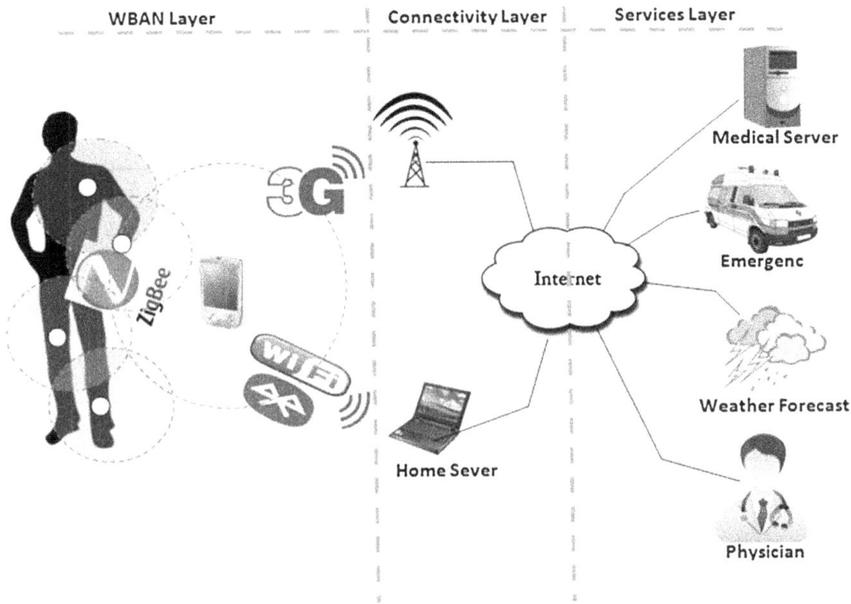

Fig. 17.8 WBAN three tier architecture

Virtual Layer/Virtual Doctor Layer (VDL)

Virtual layer is comprised of different Virtual Doctors (VD) each is specialized and store best knowledge practices in its area of specialization. Some of possible virtual doctors are described below.

(a) Virtual Dental (VDento): Teeth alignment, broken teeth and building crowns and bridges, Defective Tooth positions treatments, and supervising the duration of retainer use on the patient.
(b) Virtual cardio (VCardio): To monitor patient health parameters, predict and prevent Heart attacks.
(c) Virtual Ortho (VOrtho): To monitor broken organs and bones and to rehabilitate the patient to their routine life.
(d) Virtual Emergency (VEm): Take care of patients in emergency cases.
(e) Virtual Gynecologist (VGyno): To Monitor the fatal and pelvis activities.
(f) Virtual coach (VCo): Monitor, manage and track players exercise activities and help them in training sessions.

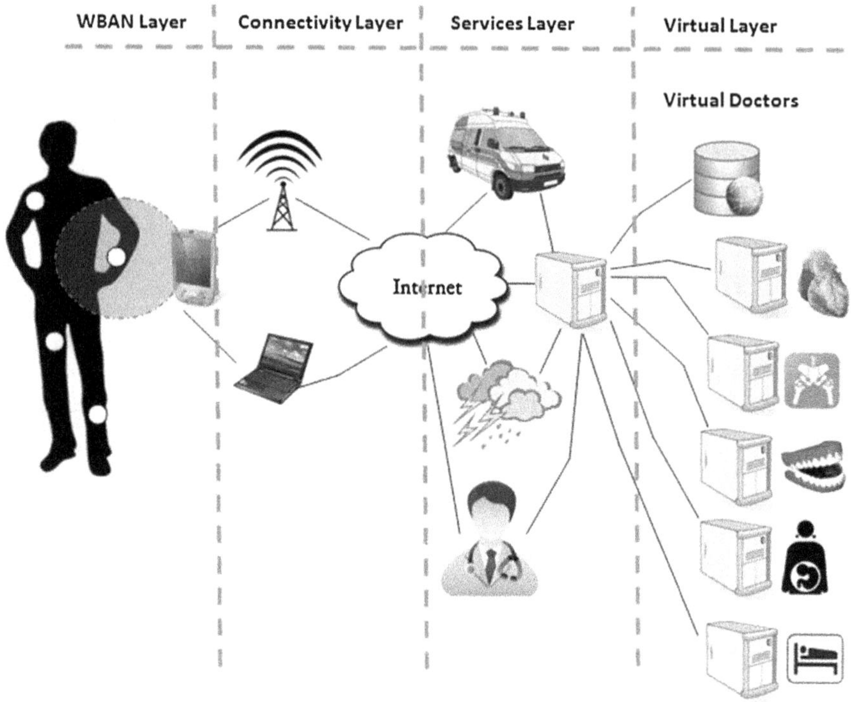

Fig. 17.9 WBAN four tier architecture virtual doctor

Virtual Doctor (VD) Specification

As described before, an extra layer called Virtual layer or Virtual Doctor Layer (VDL) is supplemented in existing WBAN architecture. VD is a special kind of computer server which simulates a doctor and can perform many tasks of the behalf of doctor such as:

- Keeps track of patients and their medicines
- Takes vital signals by using sensors installed in human body
- Gives some lifesaving drugs by using Actuator installed in human body
- Provides advices, messages and alerts for patient under treatment
- To call the Doctor / paramedic or ambulance or patient relatives if required in case of emergency
- Helps disable patients to restore their daily life.

By having a specialized VD rather than general one, more accurate and reliable health care service can be provided. For instance, VCardio may be developed to handle only cardiac patients. VCardio will be connected with all required sensors (Oxygen sensor, ECG sensor, Blood pressure sensor etc) and actuators (having reservoirs filled with lifesaving drugs) installed on human body, and equipped with a

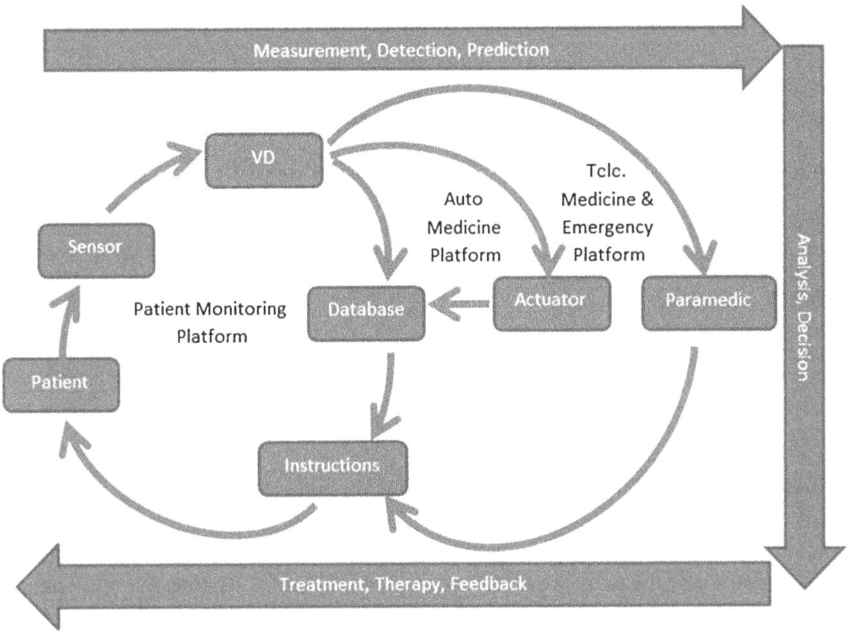

Fig. 17.10 WBAN closed loop management approach

decision support system. VCardio is to be developed and trained based upon cardiac procedures, best practices and historical data. It knows well how to and when to take vital signals of a patient and at what stage patient needs to visit the hospital/physician and what condition/state should be taken as emergency and how to handle it. VCardio will also be capable of giving some lifesaving drugs through actuator even if patient is unconscious or senseless and even before paramedic reached the patient. As cardiac patient needs to take many medicines with deferent potency continuously for longer time VCardio will remind the patient to take such medicines. At the time medicines should be taken VD will send a message on his/her cellular device about list of medicines and potency need to be taken. Patient can also inquire about his/her health condition, treatment plan or general information, and VD will answer his queries according to his vital signals. Three Loop Approach (TLP) for WBAN management of VD is suggested as shown in Fig. 17.10. These include:

1. Inner loop patient monitoring platform
2. Out loop auto medicines platform
3. Out most loop Tele. Medicine and emergency platform.

First of all patient vital signals are taken by using different sensors installed on human body then these vital signals are sent to VD, If all parameters are normal then system will follow the first loop, VD will store all information in its database and will send a message to patient about his/her health condition. If vital signals are abnormal (like blood pressure is very high/very low, sugar level is very high/low) and crosses some threshold level then VD will follow out loop and will take some action and can give some life-saving drugs through Actuator installed on human body and will inform the patient accordingly. At some certain level/stage if VD concludes that it's emergency then system will enter outermost loop and can call the doctor/nurse/ambulance/relatives as per requirements. The security issues related with WBAN are discussed below.

WBAN Security

The security concern, associated with the current WBAN is an important challenge. Security of a body area network (BAN) is unavoidable as it is mainly used for securing the life human. The security of WBAN is mainly related to:

- **Data Confidentiality:** For WBAN, the transmitted data should be strictly private and can be seen by authorized persons only, e.g. the doctor of the patient. There is a need to encrypting the data symmetrically or asymmetrically before sending.
- **Data Authentication:** It provides a means for making sure that the information is sent by the claimed sender. For this, a Message Authentication Code (MAC) is calculated using a shared secret key.
- **Data Integrity:** It makes sure that the received information has not been tampered. This can be inspected by verifying the MAC attached with the transmitted data.
- **Data Freshness:** To guarantee that the received data is recent and not outdated or belong to an old message. A solution is to add a time counter who is increased every time a message is sent.
- **Availability:** Update and accurate patient's information is always available to the doctor. The intruder can target the availability of a WBAN by disabling or capturing any node, which may cause loss of a human life. Thus, it is required to maintain continuous operation of all nodes.
- **Confidentiality of personal location information:** Location privacy is one of the major security problems in a WBAN [48]. An eavesdropper can keep track of the place and time devices are communicating. Some of the well knows Denial of Service (DoS) attacks attaches, and its counter defenses are given in Table 17.3. Major security threats and their solutions are shown in Table 17.4.

Security Paradigm in the IEEE 802.15.6 Standard

As IEEE 802.15.6 is most suitable standards for WBAN implementation, It has special security mechanism in it; this is essential as WBAN is very sensitive for security and any compromise is considered a threat of human life. IEEE 802.15.6 basic security structure has been taken from IEEE standard 802.15.4 and then modified

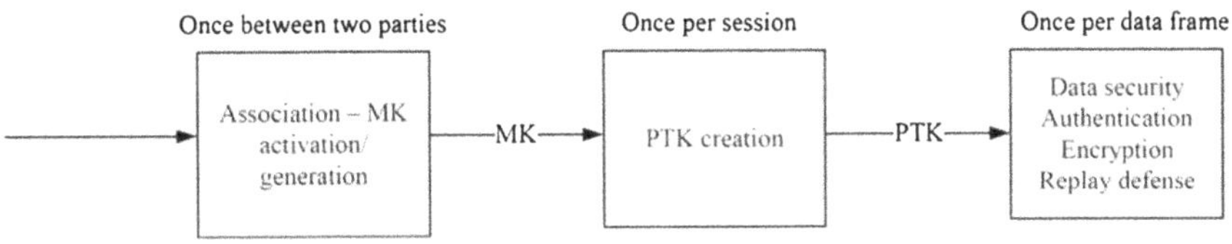

Fig. 17.11 Security mechanism for IEEE 802.15.6

according to the needs of WBAN. It defines three levels of security. Each security level has different security protection levels, properties, and frame formats.

- Level 0—unsecured communication—Lowest security levels: Where data is transmitted in unsecured frames. There is no mechanism for data integrity, authentication, privacy protection, confidentiality and replay defense.
- Level 1—authentication only—Medium security level: Where information is transmitted in secured authentication way but is not encrypted. This mode does not support privacy and confidentially.
- Level 3—authentication and encryption—Highest security level: In this mode information is transmitted in secured authentication and encryption frames. It provides solutions to all of the problems not covered by the level 0 and level 1.

The required security level is selected during the association process, i.e., when a node is joining the network. For unicast communication, a pre-shared Master Key (MK) or a new key (established via unauthenticated association) is activated. Then a Pairwise Temporal Key (PTK) is established, which is used once per session. For multicast communication, a Group Temporal Key (GTK) is shared with the corresponding multicast group. The whole security structure is given in Fig. 17.11.

Table 17.3 WBAN OSI layers and DoS attacks/defenses

Layers	DoS attacks	Defenses
Physical	Jamming	Spread-spectrum, priority messages, lower duty cycle, region mapping, mode change
	Tampering	Tamper-proof, hiding
Link	Collision	Error correcting code
	Unfairness	Small frames
	Exhaustion	Rate limitation
Network	Neglect and greed	Redundancy, probing
	Homing	Encryption
	Misdirection	Egress filtering, authorization monitoring
	Black holes	Authorization, monitoring, redundancy
Transport	Flooding	Client Puzzles
	De-synchronization	Authentication

Table 17.4 WBAN security threats and solutions

Security threats	Security requirements	Possible security solutions
Unauthenticated or unauthorized access	Key establishment and trust setup	Random key distribution
		Public key cryptography
Message disclosure	Confidentiality and privacy	Link/network layer encryption
		Access control
Message modification	Integrity and authenticity	Keyed secure hash function
		Digital signature
Denial-of-service (DoS)	Availability	Intrusion detection
		Redundancy
Node capture and compromised node	Resilience to node compromise	Inconsistency detection and node revocation
		Tamper-proofing
Routing attacks	Secure routing	Secure routing protocols
Intrusion and high-level security attacks	Secure group management, intrusion detection, secure data aggregation	Secure group communication
		Intrusion detection

Conclusion

WBAN is very useful emerging technology having immense utilities and benefits in daily life not only for medical treatment and diagnosis but also for supporting healthcare services for players training, public human safety, consumer health electronics, secure authentication and safeguarding of uniformed personnel. It is anticipated that proposed VDA of WBAN will help in implementing this emerging technology in a better way, and will provide a platform for development and integration of future devices and services. The addition of fourth layer (Virtual Layer) in existing architecture will provide an ample amount of quality of service in existing health care facilities. Dedicated virtual servers for each health facility/service will be capable of monitor/mange/serve the patient in a more reliable and accurate way.

Acknowledgments This research was partially sponsored by Sensor Networks and Cellular System Research Center, University of Tabuk, Kingdom of Saudi Arabia.

References

1. U.S. Census Bureau, "World POP Clock Projection", 2012. [Online]. Available: http://www.census.gov/population/popclockworld.html
2. BBC, "Population seven billion: UN sets out challenges".
3. U.N.O., "World Population Prospects, the 2010 Revision", 2011.

4. National Institute of Ageing and National Institute of Health, "Global Health and Aging", 2008.
5. Min Chen, Sergio Gonzalez, Athanasios Vasilakos, Huasong Cao, Victor C. Leung; "Body Area Networks: A Survey", Journal Mobile Networks and Applications archive, Volume 16 Issue 2, April 2011, Pages 171–193.
6. S. Armstrong, "Wireless connectivity for health and sports monitoring: a review", *British Journal of Sports Medicine*, vol. 41, pp. 285–289, 2007.
7. E. Chi, Dabnichki, and P.Baca, "Sensors and Ubiquitous Computing technologies in sports", *Computers in Sports*, pp. 249–268, 2008, Apr. 2008.
8. E. H. Chi, G. Borriello, G. Hunt, and N. Davies, "Guest Editors' Introduction: Pervasive Computing in Sports Technologies", *IEEE Pervasive Computing*, vol. 4, no. 3, pp. 22–25, Jul. 2005.
9. E. Preuschl, A. Baca, H. Novatchkov, P. Kornfeind, S. Bichler, and M. Boecskoer, "Mobile Motion Advisor - a feedback system for physical exercise in schools", *Procedia Engineering*, vol. 2, no. 2, pp. 2741–2747, 2010.
10. H. Novatchkov and A. Baca, "Machine learning methods for the automatic evaluation of exercises on sensor-equipped weight training machines", *Procedia Engineering*, vol. 34, pp. 562–567, Jan. 2012.
11. A. H. Mokdad, J. S. Marks, D. F. Stroup, J. L. Gerberding, "Actual causes of death in the United States, 2000", JAMA?: *the, journal of the American Medical Association*, 291(10), pp. 1238–45, Mar. 2004.
12. Y. Lim, S. Lim, J. Choi, S. Cho, C. Kim, Y.-W. L. H. Hu, H. Zhang, H. Hu, B. Xu, J. Li, and A. Ma, "A Fire Detection and Rescue Support Framework with Wireless Sensor Networks", in 2007 *International Conference on Convergence Information Technology (ICCIT 2007)*, 2007, pp. 135–138.
13. M. Bahrepour, N. Meratnia, P. Havinga, and P. S. Group, "Automatic Fire Detection?: A Survey From Wireless Sensor Network Perspective", 2007.
14. K. Sha, W. Shi, and O. Watkins, "Using Wireless Sensor Networks for Fire Rescue Applications: Requirements and Challenges", in *2006 IEEE International Conference on Electro/Information Technology*, 2006, pp. 239–244.
15. S. M. Diamond and M. G. Ceruti, "Application of Wireless Sensor Network to Military Information Integration", in *2007 5th IEEE International Conference on Industrial Informatics*, 2007, pp. 317–322.
16. H. S. L. H. S. L. Sang Hyuk Lee Sang Hyuk Lee, Soobin Lee Soobin Lee, Heecheol Song Heecheol Song, "Wireless sensor network design for tactical military applications: remote large-scale environments", in *Proceedings of the 28th IEEE conference on Military communications, MILCOM'09*, 2009, pp. 911–917.
17. M. Winkler, K.-D. Tuchs, K. Hughes, and G. Barclay, "Theoretical and Practical Aspects of Military Wireless Sensor Networks", *Journal of Telecommunications and Information Technology*, pp. 37–45, 2008.
18. B. S. Perala and C. H. Sterling, *Galvanic Skin Response as a Measure of Soldier Stress*. ARL-TR (Aberdeen Proving Ground, Md), 2007.
19. Y. -su. Seo, D. -youn. Kim, J. Cho, and B. Lee, "A WBAN MAC Protocol for Contention-based Medical and CE applications", in *International Conference on Ubiquitous Information Management and Communication (ICUIMC2010)*, 2010.
20. K. Van Laerhoven, B. P. L. Lo, J. W. P. Ng, S. Thiemjarus, R. King, S. Kwan, H. Gellersen, M. Sloman, O. Wells, P. Needham, N. Peters, A. Darzi, C. Toumazou, and G. Yang, "Medical Healthcare Monitoring with Wearable and Implantable Sensors", in *International Workshop on Ubiquitous Computing for Pervasive Healthcare Applications*, 2004.
21. L. Through and W. Technology, "Enhancing the Quality of Life Through Wearable Technology", *IEEE Engineering in Medicine and Biology Magazine*, no. June, pp. 41–48, 2003.

22. R. Paradiso, "Wearable health care system for vital signals monitoring", in *4th International IEEE EMBS Special Topic Conference on Information Technology Applications in, Biomedicine, 2003*, 2003, pp. 283–286.
23. "TinyOs". [Online]. Available: http://www.tinyos.net/
24. Microsoft, "Windows Embedded CE 6.0 R3 Development", 2012. [Online]. Available: http://www.microsoft.com/windowsembedded/en-us/develop/windows-embedded-ce-6-for-developers.aspx
25. "NesC". [Online]. Available: http://nescc.sourceforge.net/
26. Crossbow Technologies, "Mica2 Motes". [Online]. Available: http://www.xbow.com/
27. R. K. H. B. Li, K. Takizawa, B. Zhen, "Body Area Network and Its Standardization at IEEE 802.15.MBAN", in *16th IST Mobile and Wireless Communications Summit*, 2007, pp. 1–5.
28. The Institute of Electrical and Electronics Engineers, "IEEE 802.15 WPAN^{TM} Task Group 6 (TG6) Body Area Networks", 2012. [Online]. Available: http://www.ieee802.org/15/pub/TG6.html
29. ZigBee Alliance, "No Title", 2012.
30. Bluetooth SIG, "Bluetooth", 2012. [Online]. Available: http://www.Bluetooth.org
31. M. Hamalainen, A. Taparugssanagorn, R. Tesi, and J. Iinatti, "Wireless medical communications using UWB", in 2009 *IEEE International Conference on Ultra-Wideband*, 2009, pp. 485–489.
32. "Federal Communications Commission". [Online]. Available: http://www.fcc.gov/
33. IEEE, "IEEE 802.15 WPAN^{TM} Task Group 4 (TG4)". [Online]. Available: http://www.ieee802.org/15/pub/TG4.html
34. ZigBee Alliance, "ZigBee Standard". [Online]. Available: http://www.ZigBee.org/
35. IEEE, "IEEE 802.11 Wireless Local Area Networks The Working Group for WLAN Standards". [Online]. Available: http://www.ieee802.org/11/
36. J. M. Tjensvold, "Comparison of the IEEE 802.11, 802.15.1, 802.15.4 and 802.15.6 wireless standards", 2007. [Online]. Available: http://janmagnet.files.wordpress.com/2008/07/comparison-ieee-802-standards.pdf
37. Ali Katani, Deena Barakah; "Building Smart Saudi Hospitals using RFID Technologies" Proceedings of the Twelfth International Conference on Informatics and Semiotics in Organizations, ICISO 2010 - Reading, U.K., July 19–21, 2010.
38. K. S. Kwak, S. Ullah, and N. Ullah, "An overview of IEEE 802.15.6 standard", in 2010 3rd International Symposium on Applied Sciences in Biomedical and Communication Technologies (ISABEL 2010), 2010, pp. 1–6.
39. H. Richard, "Beyond Bits Health and Safety", *Designer Resource. Accelerate. Simplify.*, no. 4, 2009.
40. S. Patel, K. Lorincz, R. Hughes, N. Huggins, J. Growdon, D. Standaert, M. Akay, J. Dy, M. Welsh, and P. Bonato, "Monitoring motor fluctuations in patients with Parkinson's disease using wearable sensors".,*IEEE transactions on information technology in biomedicine*, vol. 13, no. 6, pp. 864–73, Nov. 2009.
41. Martin Brandl, Julius Grabner, Karlheinz Kellner, Franz Seifert, Johann Nicolics, Sabina Grabner, and Gerald Grabner; "A Low-Cost Wireless Sensor System and Its Application in Dental Retainers", *IEEE Sensor Journal*, Vol 9, No 3, March, 2009.
42. N. de Vicq, F. Robert, J. Penders, B. Gyselinckx, and T. Torfs, "Wireless Body Area Network for Sleep Staging", in *2007 IEEE Biomedical Circuits and Systems Conference*, 2007, pp. 163–166.
43. C. Otto, A. Milenković, C. Sanders, and E. Jovanov, "System architecture of a wireless body area sensor network for ubiquitous health monitoring", *Journal of Mobile Multimedia*, vol. 1, no. 4, pp. 307–326, 2006.
44. A. Faheem, "Wireless Body Area Sensor Network", 4th *IEEE Consumer Communications and Networking Conference CCNC*, pp. 722–726, 2007.
45. D. Kim and J. Cho, "WBAN Meets WBAN: Smart Mobile Space over Wireless Body Area Networks", in *2009 IEEE 70th Vehicular Technology Conference Fall*, 2009, pp. 1–5.

46. S. ÖZDEM R, “Remote Health Monitoring using Wireless Body Area Networks”, *ZKU Technology Journal*, vol. 11, no. 3, pp. 167–175, 2008.
47. J. Woodbridge, H. Noshadi, A. Nahapetian, and M. Sarrafzadeh, “HIP: Health integration platform”, in *2010 8th IEEE International Conference on Pervasive Computing and Communications Workshops (PERCOM Workshops)*, 2010, pp. 340–345.
48. M. Mana, M. Feham, and B. A. Bensaber, “A Light Weight Protocol to Provide Location Privacy in Wireless Body Area Network”, *International Journal of Network Security & Its Applications*, vol. 3, no. 2, pp. 1–11, 2011.

Chapter 18
Security of the Electronic Medical Record

Sokratis K. Katsikas

Abstract The shift to the networked world, that has been made possible by the explosive increase in the provision of broadband services not only to organizations but to individuals as well, allows making much better use of health information, but it also exposes this same information to a variety of threats that would not otherwise exist. These threats may, if not appropriately countered, seriously affect the security of health information and the privacy of the underlying subjects. Security and privacy technologies have grown tremendously over the past twenty years and still continue to be a field of intensive research. The result is an extensive arsenal of technological solutions to a variety of security problems. Nevertheless, healthcare organizations suffer regularly from information security breaches. This is due to the fact that security is more than erecting physical and electronic barriers; these are practically useless without an information security management system in place. This chapter presents a manager's roadmap for securing the electronic medical record.

Introduction

The proliferation of Information and Communication Technologies (ICT) in almost all aspects of our everyday life is rapidly changing our society and economy and is creating significant impact on our ways of doing things. Within the healthcare sector, the use of ICT increases at very fast rates; healthcare professionals tend to depend all the more on computerized Health Information Systems (HISs) in order to perform their everyday functions. Nowadays, healthcare professionals use HISs to assist themselves in diagnosing, to record information of a purely medical nature and to assist themselves in patient treatment in addition to the mostly administrative nature of information they once used to handle electronically.

S. K. Katsikas (✉)
Department of Digital Systems, University of Piraeus, Piraeus, Greece
e-mail: ska@unipi.gr

B. Furht and A. Agarwal (eds.), *Handbook of Medical and Healthcare Technologies*,
DOI: 10.1007/978-1-4614-8495-0_18, © Springer Science+Business Media New York 2013

Another fundamental change regarding ICT in health care is the transition from the traditional model of a stand-alone HIS, that is the HIS operating within the boundaries of a single Healthcare Organization (HO), to the networked HIS, that is a HO's HIS interconnected to HISs of other HOs or even of third parties, over national or international Wide Area Networks (WANs). Moreover, web-based e-health services are already been regularly provided and the healthcare sector has started exploiting the cloud computing paradigm [1]. Additionally, mobile devices like laptops, PDAs and even mobile phones are being increasingly used by the healthcare industry to access, store or transmit health information within the framework of providing health services [2].

This shift to the networked world, a world that provides exciting new possibilities for improving the quality of healthcare that we are provided with, including the possibility of extending diagnosing, monitoring and treating a patient outside the physical and even the logical boundaries of a HO, a shift which has been made possible by the explosive increase in the provision of broadband services not only to organizations but to individuals as well, definitely allows making much better use of health information but it also exposes this same information to a variety of threats that would not otherwise exist. These threats may, if not appropriately countered, seriously affect the security of health information and the privacy of the underlying subjects.

A google search on "Security of health information" returns about 750,000,000 results; this shows both the importance of the subject and the vast amount of information available on it. All this amount of knowledge is impossible to consolidate within the scope of a book chapter. In light of this, the purpose of this work is not to provide a complete review on the issue. Health information is a very broad term that encompasses any information related to health, be it personal (e.g. the state of health of a particular individual) or not (e.g. statistical epidemiological information). Acknowledging this fact, in order to narrow down the scope of the work herein one possible approach is to limit the extent of the health information to study; this work focuses on an organized subset of health information, namely the electronic medical record.

Note that the terms Electronic Medical Record (EMR) and electronic health record (EHR) are often used interchangeably. Yet, differences do exist and will be highlighted in the sequel.

Security and privacy technologies have grown tremendously over the past twenty years and still continue to be a field of intensive research. The result is an extensive arsenal of technological solutions to a variety of security problems. According to [3], the use of security tools and techniques like firewalls and user access controls is widespread. It appears, then, that we do have and we use the technologies to solve many of the technical problems associated with securing health information. One, however, cannot help but wonder: If this were indeed the case, then all the real security breaches [3] that we encounter everyday in healthcare organizations should not have been happening. What is, then, the problem?

The most usual problem is that, while everyone recognizes the need for securing health information, what they often neglect is the fact that security is more than erecting physical and electronic barriers. According to Bruce Schneier, "*…the fundamental problems in computer security are no longer about technology; they're about applying technology*" [4]. The strongest encryption and most robust firewall are practically worthless without an information security management system in place that—among others–articulates how these tools are to be used, managed and maintained. We thus focus herein on managing the security of the electronic medical record.

The remaining of this chapter is structured as follows: In section "Definitions" we set the scope of the subsequent discussion by giving definitions for the EMR and the EHR, of security and of privacy. Section "Threats and Security Requirements" discusses threats against the security of the EMR, as well as legal and ethical requirements to adhere to when addressing the security and privacy of EMR. Section "A Manager's Roadmap for Securing the EMR" discusses a roadmap for managing the security of EMR within an HO. Finally, section "Conclusions" summarizes our conclusions.

Definitions

As already stated, EMR and EHR, although often used interchangeably, refer to different concepts. According to [5], the Electronic Medical Record is "*An application environment composed of the clinical data repository, clinical decision support, controlled medical vocabulary, order entry, computerized provider order entry, pharmacy, and clinical documentation applications. This environment supports the patient's electronic medical record across inpatient and outpatient environments, and is used by healthcare practitioners to document, monitor, and manage health care delivery within a care delivery organization (CDO). The data in the EMR is the legal record of what happened to the patient during their encounter at the CDO and is owned by the CDO.*"

Again according to [5], the Electronic Health Record is "*A subset of each care delivery organization's EMR, presently assumed to be summaries like ASTM's Continuity of Care Record (CCR) or HL7's Continuity of Care Document (CCD), is owned by the patient and has patient input and access that spans episodes of care across multiple CDOs within a community, region, or state (or in some countries, the entire country")*. Its primary purpose is "*…to provide a documented record of care which supports present and future care by the same or other clinicians. This documentation provides a means of communication among clinicians contributing to the patient's care*" [6]. On the other hand, the Integrated Care EHR is "*a repository of information regarding the health status of a subject of care in computer processable form, stored and transmitted securely, and accessible by multiple authorized users. It has a standardized or commonly agreed logical information model which is independent of EHR systems. Its primary purpose is the support of continuing, efficient and quality integrated health care and it contains information which is retrospective, concurrent and prospective*" [7].

A related concept is that of the Personal Health Record. A personal health record (PHR) is a health record where health data and information related to the care of a patient is maintained by the patient [8].

Based on the above definitions, it can be seen that medical records of a patient may refer to PHR, EMR and EHR. A part of PHRs can be obtained from the EMR systems of different HOs and once these data are shared with other HOs they become EHR. Therefore, from a patient's point of view, there is partial overlap between all three among the PHR, the EMR, and the EHR, the degree of overlap varying with the personalized choices of each patient. More details on the differences between these concepts can be found in [5] and [9]. The main difference that concerns us here is that the EMR is managed by the HO, in contrast to the EHR and the PHR, which are managed by the patient. Thus, the responsibility for the security of the EMR lies exclusively with the HO; this is not the case with either the EHR or the PHR. Note that we distinguish between ownership and management of the records; this is because the concept of ownership may significantly differ across different legal systems.

Information security is commonly defined as the preservation of confidentiality, integrity and availability [10]. Confidentiality is preserved when information is accessed only by authorized entities; integrity is preserved when information is modified only by authorized entities; and availability is preserved when information is made available, within a reasonable time interval, to an authorized entity that requests it. Personal health information is generally agreed to be highly sensitive. The availability and integrity of such information may be crucial for the life of an individual. In addition, the confidentiality of health information is a prerequisite for the preservation of the subject's privacy and the endurance of the trustful patient-physician relationship. Unfortunately, in many cases the preservation of these three attributes of information requires taking conflicting measures and security policy makers are obliged to seek proper trade-offs [11].

Privacy has been originally defined as the right "to be let alone" [12]. In our context, privacy may be defined as the individual right of humans to determine, when, how, and to what extent information is collected about them; the right to be aware and to control the beginning of any interaction or data gathering process; and the right to choose when, how, and to what extent their personal information is made available to others [13].

A threat is defined as a potential cause of an unwanted incident, which may result in harm to a system or organization [14]. Risk is the combination of the probability of an event and its consequence [14]. An event happens when a threat materializes and exploits a vulnerability; in this way (negative) impact results on an asset. Risks are usually measured in terms of the likelihood of the threat occurring, the level of the underlying vulnerability (ies), the level of the impact and the value of the asset involved. Controls (alias safeguards or countermeasures) are means of managing risk, which can be of administrative, technical, management or legal nature.

Threats and Security Requirements

There is nothing extraordinary with personal health information that exposes it to threats different than those against other types of information. What is different is the level of vulnerabilities which threats may exploit; these are usually much higher in healthcare provision environments than in other types of environments. What is also unique to healthcare is the array of factors to be considered when assessing threats and vulnerabilities to determine the risk level [14].

With regards to confidentiality, personal health information is generally agreed to be among the most sensitive types of personal information. At the same time, it is also information that is attractive to parties who do not have a legitimate interest to access it. Often cited examples of such parties are insurance companies, employers, the pharmaceutical industry, governments and even members of the subject's family. On the other hand, personal health information needs to be shared among many parties (mostly health professionals) to ensure that the highest possible quality of health care is provided. Health professionals are bound—at least in Western cultures—by the Hippocratic oath; therefore they tend to share personal health information with fellow professionals, ignoring or neglecting the fact that they sometimes use totally insecure communication channels such as, for example, mobile phones. Conversely, healthcare personnel, be they medical, ancillary, technical or administrative, are usually—on average—more dedicated and devoted to their profession than personnel in other industry and business sectors; this may considerably reduce the likelihood of an insider threat occurring.

Lack of integrity of personal health information may result in severe consequences, including life-threatening situations. Additionally, healthcare staff often operate under stress conditions, a situation that makes humans more prone to errors and to applying procedures incorrectly. Legacy systems in healthcare often remain in use long after their useful lifetime; this practice, usually attributed to underfunding, may expose personal health information to accidental or even deliberate threats against integrity. On the other hand, technology itself may prove to inject vulnerabilities in its quest to assist clinicians in their everyday routine by enhancing user-friendliness. An example is the ability to copy-paste and drop-down menus that have been found to create serious problems with regards to preserving the integrity of the information in the EMR [15, 16].

Similarly to lack of integrity, lack of availability may also result in life-threatening situations; medical emergencies are not uncommon and the time to react to some of these does not allow for even slow responses from information systems, let alone full information unavailability. Thus, EMR systems must meet unique demands to remain operational in the face of natural disasters, system failures and denial-of-service attacks. Of course, high availability requirements are commonly found in many safety-critical systems, other than healthcare. What is unique in healthcare is that sometimes high availability conflicts with another crucial requirement of the EMR, namely the requirement of access following explicit informed consent. Again, there are of course ways of addressing this conflict in practice, usually by allowing access without proper authorization in emergencies, followed by a scrutinized audit of the actions performed during this access.

The security of the EMR, its high level of risk being unique among other, less sensitive pieces of information, must therefore be considered with special care. This rationale has also led to the formulation of an ISO/IEC standard specifically geared towards managing the security of information in healthcare environments [15]. Annex A of this standard contains an informative list of 25 types of threats that need to be considered by health organizations when they assess risks to the confidentiality, integrity and availability of health information and to the integrity and availability of related information systems, including EMR systems. These threats, re-organized into 15 more generic categories are shown in tabular form in Table 18.1.

Other studies have also addressed and categorised threats against health information systems [17] (whose EMR systems are a subset). Several studies have also addressed the issue of assessing risks in health information systems [17–19]. Given the vast amount of literature on very elaborate technical controls proposed to secure the EMR, it is astonishing—at least at a first glance—to realize that all of the above studies concur that the most critical threat that health information systems face is power failure to the servers. Of course, other high-risk threats relate to human factors, system and network failure, EMR software failure, technical obsoleteness, hardware problems etc. This is actually indicative of the fact that the preservation of the availability of health information is generally, among HO staff, believed to be far more important than the preservation of confidentiality or of integrity. This is in contrast to the feeling of the general public, who tend to believe that confidentiality is paramount.

A different view regarding the prioritization of risks is taken in [20], where the risk of failure to comply with informed consent legislation is ranked as the highest one. This highlights the importance of complying with legal requirements as well when addressing the security and privacy of the EMR.

Health information is protected by the law in several countries. In the United States, the Health Insurance Portability and Accountability Act (HIPAA) is a federal law that was designed to allow portability of health insurance between jobs. In addition, it required the creation of a federal law to protect personally identifiable health information; if that did not occur by a specific date (which it did not), HIPAA directed the Department of Health and Human Services (DHHS) to issue federal regulations with the same purpose. DHHS has issued HIPAA privacy regulations (the HIPAA Privacy Rule [21]) as well as other regulations under HIPAA, including the HIPAA Security Rule [22]. HIPAA defines privacy as an individual's interest in limiting who has access to his or her personal healthcare information and specifies that security measures must encompass all the administrative, physical, and technical safeguards in an information system [23]. HIPAA established a set of healthcare provider rules and regulations, requiring that patients be informed of their privacy rights, that uses of protected health information not needed for treatment, payment, or operations be limited, and that all employees in organizations that, in the course of providing services, come in contact with or use personal health records, be educated about privacy [24, 25]. Moreover, under the HITECH Breach notification rule [26], HIPAA covered entities and their business associates are required to provide notifi-

Table 18.1 Threat categories

No	Category	Comments
1	Masquerade	Occurs when insiders (including staff) or service providers, or outsiders (including hackers) make use of accounts that they do not own
2	Unauthorized use of health information application	Occurs either when unauthorized users use such applications or when authorized users perform unauthorized actions
3	Introduction of damaging or disruptive software	Occurs when such software (including malware) is intentionally or unintentionally introduced
4	Misuse of system resources	Occurs when authorized users use system resources for purposes not related to their work
5	Communications infiltration	Occurs when somebody tampers with the normal flow of data across a network
6	Communications interception	Occurs when somebody installs a "packet sniffer" to monitor much of the traffic on the network
7	Repudiation	Occurs when a user denies the fact that she sent a message (repudiation of origin) or that she received a message (repudiation of receipt)
8	Connection failure	Occurs when the network service is disrupted
9	Accidental misrouting	Occurs when a message is erroneously routed to an incorrect recipient
10	Hardware technical failure	Occurs when the hardware, the storage facility, the network infrastructure or the environmental support fail
11	Software technical failure	Occurs when the system software, or the network software, or the application software fail.
12	Human error	Occurs when an operator, or a person responsible for maintenance, or a user commits an error in the course of her duties
13	Staff shortage	Occurs when key personnel are absent and there is difficulty in replacing them
14	Theft	Occurs when an insider or an outsider steals information, software or hardware
15	Wilful damage	Occurs when an insider or an outsider cause physical damage to IT systems or to their supporting environment. Acts of terrorism also constitute large scale wilful damage

cation following a breach of unsecured protected health information. Similar breach notification provisions implemented and enforced by the Federal Trade Commission (FTC) [27], apply to vendors of personal health records and their third party service providers.

In Canada, the Personal Information Protection and Electronic Document Act (PIPEDA) protects personal health information against use by commercial enterprises across provincial and national boundaries. In Australia, the Privacy Act 1988 established a privacy regime that covered health information in the private sector.

The Health Records (Privacy and Access) Act 1997 was based on twelve privacy principles that have been tailored to suit the health environment. Relevant legislation exists in Victoria (Health Records Act 2001) and in New South Wales (Health Records and Information Privacy Act 2002) [28].

In the European Union, the protection of health data is legally covered by the legislation on personal data protection, health data being considered sensitive personal data. At the European level, EU directives are issued, which are addressed to the Member States, who are in turn obliged to transpose the directive into national law. The relevant directive is "Directive 95/46/EC of the European Parliament and of the Council of 24 October 1995 on the protection of individuals with regard to the processing of personal data and on the free movement of such data" [29]. Even though all Member States indeed have transposed this Directive 95/46/EC, this has not happened in a harmonized way; for instance, Article 8 on the processing of sensitive data (e.g. health data), has not been fully transposed by all Member States. This has resulted in the absence of certain legal grounds for personal health data processing in the concerned Member States, which should be present according to EU law. Moreover, diverging opinions on how to interpret the Directive and national data protection laws appeared to be another cause of the differences found [30]. An assessment of this directive and how it impacts European healthcare activities can be found in [31], whereas an analysis of legal liability of health care professionals, health care providers, system/application producers, telecommunication providers and patients when engaged in electronic health care delivery, under European law can be found in [32]. The process for reforming Directive 95/46/EC is currently underway [33].

Codes of ethics, such as the International Medical Informatics Association (IMIA) Code of Ethics for Health Information Professionals [34] and the American Health Information Management Association (AHIMA) Code of Ethics [35] also specifically address security and privacy issues.

A Manager's Roadmap for Securing the EMR

An efficient framework for managing information security is provided by the ISO/IEC 27002 standard on Information Technology—Security Techniques—Code of practice for information security management [36]. The standard is a code of practice for information security; it outlines hundreds of potential controls and control mechanisms and is also intended to provide a guide for the development of "organizational security standards and effective security management practices and to help build confidence in inter-organizational activities" [37].

Another standard, ISO 27799:2008 [14] defines guidelines to support the interpretation and implementation in health informatics of ISO/IEC 27002 and is a companion to it. ISO 27799:2008 applies to health information in all its aspects; whatever form the information takes, whatever means are used to store it and whatever means are used to transmit it [38].

The process of managing information security in an organization normally starts from identifying its security requirements. These come from three main sources [36]: one source is derived from methodically assessing risks to the organization, taking into account the organization's overall business strategy and objectives. This will not only allow the identification of threats, vulnerabilities and the likelihood of threats occurring, but will also enable the selection of security controls in a way such that the relevant expenditure is balanced against the likely business harm. Risk assessment is part of the more generic risk management process [39]; the generic methodology for information security risk management is described in ISO/IEC 27005:2011 [40].

The second source is the legal, statutory, regulatory and contractual requirements that the organization, its partners, contractors, and service providers have to satisfy, and their socio-cultural environment. These may vary with the HO's home country, as was briefly discussed in the previous section.

A further source is the particular set of principles, objectives and business requirements for information processing that an organization has developed to support its operations. In healthcare, such principles, objectives and requirements applicable to a wide range of HOs have been identified in a number of generic security policies [41].

Once the security requirements have been identified, the process continues with the selection of the appropriate security controls that will mitigate the identified risks and treat them, so that the residual risk to the organization is within acceptable levels.

There is no "cook-book solution" as to what security controls are appropriate for a particular HO's EMR system, as these will vary significantly with the results of the risk assessment exercise. However, controls that are generally considered to be common practice include the formulation of a security policy; the allocation of information security responsibilities; the formulation of information security awareness, training and education plans; the correct processing in applications; the technical vulnerability management; the business continuity management; and the management of information security incidents and improvements [36].

Security Policy

Loosely interpreted, security policies are management instructions indicating how an organization is to be run [42]. They are intended to provide guidance to those who must make present and future decisions. As such, a policy should identify the actions that people are and are not permitted to undertake. Therefore, any security policy, in order to be meaningful, should provide individuals with reasonable ability to determine whether their actions violate or comply with the policy. Security policies are mandatory; when a member of the staff of an organization wishes to take a course of action different than that specified in the policy, s/he must request special approval.

A security policy should be used as a reference for a wide variety of information security and privacy activities and is quite important to have in a HO, for a variety of reasons [43]. Such a policy for a HO should include statements on the need for health information security; the goals of health information security; the compliance scope, that defines the compliance activity in terms of people, processes, places, platforms and applications; the legislative, legal and contractual requirements and the legal and ethical responsibilities of health professionals towards information security and privacy; and arrangements for notification of information security incidents [38]. It should also be considered as an essential part of the overall information policy of the organization, a consideration that helps integrate procedural aspects within the administrative structure of the organization.

The responsibility for initiating the development of a security policy lies with the Information Security Department of an organization, or with the Computing Department. The actual development is usually carried out by staff of these departments assisted by external consultants. However, the responsibility for adopting a security policy proposal within an organization lies with the organization's management. Before any security policy can be enforced in any organization, management approval must be sought. In fact, the higher the level of management endorsing the security policy, the more efficient this policy will be, since it is likely that it will command the attention of every staff member [43].

Information Security Responsibilities

Responsibilities for the protection of individual assets and for carrying out specific security processes should be clearly identified. The assets and security processes associated with each particular system should be identified and clearly defined; the entity responsible for each asset or security process should be assigned and the details of this responsibility should be documented; and authorization levels should be clearly defined and documented [36]. Further, the duties and responsibilities of all individuals employed in or working on behalf of an HO, which are relevant to information security and privacy aspects, should be described in the written contract between the HO and each member of the staff of each contractor. Even though individuals with allocated security responsibilities may delegate security tasks to others, they remain responsible and should determine that any delegated tasks have been correctly performed.

Even though overall responsibility for security within the HO may rest with a number of managers, the practice of appointing a security officer is generally considered to be a good one. The responsibilities of such an officer include, inter alia: the support of the HO management with technical advice on security and privacy issues, as required; the implementation of security and privacy policies; the provision of advice to the HO management on training and awareness issues on security and privacy; the provision of a central point of technical conduct for HO staff and partner organizations, on security and privacy; the determination of security and privacy specifications for all software development or acquisition projects. The security officer should have expertise in the functioning and operation of health information systems; security and privacy issues and technical measures; existing and emerging information processing technologies and to be familiar with generic aspects of healthcare delivery routine; and of the pertinent legislation [44].

Information Security Awareness, Training and Education

In today's technological environment, especially within modem HOs, it is almost impossible for any employee to function properly without being at least security aware. Awareness constitutes the point-of-entry for all employees into the progression of information systems security levels. The next (training) level of the learning process aims at building knowledge, thereby producing relevant and needed security skills and competency by practitioners of functional specialties other than information systems security and, often, by individuals competent in diverse scientific disciplines. Training is required for those employees of the HO whose role in it necessitates special knowledge of security threats, vulnerabilities, policies, management and controls. Naturally, not all employees require the same level of training; this varies with the specific function of the employee, starting with baseline security training for all users and culminating in the intricate details of sophisticated technical controls for the information systems security officers. The third and last (education) level of the learning process aims at creating expertise necessary for information systems security specialists and professionals. This level applies primarily to individuals who are professionally involved with information systems security. The educated information systems security professional has the comprehensive grasp of the field required to take responsibility for her further learning in a technologically and socially ever-changing environment [45].

The HO management should identify the various target groups (general public, inpatients, outpatients, staff categories) that should be made aware of or trained in information security and privacy issues. Management should also assume responsibility for developing appropriate awareness and training programs suited to each target group. The responsibility for carrying out these programs also lies with the management [44].

A methodology for determining the training needs of staff categories within HOs with respect to information systems security is discussed in [46]; this methodology, in way of an example, is applied to a particular category of HO personnel, namely managers, whose training needs are derived. Descriptions of training courses on information systems security for different HO staff categories have been developed in [46].

Correct Processing in Applications

In order to prevent errors, loss, unauthorized modification or misuse of information in applications, appropriate controls should be designed into applications, including user developed applications to ensure correct processing. These controls should include the validation of input data, internal processing and output data. Additional controls may be required for systems that process, or have an impact on, sensitive, valuable or critical information, such as EMR systems. This further means that input data should be validated to ensure that it is correct and appropriate (e.g. boundary checks on physiological data or medication doses); applications should be designed so as to minimize the risk of loss of integrity (e.g. by incorporating validation checks to detect corruption or unauthorized modification of information); appropriate controls for ensuring message integrity within and between applications should be identified and implemented (e.g. when communication health information); and output data should also be validated (e.g. by implementing plausibility checks to ensure that data are reasonable) [36].

Technical Vulnerability Management

In order to reduce risks resulting from exploitation of published technical vulnerabilities, technical vulnerability management should be implemented. Technical vulnerability management can be viewed as a sub-function of change management and as such can take advantage of the change management processes and procedures. A current and complete inventory of assets is a prerequisite for effective technical vulnerability management. Specific information needed to support technical vulnerability management includes the software vendor, version numbers, current state of deployment, and the person(s) within the HO responsible for the software [36].

Business Continuity Management

A Disaster Recovery Plan (DRP) is a necessity for every organization that wants to "stay in business". In our particular case of interest, Health Care is a very sensitive domain because it affects human lives and health. A disaster affecting the EMR makes the delivery of medical care too difficult or even impossible. For example, to name just a few consequences, test results from microbiologists are not directly available to other departments, medication is under-serviced, several internal sectors are (logically) disconnected, and physicians cannot effectively carry out their work. Patients' health, or even their life, can be jeopardized following a fault or insufficient medical diagnoses. The treatment cost of a patient rises and the HO is in serious trouble if its EMR system cannot recover quickly. Disaster Recovery Plans should not simply be seen as a necessary burden in order to conform to standing internal or external requirements and/or regulations, such as those of the pertinent legislation. They should rather be seen as a means to benefit the HO in the event of a disaster. Indeed, an HO may benefit from the existence of such a plan in terms of reducing its costs [47].

The essential action that must be taken towards the development and establishment of a disaster recovery plan for an HO is discussed in [47], whereas the full process is described in [48, 49]. Contingency plans (covering both interim and recovery situations) should be documented, available and rehearsed to ensure that all staff members are aware of their roles if a real scenario arises [44]. A software tool specifically designed for HO environments that can define a scaled-down information system with the associated workstation structure, with which the organization can, following a disaster, achieve a scaled-down level of performance, has been proposed in [50].

Management of Information Security Incidents and Improvements

In order to ensure that information security events and weaknesses associated with information systems are communicated in a manner allowing timely corrective action to be taken, formal event reporting and escalation procedures should be in place. All employees, contractors and third party users should be made aware of the procedures for reporting the different types of event and weakness that might have an impact on the security of organizational assets. They should be required to report any information security events and weaknesses as quickly as possible to the designated point of contact [36, 44].

Moreover, in order to ensure that a consistent and effective approach is applied to the management of information security incidents, responsibilities and procedures should be in place to handle information security events and weaknesses effectively once they have been reported. A process of continuous improvement should be applied to the response to, monitoring, evaluating, and overall management of information security incidents. Where evidence is required, it should be collected to ensure compliance with legal requirements [36]. A complete guide for handling information security incidents is provided in [51].

A European Healthcare Incident Reporting Scheme (HIRS) has been proposed in [52]. A Healthcare Incident Reporting Scheme (HIRS) is defined as an information system that gathers information about the occurrence of computer security related incidents in healthcare. A HIRS processes this information and creates reports (notices) that contain specific or aggregate information about these incidents. The HIRS's clients are HOs in European countries. Information generated from the HIRS is intended to raise the awareness level on computer and communications security of its HOs' constituency.

Conclusions

Information systems (including EMR systems) in healthcare face a number of security risks that result from threats against information confidentiality, integrity and availability as well as against the patients' privacy. Legislation and regulation mandates that action is taken by healthcare organization management towards effectively mitigating these risks. A large variety of suitable technical solutions exist; however what is usually missing is a comprehensive information security management approach. Guidance towards such approaches is provided by a number of international standards. Hence, all the necessary ingredients for achieving security and privacy efficient EMR systems are there. It is up to the health professionals, the healthcare managers and their information systems staff and consultants to obtain, use and maintain their systems in ways respectful of the security of health information and of the privacy of patients, to the benefit of both patients and healthcare organizations.

References

1. http://www.transparencymarketresearch.com/healthcare-cloud-computing.html. Accessed 30 January 2013.
2. http://www.frost.com/prod/servlet/press-release.pag?docid=267265445. Accessed 30 January 2013.
3. HIMSS, 5th Annual HIMSS Security Survey, December 12, 2012, available at http://www.himss.org/content/files/2012_HIMSS_SecuritySurvey.pdf. Accessed 30 January 2013.
4. B. Schneier, Economics and Information Security, June 29, 2006, http://www.schneier.com/blog/archives/2006/06/economics_and_i_1.html. Accessed January 30, 2013.
5. D. Garets, M. Davis, "Electronic Medical Records vs. Electronic Health Records: Yes, there is a difference", A HIMSS Analytics White Paper, January 26, 2006. Available at http://www.himssanalytics.org/docs/wp_emr_ehr.pdf. Accessed 30 January 2013.
6. ISO, "Health Informatics—Requirements for an Electronic Health Record Architecture", ISO/TS 18308, 2003.
7. ISO, "Health Informatics—Electronic Health Record—Definition, scope and context", ISO/TR 20514, 2005.
8. P. Tang, J. Ash, D. Bates, J. Overhage, D. Sands, "Personal Health Records: Definitions, Benefits, and Strategies for Overcoming Barriers to Adoption", J. of American Medical Informatics Association, Vol. 13, no. 2, 2006, pp. 121–126.
9. R. Zhang, L. Liu, "Security models and requirements for healthcare application clouds", in Proceedings, 3rd International Conference on Cloud Computing (CLOUD), IEEE Press, pp. 268–275, 2010. Available at http://csrc.nist.gov/publications/nistpubs/800-12/800-12-html/index.html. Accessed 30 January 2013.
10. National Institute of Standards and Technology, An Introduction to Computer Security: The NIST Handbook, US Department of Commerce, 1995.
11. A. Pouloudi, "Focus: Conflicting concerns over the privacy of electronic medical records in the NHSnet", Business Ethics, vol. 6, no. 2, 1997.
12. S. D. Warren, L. D. Brandeis, "The right to privacy", Harvard Law Review, vol. 4, issue 193, 1890.
13. S. Katsikas, J. Lopez, G. Pernul, "The challenge for security and privacy services in distributed health settings", in B. Blobel, P. Pharow, M. Nerlich (Eds.), eHealth: Combining health telematics, telemedicine, biomedical engineering and bionfiromatics to the edge, IOS Press, 2008, pp. 113–125.
14. ISO/IEC, "Health Informatics—Information security management in health using ISO/IEC 27002", ISO/IEC 27799, 2008.
15. American Health Information Management Association, "Auditing copy and paste", Journal of American Health Information Management Association, vol. 80, issue 1, 2009, pp. 26–29.

16. L. B. Harman, C. A. Flite, K. Bond, "Electronic Health Records: Privacy, Confidentiality and Security", Virtual Mentor, Vol. 14, number 9, 2012, pp. 712–719.
17. G. Narayana Samy, R. Ahmad, Z. Ismail, "Security threats categories in healthcare information systems", Health Informatics Journal, Vol. 16, number 3, 2010, pp. 201–209.
18. I. Maglogiannis, E. Zafiropoulos, "Modeling risk in distributed healthcare information systems", in Proceedings of 28th Annual International Conference of the IEEE on Engineering in Medical and Biology Society (EMBS), 2006, pp. 5447–5450.
19. I. Maglogiannis, E. Zafiropoulos, A. Platis, C. Lambrinoudakis, "Risk analysis of a patient monitoring system using Bayesian network modelling", Journal of Biomedical Informatics, Vol. 39, 2006, pp. 637–647.
20. ENISA, Being diabetic in 2011: Identifying emerging and future risks in remote health monitoring and treatment, 2009.
21. http://www.hhs.gov/ocr/privacy/hipaa/administrative/privacyrule/index.html. Accessed 14 April 2013.
22. http://www.hhs.gov/ocr/privacy/hipaa/administrative/securityrule/. Accessed 14 April 2013.
23. http://healthcare.partners.org/phsirb/hipaaglos.htm. Accessed 14 April 2013.
24. http://www.hhs.gov/ocr/hipaa. Accessed 14 April 2013.
25. S. Kahn, V. Sheshadri, "Medical record privacy and security in a digital environment", IT Pro, March/April, 2008, pp. 46–52.
26. http://www.hhs.gov/ocr/privacy/hipaa/administrative/breachnotificationrule/. Accessed 14 April 2013.
27. http://www2.ftc.gov/opa/2009/08/hbn.shtm. Accessed 14 April 2013.
28. K. T. Win, "A review of security of electronic health records", Health Information Management, Vol. 34, no. 1, 2005, pp. 13–18.
29. http://eur-lex.europa.eu/LexUriServ/LexUriServ.do?uri=CELEX:31995L0046:en:NOT. Accessed 14 April 2013.
30. M. Verschuuren et al., "The European data protection legislation and its consequences for public health monitoring: a plea for action", European Journal of Public Health, Vol. 18, no. 6, 2008, pp. 550–551.
31. R. Clark, "Implications of the EU data protection directive and council of Europe recommendations for healthcare establishments", In The ISHTAR Consortium (Eds.), Implementing Secure Healthcare Telematics Applications in Europe, IOS Press, 2001, pp. 33–52.
32. C. Laske, "Legal liability for telemedicine and healthcare networking", in The ISHTAR Consortium (Eds.), Implementing Secure Healthcare Telematics Applications in Europe, IOS Press, 2001, pp. 53–100.
33. http://ec.europa.eu/justice/newsroom/data-protection/news/120125_en.htm. Accessed 14 April 2013.
34. http://www.imia-medinfo.org/new2/pubdocs/Ethics_Eng.pdf. Accessed 14 April 2013.
35. http://library.ahima.org/xpedio/groups/public/documents/ahima/bok1_024277.hcsp?dDocName=bok1_024277. Accessed 14 April 2013.
36. ISO/IEC, "Information technology—Security techniques—Code of practice for information security management", ISO/IEC 27002, 2005.
37. http://www.27000.org/iso-27002.htm. Accessed 14 April 2013.
38. http://www.iso.org/iso/catalogue_detail?csnumber=41298. Accessed 14 April 2013.
39. S. Katsikas, "Risk Management", in J. Vacca (Ed.), Computer and Information Security Handbook, Morgan Kaufmann, 2009.
40. ISO/IEC, "Information technology—security techniques—information security risk management", ISO/IEC 27005:2011 (E).
41. S. K. Katsikas, S. Kokolakis, "High-level Security Policies for Health Care Establishments", in B. Blobel (Ed). Health Informatics, IOS Press, 2003, pp. 98–104.
42. C. Cresson-Wood, Information Security Policies Made Easy, Baseline Software, USA, 1991.
43. S. K. Katsikas, D. G. Gritzalis, "The Need for a Security Policy in Health Care Institutions", Int. J. of Biomedical Computing, Vol. 35 (Suppl.), 1994, pp 73–81.

44. S. K. Katsikas, D. Gritzalis, "High Level Security Policy Guidelines", in Data Security for Health Care, Vols I-III, The SEISMED Consortium (Eds), IOS Press, 1996, pp. 57–81 (Vol. I), 164–188 (Vol. II), 53–77 (Vol. III).
45. S. K. Katsikas, "Health Care Management and Information Systems Security: Awareness, Training or Education?", Int. J. of Medical Informatics, Vol. 60, 2000, pp. 129–135.
46. J. Davey, "IT security training", in: ISHTAR Consortium (Eds.), in The ISHTAR Consortium (Eds.), Implementing Secure Healthcare Telematics Applications in Europe, IOS Press, 2001, pp. 149–166.
47. G. Aggelinos, S. Katsikas, "Enterprise Recovery in Health Care", in P. Bath, K. Albright, T. Norris (Eds.), Proceedings of the 12th International Symposium on Health Information Management Research - ISHIMR, 2007, pp 63–73.
48. ISO/IEC, "Information technology–Security techniques—Guidelines for information and communications technology disaster recovery services", ISO/IEC 24762:2008.
49. M. Swanson, P. Bowen, A. W. Phillips, D. Gallup, D. Lynes, Contingency Planning Guide for Federal Information Systems, NIST Special Publication 800–34 Rev. 1, available at http://csrc.nist.gov/publications/nistpubs/800-34-rev1/sp800-34-rev1_errata-Nov11-2010.pdf. Accessed 14 April 2013.
50. ISO/IEC, "Information technology—Security techniques—Information security incident management", ISO/IEC TR 18044, 2004.
51. G. Aggelinos, S. K. Katsikas, "Disaster Recovery Analysis and Management Method (DRAMM): An IT Management tool", in Proceedings, Panhellenic Conference on Informatics (PCI) 2012, Piraeus, Greece, IEEE Press, 2012.
52. D. Gritzalis, K. Mavroudakis, S. K. Katsikas, "Developing a European Computer Security Incident Reporting Service for Health Care", in The ISHTAR Consortium (Eds.), Implementing Secure Healthcare Telematics Applications in Europe, IOS Press, 2001, pp. 181–248.

Chapter 19
Towards Personalized Services in the Healthcare Domain

Maria-Anna Fengou, Georgia Athanasiou, Georgios Mantas, Ismini Griva and Dimitrios Lymberopoulos

Introduction

Healthcare services are designed for enabling the provision of medical care to the patient. The traditional healthcare services are based on the doctor-centric paradigm. Essentially, they enable healthcare providers to assess patients' health status based on information derived from medical examination and information stored in patient's electronic Medical Health Records (eMHRs) [1]. Hence, it is crucial for patient's health data to be digitalized and organized in such a way allowing their exploitation by the healthcare provider at a later point of time [2].The doctor-centric healthcare services enhance healthcare providers' diagnosing skills and enable them to give patients accurate treatment directions aiming to their earlier and safer de-hospitalization.

However, patients suffering from chronic diseases require healthcare services for prevention of emergent events before they become life-threatening. The diagnostic and treating nature of doctor-centric healthcare can not satisfy this requirement. Additionally, the doctor-centric paradigm fails on accomplishing the rising demand for the provision of low cost healthcare services to different population groups [3]. These deficiencies generated the need for adopting a different type of healthcare services in which the patient is the core entity. In consequence, the doctor-centric paradigm shifted to the patient-centric paradigm.

Patient's normal and productive life constitutes the main objective of the patient-centric paradigm. To achieve that, the deterioration of patient's health condition should always be prevented. This requirement implies the provision of personalized healthcare services to the patient at the right time, right place and right manner without

M.-A. Fengou (✉), G. Athanasiou, G. Mantas, D. Lymberopoulos
Department of Electrical and Computer Engineering, University of Patras, Rio, Patras, Greece
e-mail: afengoum@upatras.gr

I. Griva
Military Hospital Army Institute of Nursing Nimitz, Athens, Greece

B. Furht and A. Agarwal (eds.), *Handbook of Medical and Healthcare Technologies*,
DOI: 10.1007/978-1-4614-8495-0_19,

temporal and spatial limitations [4]. The continuous and uninterrupted provision of healthcare services is achieved via ubiquitous computing and networking technology. In addition, the personalization of healthcare services is achieved by exploiting the use of user profiles incorporating the preferences and the interests of the user (e.g., patient, doctor, nurse) as well as contextual and bio information related to the user. Finally, in the context of patient-centric paradigm, the notion of context-awareness is required since contextual information is essential for deployment of personalized healthcare services.

Related Work

Studying the evolution of e-health systems through last decade, it is noticed that the whole research focuses on the improvement of accurate detection of emergent events. To achieve that, the aspects of personalization and context-awareness are introduced in e-health systems. Moreover, the notion of personalization is used for effective decision making regarding the proper management of emergent events. Below, it is exposed how the feature of personalization is captured in various projects.

AMON [5, 6]

This project introduces a portable telemedical monitor providing advanced care and alert. The innovation of this project is a wrist worn device that incorporates a number of sensors and the appropriate software for online analysis and emergency detection. The feature of personalization is detected on algorithms analyzing patient's vital signs, taking into account patient's profile (age, gender, fitness and medical history) and activity information (aerobic and nonaerobic state). The result of this kind of personalized emergency detection is the reduction of false negative or positive alarms. In case an abnormality is detected, data are sent for further analysis and evaluation to Management System of Telemonitoring Center. The measured data are compared to previous medical results in order the initial diagnosis to be produced. If needed, the doctor is alerted for evaluating the initial diagnosis based on patient's profile stored on server. The patient's profile includes medical records, such as medical history, medications and other personal information like ways to contact the patient.

WEALTHY [7, 8]

In this project, research focuses on sensors. The goal of this work is the design of a wearable healthcare system which enables the simultaneous measuring of multiple vital signs and further exportation of needed parameters for alerting incidents detection. The introduced personalization in alerting functions enabled the delivery of targeting set of information. The whole procedure leads to creation of synoptic health status tables for each patient which can be used as basis for development of efficient personalized healthcare monitoring and alerting systems.

MediNet [9, 10]
In MediNet project, the concept of personalization is thoroughly explained and defined. The proposed mobile healthcare system provides a personalized self-care process to patients suffering from diabetes and cardiovascular disease. The process applied in MediNet system has been designed in the spirit of personalization. Moreover, patient's vital parameters are analyzed in personalized perspective. Finally, patient's interface has been modified in order to accomplish patient's personal preferences and needs. Regarding personalization in system's process, it is achieved in two levels. The common characteristics of patients having the same disease constitute the first level of personalization. The so-called *Group Level* personalization is defined as a macro-form of personalization enabling coarse-grained decision based on parameters such as type of disease, sex, age group and severity of disease. In a second level, personalization is confined on individual patient's characteristics. The *Individual Level* of personalization constitutes the further refined form of, where decision are made on parameters such as lifestyle, disability, socioeconomics position, prognosis, location and daily activities. Furthermore, MediNet system personalizes parameters in the dimensions of patient's profile, patient's context and location, content and goal of treatment process. Patient's interface has been developed in a personalized way as patient's personal characteristics, preference and capability are taken into consideration, besides engine's recommendations.

HeartCycle [11, 12]
This project represents a conceptual approach of a Personalized Health System (PHS). The proposed PHS system provides professional healthcare at home. The PHS is represented through two intervening closed loops corresponding to patient and healthcare provider. Essentially, the two closed loops are a patient-oriented platform in collaboration with and a healthcare provider-oriented platform. Personalization is detected on the provided services, i.e., measurement, detection and prediction, analysis and decision, therapy and feedback. The continuous reconfiguration of optimal treatment plan for each patient is the ultimate expression of personalization in this project. HeartCycle system consists of Heart Failure Management, Guide Exercise and Assessment subsystems. In these subsystems personalization is expressed through the architecture.

SEMPATH [13, 14]
In this project the concept of personalization is approached as a process continuous estimation of the best treatment scheme given patient's health status and context. The utilized technology to achieve personalization is ontology and rule-based techniques.

CHRONIOUS [15, 16]
Within the context of CHRONIOUS project, an enhanced model-platform was designed for forthcoming chronic disease management systems. Besides personalization, CHRONIOUS platform captures better the features of context-awareness and ubiquity. The CHRONIOUS project aims at the establishment of a personalized coaching healthcare system. CHRONOUS system advises users on adjusting their lifestyle to their health status requirements. In CHRONIOUS system, it is defined

that use of profile makes personalization feasible. Profiles' content is an accurate description of patient's health status. Profiles are used on identification of emergent conditions and on suggestion of proper treatment plans. The intelligent part of CHONIOUS system, i.e., Smart Assistant Device and Clinical Framework makes use of profiles, where vital signs analysis and understanding takes place. In CHRONIOUS project, the feature of personalization is enhanced regarding therapeutic plans making decisions because besides patient's vital signs, nutrition habits and drug intake are taken into consideration.

MiCARE [17]
MiCARE is a contemporary project meeting the challenges of modern healthcare. This project approaches the concept of personalization from a different point of view. By definition, personalized services are designed and provided in such a way in order to meet user's current needs and preferences. In MiCARE project, personalization is expressed in services, i.e., each personalized service is approached as a different integration and orchestration of inherited services over heterogeneous systems. However, in the context of MiCARE project, personalization is also expressed through the assignment of the roles to the appropriate medical staff given time, location and procedure.

Mobihealth [18, 19]
MobiHealth project attempts to incorporate the features of specialization, customization and personalization on the provided healthcare services as these features are widely considered as success criteria. Therefore, each provided application is targeting to a different group of patients. That is achieved as each patient is monitored by sensors specialized for his/her disease and the sensoring data are analyzed in a personalized way so as the feedback is provided. To achieve that, in MobiHealth project has been developed a context-aware service platform enabling adaptability of service delivery to user's current location, time, activity, preferences and needs. In that way, the patient takes a more active role in health process, which is the ultimate goal of personalization. The feature of personalization is introduced in the proposed platform in order to enhance the scalability of the supported services which will cover the needs of niche healthcare cases requiring simultaneous monitoring of small number of patient to large scale chronic disease management process.

OLDES [20–22]
This project aims to provide elderly people with personalized proactive and prospective health services through a proper implementation of tele-monitoring, tele-assistance, tele-healthcare and tele-medicine. OLDES project addresses the challenge of personalization through developing a health and care social platform meeting older people (i.e., user), caregiver and social network's needs and preferences. In this project, it has been studied the perspective of co-production, i.e., a socially-organized, situated driven methodology enabling open interventions of dynamically created multi-agency user communities. In order communication and information sharing between care agencies to be enhanced an advanced user profiling system, called Knowledge Management (KM) is introduced in OLDES platform.

EPI-MEDIDS (2002-2009) [23–25]
EPI-MEDICS project focuses on the development of a Personal ECG Monitoring embedding intelligent decision-making techniques for early detection of cardiac events, generation of proper alarm levels and forwarding of alarm messages to relevant healthcare providers. EPI-MEDICS is designed to the direction of ubiquitous, wearable and personalized healthcare. Decision making EPI-MEDIC system is personalized because patient's vital signs are evaluated by taking consideration of patient's risk factor stored in patient's health record. Moreover, the fact that the system interacts with the patient in order to be aware of his/her symptoms, enhances EPI-MEDIS system's personalization. EPI-MEDICS' personal monitor is supported by a web server where they are stored the patient's recorder vital signs, user information, clinical history etc. Healthcare provider while attending patient, he/she accesses EPI-MEDICS web server in order to observe the patient's personal data or to adjust decision making criteria of alarm generation. That kind of personalization entered in EPI-MEDICS system enables better handling of medium alarms.

MyHeart [26, 27]
In the context of MyHeart project, a framework for Personal Healthcare Application is being developed. In MyHeart project, personalized algorithms that take consideration of user's needs, goal and profile provide the appropriate feedback and consequently the desired personalized service.

Based on the aforementioned projects, the main objective of the current e-health systems is to assist patient on prevention, diagnosis, treatment, and lifestyle management. This enables patients to be more conscious regarding their health status without being socially isolated.

Current e-health systems are multi-state, event-driven platforms providing telemedicine services through healthcare applications [28]. The provided services which aim on prevention are characterized as proactive and those provided services which target on diagnosis and treatment are characterized as reactive [9]. Thus, healthcare monitoring and lifestyle management services under the view of prevention from emergent events are considered as proactive services. On the other hand, detection of an emergent event and activation of the appropriate treatment plans are reactive services.

Personalized Healthcare Services

The patient-centric paradigm considers the patient to be the core entity of healthcare environment. As depicted in Fig. 19.1, the healthcare environment is composed by diverse collaborating entities required for the provision of personalized healthcare services to the patient. Essentially, the health status of patient constitutes the heart of personalized healthcare services because it is the inception for their provision [29].

As defined in [28], the entities included into the healthcare environment are:

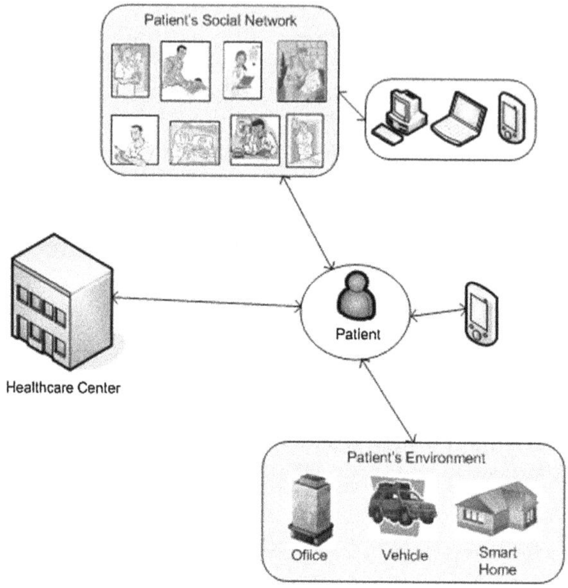

Fig. 19.1 Healthcare Environment in patient-centric paradigm [28]

- Subjects: The patient as well as a number of individuals serving pre-defined roles during the execution of the service. The group of all involved individuals for each case is referred as "patient's social network". Subjects can also be any healthcare provider taking the roles of medical professionals (e.g., doctors, nurses) and the roles of caregivers (e.g., relatives, volunteers). Each role defines the contribution of each subject on the provision of required personalized healthcare services.
- Objects: ICT (Information and Communications Technology) components deployed around the subjects. They consist of bio-sensors, context-aware sensors, GPS, mobile terminals, etc. They yield also the complementary real time information required for the provision of personalized healthcare services.
- Operational Domains: Places, where the personalized healthcare services are provided. These domains are divided into patient's personal space (e.g., homes, offices, vehicles) and medical units (e.g., healthcare centers pharmacies etc).

In the context of patient-centric paradigm, the deployment of personalized healthcare services, as depicted in Fig. 19.2, exploits information stored in the patient's profile and the profiles of any subject of patient's social network. If this information is related with real-time acquired context information (e.g., temperature, geoposition, etc) then the service is characterized as Context-Aware. Finally, the application of ubiquitous computing upon patient's context data acquired anytime and anyplace leads to the development of ubiquitous personalized healthcare services.

Especially each subject is represented by his/her corresponding user profile including his/her own attributes and properties. User profile of patient stores all information

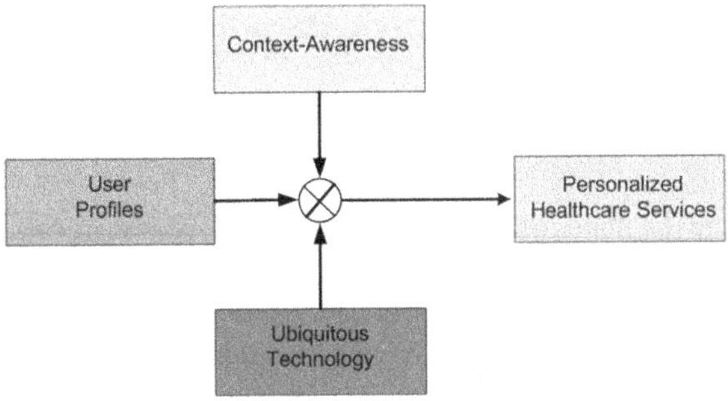

Fig. 19.2 Main features of personalized healthcare services

required for personalization of healthcare services, such as his/her health status, prevailing environmental situations, lists with preferred participants to his/her social network, carrying device's capabilities etc. User profiles of other subjects contain information determining both their capability and willingness to participate in the provision of personalized healthcare services for the patient. For instance, doctor's user profile may include information regarding his/her availability for providing healthcare service.

Context-Awareness is an enabling technology for personalized healthcare services. Essentially, context-awareness is an indispensable feature of personalized healthcare services because it guides them how to be customized [30]. A personalized healthcare system can not make the right decision for the patient's treatment without the appropriate contextual information. Usually, contextual information is captured by sensors.

Ubiquitous computing is a new technology paradigm incorporating distributed computing and mobile computing. The main objective of ubiquitous computing paradigm is to bridge the gap between virtual world and physical world integrating seamlessly information and communication technologies with people in their daily lives. Ubiquitous computing is crucial for the personalized healthcare services in order to be provided to anyone, anytime and anywhere without location and time constraints [31].

Personalization on both proactive and reactive services indicates a unique integration of different service components provided by different healthcare providers in services satisfying users' needs and preferences. This integration implies the orchestration of different healthcare providers in a treatment scheme with predefined roles delivering the treatment plan [29]. The selection of appropriate healthcare providers for the adoption of the predefined roles in the treatment scheme is a personalized procedure based on the patient's preferences and current needs.

Personalization in Patient-Centric Paradigm

Profiles in Healthcare

Profiles constitute the main mean for the expression of personalization in healthcare services. The deployment of personalized healthcare services is enabled by the use of the profiles of the participating entities that are either directly or indirectly related to the patient when an event is detected denoting that his/her health condition is critical and a ubiquitous healthcare service should be provided [29].

Based on the features of the participating entities, it is essential the existence of a profile structure for each entity. Thus, the generic healthcare profile structures are the following:

- Subject's Healthcare Profile: This profile corresponds to the patient and the patient's social network categories. In general, the Subject Healthcare Profile contains[29, 32]:
  - Personal information: data about or related to the individual (e.g., name, address, age, identifying number), which are extracted by electronic Medical Health Records (eMHRs).
  - Preferences: choices made by the individual about a given parameter (e.g., time, location) that will define or modify the behavior of the personalized service. More complex preferences can be expressed in the form of rules, activities and roles.
  - Rules: statements that can be automatically interpreted in order to define or modify the behavior of the personalized service.
  - Security: specific obligations, access policies and preferences regarding security.
  - Contextual information: Information related to patient's situation and influence on
  - Indexes: Pointers associating a subject with a patient social network.
- Operational Domain Profile: This profile corresponds to the Operational Domain category and it is distinguished to:

  ✓ The Medical Unit's Profile may contain information about [28]:

  - Identification information (e.g., name, address);
  - Critical conditions that can be handled (e.g., cardiac arrest, heart attack);
  - Available equipment and facilities;
  - Schedule of the on duty healthcare center.

  ✓ The Patient's Personal Space Profilemay contain information about [28]:

- Identification information;
- Supporting healthcare services;
- Available equipment facilities;
- Available members for support;
- Context Information.

The types of Patient's Personal Space profiles are [28]:

- Smart Home Profile: This profile corresponds to the Smart Home category;
- Office Profile: This profile corresponds to the Office category;
- Vehicle Profile: This profile corresponds to the Vehicle Profile.

Especially, the subjects move from one operational domain (situation) to another throughout the day (e.g., at home, driving, working). In each of these situations, they may have different needs for how they would like their ICT resources arranged. Thus, a subject can have several situation dependable profiles whose activation and deactivation is based on rules. [32]

Profiles Management System for Personalized Healthcare Provision

The data of the above mentioned profiles may be stored among a number of different storage locations (e.g., mobile devices, PDAs, service provider's databases) [32]. Wherever the data is stored, a profile management system will ensure that the profile data is synchronized when it is required [33].

Hence, in the healthcare domain, a profile management system is required for the efficient support and provision of personalized healthcare services to patients remotely. It is considered that each participating entity in the provision of the healthcare service has its own profile. Thus, the proposed profile management system makes use of a number of *User Healthcare Profiles* and *Patient's Personal Space Profiles* [29]. The incorporated data of each profile are stored in distributed databases.

The patients are being monitored by the system in order any critical event to be detected timely. When such an event is detected, a patient's social network profile (referred *group profile* in [28, 29]) is triggered to be created. This profile's structure allows healthcare systems to compose multiparty group-working schemes with preselected behaviors of all involved subjects [29]. In the group profile, each subject has a specific role with defined activities. The intention of each subject to participate or not is detected by his current individual profile. The dynamic creation of group profile describing the behavior and roles of all the participating entities in the group for the provision of personalized healthcare services to the patient enables the real time collaboration of the participating entities.

The main objective of the profile management system in the healthcare domain is the creation of group profiles in order to provide high quality and reliable personalized healthcare services to the patients [29]. The group profile is created based on the indexes stored in the User Healthcare Profiles. Each patient's profile contains an index to a group profile that is triggered whenever an event is detected. The events are related to the patient's health condition and they denote that the patient needs a medical advice or care due to aggravation of his/her health condition. The group is formed through certain management, scheduling and notification events [29].

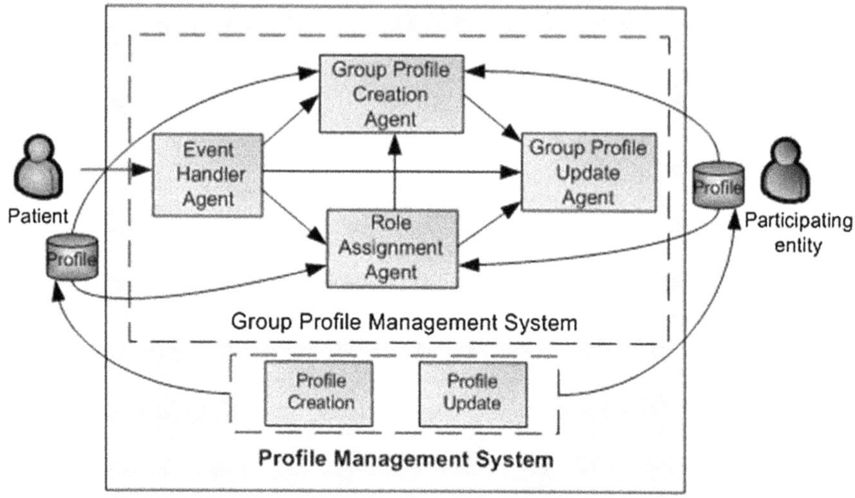

Fig. 19.3 Profile management system [29]

The profile management system integrates the following mechanisms: *Profile Creation*, *Profile Update*, *Event Handler*, *Role Assignment*, *Group ProfileCreate*, *Group Profile Update* implemented by agents as depicted in Fig. 19.3 [28].

The profile management system based on the profiles and the current context activates the appropriate mechanisms for the management of the group profile of the entities that will participate in the provision of the healthcare service to the patient.

These mechanisms deal with the context information management, as well as the individual and group profile management [28]. The deployed profiling mechanisms are based on the gathered context information, on the presence of organized and structured profiles, and the assignment of roles for the creation of group profiles [29]. Different profiling mechanisms are activated according to individual's profile, which changes, as individual's current context changes. These profiling mechanisms can be considered as simple components that can be integrated to implement personalized services [29].

The profiling mechanisms [28, 29] are described below:

- Profile Creation: Every individual is considered to have his/her profile and is added to the system as user. The profile is initially created by fundamental data that then are completed from supplementary sources. During the creation, information and preferences are also gathered from services and devices in order to populate the profile. The creation can be based on (a) explicit methods where the user actively defines the attributes, (b) implicit methods where the prefrences are inferred by monitoring user behavior or (c) combination of explicit and implicit [32]. This procedure is usually enhanced be the usage of templates in its first steps.
- Profile Update: Since the individual profile is established, it is continually maintained either manually or automatically with the usage of monitoring components,

which enable its update. Moreover, this mechanism supports services and applications to automatically suggest updates to the profile. It is important to ensure that the values of the attributes meet the user's preferences for the current context.
- Event Handler: This mechanism is responsible to detect and handle the events that trigger the creation of the group profile. These events are related to the transition of the patient's health condition from one state to another. An event can be defined as a significant change in specific bio or contextual information captured by the corresponding bio or contextual sensors. This mechanism is used to evaluate the events in order the appropriate decisions to be taken. For example, an event can denote that the patient needs a medical advice or attention and care due to aggravation of his health condition. Thus, this mechanism activates the creation of the group profile for the provision of personalized healthcare services.
- Role Assignment: This mechanism assigns roles to the potential entities of the group in order the creation of the group profile to be achieved. It defines the roles that are required and invites the potential entities in order to build the group. Each role has its competences as when a conference is convened. The patient (his health condition) and the formed group function as the convener and the participants of the session respectively.
- Group Profile Creation: This mechanism is used for the creation of the group profile. The activation of this mechanism is event-driven. Whenever an event (e.g., the patient's health condition is deteriorated) is detected by the event-handler, the group profile is created based on the pointers that are stored in the patient's profile. The entities of the group that will participate are specific. The information stored in their profiles determines whether an entity meets the conditions in order to participate. A coordinator is also defined in the group depending on the roles that participate for the provision of a UH service. For instance, if an emergency service is delivered, then a medical professional (e.g., doctor) will be responsible to coordinate the group in order all the participating entities to collaborate efficiently.
- Group Profile Update: This mechanism is used for the update of the group profile. After the activation of the group profile, collaborative actions may follow such as decision-support and profile-sharing depending on the patient's health condition. In addition, the attributes of each participant may change dynamically over time. The participants' presence is constantly verified. Moreover, if a new event is detected by the event handler, an additional role may be required and as a result another entity will be added in the already formed group.

Thus, the profile management system will enable the profiles to be [32, 33]:

- Created (mention data editing, e.g., creation templates update etc.).
- Stored: The data should be stored in a secure manner with user agreed levels of privacy applied to the availability and distribution of that data.
- Accessed: Ideally, profile data should always be available, overall networks, from all supported devices and services, including fixed and mobile services allowing service continuity and optimal user experience. The access control needs to respect principles regarding user control and legal policies.

- Synchronized: Data at different locations should be kept consistent, which may be ensured by synchronization of data and transaction security. However, although the profile data (or copies of profile data) can be distributed amongst devices and services, it should be possible to ensure that users can have the concept of centralized profiles which cover all of their devices and services.

Moreover, the profile management system:

- synchronizes all the profiles of involving entities in a provision of a personalized healthcare service.
- controls the access of different entities on patient's profile respecting his preferences and legal policies. There are general policies that define what access the entity may have to the patient's profile. However, these policies can be overwritten if the patient has defined related sharing preferences stored in his profile.

There is a variety of stakeholder entities with different objectives regarding the way they exploit/take advantage of the profile management system [33].

- End-users want to personalize their provided healthcare services in order to get the maximum of expected user experience.
- User profile providers offer all required mechanisms in order to define the users' preferences in their user profiles.
- Network providers not only take advantage of profile management system because they exploit them for personalizing their services but also they enhance profile management system functionality by providing them services such as storage and transfer of user profile and service data, data synchronization and capability negotiation.
- Service and device providers use profile management systems for personalizing their service and device, accordingly. Profile management systems, in their turn, take advantage of them for updating user profiles.

Therefore, the profile management systems provide benefit to users, primary, but also to different types of third party providers certificated by users to manage their profile content and certificated users exploiting profile information owing stakeholder.

Scenario of a Personalized Healthcare Service

In this section, we demonstrate a real world scenario depicting the way a personalized healthcare service is provided to a chronic patient. This scenario is designed to focus on the fundamentals of the personalized services without considering advanced functionality, such as the ubiquitous computing.

Christos is a 57 year old man living in Lesvos, an island of East Aegean Sea far away from the Greek mainland. 15 years ago he was diagnosed with diabetes but he was under poor glucaimic control. Besides that, 6 months ago he had a heart attack for which he was transferred and hospitalized to Hippokrateio General Hospital in Athens.

In that hospital, Christos was submitted to Coronary artery bypass surgery. He de-hospitalized 4 weeks later with instructions for strict control of his arterial pressure, blood sugar and cholesterol. Moreover, he was advised to quit smoking immediately, lose weight and in general follow a healthier way of life.

Christos' wife, Mary, contributes to his rehabilitation by helping him have a healthier nutrition and quit his bad habit as well as comply with his medical treatment.

Even if, Christos complies with medical advises, the fact that he is a diabetic patient makes him vulnerable to the appearance of a life-threatening event of silent ischemia. That is the major problem for the diabetics because it may develop while the patient has no symptoms or pain of any kind. As a result the condition goes undiagnosed and untreated and has higher probabilities for lethal.

For these reasons, Christos should be continuously and uninterrupted monitored by a system in order any critical event to be detected timely.

We consider a Smart Home to be the environment supporting the required tele-monitoring system. It is equipped with the appropriate sensors for gathering context and bio information as well as integrates the essential residential networks for the provision of requested healthcare services remotely. A bio EKG monitor could identify myocardial strain and alert the patient or his relatives at an early stage. Moreover, an acute coronary event could be diagnosed by the doctor while the patient is still on his way to the hospital providing time for early intervention such as thromvolysis. In addition blood pressure, blood sugar and cholesterol levels can be monitored at any time so that any doctor can alter the medication, providing better control for patients living far away from the general hospitals of Athens.

In addition to Mary, a number of other individuals contribute in order Christos has a healthy living. For instance, his diabetologist assesses Christos' biosignals for calibrating his glucaimic control. Obviously a social network is organized around Christos for providing him the appropriate healthcare services. Each participant in Christos' social network is represented by his/her profile which determines how it contributes on Christos' rehabilitation. Table 19.1 concentrates all participants of Christos social network and defines the actions required to be accomplished in each case.

Based on this scenario, we consider the use of Christos' profile, a number of profiles of doctors and nurses related to Christos and a set of profiles of Christos' relatives e.g., his wife.

To achieve personalized services, the e-health tele-monitoring system creates dynamically a group of eligible subjects (e.g., doctor, wife) to provide care to Christos when his health condition requires it. The proposed Profile Management System is used integrating the following mechanisms: Event Handler, Group Profile Creation, Group Profile Update.

If the current state of Christos health condition justifies the sharing of the emergency-related information from his profile, this information may be necessary to be shared with a participating entity (e.g., doctor). The sharing will be based both on general policies that define what access the participating entity may have to Christos's profile and on Christos's sharing preferences.

Table 19.1 Analysis of the scenario

Stakeholder	Relationship to client	e-health profile
Christos (patient)		• He uses a tele-health monitoring package in order to monitor his blood pressure, blood sugar and cholesterol levels in order to make alterations of his diet and medication (diabetics alter the dose of insulin based on self-monitoring) • The system alerts him, whenever acute changes of his bio markers take place including silent ischemia
Mary (Wife-caregiver)	Health profile (monitored health data, smoking condition, diet)	• She helps Christos to follow all the medical instructions • She arranges Christos special diet of low sugar, low fat, low salt • She deprives from Christos his smoking facilities • She is informed of any dangerous life threatening event so that she can transfer Christos to hospital in case of emergency • The system helps Mary to form her shopping list according to Christos' needs for low sugar, low fat, low salt diet
Diabetologist (medical professional)	Health Profile (monitored health data, smoking condition, diet)	• He supervises Christos' health condition • He makes alterations on Christos' medical treatment • He reminds Christos to make check-up twice a year
Pharmasist (medical professional)	Diet, glucose levels	• He determine Christos' needs for insulin and make arrangement for insulin supplies
Cardiologist (medical professional)	Health profile (monitored health data, smoking condition, diet)	• He diagnoses a myocardial infarction while the patient is still on his way to the hospital having time to prepare for treatment in time to prevent myocardial necrosis
Community Doctor (medical professional)	Notifications for emergent events	• He arranges Christos' transportation to a general hospital including the appropriate medical equipment

Conclusions and Future Directions

This chapter presented the basic aspects of the personalized healthcare services that are provided through the novel ICT infrastructures. The deployment of patient-centric healthcare services is a multidisciplinary task requiring the contribution of different technologies and the collaboration of many entities. From a technology point of view, personalized healthcare services exploit context-aware, user profile structures within a ubiquitous healthcare environment.

The main objectives of these services are the support of patients, especially elderly people and people with chronic diseases, in order to have an independent and safe way of life as well as the efficient collaboration of all healthcare providers involved in the treatment process. Current applied personalized healthcare services focus on facilitation of persistent patients' health status monitoring and on customization of treatment based on patient's needs and preferences. The personalized healthcare services also facilitate the self-help purposes. In addition, they facilitate the collaboration of diverse authorized subjects, objects and operational domains for the provision of accurate and timely-critical healthcare assistance.

In this chapter, we focused on the necessity of the profiles of any subject, object and operational domain involved in the establishment and provision of personalized healthcare services. Furthermore, we analyzed the structure and the functionality of a profile management system for these services. Finally, we demonstrated an operational scenario for the provision of personalized healthcare services under real world conditions.

References

1. P. Sanjoy, and S. Karthik, "On-demand health care: a new paradigm for e-health," Proceedings of the International Conference on e-Health Networking, Applications and Services (HealthCom2009), 2009.
2. R. Bali, A. Dwivedi and R. Naguib, "The Efficacy of Knowledge Management for Personalised Healthcare," Book Chapter of "Personalised Health Management Systems - The Integration of Innovative Sensing, Textile, Information and Communication technologies", IOS Press 2015, pp. 104–107.
3. L. Wilcox, D. Morris, D. Tan, J. Gatewood, "Designing patient-centric information displays for hospitals," Proceedings of the International Conference on Human Factors in, Computing Systems (CHI2010), 2010.
4. Kun-Lung Wu, C.C. Aggrawal, P.S. Yu, "Personalization with Dynamic Profiler," Proceedings of the International Workshop on, Information Systems (WECWIS2001), 2001.
5. U. Anliker, J. Ward, P. Lukowicz, G. Tröster, F. Dolveck, M. Baer, F. Keita, E. Schenker, F. Catarsi, L. Coluccini, A. Belardinelli, D. Shklarski, M. Alon, E. Hirt, R. Schmid and M. Vuskovic, "AMON: A Wearable Multiparameter Medical Monitoring and Alert System", IEEE Transactions on Information Technology in Biomedicine, Vol. 8, issue 4, 2004, pp. 415–427.
6. P. Lukowicz, U. Anliker, J. Ward, G. Troster, E. Hirt, C. Neufelt, "AMON: a wearable medical computer for high risk patients," Proceedings of the International Conference on Wearable Computers (ISWC2002), 2002.

7. R. Paradiso, G. Lorige and N. Taccini, "A Wearable Health Care System Based on Knitted Integrated Sensors," IEEE Transactions on Information Technology in Biomedicine, Vol. 9, issue 3, 2005, pp. 337–344.
8. L. Bourdon, S. Coli, G. Loriga, N. Taccini, B. Gros, A. Gemignani, D. Cianflone, F. Chapotot, A. Dittmar, R. Paradiso, "First results with the wealthy garment electrocardiogram monitoring system," Proceedings of the International Conference on, Computers in Cardiology, 2005, p. p. 615–618.
9. P. Mohan, D. Marin, S. Sultan and A. Deen, "MediNet: Personalizing the Self-Care Process for Patients with Diabetes and Cardiovascular Disease Using Mobile Telephony," Proceedings of the International Conference on Engineering in Medicine and Biology Society (EMBC2008), 2008.
10. P. Mohan, S. Sultan, "MediNet: A mobile healthcare management system for the Caribbean region," Proceedings of the International Conference on Mobile and Ubiquitous Systems: Networking and Services (MobiQuitous2009), 2009.
11. H. Reiter, N. Maglavers, "HeartCycle: Compliance and Effective in HF and CAD Closed-Loop Management," Proceedings of the International Conference on Engineering in Medicine and Biology Society (EMBC2009), 2009.
12. N. Maglavers, H. Reiter, "Towards Closed-Loop Personal Health Systems in Cardiology: the HeartCycle Approach," Proceedings of the International Conference on Engineering in Medicine and Biology Society (EMBC2011), 2011.
13. D. Alexandrou, F. Xenikoudakis, G. Mentzas, "SEMPATH: Semantic Adaptive and Personalized Clinical Pathways," Proceedings of the International Conference on eHealth, Telemedicine and Social Medicine (eTELEMED2009), 2009.
14. D. Alexandrou, C.V. Pardalis, A.D. Bouras, G. Mentzas, "SEMPATH Ontology: Modeling multi-disciplinary treatment schemes utilizing semantics," Proceedings of the International Conference on Information Technology and Applications in, Biomedicine (ITAB2010), 2010.
15. R. Rosso, G. Munaro, O. Salvetti, S. Colantonio, F. Ciancitto, "CHRONIOUS: An Open Ubiquitous and Adaptive Platform for Chronic Obstructive Pulmonary Disease (COPD), Chronic Kidney Disease (CKD) and Renal Insufficiency," Proceedings of the International Conference on Engineering in Medicine and Biology Society (EMBC2010), 2010.
16. L. Schneider, M. Brochhausen, "The CHRONIOUS Ontology Suite: Methodology and Design Principles," Proceedings of the International Conference on Biomedical Ontology (ICBO2011), 2011.
17. T.-M. Tsai, J.-T. liu, J. Y. Hsu, "MiCARE: Context-aware Authorization for Integrated Healthcare Services," Proceedings of the International Workshop on Ubiquitous Computing for Pervasive Healthcare Applications (UbiHealth2004), 2004.
18. K. Wac, R. Bults, B. van Beijnum, I. Widya, V. Jones, D. Konstantas, M. Vollenbroek-Hutten, H. Hermens, "Mobile Patient Monitoring: the MobiHealth System," Proceedings of the International Conference on Engineering in Medicine and Biology Society (EMBC2009), 2009.
19. A. van Halteren, D. Konstantas, R. Bults, K. Wac, N. Dokovsky, G. Koprinkov, V. Jones, I. Widya "MobiHealth: Ambulant Patient Monitoring Over Next Generation Public Wireless Networks," E-Health: Current Status and Future Trends, Studies in Health technology and Informatics, Vol. 106, IOS Press, 2004, pp 107–122.
20. Maniatopoulos, G, McLoughlin, I, Wilson, R, and Martin, M. "Developing Virtual Healthcare Systems in Complex Multi-Agency Service Settings: the OLDES Project." Electronic Journal of e-Government Volume 7 Issue 2, 2009, pp. 163–170.
21. D. Novak, M. Uller, S. Rousseaux, M. Mraz, J. Smrz, O. Stepankova, M. Haluzik, M. Busuoli, "Diabetes management in OLDES Project," Proceedings of the International Conference on Engineering in Medicine and Biology Society (EMBC2009), 2009.
22. D. Novak, O. Stepankova, M. Mraz, M. Haluzik, M. Bussoli, M. Uller, K. Maly, L. Novakova, P. Novak, "OLDES: New Solution for long-term diabetes compensation management," Proceedings of the International Conference on Engineering in Medicine and Biology Society (EMBC2008), 2008.

23. H. Atoui, J. Fayn, F. Gueyffier, P. Rubel, "Cardiovascular Risk Stratification in Decision Support Systems: A Probabilistic Approach. Application to pHealth," Proceedings of the International Conference on, Computers in Cardiology, 2006, p. p. 281–284.
24. F. Gouaux, L. Simon-Chautemps, J. Fayn, S. Adami, M. Arzi, D. Assanelli, MC Forlini, C. Malossi, A. Martinez, J. Placide, G.L. Ziliani, P. Rubel, "Ambient Intelligence and Pervasive Systems for the Monitoring of Citizens at Cardiac Risk: New Solutions from the EPI-MEDICS Project," Proceedings of the International Conference on, Computers in Cardiology, 2006, p. p. 289–292.
25. J. Fayn and P. Rubel, "Towards a Personal Health Society in Cardiology", IEEE Transactions on Information Technology in Biomedicine, 2012.
26. S. Guillén, P. Sala, J. Habertha, R. Schmidt, A.-T. Arredondo, "Innovative Concepts for Prevention and Disease Management of Cardiovascular Diseases," Proceedings of the International Conference on Engineering in Medicine and Biology Society (EMBC2006), 2006.
27. M. Harris, J. Habetha, "The MyHeart Project: A Framework for Personal Health Care Applications," Computers in Cardiology, 2007, p.p. 137–140.
28. M. A. Fengou, G. Mantas, D. Lymberopoulos, N. Komninos, S. Fengos and N. Lazarou, "A New Framework Architecture for Next Generation e-Health Services," IEEE Transactions on Information Technology in Biomedicine, 2012.
29. M. A. Fengou, G. Mantas, D. Lymberopoulos, "Group Profile Management in Ubiquitous Healthcare Environment," Proceedings of the International Conference on Engineering in Medicine and Biology Society (EMBC2012), 2012.
30. S. Arbanowski, P. Ballon, K. David, O. Droegehorn, H. Eertink, W. Kellerer, H. van Kranenburg, K. Raatikainen and R. Popescu-Zeletin, "I-centric Communications: Personalization, Ambient Awareness and Adaptability for Future Mobile Services," IEEE Communications Magazine, Vol. 42, issue 9, 2004, pp. 63–69.
31. U. Varshney, "Pervasive Healthcare: "Applications, Challenges And Wireless Solutions," Communications of the Association for Information Systems, AIS Electronic Library, Vol. 16, No. 1, 2005, pp. 57–72.
32. ETSI ES 642 V 1.1.1, "Human Factors (HF); Personalization of eHealth systems by using eHealth user profiles (eHealth)," ETSI Standard, 2010–09.
33. ETSI ES 202 746 V 1.1.1, "Human Factors (HF); Personalization and User Profile Management; User Profile and Information," ETSI Standard, 2010.

Chapter 20
Sensor Infrastructures for Ambient Assisted Living

Olga Murdoch, Jessie Wan, Sameh Abdalla, Michael J. O'Grady and Gregory M. P. O'Hare

Abstract The presence of people on virtual social networks, their interactions, interests and their feedback can be perceived as inputs for assistive healthcare systems to predict a certain risk or condition. In this chapter we address the modern role of Ambient Assisted Living (AAL) in daily life activities. We emphasise the significance of integrating intelligent sensor infrastructures to current AAL architectures. We describe the main features and core architecture of a sensor middleware and introduce the service gateways provided to expand the range of data inputs within AAL architectures. Finally we present a motivating scenario of a healthcare service application, (i.e., iMED), which we are employing as an example to link AAL architectures and Sensor Middlewares.

Introduction

Ambient Assisted Living (AAL) [38] refers to ICT involvements in helping elderly individuals to improve the quality of their lives, stay healthier, and to live independently for longer. AAL is a multidisciplinary research topic that includes a number of technologies and research fields such as sensor networks, pervasive computing, machine learning, ambient intelligence. Extensive research effort have been made across the world to better enhance the current advances of assisted living. Among these efforts is AALJP [2], which is a joint research activity launched in 2008 between 23 European countries with a main goal of providing cost-effective health and social care that can be delivered in the near future while ensuring growth opportunities for European businesses. AALJP has initiated over 100 projects, which are focused on the older person's mobility, social participation and interaction, as well as prevention and management of chronic conditions using ICT technologies.

O. Murdoch · J. Wan · S. Abdalla (✉) · M. J. O'Grady · G. M. P. O'Hare
CLARITY: Centre for Sensor Web Technologies, University College Dublin, Dublin, Ireland
e-mail: sameh@ucd.ie

B. Furht and A. Agarwal (eds.), *Handbook of Medical and Healthcare Technologies*,
DOI: 10.1007/978-1-4614-8495-0_20, © Springer Science+Business Media New York 2013

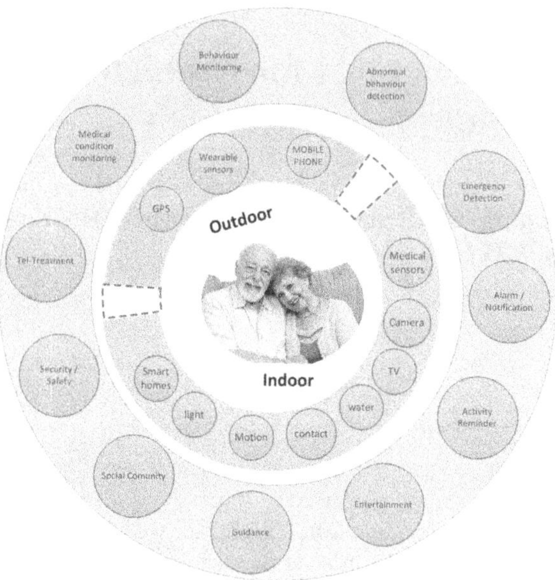

Fig. 20.1 Ambient assisted living generic framework

Sensors and sensor network technologies have been widely adopted as the enabling approach for AAL, especially for elderly people who suffer from cognitive impairment. In Fig. 20.1 we show a generic architecture and configuration of AAL systems. In general, there are two trends in developing AAL systems: one with a focus on outdoor scenarios and another that tackles indoor scenarios. Smarthomes are currently considered as the main testbed for indoor scenarios wherein large amount of sensors with heterogeneous platforms and protocols are installed. In addition, scholars are also investigating body area networks in which a number of wearable sensors can be attached on the human body and interacting with surrounding data sources. In recent years, the improved computation capability of smartphones have been drawing the attention of domain researchers to employ the increasing number of embedded sensors, such as GPS, accelerometers and light sensors, in AAL applications. Therefore, in AAL, smarphones can be perceived as sensing units and data transmission gateways.

Similar to the current advances of AAL, scholars of *Pervasive Computing* are addressing the issue of building highly responsive and self-adaptive systems which aim to increase the integration of technology into the fabric of every day living [39], e.g., smarthomes. In pervasive systems, context as referred to in [5] may comprise the information characterising the situation of any person, place, or object that is considered relevant to the interaction between a user and an application. Context data may be gathered from many sources including physical sensors deployed in the environment (sensing light or sound levels for example) and digital sources such as calendar information and data accessible via the World Wide Web (WWW). The (current) WWW encompasses diverse documents and services that produce and/or maintain real-time and static information relating to a wide range of users, places, topics, and concepts. The fusion of web-based sources of context data with that emitted from physical sensing devices will bridge the divide between the physical and the cyber world, enabling a wealth of web-based and context-aware applications.

As internet based research continues so does the evolution of the WWW where we can now access and utilize a wealth of data and services. Since the birth of social networking in particular, the WWW has become a critical source of data for context-driven applications and *Pervasive Computing* in general. User driven data sourced from real time social networks is being used to provide a richer user experience allowing applications to make recommendations based on information that can be linked to a user. More recent research incorporates context from social networks in particular, resulting in new web services, mashups and user-driven pervasive computing applications [32].

In order to provide rich yet easy-to-adopt services to end users a framework is required that can support the development and use of diverse applications. Such a framework has yet to be widely adopted as middleware and programming framework research efforts focus mainly on solving specific problems to satisfy a particular type of application. We argue that the divide between these separate and differing systems needs to be bridged in order to allow interaction and cooperation between remote systems that may be interconnected through subtle, possibly undetected means.

In order to allow such interactions the provision of a middleware architecture that supports and abstracts acquisition and use of diverse data sources is essential. While research efforts have classified context in terms of its low-level features (for example [25]), we could not find any classification or taxonomy of context in terms of the nature of context given the source it can be derived from. With this in mind, Fig. 20.2 illustrates a taxonomy of context sources and Table 20.1 classifies web-based context-sources according to this taxonomy.

The context source taxonomy not only provides a structured visualisation of how and where data is produced but it illustrates the natural flow of data accessible via the

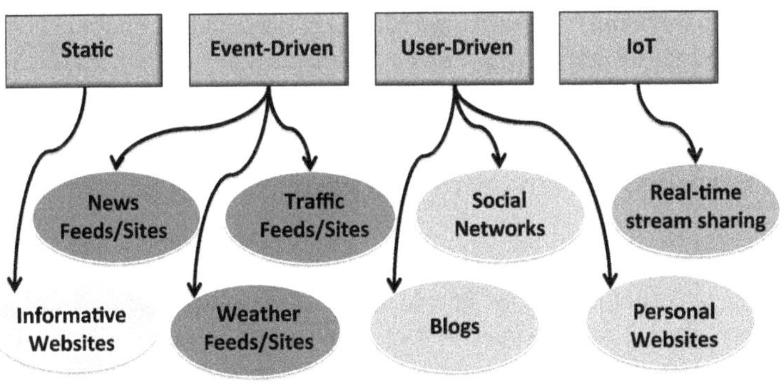

Fig. 20.2 Taxonomy of web-based sources of context

Table 20.1 Classification of web-based context sources

Type	Definition	Examples
Static	Knowledge or fact	Informative or factual documents, Web 1.0
User driven	User provided data where user desire to updates instigates the change	Microblogging, social networks
Event driven	Autonomous or manual reporting as response to event or schedule	Weather websites/API's, news
IoT	Live data stream from remote networks or devices	Pachube, thing speak
Service	Combination of context and application logic to learn more about a data	Klout, peer index

WWW. Whether data is produced by measuring physical elements (using physical sensing devices), web users providing updates, or real time information disseminated about events as and when they occur, this context data can now be passed through various services, transforming "low-level" sensed data into abstract knowledge that can be used to drive applications.

The SIXTH middleware framework adopts this approach in it's provision of cyber sensors and services for use by application developers. A description of SIXTH and explanation of how it is used in the development of diverse context-driven systems follows.

This chapter is organized as follows: In section "AAL literature Review: Sensors Perspective" we review the literature of Ambient Assisted Living (AAL) from Sensors perspective. In section "The Sensor Infrastructure" we present a sensor infrastructure that will have a social impact on common AAL scenarios. In section "Motivating Scenario: iMED" we introduce a service application, (i.e., iMED), that brings together inhabitants of smarthomes, pharmacies, medicines distributors, pharmaceutical companies, navigation systems, and lightweight computing devices (e.g., smartphones). In the final section we introduce a possible integration between the earlier introduced sensor infrastructure and a healthcare service application (Fig. 20.3).

AAL Literature Review: Sensors Perspective

Alzheimer, as a common case of Dementia, is one of the most frequent chronic disease that affects older people. People who suffer from dementia gradually lose skills of everyday life, such as memory loss, wandering, sleeping and eating disorder, depression and so on. Extensive research efforts have been made to discover the nature of Alzheimer's behaviour [15]. However, the early stage of Dementia is commonly seen as normal part of the aging process, as a consequence, the best time for treatment

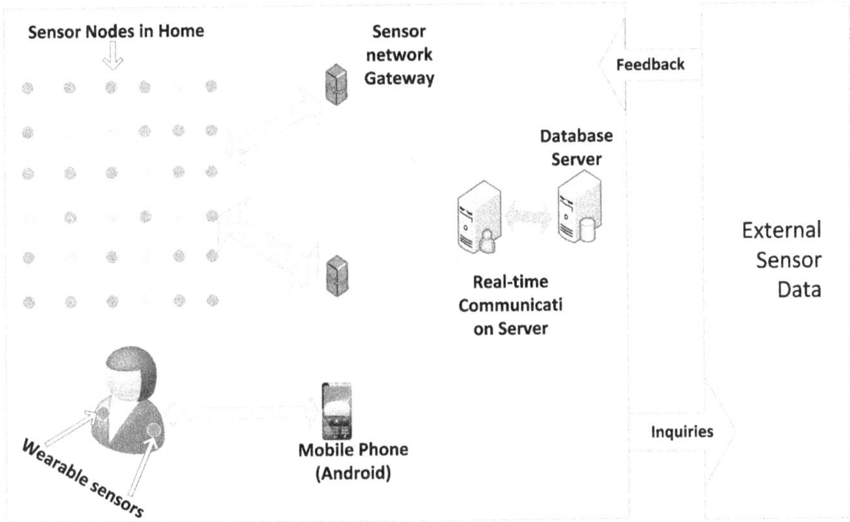

Fig. 20.3 Architecture of sensor embedded ambient assisted living system

is often missed. Thus, it becomes extremely important that the behaviour of elderly in general and Dementia patients in particular can be monitored and managed.

Information and Communication Technologies (ICT) have been widely prompted to enhance the smart, comfortable and cost-effective behaviour monitoring, as well as pervasive healthcare services. Depending on the symptoms of Alzheimer various circumstances must be considered, these circumstances are:

- Elderly, especially people with mental illness, are not able to and not willing to learn and use new technologies, and they are usually afraid of new technologies too.
- Elderly are usually more concerned about their privacy, and desire of dignity.
- Alzheimer's patients suffer from depression, anxious and emotional disorder more often and ordinary elderly.

Smart living [33, 34] is a multidisciplinary research topic that envisage a number of research sub-disciplines, which include Ambient Intelligence, smart environments, pervasive computing, machine learning, social media, activity and situation recognition, intelligent user interfaces as well as adaptive personalisation. Smart living is frequently synonymous with the smart home, where information on the home and its occupier are perceived, behaviours can be captured, and intelligent and personalised services delivered [28].

A number of leading smart home projects around the world have been proposed or already deployed (for an overview [14]). One of the main objectives of the smart homes is related to the improvement of comfort, dealing with medical rehabilitation, monitoring mobility and physiological parameters, and delivering therapy assistance or alarms [8]. Sensors and sensor networks have been commonly integrated with many smart homes, as well as cameras, microphones, TVs, and a number of smart appliances. User monitoring is the fundamental element in the vast majority of the smart home projects. A combination of technologies have been involved, such as artificial neural networks, context decision computing, artificial intelligence, computer version, statistical analysis, detection of human behaviour and actions, location recognition, case-based reasoning, home automation and many other areas of research [9].

Considerable amount of healthcare-driven smart homes have been developed are currently under investigation, such as MavHome [12], the GatorTech Smart House [16], the AwareHome [19], Easy Living [7], a fuzzy base reasoning system for healthcare [40], multimedia based smart medical home [4, 20] and so forth. Additionally, [13] presents a formal approach for situation awareness and the detection of abnormal behaviours of cognitive impaired people, in the smart space.

One of the major purposes of building a smart home in the healthcare domain is that patients behaviours and situations can be monitored and recognized. This has been confirmed to be extremely important for delivering proper treatments for patients [36, 35]. Human behavior and situation recognition has been studied extensively in recent years, especially in the smart home environment [26, 37]. Recent research on activity recognition has made significant progress. Nevertheless, in line with the sensing devices that are installed in the smart home, technologies and methodologies for recognizing activities may vary.

The idea of adopting sensors and sensor networks for activity monitoring and recognition has been prevalent for couple of decades [1, 11]. A range of sensors have been made available and deployed to enable smart monitoring. One of the earliest activity recognition frameworks is concerned with adding a number of accelerometers to the human body to recognize complex activity by monitoring the movement of different parts of human body. Attaching sensing devices to one's body can be annoying unless the sensors are as tiny as invisible that can be added to the outfits one's wear without obstructing presence. Therefore, contact sensor based approaches becoming more prevalent, whereas sensors are attached to objects of everyday life, such as cabinets, wardrobes, fridges, books, and so on. Additionally, ambient environmental sensors also play an essential role, such as monitoring the temperature, humidity, dust, noise, water flow, smoke, gas and so forth. However, sensor data only is not sufficient for recognizing complex activities and behaviours. Thus several techniques and approaches can be combined to improve the performance of recognition, which are the specification-based approach and learning based approach.

Extensive research efforts have been made in the acceleration based motion and gesture detection. One or more accelerometer sensors can be adhered on human body, which are usually located on the arm, ankle, thigh, wrist, hip and so on. A few motions can be captured as determined by 2-axis or 3-axis accelerometer data, such as walking, sitting, standing, running, stretching, scrubbing, cycling, etc. In addition, the number of accelerometer sensors and the position where the sensors are mounted are carefully considered, which significantly contributes to the accuracy of the recognition performance. Furthermore, learning based approaches are widely applied, such as Naïve Bayes, decision tree etc. Additionally, to interpret the acceleration data, mean and standard deviations are commonly calculated.

[3] presents a system that is able to detect numerous motions and activities using the user mounted acceleration data from a number of on-body accelerometers, which include walking, sitting and relaxing, standing still, watching TV, Running, scrubbing, folding laundry, brushing teeth, riding elevator, walking carrying items, working on computer, eating or drinking, reading, cycling, strength-training, vacuuming, lying down and climbing stairs. Another motion detection application is described in [31], where one single accelerometer is worn on the subject's pelvis, to recognise a number of gestures include standing, walking, running, claiming up stairs and so on. uWave [24] develops an recognition algorithms that recognising eight personalised gestures using a single accelerometer sensor. It achieves very high accuracy of 98.6 % by using a large amount of training example. Countless applications have been documented, which includes [17, 21, 27, 29, 30]. Furthermore, another widespread utility of acceleration data is fall detection, which is extremely important for elderly health monitoring, and numerous such system have been proposed [6, 10, 18, 22, 23].

The Sensor Infrastructure

Through the SIXTH middleware platform context driven applications are abstracted away from the underlying sensing network, enabling developers to achieve more with less effort. While this paper focusses on the use of high-level SIXTH components, it is important to understand the SIXTH architectural concepts that provide support for the plug-and-play interactions that form the core of this research. Here we provide a high level description of these concepts and motivate their use by enumerating goals that the SIXTH Middleware aim to achieve.

The SIXTH architecture is agnostic to the sources of data it supports. This is achieved through the provision of Adaptor Templates that enable a developer to easily create a custom adaptor for their data source, be it a web-based source, a new physical sensing device or an existing cyber/physical network operating on a different platform. The SIXTH architecture combines the use of a set of "generic" concepts, i.e., modules that can be replaced and/or combined in a plug-and-play manner. These modules are:

- **Adaptors**: provide seamless interaction with heterogeneous cyber and physical sensor platforms.
- **Receivers**: conduits for received data - sensor data, middleware events, (re)tasking events etc.
- **Query**: specifies a filter on captured sensor data.
- **Notifiers**: deliver filtered data notification based upon a set query.
- **Discovery**: controls data dissemination, the data retention policy and access to re-taskable components.

This framework's goals are: (1) Support the rapid development of a diverse range of context driven applications. (2) Enable a zero-configuration (plug-and-play) philosophy. (3) Minimal system programming for deployment. (4) Transparent sensor network deployments (achieved through adaptors and services) in network intelligence. (5) dynamic (re)tasking of sensors and sensor networks. And (6) treat physical and cyber sensor networks as equals.

SIXTH Cyber Sensing Architecture

The SIXTH Cyber Sensing architecture (see Fig. 20.4) provides data acquisition and interaction capabilities that enables uniform use of context and contextual services in a plug-and-play manner. Such an architecture supports context-driven application development through the provision of interchangeable components that can be combined according to application specific demands. The core abstractions are cyber sensors and services. SIXTH Adaptors and Service Factories control the production and configuration of cyber sensors (and cyber sensor facades for physical sensing devices) and high-level services, which can be achieved at run-time without causing disruption to the network. These features enable SIXTH to fully support self-adaptive and autonomous systems where the requirements and demands change dynamically during the lifetime of the network.

A working SIXTH deployment consists of interchangeable bundles where each bundle is classified as either an Adaptor or a Service Factory. Each diverse environment to be monitored requires its own adaptor bundle (e.g., for a particular Social Network). SIXTH provides a bundle which contains services that do not use externally sourced techniques (such as web services). This bundle can be utilized and extended according to the developers needs. All services that utilize external sources require a Service Factory bundle of their own in order for the relevant abstractions to be made.

The architecture was designed with simplicity in mind. Each component should be as basic as its purpose allows while enabling a generic solution to the problem it is solving. For example, a sensor monitoring a Twitter User should only monitor the user and not perform any additional functionality. This simplicity mimics the behaviour of resource constrained physical sensing devices where simplicity is enforced due to limited resources.

Adaptors and Cyber Sensors

As previously described, an adaptor is a SIXTH component that is responsible for enabling seamless interaction with diverse sensor platforms. In terms of a physical sensing device this means providing the required abstractions that enable the adaptor to produce a cyber sensor facade for use by developers. This facade enables physical and cyber sensed data to be treated uniformly by application developers and end users.

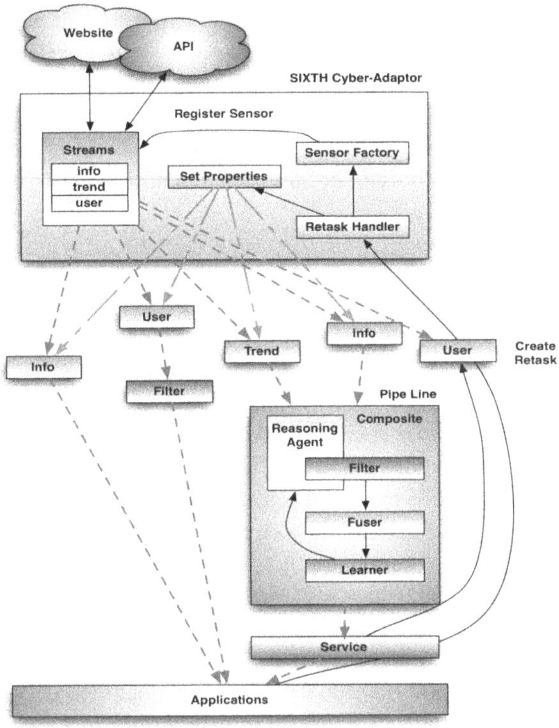

Fig. 20.4 SIXTH cyber sensing architecture

Cyber sensor facades also provide an abstraction that allows cyber sensor instances to be created and (re)tasked dynamically regardless of whether the underlying source is physical or web-based. From hereon in the term cyber sensor can refer to a sensor monitoring a web-based environment or a cyber sensor facade, unless otherwise specified.

Adaptors have the ability to produce cyber sensors of differing types according to the source they are monitoring. For example, the SIXTH Twitter Adaptor can produce a TwitterInfoSensor (tweets relating to specific users, keywords or from specific places), a TwitterTrendSensor (monitors twitter trends) and a TwitterUserSensor (monitors a particular user).

A SIXTH Cyber Adaptor is composed of the following core components:

- Retask Handler: resolves messages sent from applications/services and delegates the task to the appropriate component (sensor factory or properties delegator).
- Cyber Sensor Factory: produces Cyber Sensors of a specified type with unique ID's.
- Properties Delegator: instructs each sensor to configure themselves according to the properties specified by a user.
- Adaptor Stream: performs the work necessary to acquire the relevant data for all sensors attached to this adaptor.

The adaptor stream component enables the acquisition of data for numerous cyber sensors without overloading the source with duplicate requests. The adaptor stream either senses at a frequency determined by the source (e.g., when using a streaming API the frequency is sometimes not configurable) or calculates the frequency based on that while each individual sensor has been configured to use). The adaptor stream pushes each piece of sensed data to the appropriate sensor which in turn streams data according to its own frequency.

Cyber Sensor Capabilities

When a cyber sensor is created in an adaptor it is assigned a unique identifier that is sent to the application that requested its creation. Using this ID, the developer can then configure their cyber sensor according to their needs. Each cyber sensor provides very basic abstractions that unify the interactions a developer makes with diverse types of sensors. For example, a source such as Twitter requires location be specified as a bounding box. Utilizing services implemented as SIXTH bundles, cyber sensors that support location configuration can be (re)tasked by a developer using the format of his or her choice, e.g., String name, geographical coordinates, or a unique identifier such as Yahoo!'s WOEID. Deployments that do not contain these bundles will function as normal but without these helpful abstractions. Every cyber sensor can be configured according to the properties it supports. Typical properties to expect in cyber sensors include location, keyword, time, etc.

Service Factories and High-Level Services

While SIXTH Adaptors and Cyber Sensors are responsible for real time acquisition of customised data streams, SIXTH high-level services can be applied to these data streams interchangeably, enabling the transformation from data to abstract knowledge.

SIXTH Pipe Services

SIXTH Pipes constitute the most basic type of high-level service. They are software components that can be applied to individual sensors at runtime. The purpose of a pipe is to perform some action using the data that passes through it. A pipe is used by applying it to a cyber sensor using the same configuration mechanism as any other property the sensor supports. What happens to or because of the values contained in the data that passes through a pipe is dependent on the type of pipe and the logic contained within it.

Before sensor data is received by an application it passes through all (if any) pipes that have been applied to it. Every pipe is configured (by the user) to focus on a particular part (modality) of the sensor data.

Filter Pipe

The purpose of a filter pipe is to prevent sensor data that does not satisfy a configurable threshold from being sent on to an application. For example an application may only be Social Network users who's influence score is above a minimum threshold. A SIXTH filter pipe takes a sensor data object as its input and outputs either the same sensor data object or null, depending on whether the data satisfied the filter requirements.

Fuser Pipe

The purpose of a fuser pipe is to perform simple data fusion. Additional knowledge relating to a specified modality is either retrieved or calculated and is added to the original data. Nothing from the original data is overwritten or lost. For example, any sensor data that includes a twitter screen name can have klout data relating to that user added to the packet. A SIXTH fuser pipe takes a sensor data object as its input, adds additional values related to its existing data, and outputs the updated sensor data.

Learner Pipe

The purpose of a learner pipe is to gain some knowledge from the data that passes through it. For example,a learner pipe could be used to identify a pattern in temperature increase/decrease based on the temperature modality of the sensor data objects as they pass through. A SIXTH learner pipe takes a sensor data object as input and outputs the same object unchanged.

Transformer Pipe

The purpose of a transformer pipe is to convert part of the sensor data into another format. For example, an application might receive location data as a string name but would prefer it as geographical coordinates. A SIXTH transformer pipe takes a sensor data object as its input, replaces the specified modality value with its converted version, and outputs the updated sensor data.

Composite Pipe

The purpose of a composite pipe is to manage and control individual pipes internally within it. The composite pipe may reason on the results of internal pipes and can effect changes according to its overall state (changes can only be made within the composite pipe and its internal pipes).

SIXTH Application Services

Every application service has the potential to become a composite service by utilizing other services as well as cyber sensors. Since any SIXTH powered application can be embedded as a SIXTH application service, the limits in terms of how SIXTH can be extended are directly connected to our own limits as researchers and developers.

Motivating Scenario: iMED

Interoperability among diverse technologies is an approach to innovation when it comes to end-users' service provisioning. This section investigates the possibility to integrate the initial schema of a service provisioning application, (i.e., iMED), and the SIXTH framework introduced in previous section. The iMED service brings together inhabitants of smarthomes, pharmacies, medicines distributors, pharmaceutical companies, navigation systems, and lightweight computing devices (e.g., smartphones).

The general system architecture of iMED after considering the SIXTH framework is presented in Fig. 20.5. The iMED system architecture consists of four interaction layers that represent the system players. These layers are:

- **Users Layer**: This layer represents the main players in the system architecture such as application users and pharmacists.
- **Interfacing Layer**: This layers contains the iMED mobile application and back-end terminal. The iMED mobile client application was originally developed for PDAs. A user will interact with this layer to go through a questionnaire and find the exact medicine or location-aware alternatives. A user may also login into his/her personal profile where saved data exist and retrieve medicines he saved before.
- **Supplying Layer**: In this layer only companies related to the production and the distribution of a medicine are involved. The distributed companies are informed about the stock status of a particular medicine at pharmacies. In this phase the production companies are also getting involved. They are required to provide to distributing companies those medicines of critical stock status.
- **Backoffice Layer**: This separate block has an overlapping functions. It must be connected to all layers in order to deliver data required for the particular participant. These databases play various functions for every participant:

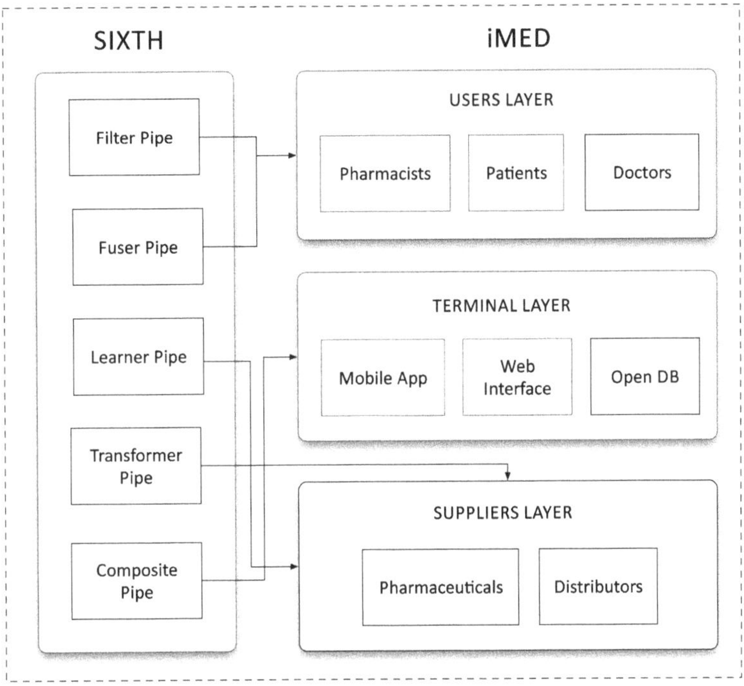

Fig. 20.5 General iMED system architecture

1. **iMED User**—using a Mobile Application a user can have access to a huge number of available medicines, to find a closest pharmacy, to perform the request of needed medicine in this pharmacy and store his/her history profile, that can be available at any moment and any place.
2. **Pharmacist**—can update the information about the medicine situation in a pharmacy, manage the structure of a pharmacy, retrieve data about unknown medicine and possible local alternatives, and perform request to distributing companies.
3. **Distributing Companies**—retrieve data about the situation in serviced pharmacies, receive requests from pharmacies, update dates of delivery.
4. **Industrial Companies**—update information about the medicine, adding data about released medicine.

Interactions of Different Components

The Mobile-Based iMED

iMED Mobile-based application is mobile service client application that is installed on a user device. This application provides number of questions that leads a user to the correct choice of the required medicine. This choice based on the local pharmaceutical databases and can be verified by pharmacist. The exact address of a nearby pharmacy is provided by the used terminal as well as the path to it from current location using GPS service.

There are different scenarios in which a user is expected to use the iMED mobile application, these scenarios are:

Scenario I: A user feels unwell. He goes through a provided wizard in order to determine the medicine that fulfills his requirements. Based on the result of this test, further actions will be considered and performed. During this scenario a user communicates with the application by means of question/answer scheme which leads to the proper choice of *local* available medicine. The core of this scenario is to provide preliminary illness identification with following choices of the treatment. It can then be seen that basic input parameter is a query coming from a user, based on the answers the system starts to search for the matching medicine in the general database. This database provides information about the medicine from the home country of a user and also the analogues names related to the current location of a user. Moreover, the descriptions of analogues are shown on the languages of a user, that was determined at the beginning of the application run. Among with the recommended medicine information about the pharmacy (closest) where this medicine (analogues for the current country) is available can be provided. The exact address and the open hours are included into that information. Also, a user can request the path to this pharmacy according to his/her current location. In this case mobile device must establish connection to GPS and direct a user.

Scenario II: A user is determined about the kind of medicine he requires but not the corresponding one in current location. The user uses the provided search engine to check the name of the medicine, find the alternative one in that country where he is right now. In addition, it's also possible to see the same medicine in different countries and check the compatibility with other types of medicines and herbal drugs.

Scenario III: A user requests information about the closest pharmacy, open hours of it and directions. Chosen this option a user can retrieve useful information about the pharmacy that is near by and in the neighbourhood, also user can see the open hours of selected items and check if they have night opening time. After all a user can issue the request to the selected pharmacy to order the chosen medicine asking to prepare it or to deliver it to user's place.

The iMED Software Application

Using Personal Computers (PCs) the iMED software application can be downloaded from the internet, customised and installed as any other common software. This application is oriented for fixed users and it has the same set of functions as the Mobile version of iMED. Also, this application is continuously updated through the Internet and it links service users with the nearest pharmacies and available doctors if a prescription is required. The iMED as a software application consists of two main side of the service, the Client and Server sides. There are two main users of the Client side: the iMED User and the Pharmacist. On the server side a Data Feeding Applications are running to ensure the fulfilling and matching of all pending requests/inquiries.

On the Pharmacist side, the iMED interface provides the list of all medicines currently available, their description, and the alternative brands or names of the very same medicine that are available in other countries. These later descriptions are also available in many languages and displayed according to the pharmacist's preferences. Using this service interface the pharmacist is then aware about the medicine he has and their alternative in different countries depending on the patient's background. In addition, the iMED application allows pharmacists to proceed with the iMED User order online and request a destination delivery if required. Among other several features, the pharmacist would be able to perform medicines database updates of his own pharmacy stock, read reviews left by customers and right more attracting information about his pharmacy. Pharmacists using iMED would also be able to interact with the distributing companies to make an online order all through the application interface, and cooperates with industrial companies to get an information about new released medicine.

From a server standpoint the iMED application can provide the following:

- The database of the all available medicine in a current country and their analogues in other countries with corresponding descriptions.
- The list of the questions leads an iMED User closer to the illness identification (release in TEXT and AUDIO view).
- Database with detailed description of pharmacy location and open hours.
- Bridging system to the database of the Distributing Companies and Industrial Companies.
- Personal iMED User space to store his/her history of medical actions, to keep important information about taken injections and possible allergies.

Conclusions

In this chapter we presented an extensive literature review of Ambient Assisted Living (AAL) while addressing the significance of AAL integrations in our daily life activities. We emphasized the importance of integrating intelligent sensors infrastructures to current AAL architectures. We described the main features and core architecture of the SIXTH sensor middleware. We then briefly presented iMED that is a healthcare service application that we are currently investigating as a linking case-study between common AAL architectures and Sensor Middlewares.

Acknowledgments Authors of this chapter would like to acknowledge the support of the Science Foundation Ireland (SFI) under grant 07/CE/I1147 as well as the European regional Development Fund (ERDF) for supporting the SC project through the Ireland Wales Program (INTERREG 4A).

References

1. I.F. Akyildiz, Weilian Su, Y. Sankarasubramaniam, and E. Cayirci. A survey on sensor networks. *IEEE Communications Magazine*, 40(8):102–114, Aug 2002.
2. Ambient Assisted Living Joint Programme. (AAL JP). http://www.aal-europe.eu/new-website-launch-rebranding-the-aaljp/. Accessed: March 2013
3. Ling Bao and Stephen Intille. Activity recognition from user-annotated acceleration data. In Alois Ferscha and Friedemann Mattern, editors, *Pervasive Computing*, volume 3001 of *Lecture Notes in Computer Science*, pages 1–17. Springer Berlin / Heidelberg, 2004.
4. Juan A. Botia, Ana Villa, and Jose Palma. Ambient assisted living system for in-home monitoring of healthy independent elders. *Expert Systems with Applications*, 39(9):8136–8148, 2012.
5. Khouloud Boukadi, Chirine Ghedira, Sodki Chaari, Lucien Vincent, and Emad Bataineh. Cwsc4ec: how to employ context, web service, and community in enterprise collaboration. In *Proceedings of the 8th international conference on New technologies in distributed systems*, NOTERE '08, pages 6:1–6:12, New York, NY, USA, 2008. ACM.
6. AK Bourke, JV O'brien, GM Lyons, et al. Evaluation of a threshold-based tri-axial accelerometer fall detection algorithm. *Gait & posture*, 26(2):194–199, 2007.
7. Barry Brumitt, Brian Meyers, John Krumm, Amanda Kern, and Steven Shafer. Easyliving: Technologies for intelligent environments. In Peter Thomas and Hans-W. Gellersen, editors, *Handheld and Ubiquitous Computing*, volume 1927 of *Lecture Notes in Computer Science*, pages 97–119. Springer Berlin/Heidelberg, 2000.
8. Barry Brumitt, Brian Meyers, John Krumm, Amanda Kern, and Steven A. Shafer. Easyliving: Technologies for intelligent environments. In *Proceedings of the 2nd international symposium on Handheld and Ubiquitous Computing*, HUC '00, pages 12–29, London, UK, UK, 2000. Springer-Verlag.
9. Marie Chan, Daniel Estève, Christophe Escriba, and Eric Campo. A review of smart homes-present state and future challenges. *Comput. Methods Prog. Biomed.*, 91:55–81, July 2008.
10. J. Chen, K. Kwong, D. Chang, J. Luk, and R. Bajcsy. Wearable sensors for reliable fall detection. In *The 27th Annual International Conference of the Engineering in Medicine and Biology Society, 2005. IEEE-EMBS.*, pages 3551–3554. IEEE, 2006.
11. L. Chen, J. Hoey, C. D. Nugent, D. J. Cook, and Z. Yu. Sensor-based activity recognition. *IEEE Transactions on Systems, Man, and Cybernetics, Part C: Applications and Reviews*, PP(99):1–19, 2012.
12. D.J. Cook, M. Youngblood, III Heierman, E.O., K. Gopalratnam, S. Rao, A. Litvin, and F. Khawaja. Mavhome: an agent-based smart home. In *Pervasive Computing and Communications, 2003. (PerCom 2003). Proceedings of the First IEEE International Conference on*, pages 521–524, March 2003.
13. Antonio Coronato and Giuseppe De Pietro. Situation awareness in applications of ambient assisted living for cognitive impaired people. *Mobile Networks and Applications*, pages 1–10, 2012.

14. Liyanage C. De Silva, Chamin Morikawa, and Iskandar M. Petra. State of the art of smart homes. *Eng. Appl. Artif. Intell.*, 25(7):1313–1321, October 2012.
15. Kirstie Hawkey, Kori M. Inkpen, Kenneth Rockwood, Michael McAllister, and Jacob Slonim. Requirements gathering with alzheimer's patients and caregivers. In *Proceedings of the 7th international ACM SIGACCESS conference on Computers and accessibility*, Assets '05, pages 142–149, New York, NY, USA, 2005. ACM.
16. S. Helal, W. Mann, H. El-Zabadani, J. King, Y. Kaddoura, and E. Jansen. The gator tech smart house: a programmable pervasive space. *Computer*, 38(3):50–60, March 2005.
17. Do-Un Jeong, Se-Jin Kim, and Wan-Young Chung. Classification of posture and movement using a 3-axis accelerometer. In *International Conference on Convergence Information Technology, 2007*, pages 837–844, Nov. 2007.
18. M. Kangas, A. Konttila, P. Lindgren, I. Winblad, and T. Jämsä. Comparison of low-complexity fall detection algorithms for body attached accelerometers. *Gait & Posture*, 28(2):285–291, 2008.
19. Cory Kidd, Robert Orr, Gregory Abowd, Christopher Atkeson, Irfan Essa, Blair MacIntyre, Elizabeth Mynatt, Thad Starner, and Wendy Newstetter. The aware home: A living laboratory for ubiquitous computing research. In Norbert Streitz, Jane Siegel, Volker Hartkopf, and ShinGichi Konomi, editors, *Cooperative Buildings. Integrating Information, Organizations, and Architecture*, volume 1670 of *Lecture Notes in Computer Science*, pages 191–198. Springer Berlin / Heidelberg, 1999.
20. Jinman Kim, Zhiyong Wang, Tom Weidong Cai, and David Dagan Feng. 23 - multimedia for future health : Smart medical home. In David Dagan Feng, editor, *Biomedical Information Technology*, pages 497–512. Academic Press, Burlington, 2008.
21. Seon-Woo Lee and K. Mase. Activity and location recognition using wearable sensors. *IEEE Transactions on, Pervasive Computing*, 1(3):24–32, 2002.
22. Q. Li, J.A. Stankovic, M.A. Hanson, A.T. Barth, J. Lach, and G. Zhou. Accurate, fast fall detection using gyroscopes and accelerometer-derived posture information. In *Wearable and Implantable Body Sensor Networks, 2009. BSN 2009. Sixth International Workshop on*, pages 138–143. IEEE, 2009.
23. U. Lindemann, A. Hock, M. Stuber, W. Keck, and C. Becker. Evaluation of a fall detector based on accelerometers: A pilot study. *Medical and Biological Engineering and Computing*, 43(5):548–551, 2005.
24. Jiayang Liu, Zhen Wang, Lin Zhong, J. Wickramasuriya, and V. Vasudevan. uwave: Accelerometer-based personalized gesture recognition and its applications. *Pervasive and Mobile Computing*, 5(6):657–675, 2009.
25. Robert Lokaiczyk and Manuel Goertz. Extending low level context events by data aggregation. In *Proceedings of I-KNOW08 and I-MEDIA'08*, Graz, Austria, 2008.
26. F. Mastrogiovanni, A. Sgorbissa, and R. Zaccaria. Activity recognition in smart homes: from specification to representation. *J. Intell. Fuzzy Syst.*, 21(1, 2):33–48, April 2010.
27. U. Maurer, A. Smailagic, D.P. Siewiorek, and M. Deisher. Activity recognition and monitoring using multiple sensors on different body positions. In *International Workshop on Wearable and Implantable Body Sensor Networks, 2006. BSN 2006*, pages 110–116, April 2006.
28. Michael OGGrady, Conor Muldoon, Mauro Dragone, Richard Tynan, and Gregory OGHare. Towards evolutionary ambient assisted living systems. *Journal of Ambient Intelligence and Humanized Computing*, 1:15–29, 2010. 10.1007/s12652-009-0003-5.
29. J. Parkka, M. Ermes, P. Korpipaa, J. Mantyjarvi, J. Peltola, and I. Korhonen. Activity classification using realistic data from wearable sensors. *IEEE Transactions on Information Technology in Biomedicine*, 10(1):119–128, January 2006.
30. S.J. Preece, J.Y. Goulermas, L.P.J. Kenney, and D. Howard. A comparison of feature extraction methods for the classification of dynamic activities from accelerometer data. *IEEE Transactions on Biomedical Engineering*, 56(3):871–879, March 2009.
31. N. Ravi, N. Dandekar, P. Mysore, and M.L. Littman. Activity recognition from accelerometer data. In *Proceedings of the National Conference on Artificial Intelligence*, volume 20, page 1541. Menlo Park, CA; Cambridge, MA; London; AAAI Press; MIT Press; 1999, 2005.

32. A. Rosi, M. Mamei, F. Zambonelli, S. Dobson, G. Stevenson, and Juan Ye. Social sensors and pervasive services: Approaches and perspectives. In 2011 *IEEE International Conference on Pervasive Computing and Communications Workshops (PERCOM Workshops)*, pages 525–530, March 2011.
33. Kimiko Ryokai, Stefan Marti, and Hiroshi Ishii. Designing the world as your palette. In *CHI '05 Extended Abstracts on Human Factors in Computing Systems*, CHI EA '05, pages 1037–1049, New York, NY, USA, 2005. ACM.
34. Itiro Siio, Jim Rowan, and Elizabeth Mynatt. Peek-a-drawer: communication by furniture. In *CHI '02 Extended Abstracts on Human Factors in Computing Systems*, CHI EA '02, pages 582–583, New York, NY, USA, 2002. ACM.
35. Janani C. Sriram, Minho Shin, Tanzeem Choudhury, and David Kotz. Activity-aware ecg-based patient authentication for remote health monitoring. In *Proceedings of the 2009 international conference on Multimodal interfaces*, ICMI-MLMI '09, pages 297–304, New York, NY, USA, 2009. ACM.
36. Myung-kyung Suh, Lorraine S. Evangelista, Chien-An Chen, Kyungsik Han, Jinha Kang, Michael Kai Tu, Victor Chen, Ani Nahapetian1, and Majid Sarrafzadeh1. An automated vital sign monitoring system for congestive heart failure patients. In *Proceedings of the 1st ACM International Health Informatics Symposium*, IHI '10, pages 108–117, New York, NY, USA, 2010. ACM.
37. Emmanuel Munguia Tapia, Stephen S. Intille, and Kent Larson. Activity recognition in the home using simple and ubiquitous sensors. In *Pervasive*, pages 158–175, 2004.
38. G. Van Den Broek, F. Cavallo, and C. Wehrmann. *AALIANCE ambient assisted living roadmap*, volume 6. Ios PressInc, 2010.
39. Mark Weiser. The computer for the 21st century. *Sigmobile Mobile Computing and Communications Review*, 3(3):3–11, July 1999.
40. Bingchuan Yuan and John Herbert. Fuzzy cara - a fuzzy-based context reasoning system for pervasive healthcare. *Procedia Computer Science*, 10(0):357–365, 2012.

Chapter 21
Improving Safety in Medical Devices from Concept to Retirement

Martin McHugh , Fergal McCaffery, Silvana Togneri MacMahon and Anita Finnegan

Introduction

As with many domains the use of software within the healthcare industry is on the rise [1, 2] within the last 20 years. The use of this software ranges from performing administrative tasks such as patient registration to life sustaining tasks such as within a pacemaker. Prior to this, medical devices primarily consisted of hardware with a software component. A significant shift has occurred with medical device manufacturers realizing that functionality can be added to a medical device through the use of software. As the functionality of the medical device grows, so does the complexity and therefore the risk. The risk associated with this complexity applies to both the use of software in standalone devices and also medical devices designed for incorporation into a medical IT network. The incorporation of a medical device into an IT network can introduce risk to the safety, effectiveness and security (data and system) of the device. With an increase in complexity there is an increased risk of harm to the patient, clinician or third party.

The most famous failure of software resulting in harm to a patient within a medical device was with Therac-25 [3]. Therac-25 was a radiation therapy machine which used software to control when a beam spreader plate moved into position to reduce a patient's exposure to radiation. As a result of a failure within the software, this spreader plate did not always move into position when necessary and as a result of this failure, four people died and two were left permanently disfigured. In light of this failure and other significant failures of medical devices as a result of software malfunctions, regulatory bodies introduced regulations to ensure safe and reliable performance of medical devices consisting of software [4].

Within the United States (US) medical devices are regulated by the Food and Drug Administration (FDA). Within the European Union, they are regulated through the

M. McHugh (✉) · F. McCaffery · S. T. MacMahon · A. Finnegan
Department of Computing and Mathematics, Dundalk Institute of Technology, County Louth, Ireland
e-mail: martin.mchugh@dkit.ie

B. Furht and A. Agarwal (eds.), *Handbook of Medical and Healthcare Technologies*, DOI: 10.1007/978-1-4614-8495-0_21, © Springer Science+Business Media New York 2013 awarding of the CE mark, which can be awarded by notified bodies within each of the EU member states. Within Canada, medical devices are regulated by Health Canada. Whilst regulations vary between regions, the standards followed for the development of medical device software are typically universal. These standards include EN ISO 13485:2003—Medical Devices—Quality Management Systems [5], EN ISO 14971:2012: Medical Devices—Application of Risk Management to medical devices [6] and IEC 62304:2006—Medical Devices—Software Lifecycle Processes [7]. The primary concern of regulatory bodies is that medical devices are safe and reliable. To achieve this, all medical devices, regardless of safety classification marketed for use in the EU, US or Canada, must be developed in accordance with a Quality Management System (QMS). Within the EU and Canada, regulatory bodies recommend that medical device manufacturers develop their devices in accordance with EN ISO 13485. Prior to July 2012, medical devices manufacturers wishing to market a device for use within the US were required to adhere to the FDA Quality System Regulations (QSR) known as FDA 21 CFR Part 820 [8]. However, from July 1, 2012, the FDA began a pilot program in which they offer device manufacturers the option of submitting their quality system audits which are compliant with EN ISO 13485 [9]. This is seen as a step towards a harmonization between FDA regulations and Health Canada; however, it has the knock-on effect of being more beneficial to manufacturers who adhere to EU regulations.

Whilst medical device manufacturers are compliance centric, there is also a shift towards following industry best practices in order to further enhance development practices. However, current frameworks for software development best practices are not domain specific and don't address practices which are specific to the development of medical device software. Therefore, there is a need for a medical device software development specific framework, which aims to combine industry best practices for the entire development and maintenance lifecycles of medical device software with necessary regulations which medical device manufacturers must adhere to.

Section "Types of Software Used in Healthcare" provides a description of the different types of software used within the healthcare domain. Section "Regulating Software in Healthcare" provides details of the regulations to which medical device manufacturers must adhere when developing medical device software. Section "Developing Software for Use in Healthcare" details how medical device software organizations can develop safer and more reliable software by following Capability Maturity Models and discusses the development of a medical device software specific Process Assessment Model (PAM) and Process Reference Model (PRM). This PAM and PRM combine regulations with software development industry best practices that medical device software organizations can follow when developing regulatory compliant software. Section "Risk Management of IT Networks Incorporating Medical Devices" focuses on the development of a PRM and PAM to manage the risks associated with the incorporation of a medical device into a hospital IT network. Section "Security Assurance of Medical Devices" discusses the development of a Security Assurance PRM and PAM which aims to assess the development process of a medical device and also establish a security capability level for the developed product and finally

Sect. "Conclusions and Summary" presents the summary and conclusions of this chapter.

The primary contribution of this chapter is to provide medical device organizations with information relating to the regulations to which they must adhere and the standards they are recommended to follow. These standards and regulations cover areas including medical device software development, the application of risk management to devices connected to a healthcare network and security use cases for medical devices. Also information regarding the frameworks which combines the requirements of regulations, the guidance of the standards and industry best practices is presented.

Types of Software Used in Healthcare

Software was first used in healthcare in the 1960s to perform administrative tasks. It was soon realized that introducing software into healthcare could decrease costs, increase patient satisfaction and improve hospital processes which improves patient care. However, since its introduction the use of software has grown exponentially [2]. Whilst the first software used in healthcare was limited to administrative tasks, modern software can be used to perform various tasks ranging from registering patient details on admission into a hospital to controlling a life sustaining device such as defibrillators. As the range of tasks which software could perform was so vast, categorization of that software was required. This categorization is based upon the intended use of the software and in accordance with regulatory requirements. These categories are:

- Software as an accessory to a medical device;
- Software as a medical device in its own right;
- Software as a medical device data system (MDDS); or
- Software currently unclassified and not subject to specific regulations.

Software as an Accessory to a Medical Device

An accessory to a medical device is an item which in itself is not a medical device but when connected to a medical device assists the medical device to perform its intended function.

The EU regulations define an accessory to a medical device as [10]:

"an article which whilst not being a device is intended specifically by its manufacturer to be used together with a device to enable it to be used in accordance with the use of the device intended by the manufacturer of the device"

Crumpler and Rudolph provided two definitions of software as an accessory to a medical device based upon the FDA's written guidance [11]:

(1) *"a (software) accessory is a (software) unit which is intended to be attached to or used in conjunction with another finished device": or*
(2) *"a software accessory to a medical device either accepts data from the user and modifies it for input to a medical device, or takes the data from a medical device modifies it for presentation to the user".*

It can be seen that whilst the wording between the EU and FDA regulations varies, the definitions are very similar. In essence software is defined as being an accessory to a medical device when it is connected to a medical device to facilitate the operation of that medical device. For example, if a spreadsheet application receives input from a heart rate monitor and calculates averages heart rate over a period of time it is considered an accessory to a medical device.

The key point to note is; where software meets the criteria of an accessory, it assumes the safety classification of the parent device to which it is connected. In our previous example, if the heart rate monitor received a Class III safety classification then the spreadsheet application would automatically assume the Class III safety classification and would undergo the same level of regulatory scrutiny as the heart rate monitor.

Software as a Medical Device in its Own Right

Software is defined as being a medical device if its intended function meets the definition of a medical device. In the EU the definition of medical device is [12]:

"any instrument, apparatus, appliance, software, material or other article, whether used alone or in combination, including the software intended by its manufacturer to be used specifically for diagnostic and/or therapeutic purposes and necessary for its proper application"

The FDA defines a medical device as:

"...an instrument, apparatus, implement, machine, contrivance, implant, in vitro reagent, or other similar or related article, including a component part, or accessory which is: recognized in the official National Formulary, or the United States Pharmacopoeia, or any supplement to them, intended for use in the diagnosis of disease or other conditions, or in the cure, mitigation, treatment, or prevention of disease, in man or other animals, or intended to affect the structure or any function of the body of man or other animals, and which does not achieve any of its primary intended purposes through chemical action within or on the body of man or other animals and which is not dependent upon being metabolized for the achievement of any of its primary intended purposes."

Health Canada provides a specific definition as to when software is considered a medical device [13]:

"Software regulated as a medical device;

(1) *Provides the only means and opportunity to capture or acquire the data from a medical device for aiding directly in diagnosis or treatment of a patient; or*
(2) *Replaces a diagnostic or treatment decision made by a physician."*

Software as a Medical Device Data System

In 2011, the FDA released its rule regarding MDDS known as CFR 21 Part 880.6310 [14]. As part of this rule the FDA released its definition of a MDDS:

"A device that is intended to provide one or more of the following uses, without controlling or altering the functions or parameters of any connected medical devices:

(i) *The electronic transfer of medical device data;*
(ii) *The electronic storage of medical device data;*
(iii) *The electronic conversion of medical device data from one format to another format in accordance with a pre-set specification; or*
(iv) *The electronic display of medical device data."*

Prior to this rule being introduced by the FDA, software performing any of the functions outlined in the definition of a MDDS was either regarded as an accessory to a medical device which assumed the safety classification of the parent device or was considered a medical device in its own right and was required to undergo a separate process of achieving regulatory approval. However, since the introduction of this rule, if software exclusively performs one or more of the functions as outlined in the definition of a MDDS will automatically receive a Class I safety classification. The FDA has determined that any risk posed by a MDDS would potentially come from inadequate software quality or incorrect functioning of the device. It is expected that potential issues such as these would be resolved by the use of a QMS in accordance with FDA regulations [15].

There is, however, an exception to this rule. If software exclusively performs one or more of the functions outlined in the definition of a MDDS and is used for active patient monitoring then it cannot be considered a MDDS and must be considered an accessory or medical device.

Software Currently Unclassified and Not Subject to Specific Regulation

The previous sections have discussed software that is used directly and indirectly with patient care and the category into which they fall. However, there are software applications that are used in healthcare that are currently unclassified and not subject to specific regulation.

Software used within Hospital Information Technology (HIT) which is only used for administrative purposes is currently unclassified [12]. Regulations are primarily concerned with patient safety and as there is no potential risk to patient safety as result of a defect in administrative software, if falls beyond the scope of regulatory scrutiny.

Also Electronic Health Records (EHR) and Computerized Physician Order Entry (CPOE) systems are currently unclassified. Upon reading the functions which these systems perform they do appear to fall into one of the categories previously mentioned. However, regulatory bodies have recognized that in the future these systems have the ability to automatically order tests for patients, therefore initiating the generation of clinical data and as a result would meet the definition of being a medical device [15].

Regulating Software in Healthcare

As medical devices can have a direct impact on a person's wellbeing, necessary controls are put in place to ensure the safe and reliable performance of the device. These controls take the form of regulations. Medical device manufacturers wishing to market a device into a region must adhere to the regulations of that region. In this section we describe the regulations within the EU, US and Canada which impact the development of software for use within the healthcare domain.

European Union Regulations

Medical devices marketed within the EU must carry the CE mark. The awarding of this mark certifies that the device has been developed in accordance with all of the applicable EU regulations. The CE mark is awarded by notified bodies within EU member states and once a device manufacturer receives a CE mark in any member state they are permitted to market their device in all of the member states.

Medical device manufactures must adhere to the Medical Device Directive (MDD) and its latest amendment to achieve the CE mark [16]. The MDD (93/42/EEC) has been amended 5 times with the latest amendment (2007/47/EC) being released in 2007. As part of this amendment, there were 14 significant amendments to the original directive [17]. The most significant of these amendments to impact software is the inclusion of software into the definition of being a medical device. Whilst previous amendments did allow for software to be a component of a medical device, they did not extend to standalone software being recognized as an active medical device. An active medical device is defined in the amendment to the MDD as:

"any medical device operation of which depends on a source of electrical energy or any source of power other than that directly generated by the human body or gravity and which acts by converting this energy.....Stand-alone software is considered to be an active medical device"

As a result of the inclusion of this wording into the amendment, situations may now arise where software can be the only component of a medical device used in a healthcare setting, subject to regulatory scrutiny. Prior to this amendment software was always seen as a component of a hardware device. To ensure the safety of the healthcare software the latest amendment to the MDD states:

"For devices which incorporate software or which are medical software in themselves, the software must be validated according to the state of the art taking into

account the principles of development lifecycle, risk management, validation and verification."

However, the amendment to the MDD does not clarify what is meant by "state of the art", but it is generally accepted that state of the art is referred to as best practice and best practice for medical device software development is achieved by following IEC 62304 and its aligned standards. To accompany this, the EU regulations require that all medical devices are developed in accordance with a Quality Management System (QMS), such as ISO 13485 and in accordance with a risk management standard such as ISO 14971. These standards are harmonized for use within the EU [18].

When the latest amendment to the MDD was released, confusion arose as to when software would be considered an active medical device. The only clarification provided as part of the amendment was that software used in healthcare for administrative purposes is considered not to be a medical device. It was not until January 2012 when the European Council released the MEDDEV [10] document to accompany the amendment to the MDD that clarified which type of software was subject to regulatory scrutiny.

FDA Regulations

Medical devices marketed in the US must meet the FDA requirements. Unlike the EU, the FDA is the only regulatory body with the authority to approve a medical device for use within the US. Also unlike the EU the FDA does not specifically regulate software used in healthcare. Rather, if the software meets the definition of being a medical device then it is regulated in the same way as a hardware device that meets the same definition. All medical devices regardless of safety classification marketed in the US must adhere to either the FDA's Quality System Regulations (QSR) or to ISO 13485. However, since the Therac-25 incident, the FDA has recognized the increasingly significant role which software plays in healthcare and as a result has commissioned guidance documents which medical device software organizations can follow. These guidance documents include:

- Design Controls Guidance for Medical Device Manufacturers [19];
- General Principles of Software Validation [20];
- Guidance for Industry and Food and Drug Administration—Mobile Medical Applications [21];
- Guidance for Industry and FDA Reviewers and Compliance on Off-The-Shelf Software use in Medical Devices [22].

Also in conjunction with the regulations and the guidance documents the FDA releases rules. The most recent of these rules which impact on the development of software is the rule on Medical Device Data Systems. Figure 21.1, shows the relationship between the regulations, guidance documents and rules. As with the EU, the FDA recognizes that IEC 62304 is considered to be medical device software development best practice and has been a consensus standard under FDA guidelines

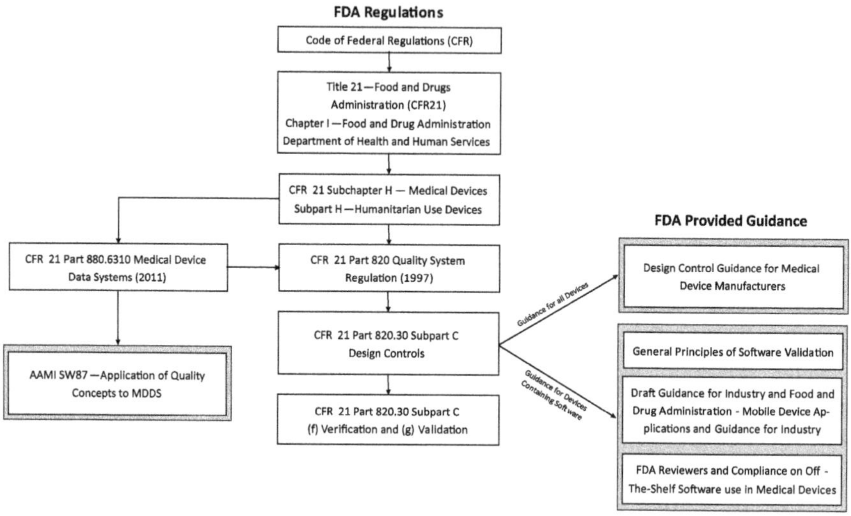

Fig. 21.1 FDA regulations, guidance documents and rule

since September 2008. One advantage of following IEC 62304 is that medical device software development organizations following IEC 62304 are not obliged to describe their processes in detail when seeking regulatory approval [23].

Health Canada Regulations

Health Canada regulates medical devices through its Medical Device Regulations Document SOR/98-282 [24]. Health Canada requires medical device organizations to validate the performance of the software to ensure it performs as intended. Medical device software organizations are required to submit validation studies when seeking regulatory approval. As with the EU, Canada recognizes that software can be a medical device in its own right and as so necessary controls must be put in place to ensure the safe and reliable performance of that medical device software. To achieve this all medical devices marketed in Canada must be developed in accordance with ISO 13485. Health Canada has also released guidance as to when software used in healthcare is considered to be a medical device.

Safety Classifications

Each region also categorizes medical devices based upon the potential risk the device poses. Table 21.1, shows the risk classification defined by each region and also shows

Table 21.1 Safety classification of medical devices

Risk	Low	Medium		High
EU	Class I	Class IIa	Class IIb	Class III
Canada	Class I	Class II	Class III	Class IV
US	Class I	Class II		Class III

how the risk classification of each region relates to the classification of the other regions.

The level of risk a device poses will determine the level of regulatory scrutiny applied to the device. For example, in the US class I devices are subject to the least amount of regulatory control. They are subject to "General Controls" which includes provisions that concern issues such as misbranding and premarket notification. Class II devices are subject to "General Controls" also, however they are subject special controls such as adherence to mandatory performance standards and post market surveillance. Post market surveillance is the practice in which the FDA monitors the device once it has been released onto the market. Finally, class III devices must adhere to "General Controls" and special controls as with Class II, however devices marketed as class III devices must also request premarket approval. The process of achieving premarket approval involves the FDA evaluating the safety of the device prior to it being released onto the market [25].

Developing Software for Use in Healthcare

The safety of medical device software is determined by the processes followed during development [26]. As a result medical device software manufacturers are advised to follow defined pathways when developing software. The Software Process Improvement (SPI) is gaining momentum in the generic software development industry, but has yet to be widely adopted in the medical device software development industry [27]. SPI methods such as agile software development have shown significant benefits where they have been embraced.

Capability Maturity Models in Medical Device Software

SPI models exist including the Capability Maturity Model Integration (CMMI®) [28] and ISO 15504-5:2006 [29] (SPICE), but these do not provide sufficient coverage of medical device regulations and standards [30]. In order to address the requirement for a medical device software process assessment and improvement model the Regulated Software Research Group (RSRG) at Dundalk Institute of Technology (DkIT) commenced the development of Medi SPICE a medical device specific SPI model which is being developed in collaboration with the SPICE User Group. This model is being developed similarly to Automotive SPICE [31], which is a domain specific SPI model for the automotive industry.

What is Medi SPICE?

Medi SPICE is based upon the latest versions of ISO/IEC 15504-5 and ISO/IEC 12207:2008 [32]. It provides coverage of the relevant medical device regulations, standards, technical reports and guidance documents. These include IEC 62304:2006 and its aligned standards, the FDA regulations [33] and guidance documents, and the amendment to the European Medical Device Directive and guidelines. The objective of undertaking a Medi SPICE assessment is to determine the state of a medical device organization's software processes and practices in relation to the regulatory requirements of the industry and to identify areas for process improvement [34]. It can also be used as part of the supplier section process when an organization wishes to outsource part or all of their medical device software development to a third party or a remote division [35].

Medi SPICE contains a Process Reference Model (PRM) which consists of forty two processes and twelve subprocesses which are fundamental to the development of regulatory compliant medical device software. Each process has a clearly defined purpose and outcomes that must be accomplished to achieve that purpose. Medi SPICE also contains a Process Assessment Model (PAM) which is related to the PRM and forms the basis for collecting evidence and the rating of process capability. This is achieved by the provision of a two-dimensional view of process capability. In one dimension, it describes a set of process specific practices that allow the achievement of the process outcomes and purpose defined in the PRM; this is termed the process dimension. In the other dimension, the PAM describes capabilities that relate to the process capability levels and process attributes, this is termed the capability dimension.

In line with ISO/IEC 15504-2:2003 [36] Medi SPICE process capability is defined over six levels:

- Level 0 Incomplete;
- Level 1 Performed;
- Level 2 Managed;
- Level 3 Established;
- Level 4 Predictable;
- Level 5 Optimizing.

The Medi SPICE PRM and PAM are being released in stages and each stage is extensively reviewed by interested parties from the SPICE User Group, representatives from international medical device standards bodies (i.e. IEC SC62A JWG3) and industry experts. This collaborative approach is seen as a key element in the development of Medi SPICE to ensure coverage of both the SPI and medical device software regulatory requirements [34]. The overall objective of Medi SPICE is to provide a conformity assessment scheme to support first, second or third party assessments. It is envisaged that results from these assessments may be recognized by the relevant regulatory bodies.

Assessing Against Medi SPICE

Like other SPI assessments models i.e. CMMI® and IEC 15504-5:2006, a full Medi SPICE assessment will require considerable planning and resources to successfully undertake. While Medi SPICE is being developed with the objective of being as efficient as possible the necessity for rigor dictates the level of planning, resources and analysis required for its successful implementation. While the need for and importance of Medi SPICE is understood [37], it was also appreciated by the RSRG that there was a specific requirement for lightweight assessment methods in the medical device software industry [38]. In particular there was industry led demand for a lightweight assessment method based on Medi SPICE. This was communicated directly to the RSRG by numerous medical device organizations. To address this specific requirement Medi SPICE-Adept was developed. There were two additional objectives in undertaking this task. The first was the opportunity to leverage the extensive research [39] and level of detail which developing Medi SPICE provided. The second was the opportunity to identify and facilitate the use of agile and lean methods. The use of agile and lean methods for medical device software development is an area that the RSRG are also currently researching to assist organizations increase the efficiency of their software development practices [40].

To be effective Medi SPICE-Adept required the employment of a lightweight approach for undertaking software process assessment and improvement. This included the use of a limited number of personnel to carryout and participate in the assessment while also maximizing the benefit of the time and effort of those involved. It was envisaged that Medi SPICE-Adept would eventually encompass all the Medi SPICE processes. It was therefore recognized that an assessment could take place either over 1 day or a number of days depending on how many processes were being assessed. It was also important that organizations could select the specific processes which were of most benefit for achieving their business goals. The focus of the method was on the evaluation of the essential practices, key work products and the achievement of the outcomes which were necessary for the attainment of the specific process purpose being assessed. Medi SPICE-Adept therefore needed to be process dimension centric in its focus.

Finally, the objective of undertaking a Medi SPICE-Adept assessment is not to receive formal certification or a rating, but rather to identify an organization's strengths and weaknesses and to facilitate process improvement. Having defined the criteria which had to be met the next step was to undertake the development of Medi SPICE-Adept.

Assessing Against Medi SPICE Using Lightweight Assessment Models

The RSRG have previously developed and implemented three lightweight software process assessment methods Adept [41], Med-Adept [42] and Med-Trace [43] the objective was to leverage that experience and utilize it for the development of Medi SPICE-Adept. It was in this context that work commenced on the development of Medi SPICE-Adept. It was recognized that this assessment method needed to cover more processes and provide more detailed analysis than those methods which had been previously developed. While this was the case Medi SPICE-Adept was still required to be lightweight to fulfill its purpose. The first task was to identify the initial Medi SPICE processes that would be utilized. The goal was to select a limited number of processes that would be most beneficial and relevant to industry. To achieve this, industry experts were consulted and ten processes were selected:

- Requirements Elicitation;
- System Architectural design;
- Systems Requirements Analysis;
- Software Requirements Analysis,
- Software Construction;
- Software Integration;
- Software Testing;
- Configuration Management;
- Change Request Management;
- Verification.

While these were the initial processes selected Medi SPICE-Adept will additionally provide coverage of all the Medi SPICE processes and subprocesses.

The Medi SPICE PAM had been developed for each of the initial processes which were based on best practice as outlined by the latest version of ISO/IEC 15504-5 and the specific requirements of the medical device regulations, standards, technical reports and guidance documents. As a result each process had a defined purpose and outcomes, specific practices and work products were also included for the achievement of these outcomes and purpose. Additionally, each outcome and specific practice was mapped to the regulations, standards etc. on which it was based. To facilitate the assessment each of the initial processes were evaluated and specific questions identified based on the Medi SPICE PAM. Questions relating to the current or potential use of agile and lean software methods were also identified and included. This work was undertaken by five members of the RSRG team with extensive experience of SPI and knowledge of medical device software development and included two experts in the area of lean and agile methods. The next step was to develop the specific procedure for implementing a Medi SPICE assessment.

Implementing a Medi SPICE Assessment

Based on the RSRG's previous experience of developing and undertaking lightweight software process assessments [38] a seven stage procedure for undertaking a Medi SPICE Assessment was defined. The assessment team should normally consist of two assessors who share responsibility for conducting the assessment. The seven stages of the procedure are as follows: Prior to undertaking an assessment a preliminary meeting between the lead assessor and the company takes place. This is the first stage in the procedure and during this meeting the lead assessor discusses the main drivers for the company wishing to undertake an assessment. In this context the expectations regarding what can be realistically achieved are discussed and the procedure for undertaking the assessment is outlined. Then a schedule is developed. At the second stage the lead assessor meets with the staff and management from the company who will be participating in the assessment. Here an overview of the Medi SPICE assessment method is presented and details of what staff participation will involve. The onsite assessment is the third stage in the procedure. During the onsite assessment the lead assessor conducts interviews with relevant staff based on scripted Medi SPICE-Adept questions. The second assessor who also participates in the interviews prepares interview notes and may ask additional questions when clarification is required. Work products may also be requested and briefly reviewed at this stage. A maximum of five processes are assessed in a single day with the interviews for each process taking approximately one hour. At the fourth stage the findings report is prepared off-site based on the data gathered at stage three. Each process is reviewed in turn and where relevant particular strengths and issues (weaknesses) are identified based on the evaluation and interview notes. Suggested actions to address these issues are then outlined and discussed. The possibility for the use of appropriate agile and lean practices is also considered. These are then documented and included in the findings report. This is a joint effort between the assessors and may include other SPI and/or lean and agile experts if required. The findings report is then presented to the management and staff who took part in the assessment which is the fifth stage in the procedure. Having provided adequate time for the findings report to be read and considered by the organization at the sixth stage the contents of the report is discussed in detail with the relevant management and staff. At this point specific objectives for process improvement are collaboratively defined based on the findings report which results in the development of a process improvement plan. Given the lightweight nature of Medi SPICE-Adept improvements that offer the greatest benefits in terms of compliance, quality and the achievement of business goals are selected for inclusion in this plan. At the seventh stage in the procedure the organization having implemented the process improvement plan have the opportunity of having the processes reassessed. Based on this, a final detailed report is prepared which highlights what has been achieved and an updated improvement plan is also provided.

Risk Management of IT Networks Incorporating Medical Devices

Traditionally, when medical devices were connected to a network, the network would be a proprietary network that would be provided, installed and supported by the medical device vendor. This allowed the medical device vendor to have control over configuration such as IP addressing which made support and service of the network easier. With the medical device vendor providing the network, this relieved the hospital of the responsibility of supporting life critical applications themselves. However use of proprietary networks in this way presented a number of disadvantages in that, as medical devices increasingly were designed to be incorporated into a network, the result was a proliferation of these networks resulting in the situation where large hospitals could have a large number of private networks. The maintenance of a large number of private networks is impractical and increasingly devices are being designed to be incorporated into a hospitals general IT network. General hospital IT networks are highly flexible and highly configurable. Incorporating a medical device into a general IT network can introduce additional risks that are particular to the incorporation of the device into the IT network and which may not have been considered during the design and manufacture of the device [44].

In order to address these risks, IEC 80001-1: Application of risk management for IT-networks incorporating medical devices [45] was published in 2010 which outlines the roles, responsibilities and activities that are required for the risk management of a medical IT network. IEC 80001-1 advocates a life cycle approach to risk management. The standard looks at the medical IT network from the perspective of maintaining three key properties of the network—Safety, Effectiveness and (Data and System) Security. Safety deals with ensuring that the device does not cause harm to the patient, the user of the device or the environment. Effectiveness is concerned with ensuring that the device continues to provide the intended result for the patient and the Responsible Organization. A Responsible Organisation is defined within the standard as an entity accountable for the use and maintenance of a medical IT network. Data and System Security ensures that information assets are reasonably protected from degradation of confidentiality, integrity, and availability. A medical IT network is defined within IEC 80001-1 as an "an IT network that incorporates at least one medical device".

Assessment Against IEC 80001-1

While IEC 80001-1 outlines the roles, responsibilities and activities that are required for risk management, there is currently no method which allows for assessment against IEC 80001-1. In order to address this, a Process Assessment Model (PAM) has been developed to allow for assessment against IEC 80001-1. The PAM was developed in accordance with the requirements for Process Assessment as described in ISO/IEC 15504-2 [46]. According to these requirements a PAM must be developed by extending a Process Reference Model (PRM) with the addition of a measurement framework. This measurement framework is described in ISO/IEC 15504-2 and contains 6 capability levels ranging from "incomplete" to "optimized".

Once the requirements for the development of PRMs and PAMs as described in ISO/IEC 15504-2 had been reviewed, it was necessary to determine an approach to the development of the PRM and PAM for assessment against IEC 80001-1. In order to do determine this approach, a review of standards similar to IEC 80001-1 was undertaken in order to determine what assessment methods were available for assessment against these standards and to determine how these assessment methods were developed. The research focused on ISO/IEC 20000-1 [47] which is a generic Service Management standard which is identified in Annex D of IEC 80001-1 as being similar to IEC 80001-1. While a medical IT network is set up to fulfill a specific purpose, it shares a number of characteristics with a general IT network [48]. Recognising this, in Annex D of IEC 80001-1 the requirements of ISO/IEC 20000 were reviewed to see if they could fulfill the requirements of IEC 80001-1. While it was recognized that IEC 20000-1 could not fulfill all of the requirements of IEC 80001-1, Annex D highlights areas where there are common processes between the two standards and areas where though the terminology is different, the underlying role, document or process is similar. The research focused on the Tudor IT Service Management Process Assessment (TIPA)[49] method which can be used to assess against ISO/IEC 20000-1 and another Service Managements standard, the Information Technology Infrastructure Library (ITIL) [50].

During the development of the TIPA assessment method it was noted that while ISO/IEC 15504-2 is clear in its requirements for process assessment in terms of the development of PRMs and PAMs, it does not provide guidance on how to transform the input or the domain requirements into the output or the PRM and PAM [51]. To address this need the TIPA transformation process, a goal oriented requirements engineering technique, was developed to give guidance ion the development of PRMs and PAMs which are consistent with the requirements as expressed in ISO/IEC 15504-2. The TIPA transformation technique also ensures that the processes within the PRM and PAM are described in a way which is consistent with ISO/IEC TR 24774 [52] which gives guidelines for process description. Given the similarities between ISO/IEC 20000-1 and IEC 80001-1 as previously discussed, the TIPA transformation process was used in the development of the PRM and PAM for assessment against IEC 80001-1. The transformation process was used in the development of the PRM which was then extended with the addition of a measurement framework to form the PAM. The PRM and PAM for assessment against IEC 80001-1 is discussed in the next section.

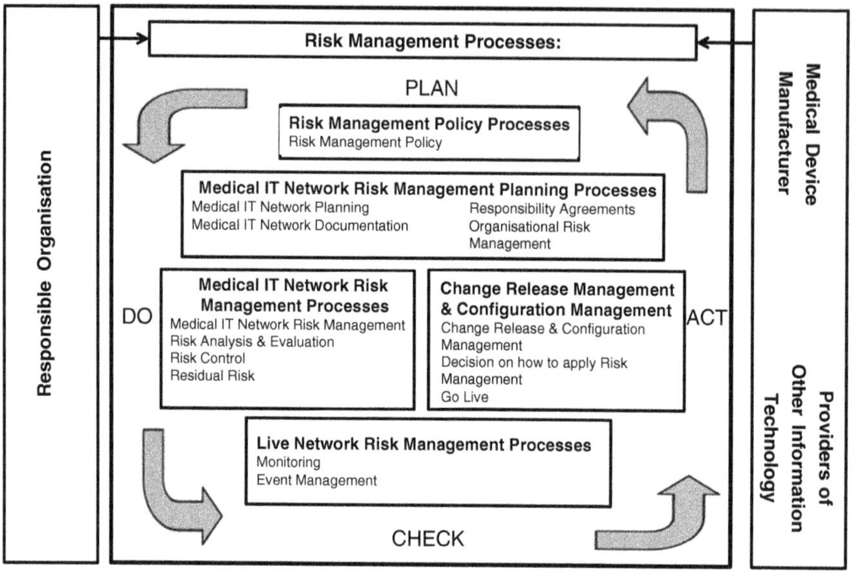

Fig. 21.2 IEC 8001-1 PRM process map

IEC 80001-1 Process Reference Model and Process Assessment Model

The PRM for assessment against IEC 80001-1 contains two main process categories—Primary Processes and Organizational Processes. The Primary Processes category is concerned with the performance of risk management activities and contains three process groups which contain nine processes in total. The process groups in the Primary Processes category are Medical IT Network Risk Management Process Group, Change Release Management and Configuration Management Process Group and finally the Live Network Risk Management Process Group. The Organizational Process category is concerned with the planning and management or risk management activities and contains a single process group called the Medical IT Network Documentation and Planning Process Group which contains 5 Processes. The PRM maintains the "Plan, Do, Check, Act" approach which is used in ISO/IEC TR 20000-4 [53] (which is the PRM for ISO/IEC 20000-1). The 14 processes as defined in the PRM are shown below.

The descriptions of the processes shown in Fig. 21.2 were extended to include base practices and work products which together with the addition of the measurement framework formed the PAM.

Future Validation and Development of the Assessment Framework

The next stage once complete will allow for assessment against IEC 80001-1 using an assessment method. The assessment method will be follow a staged process which will deal with aspects of the management of the assessment and which will provide a comprehensive list of questions related to each process within the PAM which will allow the assessor to establish the capability level associated with each process which will be the main stage of the assessment method. On the basis of this stage of the assessment, areas for improvement will be identified which will be communicated. A plan for these improvements will be delivered and a further assessment against this plan will be completed at a later date. Work on the development of this assessment method is ongoing.

The PRM and PAM which have been developed are currently being validated. Validation will be carried out in three ways. The PRM and PAM which are described in this chapter will be reviewed by the developers of the TIPA framework who will review the PRM and PAM in terms of their conformance with the requirements of ISO/IEC 15504-2 using experience gained during the development of a ISO/IEC 15504-2 compliant PAM for assessment against ISO/IEC 20000-1.The PAM has been raised as a new work item proposal for inclusion in the IEC 80001 family of standards. In the second stage of validation, the PAM will be reviewed by members of the international standards community, who have developed the IEC 80001-1 standard, in terms of its ability to assess against the requirements contained within IEC 80001-1. The final stage of validation will be the use of the PAM and assessment method within a hospital environment. The validated PAM and assessment method will then be used to perform a trial assessment within another hospital. The final PRM, PAM and assessment method will allow for assessment against IEC 80001-1. The PAM will be included in the IEC 80001 family of standards and as an international standard will provide an internationally recognized way to assess against the requirements as outlined in the IEC 80001-1 standard.

Security Assurance of Medical Devices

In the last number of years, there has been substantial advancement in the design and functionality of medical devices to offer patients a more sophisticated, reliable means of medical care. These advancements are mainly due to the growing use of software in medical devices. With the inclusion of software in medical devices, the next step in advancement came with the introduction of interoperable and connected medical devices incorporating technology to communicate wirelessly and across networks. The advantage of this development in medical device design is that patients can now receive around the clock monitoring and real-time treatment outside the healthcare environment without a consultant present. As for the healthcare providers, these devices alleviate the need for additional resources to monitor and administer the care or treatment to their patients. The downside to this is that while these design advancements do benefit the healthcare industry and patient care in many ways, it also introduces new risks to patient safety. These are security risks, vulnerabilities and threats.

Traditionally medical devices were designed to be stand-alone devices but we see many different types of devices that communicate wirelessly and over networks in today's world with each device type presenting different security concerns. While there have been no malicious attacks on medical devices recorded to date there have been a number of controlled hacks on medical devices. Implantable medical devices (IMDs) have been targets of some of the controlled hacks in the last year or so. One such incident was at the Black Hat Security Conference in Las Vegas in 2011. The diabetic security researcher carried out a controlled hack on his own insulin pump during his presentation and gained sufficient access to allow him to increase and decrease the insulin dosage. On both occasions, there was no warning that the device had been tampered with and there was no warning that the patient could possibly die. External medical devices also pose problems with regard security. Many devices have built in commercial operating systems, which were designed by software developers but, because these are widely used operating systems, they are more susceptible to malicious attacks. The other types of medical devices which are of concern are the increasingly portable medical devices and Bring Your Own Devices (BYODs). More and more practitioners are using smartphones and iPads to retrieve electronic patient health information (EPHI) in patient consultations [54].

The age of interoperability and connected medical devices has just begun and so the area of security in such devices is not fully exploited as yet by the medical device community and researchers but more worryingly by malicious attackers. As of yet, there is no formal governance for the assessment of such medical devices process capability or for the establishment of medical device product capability with regard security. Over the last number of years there has been a lot of concern among the medical device community in regard to interoperable and connected medical devices and their communication abilities in terms of security vulnerabilities, threats and risks. This has been reflected through the many publications, technical reports and guidance documents released such as IEC/TR 80001-2-2 [55]. In August 2012, the Government Accountability Office (GAO) published a report [56] that clearly indicated the need for the FDA to enhance their assessment of security medical devices and concluded with the recommendation that the FDA address these issues.

This section discusses research that sets out to address this problem by establishing a methodology to assure the security of connected and interoperable medical devices on IT networks. Figure 21.3 outlines the architecture of the solution that is discussed in more detail in the following sections.

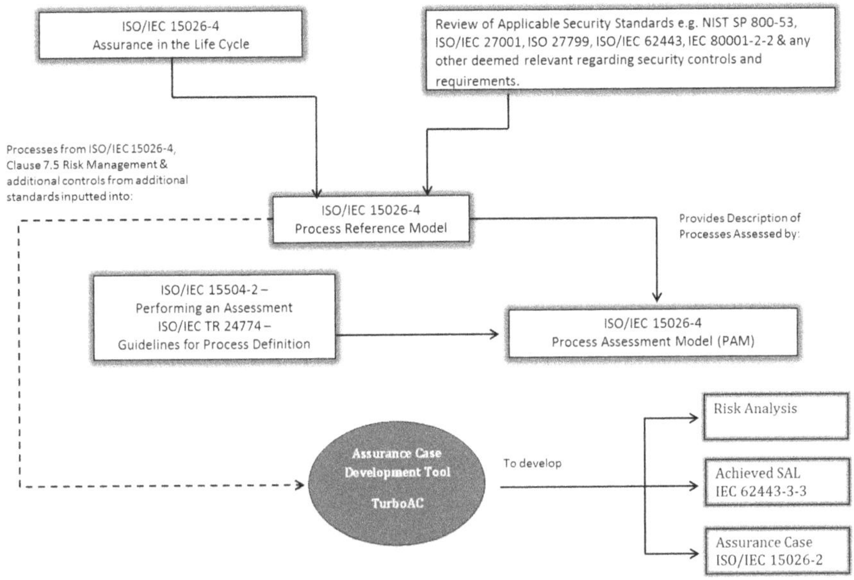

Fig. 21.3 Approach overview

Establishing Meaningful Security Controls

The first step in developing this model is to conduct a comprehensive review of existing security standards and guidance documents. These will include ISO/IEC 27001 [57], ISO/IEC 27799 [58], ISO 15408 [59], IEC 62443-3-3 [60], and NIST SP 800-53 [61]. Each of these standards and guidance documents similarly present security classes and controls. A list of applicable security controls to be addressed during the development risk assessment process will be derived from the previously mentioned sources through the use of expert opinion. The FDA and carefully selected expert users will validate this derived set of controls. The outcome of this will be a published technical report with a cross-standard mapping of security controls to be considered in regard to interoperable medical devices communicating over an IT network.

IEC/TR 80001-2-2 [55] is a technical report that sets out to promote the communication of security controls, needs and risks of medical devices to be incorporated into IT networks between Medical Device Manufacturers (MDMs), IT vendors and Healthcare Delivery Organisations (HDOs). This technical report presents 20 security capabilities (See Table 21.2). It is anticipated that the upcoming technical report outlining a set of mandatory security controls will be reflected in a new revision of IEC 80001-2-2 should the technical report highlight gaps with the existing 20 security capabilities.

Table 21.2 IEC/TR 80001-2-2 capabilities

	Security capability	Code
1	Automatic Logoff	ALOF
2	Audit Controls	AUDT
3	Authorization	AUTH
4	Configuration of Security Features	CNFS
5	Cyber Security Product Upgrades	CSUP
6	Data Backup and Disaster Recovery	DTBK
7	Emergency Access	EMRG
8	Health Data De-Identification	DIDT
9	Health Data Integrity and Authentication	IGAU
10	Health Data Storage Confidentiality	STCF
11	Malware Detection/Protection	MLDP
12	Node Authentication	NAUT
13	Person Authentication	PAUT
14	Physical Locks on Device	PLOK
15	Security Guides	SGUD
16	System and Application Hardening	SAHD
17	Third-Party Components in Product Lifecycle Roadmaps	RDMP
18	Transmission Confidentiality	TXCF
19	Transmission Integrity	TXIG
20	Unique User ID	UUID

Process Assurance

This research presents a methodology to address security concerns in the medical device domain specifically looking at networked medical devices. As a way to assure medical devices, the methodology takes an approach from the development process capability and also the final product quality assurance. In establishing a process capability level for the development of a medical device, MDMs gain better control over their processes and output. This also proves beneficial from a compliance assessment point of view when there are clearly defined and measurable processes in place.

For the problem solution a PAM will be used. These are widely used in software/I.T. businesses to measure the capability of an organization to achieve particular processes. The two most widely used models are CMMI [62] and the ISO/IEC 15504 family. We have selected the international standard for process assessment, ISO/IEC 15504-2 [63] that sets out requirements for defining process assessment models and for performing process assessments.

In using this standard, the two major outcomes will be a PRM and PAM. A PAM contains two dimensions; these are the Process Dimension and the Capability Dimension. The Process Dimension is developed from an external PRM that provides the processes for assessment in terms of 'Purpose' and 'Outcome'. The PAM expands the PRM with the use of Performance Indicators called Base Practices and Work Products. Work Products are both the inputs and outputs to each process and the

Base Practices describe the process activities that convert these inputs to process outputs.

The Capability Dimension is based upon six capability levels ranging from Level 0 'Incomplete' to Level 5 'Optimizing'. Achievement of a capability level is based upon the achievement of Process Attributes (of which there are a total of nine) for Capability Levels 1 through to 5. A Process Attribute is the measurement characteristic of each process. For example, in achieving capability level 1, 'Performed', the Process Attribute is Process Performance, for capability level 2, 'Managed', one Process Attribute is Process Management, and so on.

ISO/IEC 15504-6 [64] describes an exemplar PAM and will form the foundation of the model as it utilizes ISO/IEC 15288 [65] as the PRM. This international standard (ISO/IEC 15288) has been selected as it addresses system life cycle processes. As these networked medical devices can contain a combination of hardware, software, people, processes etc. it is deemed the most suitable foundation for the PAM. ISO/IEC 15288 is a framework to improve the communication and cooperation among parties that design, develop, use and maintain systems. It covers the entire life cycle of systems development from concept straight through to retirement and also including acquisition and supply processes.

Due to the criticality of networked medical devices, this PAM will be extended to include additional processes from ISO/IEC 15026-4 [66]. This is yet another international standard specifically addressing assurance in the life cycle. ISO/IEC 15026-4 is mainly utilized where additional assurance for a critical property, such as dependability, safety or security, is required for a system or software. The standard is used as an add-on to an already existing life cycle process standard such as that of ISO/IEC 15288. Therefore, this extension of the PAM lines up with ISO/IEC 15504-6 building upon existing processes addressed here.

Finally, the PAM will be further extended to include the 20 security capabilities presented in IEC/TR 80001-2-2 (Table 21.2). This will be included in the system risk management process. In developing a networked medical device, MDMs will be required to specifically address all 20 security capabilities and determine which of those are applicable to the medical device. Justification of non-applicable security capabilities will be required.

Product Assurance

Having established the process assurance for the development of medical devices to be incorporated into an IT network, the research will further assure the medical device by addressing the security assurance of the deliverable. This means assurance starts at the beginning of the acquisition process between the HDO and the MDM. In support of IEC/TR 80001-2-2, the outcome of this methodology will be the communication of the target security capability requirement of a device by the HDO to the MDM and then a justification of an achieved security capability requirement from the MDM to the HDO. This is the first input in the product assurance strategy

Table 21.3 Security capability requirements for ALOF

Implementation identifier	Capability
ALOF.01	A screensaver starts automatically 5 min after last key-stroke/mouse movement operation
ALOF.02	The screensaver clears all displayed health data from the screen
ALOF.03	The screensaver does not log-off the user/does not terminate the session
ALOF.04	User has to log-in after occurrence of the screensaver
ALOF.05	The user-session terminates automatically 60 min after last key-stroke/mouse movement/touchscreen operation.

of this model. In communicating this information a vector schema will be utilised. Table 21.2 presents the security capabilities. In order to better define the requirements of the HDO this will be further broken down. Each security capability will have a sub set of requirements. Table 21.3 shows an example break down for security capability *Automatic Logoff*(ALOF). Each of the security capability requirements will be displayed on a vector as follows:

$$T{-}ALOF = \{1, 0, 1, 1, 0\}$$

This vector indicates the HDO's target security capability requirement (T) for *Automatic Logoff* to have in place the sub requirements ALOF.01, ALOF.03 and ALOF.04. Zero on the vector indicates that that particular sub requirement is not required. This format will be used for all security capabilities and their sub requirements. During the risk management process, required security controls will be identified. These controls will be the second input to the product assurance element of this methodology. This will be achieved through the utilisation of a tool. This tool will be used to further build on the risk management processes. Each security capability will be addressed in the FMEA or risk analysis builder within the tool. In turn the tool will automatically build an assurance case and outline in detail the evidence gathered to support the achievement of each security assurance level. To date, assurance cases have mainly be used within in the medical device domain to address safety and are recommended to MDMs as part of the infusion pump initiative [67]. A similar type methodology will be adapted here addressing security as the critical property.

ISO/IEC 15026-2 [68] defines requirements for the structure and content of an assurance case. An assurance case is a body of evidence organized into an argument demonstrating some claim that a system holds i.e. is acceptably secure. An assurance case is needed when it is important to show that a system exhibits some complex property such as safety, security, or reliability. Security assurance cases are often compared with a legal case where there are two elements to the case, the argument and the evidence to support a claim. For an assurance case to be effective it must satisfy the following points:

- Must make a claim or set of claims about a property of a system;
- Produce the supportive evidence;

- Provide a set of arguments;
- Make clear the assumptions and judgements underlying the arguments;
- Associate different viewpoints and level of detail.

Upon completion of the risk management process, the MDM will have established the achieved security capability requirements for the product and developed a security assurance case with proof, through evidence, of the security assurance of the networked medical device. This will be detailed on the security assurance case, which will be held by the MDM for third party regulatory assessment. It may be the communication article between the MDM and the HDO in which, the HDO IT Administration staff may include in their risk management file should the medical device be installed into their IT network. Upon completion of the security assurance case, the MDM will then follow the same format as the HDOs to highlight the security capability requirements as was done at the start of the acquisition process by the HDO. They too will use a vector format to present the achieved security capability requirements of the medical device. Using the previous example, the achieved security capability requirements (A) for *Automatic Logoff* could be as shown below. This example shows that ALOF.02, although not stated as a target security capability requirement, is also shown as being implemented. Again, for each of the 20 security capabilities, the achieved security capability requirements will be communicated to the HDO.

$$A\text{–}ALOF = \{1, 1, 1, 1, 0\}$$

Conclusions and Summary

Medical devices have a direct impact on an individual's wellbeing. Therefore to ensure the safe and reliable performance of medical devices regulations have been put in place. These regulations dictate what information a medical device manufacturer should produce as evidence as to how safe the device is. However, regulatory bodies do not provide comprehensive guidance as to how this objective evidence must be produced.

Traditionally, a medical device was considered a hardware device with a software component. In this case, the safety of the device could be proved through the hardware functioning of the device. However, recent changes to regulations now mean that a medical device may consist solely of software. As a result there is no hardware element which can produce evidence to support the safety of the device. To overcome this, medical device software organizations are recommended to follow the latest state of the art development processes and standards such as IEC 62304; however, IEC 62304 has not been updated since the recent changes to regulations and as a result it is not sufficiently comprehensive to provide coverage of all of the necessary stages of development.

To fill this void and to draw upon the software industry best practices, Medi SPICE is currently under development by the RSRG. Medi SPICE will act as a single point of reference for medical device software organizations when developing regulatory compliant software. Medi SPICE combines international regulations, medical device software standards and software development best practices to a single point. Medi SPICE aims to provide coverage of all of the stages of medical device software development and maintenance.

While Medi SPICE is under development to respond to the needs of the medical device software industry an emerging area causing concerns regarding medical device safety, is the connecting of medical device to networks. This creates a new level of concern with regards to the impact other devices on the same network will have on the medical device and also the potential security implications of a device being accessed by an unauthorized user. To address these risks two frameworks are currently under development by the RSRG which aim to address these risks.

IEC 80001-1 takes a life cycle approach to risk management of IT networks which incorporate medical devices. The incorporation of a device into an IT network can introduce risks that may not have been considered during the design and manufacture of the medical device. While HDOs may perform risk management activities, there is no method that exists to allow a HDO to assess the capability of their risk management processes against the requirements of IEC 80001-1 which outlines risk management activities which are specific to the incorporation of a medical device into an IT network. Research to date has focused on the development of a PRM and PAM for assessment against IEC 80001-1. The PRM and PAM have been raised as a new work item proposal and will be part of a technical report within the IEC 80001-1 family of standards. When an assessment is performed using the IEC 80001-1 PAM, this will allow the HDO to assess the capability of risk management processes and will provide an insight into areas where process improvement can take place and a higher capability level can be achieved. IEC/TR 80001-2-2 defines the security capabilities that a MDM or IT vendor must communicate to the HDO in order to enhance knowledge of security risks and controls the HDO IT administration staff should consider and vice versa. The outcome of this research will provide many benefits for both the HDOs and the MDMs. For the HDOs some of the benefits will include:

1. A common framework to assist in the selection of suppliers through process capability levels.
2. Guidance for the communication of medical device security needs.
3. Better understanding of the security capability of the devices.
4. Knowledge of the security assurance of the device through the use of a vector for the target and achieved security capability requirements.

The MDMs also benefit through:

1. Better knowledge of the capability level of their life cycle processes with clear insight for process improvement.
2. A method to add additional assurance to their processes through the extension of the PRM using the international standard ISO/IEC 15026-4, Assurance in the Life Cycle.

3. A focused security risk management process with the inclusion of a defined set of security capabilities and further requirements.
4. A method and tool for the automatic development of security assurance cases

Currently, there is no methodology to address both the development processes and the product capabilities of medical devices in terms of security. Hence, it is envisaged that the output of our research will positively impact the medical device domain in both the EU and the US by building awareness of security vulnerabilities, threats and related risks between the HDO and the MDM [69].

Whilst the research presented in this chapter is on-going, there is a clear need for the models which have been presented. This need has been identified through collaboration with the medical device industry, the standards community and regulatory bodies such as the FDA. Once completed, each of the models presented will have a direct impact on the safe and reliable performance of medical devices which are also secure.

References

1. I. Lee and O. Sokolsky, "Medical cyber physical systems," presented at the 47th Design Automation Conference, Anaheim, California, 2010.
2. R. K. Bhaskar and G. Somu, "Adoption Of Information Technology (IT) In Healthcare Delivery-Experience At A Tertiary Level Hospital" *International Journal of Medical Informatics*, vol. 5, 2011.
3. L. Ash, *The Web Testing Companion: The Insider's Guide to Efficient and Effective Tests*. New York: John Wiley & Sons, 2003.
4. N. Leveson, *Safeware: System Safety and Computers*: Addison Wesley, 1995.
5. ISO, "*ISO/IEC 13485:2003 Medical devices - Quality management systems - Requirements for regulatory purposes*," ed. International Organisation for Standards - Geneva, Switzerland, 2003.
6. ISO, "*ISO/IEC 14971:2007 Medical devices - Application of risk management to medical devices*," ed. International Organisation for Standards - Geneva, Switzerland 2007.
7. AAMI, "ANSI/AAMI/IEC 62304, Medical device Software - Software life cycle processes," ed. Association for the Advancement of Medical Instrumentation, 2006.
8. FDA, "Title 21-Food and Drugs Chapter I -Food and Drug Administration Department of Health and Human Services subchapter h-Medical Devices part 820 Quality System Regulation," ed: *U.S. Department of Health and Human Services*, 2007.
9. *Guidance for Industry, Third parties annd Food and Drug Administration Staff, Medical Device ISO 13485:2003 Voluntary Audit Report Submission, Program*, 2012.
10. *Medical Devices Guidance Document - Qualification and Classification of stand alone software MEDDEV 2.1/6*, 2012.
11. E. S. Crumpler and H. Rudolph, "FDA Software Policy and Regulation of Medical Device Software," *Food and Drug Law Journal*, vol. 52, 1997.
12. *Directive 2007/47/EC of the European Parliament and of the Council of 5 September 2007*, 2007.
13. Health Canada. (2011, 10/01/2013). *Software Regulated as a Medical Device* Available: http://www.hc-sc.gc.ca/dhp-mps/md-im/activit/announce-annonce/md_qa_software_im_qr_logicels-eng.php
14. FDA, "21 CFR Part 880 Medical Devices; Medical Device Data Systems Final Rule." *Federal Register* vol. 76, pp. 8637–8649, 2011.

15. M. McHugh, F. McCaffery, and V. Casey, "US FDA releases final rule on Medical Device Data Systems - What does this mean for device manufacturers," *Journal of Medical Device Regulation*, vol. 8, pp. 35–40, 2011.
16. M. Klumper and E. Vollebregt, "The Regulation of Software for Medical Devices in Europe," *Journal of Medical Device Regulation*, vol. 7, pp. 5–13, 2010.
17. M. McHugh, F. McCaffery, and V. Casey, "Changes to the International Regulatory Environment," *Journal of Medical Devices*, vol. 6, 2012.
18. *Commission communication in the framework of the implementation of the Council Directive 93/42/EEC of 14 June 1993 concerning medical devices (Publication of titles and references of harmonised standards under the directive)*, 2010.
19. *FDA Design Control Guidance for Medical Device Manufacturers*, 1997.
20. FDA, "General Principles of Software Validation: Final Guidance for Industry and FDA Staff," ed: *Centre for Devices and Radiological Health*, 2002.
21. FDA, "Draft Guidance for Industry and Food and Drug Administration - Mobile Device Applications," ed: *Centre for Devices and Radiological Health*, 2011.
22. FDA, "Guidance for Industry, FDA Reviewers and Compliance on Off-The-Shelf Software use in Medical Devices," ed: *U.S. Department of Health and Human Services*, 1999.
23. P. Jordan, "Standard IEC 62304 - Medical Device Software - Software Lifecycle Processes," presented at the The Institution of Engineering and Technology Seminar on Software for Medical Devices London, 2006.
24. Minister of Justice, "Medical Device Regulations SOR/98-282," in http://laws-lois.justice.gc.ca, ed, 2012.
25. D. M. Zuckerman, P. Brown, and S. E. Nissen, "Medical device recalls and the fda approval process," *Archives of Internal Medicine*, vol. 171, pp. 1006–1011, 2011.
26. P. L. Jones, J. Jorgens, A. R. T. Jr, and M. Weber, "Risk Management in the Design of Medical Device Software Systems," *Biomedical Instrumentation & Technology: July 2002*, vol. 36, pp. 237–266, 2002.
27. C. Denger, R. L. Feldman, M. Host, C. Lindholm, and F. Schull, "A Snapshot of the State of Practice in Software Development for Medical Devices," presented at the First International Symposium on Empirical Software Engineering and Measurement, 2007. ESEM 2007, Madrid, 2007.
28. *Capability Maturity Model® Integration for Development Version 1.2*, 2006.
29. ISO/IEC 15504–5:2006, "Information technology - Process Assessment - Part 5: An Exemplar Process Assessment Model," ed. Geneva, Switzerland: ISO, 2006.
30. F. Mc Caffery and A. Dorling, "Medi SPICE Development," *Software Process Maintenance and Evolution: Improvement and Practice Journal* vol. 22 pp. 255–268, 2010.
31. Automotive SIG, "Automotive SPICE Process Assessment V 2.2," ed, 21 August 2005.
32. ISO/IEC 12207:2008, "Systems and software engineering - Software life cycle processes," ed. Geneva, Switzerland: ISO, 2008.
33. US FDA, "21 CFR Part 820 Quality System Regulations," *Code of Federal Regulations, Title 21*, vol. 8, Revised April 1, 2011.
34. F. Mc Caffery, A. Dorling, and V. Casey, "Medi SPICE: An Update," in *International Conference on Software Process Improvement and Capability Determinations (SPICE)*, Pisa, Italy, 2010, pp. 195–198.
35. V. Casey, "Virtual Software Team Project Management," *Journal of the Brazilian Computer Society*, vol. 16, pp. 83–96, August 2010 2010.
36. ISO/IEC 15504–2:2003, "Software engineering - Process assessment - Part 2: Performing an assessment," ed. Geneva, Switzerland: ISO, 2003.
37. F. Mc Caffery and A. Dorling, "Medi SPICE: An Overview," *in International Conference on Software Process Improvement and Capability Determinations (SPICE)*, Turku, Finland, 2009, pp. 34–41.
38. F. Mc Caffery, V. Casey, and M. Mc Hugh, "How Can Software SMEs become Medical Device Software SMEs," in *European Systems & Software Process Improvement and Innovation Conference, (EuroSPI)*, Copenhagen 2011, pp. 247–258.

39. F. Mc Caffery, J. Burton, V. Casey, and A. Dorling, "Software Process Improvement in the Medical Device Industry," in *Encyclopedia of Software Engineering*. vol. 1, P. Laplante, Ed., ed New York: CRC Press Francis Taylor, Group, 2010, pp. 528–540.
40. O. Cawley, I. Richardson, and X. Wang, "Medical Device Software Development - A Perspective from a Lean Manufacturting Plant," *in 11th International SPICE Conference on Process Improvement and Capability dEtermination 2011, Dublin City University, Ireland, 2011*, pp. 84–96.
41. F. Mc Caffery, I. Richardson, and G. Coleman, "Adept - A Software Process Appraisal Method for Small to Medium-sized Irish Software Development Organisations," in *European Systems & Software Process Improvement and Innovation (EuroSPI 2006), Joensuu, Finland*, 2006, pp. 7.12-7.21.
42. F. Mc Caffery and V. Casey, "Med-Adept: A Lightweight Assessment Method for the Irish Medical Device Software Industry," in *European Systems & Software Process Improvement and Innovation Conference, (EuroSPI)*, Grenoble, France, 2010, pp. 1.9 - 1.16.
43. V. Casey and F. Mc Caffery, "A lightweight traceability assessment method for medical device software," *Journal of Software Maintenance and Evolution Research and Practice*, October 2011 2011.
44. T. Gee. (2008, 27/1/2012). *Medical Device Networks Trouble Industry*. Available: http://medicalconnectivity.com/2008/12/18/medical-device-networks-trouble-industry/
45. IEC, "IEC 80001–1 - Application of Risk Management for IT-Networks incorporating Medical Devices - Part 1: Roles, responsibilities and activities," ed. Geneva, Switzerland: International Electrotechnical Commission, 2010.
46. ISO/IEC, "ISO/IEC 15504–2:2003 - Software engineering – Process assessment – Part 2: Performing an assessment," ed. Geneva, Switzerland, 2003.
47. ISO/IEC, "ISO/IEC 20000–1:2011 - Information technology –Service management Part 1: Service management system requirements," ed. Geneva, Switzerland, 2011.
48. M. Janssen and R. Schrenker, "Guidelines From 80001: Maintaining a Medical IT Network," *Biomedical Instrumentation & Technology*, vol. 45, pp. 295–299, 2011/07/01 2011.
49. B. Barafort, V. Betry, S. Cortina, M. Picard, M. St Jean, A. Renault, O. Valdés, and P. R. C. H. Tudor, *ITSM Process Assessment Supporting ITIL : Using TIPA to Assess and Improve your Processes with ISO 15504 and Prepare for ISO 20000 Certification* vol. 217. Zaltbommel, Netherlands: Van Haren, 2009.
50. The Cabinet Office, "ITIL 2011 - Summary of Updates," ed. Norfolk, England: Crown Copyright, 2011.
51. B. Barafort, A. Renault, M. Picard, and S. Cortina, "A transformation process for building PRMs and PAMs based on a collection of requirements - Example with ISO/IEC 20000," presented at the SPICE Nuremberg, Germany, 2008.
52. ISO/IEC, "ISO/IEC TR 24774:2010 - Systems and software engineering – Life cycle management – Guidelines for process description," ed. Geneva, Switzerland, 2010.
53. ISO/IEC, "ISO/IEC TR 20000–4:2010 - Information technology – Service management - Part 4: Process reference model," ed. Geneva, Switzerland, 2010.
54. DHS, "Attack Surface: Healthcare and Public Heath Sector," 2012.
55. IEC, "TR 80001–2-2 - Application of risk management for IT-networks incorporating medical devices - Guidance for the disclosure and communication of medical device security needs, risks and controls," ed: International Electrotechnical Committee, 2011, p. Page 30.
56. Government Accountability Office, "Medical Devices, FDA Should Expland Its Consideration of Information Security for Certain Types of Devices," 2012.
57. ISO/IEC, "27001 Information Technology - Security Techniques - Information Security Management Systems - Requirements," ed, 2005.
58. ISO, "EN ISO 27799:2008 Health informatics. Information security management in health using ISO/IEC 27002," ed, 2008.
59. ISO/IEC, "15408-2 Information Technology - Security Techniques - Evaluation Criteria for IT Security," in *Security Functional Components*, ed, 2008.

60. IEC, "62443-3-3 - Security for industrial automation and control systems - Network and system security - System security requirements and security assurance levels Introductory," ed, 2011.
61. NIST, "800-53 Recommended Security Controls for Federal Information Systems and Organisations," U. S. D. o. Commerce, Ed., Revision 3 ed, 2009.
62. SEI, "CMMI for Development," 2006.
63. ISO/IEC, "15504-2: 2003 Software Engineering - Process Assessment - Performing an Assessment," ed, 2003.
64. ISO/IEC, "15504-6:2008 Information technology – Process assessment – An exemplar system life cycle process assessment model," ed, 2008.
65. ISO, "Systems and software engineering - System life cycle processes," ed, 2008.
66. ISO/IEC, "15026-4: Systems and Software Engineering - Systems and Software Assurance - Assurance in the Life Cycle," ed, 2012.
67. FDA, "Total Product Life Cycle: Infusion Pump - Premarket Notification [510(k)] Submissions - Draft Guidance," ed, 2010.
68. ISO/IEC, "15026-2: 2011 Systems & Software Engineering, Systems & Software Assurance, Part 2: Assurance Case," ed, 2011, p. 28.
69. A. Finnegan, F. McCaffery, and G. Coleman, "Development of a process assessment model for assessing security of IT networks incorporating medical devices against ISO/IEC 15026–4," presented at the Healthinf 2013, Barcelona, Spain.

Chapter 22
Wearable and Implantable Technologies for Cardiovascular Health Informatics

Yali Zheng, Carmen C. Y. Poon and Yuan Ting Zhang

Introduction

Though modern medical technologies have been progressed significantly in this century, cardiovascular disease (CVD) is still one of the leading causes of death worldwide. The number of patients with CVD in China is around 230 million, and about 3 million die from CVD annually, which accounts for 41 % of all-cause death [1]. In the United States, CVD-related death account for more than one-third of all deaths. CVD are posing great economic challenges worldwide. In 2010, the global cost of CVD is estimated at US$ 863 billion [2].

Some major problems in the present cardiovascular healthcare practice cause the condition of high mortality and morbidity as well as high expenses. Firstly, the clinicians often use the traditional risk factors for CVD risk stratification, such as age, office blood pressure, smoking habits and diabetes. It can only identify the diseases at late stage when the subject presented significant symptoms, and therefore makes the treatment costly and ineffective. Secondly, the present healthcare system is unable to provide early interventions when emergent events occurred out of hospital. Therefore, these situations are calling for a new healthcare system which emphasizes on preventing and predicting diseases before the emergence of significant disease symptoms and also providing pervasive and pre-emptive healthcare.

Y. Zheng · C. C. Y. Poon · Y. T. Zhang
Joint Research Center for Biomedical Engineering (JCBME),
Department of Electronic Engineering, The Chinese University of Hong Kong,
Hong Kong SAR, China

C. C. Y. Poon
Department of Surgery, The Chinese University of Hong Kong, Hong Kong SAR, China

Y. T. Zhang (✉)
Key Laboratory for Health Informatics of Chinese Academy of Science (HICAS),
Shenzhen, China
e-mail: ytzhang@ee.cuhk.edu.hk

B. Furht and A. Agarwal (eds.), *Handbook of Medical and Healthcare Technologies*, 481
DOI: 10.1007/978-1-4614-8495-0_22, © Springer Science+Business Media New York 2013

Health informatics is an area which deals with the Acquisition, Transmission, Processing, Storage and Retrieval (p-STAR) of multi-modal health and biomedical information to help improving healthcare management and medical decision making. Sensing is one of the major technologies to acquire health and medical information from healthy people or patients. The sensor-based devices can be either wearable or implantable which depends on the location of the sensing elements: in body or on body. The health information collected from the sensors will then be wirelessly transmitted to a data collector such as a cellphone and relayed to the remote database server for storage and processing. If expert system is included, feedback will be delivered for treatment.

Some advantages of wearable and implantable technologies are expected to significantly improve the quality, effectiveness and efficiency of cardiovascular healthcare. Firstly, they can be used to collect long-term and continuous health information for tracking the progressive development of chronic diseases for early diagnosis and treatment. In addition, it can provide unobtrusive monitoring in a natural environment for the convenient of use.

This chapter will discuss the two sensing technologies, i.e., wearable and implantable technologies. Firstly, the state-of-the-art of wearable and implantable technologies will be introduced. Then the key technologies in developing wearable and implantable systems will be discussed, such as modeling techniques for accurate wearable sensing, motion artifacts reduction and low power system design for wearable systems together with wireless power transfer techniques for implantable systems. Moreover, the critical challenges and some potential solutions will be mentioned.

Wearable Technologies

Many wearable sensors have been designed to monitor different aspects of the cardiovascular system, from which some important cardiovascular parameters can be derived or estimated, such as heart rate (HR), blood pressure (BP), blood oxygen saturation (SpO2), respiration rate and tidal volume. Here we will firstly introduce some of these wearable sensors and their recent advancement, and then review the state-of-the-art of wearable health monitoring systems for measuring multiple parameters.

Wearable Sensors

(1) *Electrocardiogram*

Electrocardiogram (ECG) is the most commonly monitored physiological signal for CVD patients. It describes the electrical activity of the heart, providing important information about the presence of coronary artery diseases, heart arrhythmias, and other cardiac failures. The commonly used ECG electrodes are the wet silver/silver chloride (Ag/AgCl) type, which are directly affixed to body and may cause skin irritation in long-term monitoring. Some contactless ECG electrodes have been developed to overcome this problem. For example, conductive textiles were adopted as ECG electrodes to record the electrical signal through clothing using the concept of displacement current through capacitive coupling [3, 4]. Another problem with the Ag/AgCl electrode is that the signal may degrade due to the dehydration of Ag/AgCl electrodes. Some dry ECG electrodes were developed, such as the PDMS-based surface electrode [5] and planar-fashionable circuit board electrodes on shirt [6], which not only solved the signal degradation problem, but also were designed with flexible base to form good contact with the body. To improve the signal quality, active ECG electrodes with functional electronics for signal amplification, noise reduction and filtering were also developed [7].

(2) *Photoplethysmogram*

Photoplethysmogram (PPG) is detected by an optical measurement technique and reflects the blood volume changes in the microvasuclar bed of tissue. It has been broadly applied in various clinical settings [8]. In the application of wearable hemodynamic monitoring, it has been used for monitoring parameters such as blood oxygen saturation [9], blood pressure by a cuff-less approach [10] and cardiac output [11]. A PPG measurement system often consists of a light emitting diode (LED) in the red or near infrared red range, photodiode and processing electronics. It can work in reflective mode where the light reflected from the tissue will be detected or in transmission mode where the transmitted light passing through the tissue will be detected. PPG can be measured at different sites of the body, such as ear, finger and toe. Recently, the author's group designed an eyeglasses-based device to measure PPG at the nose bridge [12]. Compared to those designs at finger or ear site, no clip is needed during monitoring, which makes the design very suitable for long-term use. The most challenging issue of PPG measurement is the high power consumption of LED. Duun et al. [13] recently designed a ring shaped backside silicon pn photodiode as shown in Fig. 22.1, which is capable of giving optimal gathering of light and therefore significantly reduce the driving currents for LED.

(3) *Blood pressure*

As the important risk factor of CVD, blood pressure (BP) is measured by means of sphygmomanometer clinically. Conventional blood pressure meters, which are designed with an inflatable cuff, may cause discomfort to the users when used frequently and are unsuitable if not impossible for long-term and wearable monitoring. Pulse transit time (PTT) which is the time delay between the R-peak of ECG waveform and foot or peak of the PPG waveform, as shown in Fig. 22.2a, is correlated with arterial blood pressure through Moens-Korteweg equation which describes the quantitative relationship of pulse wave velocity (PWV) and the elasticity of arteries. PTT and BP have been found closely related in extensive studies [10, 14]. Since PTT can be easily measured from ECG and PPG by wearable devices, this PTT-based BP

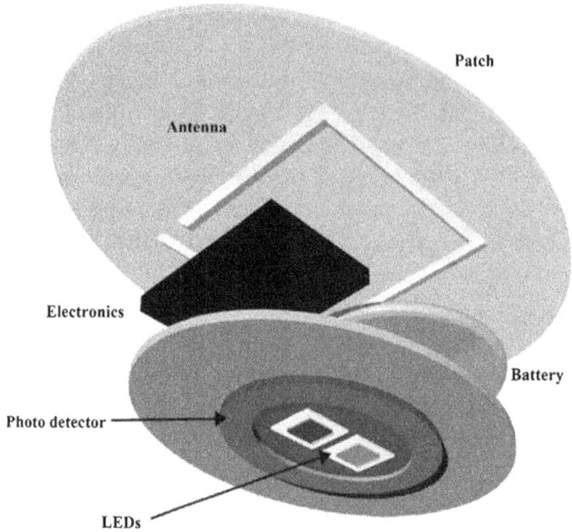

Fig. 22.1 Illustration of a novel PPG sensor which consists of commercial LEDs and a ring-shaped photodiode, the signal processing electronics, wireless radio communication and coin cell battery [13]

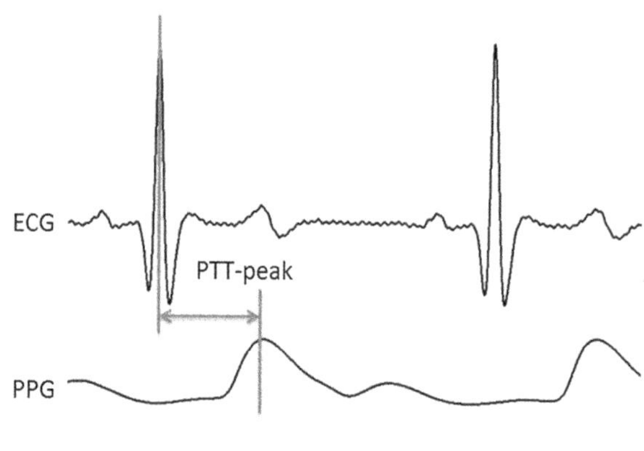

Fig. 22.2 PTT is defined as the delay between the R-peak of ECG waveform and foot or peak of the PPG waveform

estimation method is very promising for long-term and continuous BP monitoring. However, the major problem with this PTT-based BP estimation method compared with cuff-based methods is that it needs calibration to determine the individual parameters in the function of PTT and BP. To avoid individual calibration, Chen et al. recently proposed a new function of PTT and BP by adding an age-and-gender-related parameter based on assumption that the elasticity of the blood vessels changes with age and gender [15]. The major challenge of PTT-based BP estimation method is that some subjects showed high correlation between systolic BP (SBP) and PTT ($r > 0.5$), but some others showed low correlation ($r > 0.5$) [14]. The underlying mechanism is still not fully understood. Some studies presumably attributed this to the change of vessel state during dynamic state, i.e., vasodilation or vasoconstriction [14]. Other studies reported that it may be the contribution of pre-ejection period [16].

(4) *Respiration*

Respiratory inductive plethysmography (RIP) has been considered as the most promising technique for long-term and unconstrained monitoring of respiration. RIP was firstly introduced to clinical medicine in 1978 and it mainly consists of two sensors (sinusoidal arrangement of electrical wires) placed around the level of rib cage (RC) and abdomen (AB), an oscillator, a frequency demodulator and a microprocessor. During inspiration and expiration, the cross-sectional area of RC and AB changes and induces the change of the inductance of the two sensors, which thus modulates the frequency of the oscillatory signal. Through demodulation, the respiratory waveform from RC and AB can be obtained respectively and the amplitude of each waveform is proportional to the inspiratory or expiratory volume. From the respiratory waveform, the tidal volume (TV) and respiration rate can be derived. To calculate TV, calibration is needed to identify the calibration coefficients in the following equation:

$$\Delta V_a = \alpha \cdot \Delta RC + \beta \cdot \Delta AB, \tag{22.1}$$

where, ΔVa is the change of the volume at mouth, ΔRC and ΔAB are changes in RIP signals from RC and AB, respectively. α and β are the calibration coefficients. Recently, an improvement has been made on RIP to reduce the power consumption [17]. Each RIP sensor was excited by a momentary and periodical current signal with excitation duration of 100 µs. By introducing this pulse amplitude modulation method, the power consumption of RIP sensors can be reduced to 1/10000 of the original consumption. The improved design of RIP sensors were integrated into a garment for continuous ambulatory monitoring of respiratory parameters, such as tidal volume and respiration rate. A novel approach for long-term monitoring of respiration based on mechanism of pressure sensing was developed in [18]. The textile capacitive pressure sensor worked as a plate capacitor and was formed by two opposed conductive textiles which were kept apart by a layer of 3D textile in the middle. The sensor was protected from moisture by a layer of water-repellent textile. The construction of this textile capacitive pressure sensor is shown in Fig. 22.3a and the placement of the four sensors on the chest of body to perform wearable monitoring of respiration pattern is shown in Fig. 22.3b. An additional layer of conductive fabric connected to ground and water-repellent fabric were applied to resist some external influences such as body motion and external fields.

State-of-the-art of Wearable Health Monitoring Systems

The wearable health monitoring systems (WHMSs) mainly contains four basic components: sensors, processing electronics, communication and power management units. The feature of WHMSs can be summarized as MINDS: Miniaturized, Intel-

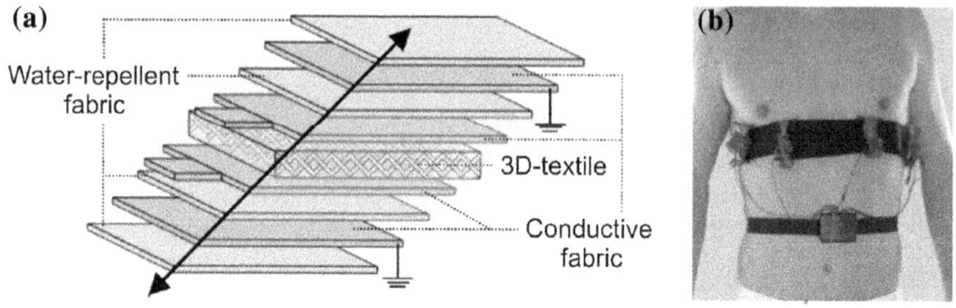

Fig. 22.3 **a** The construction of the textile capacitive pressure sensor; **b** The placement of the four textile sensors on the body [18]

ligent, Networked, Digitalized and Standardized [19]. A number of prototypes of WHMSs embedded into the accessories or clothing have been developed in the past years, such as earring sensor and wireless earpiece for PPG sensing [20], a wrist-type device AMON for ECG, SpO2, BP, physical activity monitoring [21], a glove-type pulse oximeter [22], a waist-worn biofeedback device for ECG, heart rate, respiration monitoring [23], a watch for cuff-less BP and heart rate monitoring [24] and a health shirt for ECG, PPG and cuff-less BP monitoring [25].

One of the most important issues in designing these systems is to consider the comfort of use to improve the acceptability of the devices to the users. In the following, we will introduce some cutting-edge design of WHMSs.

(1) *Single-site multi-sensor micro-integration platform*

At present, most of the multi-parameter wearable monitoring systems are designed with sensors connected through wires [26] or through conductive fibers integrated in clothing [27]. Chuo et al. developed a flexible single-site multi-sensor wearable monitoring platform [28, 29] to record cardiac vibrations and potentials simultaneously from the chest and further derived multiple physiological parameters such as body motion, activity intensity, tilt, respiration, cardiac vibration, heart rate for CVD health care applications. The biopotential electrodes were integrated with the vibration sensor and all electronics on a flexible polyimide substrate. The interconnects were also implemented into the platform through microfabrication process, as shown in Fig. 22.4.

Due to its high integration, the single-site platform would greatly improve the comfort of use in long-term monitoring. In addition to this advantage, the simultaneous recording of electrical and mechanical activities has great potential to provide additional insight for early diagnostics of certain cardiac diseases [30]. Though high integration of the components indeed brings convenience during wearable monitoring, it has limitations in extending to the measurement of other physiological parameters, such as blood pressure which needs signal recordings from different sites of the body.

(2) *Textile-based multi-parameter wearable health monitoring system*

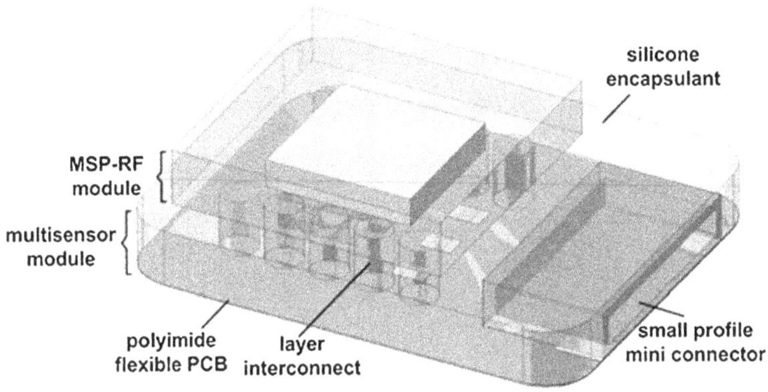

Fig. 22.4 Illustration of different layers of the multi-sensor platform [28]

Smart textile-based wearable health monitoring systems (T-WHMSs) is very suitable for wearable health monitoring for at least two reasons: (1) textile-based sensors can improve the comfort of use and enable long-term monitoring; (2) it provides a solution to seamlessly integrate the entire system into clothing which is part of our daily lives and thus realize measurement of multiple biomedical parameters unobtrusively. Recently, as shown in Fig. 22.5, Coyle et al. [31] developed a textile-based wearable sensing garment (BIOTEX), which can measure a number of physiological signals and parameters such as ECG, heart rate, blood oxygenation and respiration. Three textile electrodes for ECG recording, the optical fiber for the blood oxygenation measurement and the piezoresistive sensor for respiration monitoring were all integrated into the garment by a knitting-dedicated machine.

(3) *Epidermal electronic systems for wearable health monitoring*

The emerging area of flexible electronics provides a brand new approach on the design of WHMSs. Unlike the traditional wafer or PCB-based technologies, these devices, namely "Epidermal Electronic Systems (EES)", are of ultra-thin (around 5 μm), ultra-light (around 1 mg/cm^2) and ultra-low modulus (around 5 kPa) [32]. The advantageous mechanical properties of EES make it possible to be robustly adhesive to the skin without any extra fixturing hardware. Moreover, it is tolerant to large strain deformation. EES can be used to monitor any electrophysiological signals on the body. Figure 22.6 shows the multifunctional EES on the skin under compression and tension [32].

The major challenge of designing such EES is to form good adhesion between the device and skin, i.e., the mechanical properties (i.e., elastic moduli, bending stiffness, and areal mass densities) of EES should match very well with that of epidermis. To achieve this, mechanics models have been established to investigate the effects of some factors on adhesion, such as interfacial delamination under tension/compression, skin roughness, device thickness and size [32]. The results con-

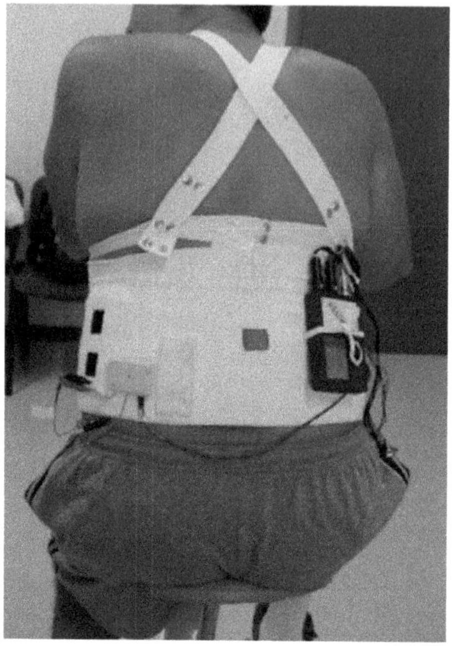

Fig. 22.5 BIOTEX integrated with textile sensors including ECG electrodes, pulse oximetry and respiration sensors [31]

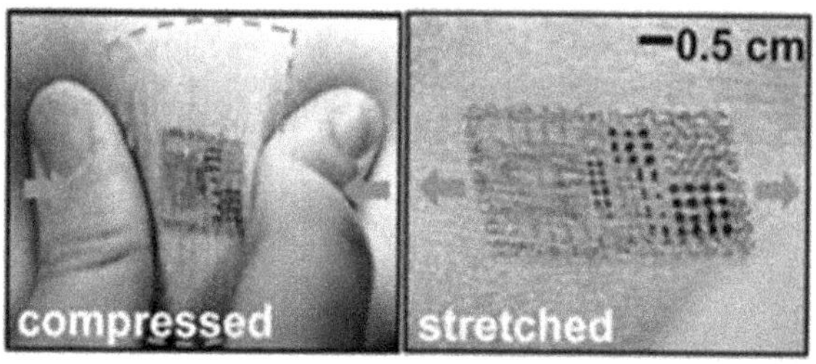

Fig. 22.6 Multifunctional EES on skin: compressed (*left*), stretched (*right*) [32]

firmed that the critical tensile and compressive strain decreased with the increase of the PDMS thickness and modulus.

Some important features of EES enable it very competitive in wearable health monitoring, including: flexible structure to form good contact with body and reduce motion artifacts, small size and light weights to ensure comfort of use in natural settings as well as biocompatible materials to avoid skin irritation.

Key Technologies for Developing WHMSs

Some practical concerns must be solved before WHMSs can be widely used in real-life scenarios, including accuracy and standardization of wearable sensing, removal of segments with motion artifacts and low power design for long-term usage. Here we will discuss the major enabling technologies in developing WHMSs.

(1) *Modeling techniques for accurate wearable sensing*

Due to the noninvasive nature of wearable monitoring, some parameters, such as arterial BP, cardiac output and tidal volume, are difficult to be measured directly. Therefore, physiological-based models are needed in these situations to quantitatively describe the relationship between the targeted parameters and what can be measured or calculated directly from the recorded signals.

The model for PTT and BP has been discussed above; here we will give another example about how to use modeling technique to estimate the tidal volume from textile capacitive force sensor. For the respiration monitoring system we discussed in Fig. 22.3 [18], the respiration volume (ΔV) should be estimated from the capacitance (C) which can be directly measured by the capacitive pressure sensor attached on the chest. Some assumptions are needed before modeling:

(1) The lung is assumed as a ball, so its volume is proportional to the third power of the radius. Then the respiration volume (ΔV) can be represented as:

$$\Delta V = V_2 - V_1 = \frac{4}{3}\pi\left(r_2^3 - r_1^3\right) \tag{22.2}$$

(2) During the expansion of the thorax, the change of the radius (Δr) is assumed to be equal to the change of the thickness (Δd) of the capacitive sensor. the respiration volume can be estimated as:

$$\Delta\tilde{V} = V_2 - V_1 = 4/3\pi\left((r_1 + \Delta d)^3 - r_1^3\right), \tag{22.3}$$

Based on the formula, $C = \varepsilon_0\varepsilon_r\frac{A}{d}$, Eq. (22.3) can be rewritten as:

$$\Delta\tilde{V} = 4/3\pi\left((r_1 + \varepsilon_0\varepsilon_r A(\frac{1}{C_1} - \frac{1}{C_2}))^3 - r_1^3\right),$$

where r_1, r_2 are the radiuses of the lung before and after inspiration respectively, ε_0 is the permeability in vacuum, ε_r is the relative permeability of the capacitor, and A is the area of the capacitor. Using this model, the respiration volume can be roughly estimated.

On the other hand, modeling techniques can be used to investigate the influence of some external factors on the accuracy of sensing. For example, the contact force between the sensors and the measurement site may change the contact impedance of the ECG electrode which may affect the quality of the ECG signal. Beckmann gave

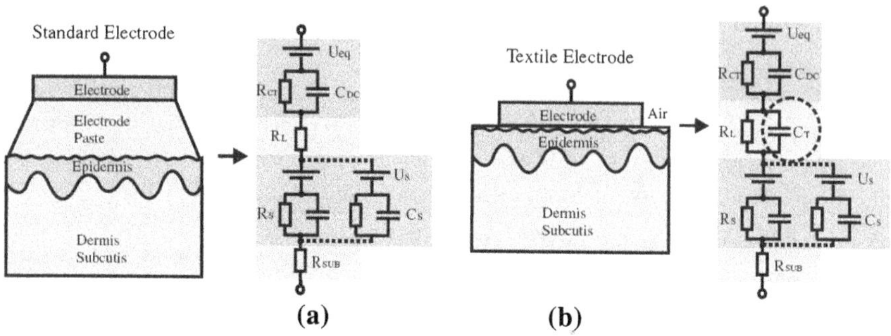

Fig. 22.7 **a** Equivalent circuit of a standard electrode–electrolyte skin interface; **b** Equivalent circuit of a textile electrode–electrolyte skin interface [33]

the electrical modeling of the interface between the textile electrode and skin [33]. Being different from a standard electrode–electrolyte skin interface in Fig. 22.7a, the electrode paste layer was replaced by the air layer due to lack of the hydrogel in a textile electrode–electrolyte skin interface as shown in Fig. 22.7b, which reflected on the equivalent circuit was the addition of an capacitance C_T.

The overall impedance of textile electrode-electrolyte skin interface can be represented as:

$$Z_{Textile} = \frac{R_cT}{1 + jwR_{CT}C_{DC}} + \frac{R_L}{1 + jwR_LC_T} + \frac{R_s}{1 + jwR_sC_s} + R_{SUB}. \tag{22.4}$$

Based on this model, factors that may influence the contact impedance can be investigated quantitatively. For example, when a higher contact force is applied, the distance between the electrode and the skin will decrease, which will increase the interface capacitance and decrease the contact impedance according to Eq. (22.5),

$$Z \approx \frac{1}{C} = \frac{1}{\varepsilon_0\varepsilon_r} \cdot \frac{d}{A}, \tag{22.5}$$

The contact area between the electrode and the skin will also increase as another contributor to the decrease of the contact impedance. The results indicate that good contact can help to decrease the contact impedance and therefore improves signal transmission.

Another example of the application of modeling was shown in [34]. The effect of contact force between the photoplethysmographic sensor and the fingertip was investigated based on a theoretical model by taking into account the nonlinear biomechanical properties of vessel wall. The results showed that PTT increased with the applied contact force, but after reaching the maximum at zero transmural pressure, PTT remained at a constant level at negative transmural pressure. This results imply that attention should be paid on the interpretation of PTT in clinical settings or when it is used for BP estimation [10] since it changes with the contact force.

In summary, modeling techniques can be broadly applied into the area of wearable sensing. Based on modeling, new methods of wearable measurement can be proposed or theoretical guidance can be given about the design of system or clinical interpretations of measurement.

(2) *Motion artifacts removal*

Motion artifacts are one of the major bottlenecks that constrain the practical use of the wearable devices in real-life. Many different solutions have been proposed to remove or reduce motion artifacts, which can be summarized into two types: (1) motion-tolerant firmware design and (2) adaptive signal processing techniques. Design with lightweight can help reduce the motion artifacts induced by sensor shift. Another strategy is to design the sensor to keep good contact with the skin. For example, a neodymium magnet was introduced on one side of earpiece to hold the sensor which was placed on the opposite side of earpiece for motion-tolerant PPG measurement [20]. Adaptive noise cancellation (ANC) introduced an additional sensing element (i.e., accelerometer) to generate artifact reference signal, which was then processed by an adaptive filter to produce the estimation of the motion-induced noise signal. The filter would be re-adjusted to minimize the error between the estimation and the real noise signal when the real noise changed. In [35], it gave detailed illustration on this method.

(3) *Low power system design*

Low power design is imperative for WHMSs for long-term use. In addition to those typical low power circuit design techniques, such as sub-threshold circuits [36] and low voltage circuit design [37], some *system level* low power strategies have been proposed recently to optimize the power consumption of WHMSs. For example, non-uniform data sampling was presented in [38] where the sample rate dynamically varied based on signal activity determined by the second derivative of the input voltage.

Moreover, the promising technology of energy harvesting has also been applied in this area. It harvests energy from environment and converts it into energy to store. The major sources of energy are environmental vibrations and motion of biological systems which can be made use of by piezoelectric materials to power wearable systems. A nanogenerator with unique hybrid piezoelectric structure has recently been demonstrated in [39]. The hybrid-fiber nanogenerator was composed of ZnO nanowire array and poly-vinylidene fluoride (PVDF) polymer around a conducting fiber, as shown in Fig. 22.8a. The nanowire enhanced the surface-contact area, and the PVDF acted as a protective material for high durability under deformation. Under folding-releasing of an elbow as shown in Fig. 22.8b, the mechanical energy can be converted into electricity through the hybrid fiber. The results showed that the nanogenerator can reach electrical outputs of similar to 0.1 V and similar to 10 nA cm^{-2}.

Summary of Wearable Technologies for CV Health Informatics

It is expected that WHMSs will be designed without cumbersome wires by making use of new materials and technologies such as textile and flexible electronics. These

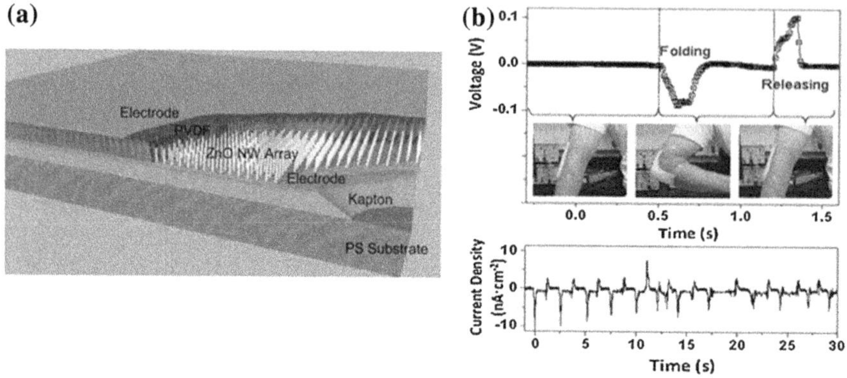

Fig. 22.8 **a** Schematic 3D diagram depicting the structure of the hybrid generator in plane-shape; **b** Open-circuit voltage output of a fiber device depending on the folding and releasing of the elbow [39]

new technologies will significantly improve the comfort of use and increase the acceptability of WHMSs to users.

Implantable Technologies

Thanks to the rapid development of microsystem technology, a number of cardiovascular implantable devices (CIDs) have been developed for the diagnosis and treatment of CVDs. CIDs have gained great interest of academic and industrial area since their first introduction in 1958. Traditional CIDs such as pacemaker, implantable cardioverter-defibrillator and cardiac resynchronization devices were mainly designed to monitor the condition of the atrial and ventricular rhythm to initiate therapies. However, the emerging technologies begin to focus on providing continuous monitoring of more health information through implantable sensors, such as heart rate, intracardiac and intravascular pressure and other CVD related parameters. This type of CIDs can be termed as implantable cardiovascular monitor (ICM).

ICMs are mainly used to measure long-term and ambulatory cardiovascular health information at home or clinic. It is expected to be integrated into telemedicine system for remote healthcare management to greatly improve the quality of life of CVD patients. In addition, ICMs have great potential to reduce CVD-related medical expenses. In a recent clinical trial, it showed that implantable hemodynamic monitoring systems may reduce rates of hospitalization by 37 % in patients with New York Heart Association (NYHA) class III heart failure [40]. Moreover, the long-term monitoring of some important hemodynamic parameters by ICMs may be able to provide valuable information for gaining pathophysiological insights of CVDs and tracking the responses to treatments for optimized therapies [41].

In the following, we will introduce the current state of ICMs and the major challenges in developing ICMs.

Current State of Implantable Cardiovascular Monitor

At present, some commercially available ICMs were developed for different applications, such as *HeartSensor* and *RemonCHF* for heart failure management, *EndoSure* [42] for aneurysm sac pressure monitoring, etc. Generally, these devices consist of an implantable sensor to record CVD-related health information and a wearable external device to power the implant, receive and send health information to a secure remote server.

The design of the implanted sensor is the most challenging part due to the strict requirements on miniaturization, low power consumption and biocompatibility for long-term use. In 2006, CardioMEMS Inc. developed the first wireless and implantable pressure sensor known as *HeartSensor*. The implant were packaged within a hermetically sealed capsule, including a pressure sensitive capacitor which measures resonant frequency shift with changes in pressure, a 3-dimensional coil and electronics. Two wired nitinol loops were attached with the capsule to avoid sensor distant migration. There were no batteries in the implant which was powered by external power source through the coil. After implantation into the distal branch of the pulmonary artery, continuous pulmonary artery pressure can be recorded. The safety and efficiency of *HeartSensor* has been validated in a recent clinical trial [43].

Chow et al. recently developed a stent-based cardiovascular pressure monitor, where the stent was used as both the package substrate and radiating structure for wireless power and data transmission [44]. By integrating the stent transmitter with a MEMS capacitor for pressure sensing, ASIC processing electronics and RF powering circuits, the stent-based monitor can be implanted in any vessel or body conduit.

Bingger et al. designed an *extravascular* implantable pressure sensor based on a flexible silicon strip [45]. By wrapped around a blood vessel, it measures the vessel's diameter and the arterial blood pressure can be estimated accordingly. Unlike other rigid extravascular devices, it would not constrict the blood vessel during measurement.

Wireless Power Transfer for Implantable Cardiovascular Monitor

Powering is the most challenging issue in the design of implantable devices. Powering through wire is not desirable since it may bring inconvenience and cause infection for long-term use. Battery not only occupies additional space but also needs to be replaced through surgery when it is depleted. Wireless powering is the most promising method in the area of biomedical applications. There are mainly two kinds of wireless power transfer techniques: *inductive coupling* and *electro magnetic radiation*. The key issue in the design of wireless power transfer system is to optimize the power transfer efficiency. In the following, some methods to improve the power transfer efficiency will be introduced.

(1) *Inductive coupling*

Inductive coupling has been applied in biomedical area for wireless power transmission for decades. It contains two coils: the external coil and implanted coil. The implanted coil receives the energy transmitted from the external coil within very near distance through magnetic field, and therefore named "near field transmission". The coupling coils operate at a few MHz to minimize the power absorption by the tissues. The power transfer efficiency of a typical two-coil inductively coupled wireless power transfer system was derived to be:

$$\eta = \frac{k_{12}^2 Q_1 Q_2}{1 + k_{12}^2 Q_1 Q_2}, \tag{22.6}$$

where Q_1 and Q_2 are the quality factor of the external and implanted coil, respectively, and k_{12} is the coupling coefficient of the coil pair which increases with the size of the coil pair and decreases with the separation between coil pair. Due to the strict geometry limitations in implantable applications, the major solution to optimize the power transfer efficiency should be maximizing Q of the coil pair.

Yang et al. [46] firstly developed a distributive model of a coil and the closed form analytical solution of self-resonant frequency (f_{self}) and Q of the coil was derived in the following equations:

$$Q(f) \approx 2\pi fL\left(1 - \frac{f^2}{f_{self}^2}\right)/R_{DC}\left(1 + \frac{f^2}{f_h^2}\right), \text{ and} \tag{22.7}$$

$$f_{self} = \frac{1}{2\pi\sqrt{LC_{self}}}, \tag{22.8}$$

where f_h is the frequency at which the AC power dissipation is twice the DC power dissipation, R_{DC}, L, C_{self} is the DC resistance, the inductance and the total equivalent parasitic capacitance of the coil, and f is the operation frequency.

Based on these equations, design parameters of coil such as the inner diameter, winding sequence, the number of strands per turn, and the diameter of an individual strand to achieve maximal Q can be optimized. For example, Q of two coils (coil I and II) with different separation between layers were compared, as shown in Fig. 22.9. It can be seen that Q of coil II was much lower than coil I at high frequency since the separation between layers decreased C_{self}, thus increased f_{self} and Q.

Recently, a four-coil power transfer system was designed to improve power efficiency [47]. As shown in Fig. 22.10a, by inserting another couple of coils, i.e., the primary (coil 2) and secondary coil (coil 3) between the driver (coil 1) and load coil (coil 4), the power transfer efficiency of the system can be derived as:

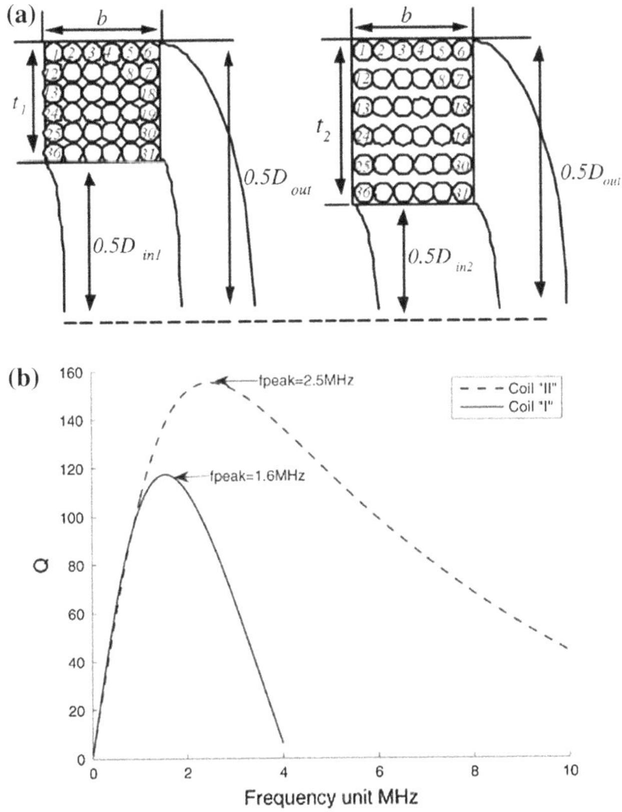

Fig. 22.9 **a** Coils' cross sections: the *left* (Coil I) is tightly wound and the *right* (Coil II) is loosely wound; **b** Q versus Frequency curves of coils [46]

$$\eta = \frac{k_{23}^2 Q_2 Q_3}{1 + k_{23}^2 Q_2 Q_3}, \tag{22.9}$$

where Q_2 and Q_3 are quality factors of coil 2 and coil 3, respectively. Equation (22.9) has a similar form as Eq. (22.6), and the only difference is that the power transfer efficiency was determined by quality factor of the primary and secondary coil, not Q of driver and load coil, i.e., Q_1 and Q_4. Since Q_1 and Q_4 were limited by the source resistance and load resistance of the system, while Q_2 and Q_3 were not, the power transfer efficiency can be improved. Another advantage of the four-coil system is that the power efficiency of two-coil system decreased significantly with respect to the distance between the two coils. From Fig. 22.10b, the efficiency can maintain 80 % when the distance increased to 20 mm and 30 % at the distance of 30 mm. However, the cost for these advantages would be the additional space for the additional coils, which needs careful design, especially for the implanted part.

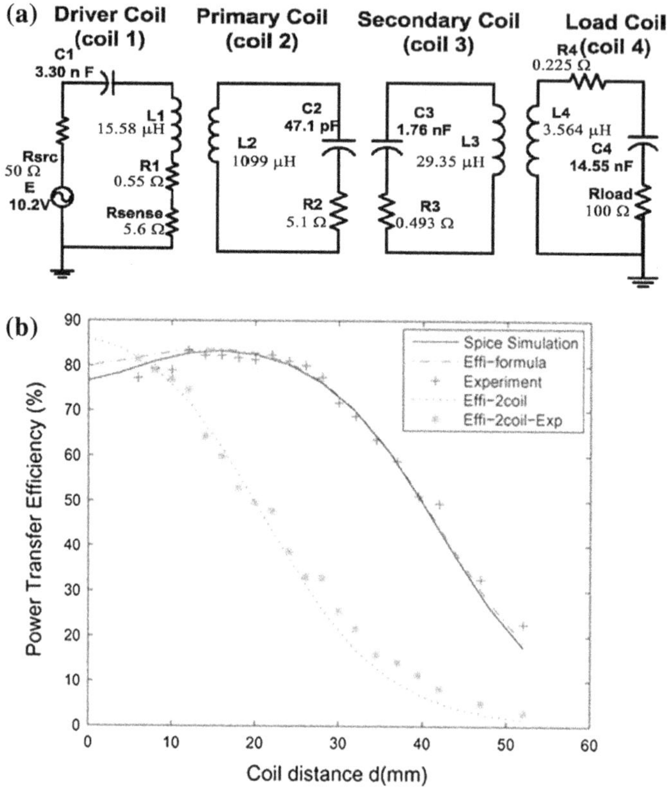

Fig. 22.10 **a** Electrical model of the four-coil power transfer system; **b** The simulation and experimental result of power transfer efficiency versus coil distance in a two-coil and four-coil power transfer system [47]

In addition to these methods of optimizing quality factor of the coil, Kurs et al. [48] presented a quantitative model of two self-resonant coils and theoretically proved that the energy transfer efficiency can be maximized when the coil pair were on resonant. Nevertheless, the miniaturization of coils remains a challenge for implantable applications.

(2) *Electromagnetic radiation*

Electromagnetic (EM) radiation method can transmit power in further distance through EM field, i.e. "far-field transmission". The antenna design is very challenging due to its interaction with the surrounding biological tissues. Some factors such as the implanted depth of the antenna and the thickness of the tissue layer could have an effect on the power propagation of the wireless link [49]. Therefore, it is necessary to model the antenna and the surrounding tissue to simulate the effect of these factors on the radiating properties of the antenna for optimization of the link.

For example, the radiation properties of the stent-based antenna was quantitatively evaluated in [50]. The stent was modeled as a hollow stainless-steel cylinder, which

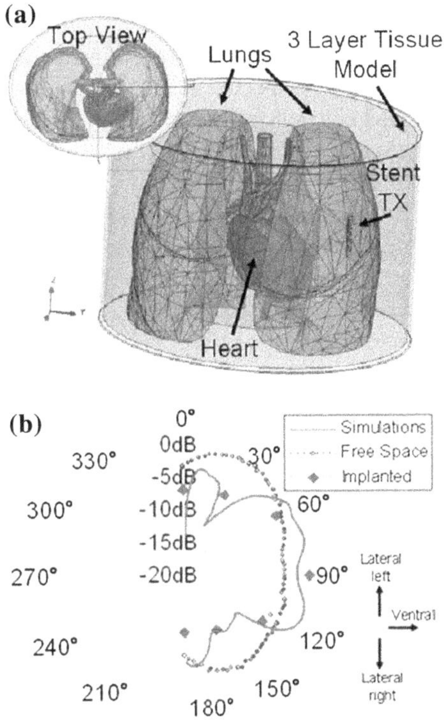

Fig. 22.11 **a** Model of the chest containing major organs, vessels and a custom three-layer cylindrical tissue; **b** Antenna patterns from simulation and measurements in free space and implanted settings [50]

was simple but sufficient to characterize properties of the antenna since the size of the stent was in sub-wavelength dimensions at 2.4 GHz. The upper chest region was modeled as a cylindrical shape and simplified to contain lungs, parts of the respiratory tract, heart and major veins and arteries as shown in Fig. 22.11a. A custom three-layer tissue model was used to model the remaining chest volume, and the layers were set with appropriate dielectric properties [50]. By integrating the stent-based antenna model with the body model, the radiation properties of the antenna after implantation can be simulated. The simulation and *in vivo* measurement results in Fig. 22.11b matched reasonably well, which indicates that the model was sufficient.

Challenges in Developing ICM

(1) *Miniaturization*

Most present studies prefer to design the wireless link operated at frequency of lower than 10 MHz to minimize power consumption caused by tissue absorption and yield high power transfer efficiency. This would, however, result in large antenna size. Some efforts have been devoted to the miniaturization of the implant. Recently, Ada et al. theoretically proved that high power transfer efficiency can also be achieved with EM radiation method at GHz. To find the optimal frequency, the biological tissue was modeled as a dispersive dielectric in a homogeneous medium, and power link was modeled as a generalized two-port network. Full-wave analysis based on Maxwell's equation was performed. It was found that the optimal frequency was 2 order of magnitude higher than that are used today, which would significantly promote the miniaturization of the implant [51]. In addition to the miniaturization of antenna, nanotechnology also helps advance the miniaturization of driving electronics and power electronics for implantable devices, such as carbon nanotubes, nanowires for interconnects [52], assembly techniques [53], nanogenerator and nanopiezotronics for energy harvesting [54].

(2) *Foreign body response*

Some implants of ICM are stent-like to facilitate implantation into vessels. However, restenosis is the most challenging issue faced by cardiovascular stents after long-term implantation. The surface of the stent becomes fouled with proteins and cells due to tissue inflammation or foreign body response within a short period of time after sensor implantation [55]. This undesirable process will result in difficulty and inaccuracy of sensing. To solve this, metallic stents with biocompatible coatings, such as polymer-coated drug-eluting stents (DES) [56] have been used clinically to alleviate restenosis, but it would cause new clinical problems, such as late stent thrombosis due to the lack of endothelial cell coverage over the inner stent wall. Recently, nanotechnology plays an important role in this area by providing nanostructure materials, which can modify the surface of the implantable sensors and thus relieve the adverse effect from implantation. It is suggested that due to the different contact angle and therefore different degree of hydrophobicity or hydrophilicity, nanostructured coatings are able to improve the sensing performance *in vivo* [55]. Based on this, some nanostructure-coated stents have been developed, such as nanoparticle-eluting stents [57] and bare metal coronary stent with plasma-induced nanopillars on surface [58]. For more information about the application of nanotechnology on cardiovascular stent design, readers may refer to [59].

Particular care should be taken on that nanoparticles may leak out of the implants and enter into the body to cause health risks. It is suggested that investigation into the effects of nanoparticles size on its movement in the body may help deduce a critical size of particles and thus reduce this adverse effect [55].

Summary of Implantable Technologiesfor CV Health Informatics

In summary, by combining nanotechnologies, ICMs will step forward towards smaller, more biocompatible and power efficient to implement long-term monitoring in real life.

Conclusion

In this chapter, the wearable and implantable technologies have been discussed, which can be interconnected by body sensor network aiming to provide long-term and continuous monitoring of health status ubiquitously for the healthy or patients with cardiovascular diseases. With efforts and collaboration from different areas of engineering and medicine, it is expected that cardiovascular health care will be significantly improved by wearable and implantable technologies in terms of quality and efficiency in the future.

References

1. S. S. Hu, L. Z. Kong, R. L. Gao, M. L. Zhu, W. Wang, Y. J. Wang, Z. S. Wu, W. W. Chen, and M. B. Liu, "Outline of the Report on Cardiovascular Disease in China, 2010," Biomedical and Environmental Sciences, Vol. 25, No. 3, 2012, pp. 251–256.
2. D. E. Bloom, E. T. Cafiero, E. Jané-Llopis, S. Abrahams-Gessel, L. R. Bloom, S. Fathima, A. B. Feigl, T. Gaziano, M. Mowafi, A. Pandya, K. Prettner, L. Rosenberg, B. Seligman, A. Z. Stein, C. Weinstein, The Global Economic Burden of Non-Communicable Diseases: Geneva: World, Economic Forum, 2011.
3. H. Baek, G. Chung, K. Kim, and K. Park, "A Smart Health Monitoring Chair for Nonintrusive Measurement of Biological Signals," IEEE Transactions on Information Technology in Biomedicine, Vol. 16, No. 1, 2012, pp. 150–158.
4. K. F. Wu, C. H. Chan, Y. T. Zhang, "Contactless and Cuffless Monitoring of Blood Pressure on a Chair Using E-Textile Materials," in 3rd IEEE/EMBS International Summer School on Medical Devices and, Biosensors, 2006.
5. J. Y. Baek, J. H. An, J. M. Choi, K. S. Park, and S. H. Lee, "Flexible Polymeric Dry Electrodes for the Long-Term Monitoring of Ecg," Sensors and Actuators a-Physical, Vol. 143, No. 2, May 2008, pp. 423–429.
6. J. Yoo, Y. Long, L. Seulki, K. Hyejung, and Y. Hoi-Jun, "A Wearable Ecg Acquisition System with Compact Planar-Fashionable Circuit Board-Based Shirt," IEEE Transactions on Information Technology in Biomedicine, Vol. 13, No. 6, 2009, pp. 897–902.
7. T. H. Kang, C. R. Merritt, E. Grant, B. Pourdeyhimi, and H. T. Nagle, "Nonwoven Fabric Active Electrodes for Biopotential Measurement During Normal Daily Activity," IEEE Transactions on Biomedical Engineering, Vol. 55, No. 1, Jan 2008, pp. 188–195.
8. A. John, "Photoplethysmography and Its Application in Clinical Physiological Measurement," Physiological Measurement, Vol. 28, No. 3, 2007, p. R1.
9. R. G. Haahr, S. B. Duun, M. H. Toft, B. Belhage, J. Larsen, K. Birkelund, and E. V. Thomsen, "An Electronic Patch for Wearable Health Monitoring by Reflectance Pulse Oximetry," IEEE Transactions on Biomedical Circuits and Systems, Vol. 6, No. 1, Feb 2012, pp. 45–53.
10. C. C. Y. Poon and Y. T. Zhang, "Cuff-Less and Noninvasive Measurements of Arterial Blood Pressure by Pulse Transit Time," in 27th Annual International Conference of the IEEE Engineering in Medicine and Biology Society 2005.
11. L. Wang, C. C. Y. Poon, and Y. T. Zhang, "The Non-Invasive and Continuous Estimation of Cardiac Output Using a Photoplethysmogram and Electrocardiogram During Incremental Exercise," Physiological Measurement, Vol. 31, 2010, p. 715.
12. Y. L. Zheng, B. Leung, S. Sy, Y. T. Zhang, and C. C. Y. Poon, "A Clip-Free Eyeglasses-Based Wearable Monitoring Device for Measuring Photoplethysmograhic Signals," in 27th Annual International Conference of the IEEE-EMBS, 2012.

13. S. B. Duun, R. G. Haahr, K. Birkelund, and E. V. Thomsen, "A Ring-Shaped Photodiode Designed for Use in a Reflectance Pulse Oximetry Sensor in Wireless Health Monitoring Applications," IEEE Sensors Journal, Vol. 10, No. 2, 2010, pp. 261–268.
14. M. Y. M. Wong, E. Pickwell-MacPherson, and Y. T. Zhang, "The Acute Effects of Running on Blood Pressure Estimation Using Pulse Transit Time in Normotensive Subjects," European Journal of Applied Physiology, Vol. 107, No. 2, 2009, pp. 169–175.
15. Y. Chen, C. Wen, G. Tao, M. Bi, and G. Li, "Continuous and Noninvasive Blood Pressure Measurement: A Novel Modeling Methodology of the Relationship between Blood Pressure and Pulse Wave Velocity," Annals of Biomedical Engineering, Vol. 37, No. 11, 2009, pp. 2222–2233.
16. J. Muehlsteff, X. L. Aubert, and M. Schuett, "Cuffless Estimation of Systolic Blood Pressure for Short Effort Bicycle Tests: The Prominent Role of the Pre-Ejection Period," in 28th Annual International Conference of the IEEE Engineering in Medicine and Biology Society (EMBC), 2006.
17. Z. B. Zhang, Y. H. Shen, W. D. Wang, B. Q. Wang, and J. W. Zheng, "Design and Implementation of Sensing Shirt for Ambulatory Cardiopulmonary Monitoring," Journal of Medical and Biological Engineering, Vol. 31, No. 3, 2011, pp. 207–215.
18. T. Hoffmann, B. Eilebrecht, and S. Leonhardt, "Respiratory Monitoring System on the Basis of Capacitive Textile Force Sensors," IEEE Sensors Journal, Vol. 11, No. 5, 2011, pp. 1112–1119.
19. C. C. Y. Poon, W. B. Gu, and Y. T. Zhang, "Health Informatics for Low-Cost and High-Quality Health Care," in 2010 Annual International Conference of the IEEE Engineering in Medicine and Biology Society (EMBC), 2010.
20. M. Z. Poh, N. C. Swenson, and R. W. Picard, "Motion-Tolerant Magnetic Earring Sensor and Wireless Earpiece for Wearable Photoplethysmography," IEEE Transactions on Information Technology in Biomedicine, Vol. 14, No. 3, 2010, pp. 786–794.
21. U. Anliker, J. A. Ward, P. Lukowicz, G. Troster, F. Dolveck, M. Baer, F. Keita, E. B. Schenker, F. Catarsi, L. Coluccini, A. Belardinelli, D. Shklarski, M. Alon, E. Hirt, R. Schmid, and M. Vuskovic, "Amon: A Wearable Multiparameter Medical Monitoring and Alert System," IEEE Transactions on Information Technology in Biomedicine, Vol. 8, No. 4, 2004, pp. 415–427.
22. M. Rothmaier, B. Selm, S. Spichtig, D. Haensse, and M. Wolf, "Photonic Textiles for Pulse Oximetry," Optics Express, Vol. 16, No. 17, Aug 2008, pp. 12973–12986.
23. G. Z. Liu, B. Y. Huang, and L. Wang, "A Wearable Respiratory Biofeedback System Based on Generalized Body Sensor Network," Telemedicine and e-Health, Vol. 17, No. 5, 2011, pp. 348–357.
24. C. C. Y. Poon, Y. M. Wong, Y. T. Zhang, "M-Health: The Development of Cuff-Less and Wearable Blood Pressure Meters for Use in Body Sensor Networks," presented at the IEEE/NLM Life Science Systems and Applications, Workshop, 2006.
25. Y. T. Zhang, C. C. Y. Poon, C. H. Chan, M. W. W. Tsang, K. F. Wu, "A Health-Shirt Using E-Textile Materials for the Continuous and Cuffless Monitoring of Arterial Blood Pressure," in 3rd IEEE/EMBS International Summer School on Medical Devices and, Biosensors, 2006.
26. C. W. Mundt, K. N. Montgomery, U. E. Udoh, V. N. Barker, G. C. Thonier, A. M. Tellier, R. D. Ricks, R. B. Darling, Y. D. Cagle, N. A. Cabrol, S. J. Ruoss, J. L. Swain, J. W. Hines, and G. T. A. Kovacs, "A Multiparameter Wearable Physiologic Monitoring System for Space and Terrestrial Applications," IEEE Transactions on Information Technology in Biomedicine, Vol. 9, No. 3, Sep 2005, pp. 382–391.
27. P. Castiglioni, A. Faini, G. Parati, and M. Di Rienzo, "Wearable Seismocardiography," in 29th Annual International Conference of the IEEE Engineering in Medicine and Biology Society, 2007.
28. Y. Chuo and B. Kaminska, "Sensor Layer of a Multiparameter Single-Point Integrated System," IEEE Transactions on Biomedical Circuits and Systems, Vol. 3, No. 4, 2009, pp. 229–240.
29. Y. Chuo, M. Marzencki, B. Hung, C. Jaggernauth, K. Tavakolian, P. Lin, and B. Kaminska, "Mechanically Flexible Wireless Multisensor Platform for Human Physical Activity and Vitals Monitoring," IEEE Transactions on Biomedical Circuits and Systems, Vol. 4, No. 5, Oct 2010, pp. 281–294.

30. W. P. S. McKay, P. H. Gregson, B. W. S. McKay, and J. Militzer, "Sternal Acceleration Ballistocardiography and Arterial Pressure Wave Analysis to Determine Stroke Volume," Clinical and Investigative Medicine, Vol. 22, 1999, pp. 4–14.
31. S. Coyle, K. T. Lau, N. Moyna, D. O'Gorman, D. Diamond, F. Di Francesco, D. Costanzo, P. Salvo, M. G. Trivella, D. E. De Rossi, N. Taccini, R. Paradiso, J. A. Porchet, A. Ridolfi, J. Luprano, C. Chuzel, T. Lanier, F. Revol-Cavalier, S. Schoumacker, V. Mourier, I. Chartier, R. Convert, H. De-Moncuit, and C. Bini, "Biotex-Biosensing Textiles for Personalised Healthcare Management," IEEE Transactions on Information Technology in Biomedicine, Vol. 14, No. 2, Mar 2010, pp. 364–370.
32. D. H. Kim, N. Lu, R. Ma, Y. S. Kim, R. H. Kim, S. Wang, J. Wu, S. M. Won, H. Tao, A. Islam, K. J. Yu, T.-i. Kim, R. Chowdhury, M. Ying, L. Z. Xu, M. Li, H. J. Chung, H. Keum, M. McCormick, P. Liu, Y. W. Zhang, F. G. Omenetto, Y. G. Huang, T. Coleman, and J. A. Rogers, "Epidermal Electronics," Science, Vol. 333, No. 6044, August 12, 2011 2011, pp. 838–843.
33. L. Beckmann, C. Neuhaus, G. Medrano, N. Jungbecker, M. Walter, T. Gries, and S. Leonhardt, "Characterization of Textile Electrodes and Conductors Using Standardized Measurement Setups," Physiological Measurement, Vol. 31, 2010, pp. 233–247.
34. X. F. Teng and Y. T. Zhang, "Theoretical Study on the Effect of Sensor Contact Force on Pulse Transit Time," IEEE Transactions on Biomedical Engineering, Vol. 54, No. 8, 2007, pp. 1490–1498.
35. S. Yoon, S. Min, Y. Yun, S. Lee, and M. Lee, "Adaptive Motion Artifacts Reduction Using 3-Axis Accelerometer in E-Textile Ecg Measurement System," Journal of Medical Systems, Vol. 32, No. 2, 2008, pp. 101–106.
36. J. Kim, M. S. Chae, and W. Liu, "A 220nw Neural Amplifier for Multi-Channel Neural Recording Systems," in IEEE International Symposium on Circuits and Systems, 2009.
37. E. Villegas, "A Low-Power Wide Range Transimpedance Amplifier for Biochemical Sensing," in 29th Annual International Conference of the IEEE Engineering in Medicine and Biology Society, 2007.
38. R. Rieger and S. H. Nian, "Integrated Control Circuit for Adaptive Sampling," Analog Integrated Circuits and Signal Processing, Vol. 72, No. 1, Jul 2012, pp. 227–235.
39. M. Lee, C. Y. Chen, S. Wang, S. N. Cha, Y. J. Park, J. M. Kim, L. J. Chou, and Z. L. Wang, "A Hybrid Piezoelectric Structure for Wearable Nanogenerators," Advanced Materials, Vol. 24, No. 13, Apr 2012, pp. 1759–1764.
40. W. T. Abraham, P. B. Adamson, R. C. Bourge, M. F. Aaron, M. R. Costanzo, L. W. Stevenson, W. Strickland, S. Neelagaru, N. Raval, S. Krueger, S. Weiner, D. Shavelle, B. Jeffries, and J. S. Yadav, "Wireless Pulmonary Artery Haemodynamic Monitoring in Chronic Heart Failure: A Randomised Controlled Trial," The Lancet, Vol. 377, No. 9766, 2011, pp. 658–666.
41. M. R. Zile, T. D. Bennett, M. S. J. Sutton, Y. K. Cho, P. B. Adamson, M. F. Aaron, J. M. Aranda, W. T. Abraham, F. W. Smart, L. W. Stevenson, F. J. Kueffer, and R. C. Bourge, "Transition from Chronic Compensated to Acute Decompensated Heart Failure - Pathophysiological Insights Obtained from Continuous Monitoring of Intracardiac Pressures," Circulation, Vol. 118, No. 14, Sep 2008, pp. 1433–1441.
42. CardioMEMS. (2007). Announces Fda Clearance of the Endosure^TM Wireless Aaa Pressure Measurement System for Measuring Intrasac Pressure During Thoracic Aortic Aneurysm (Taa) Repair. Available: http://www.cardiomems.com/content.asp?display=news&view=9.
43. P. B. Adamson, W. T. Abraham, M. Aaron, J. M. Aranda Jr, R. C. Bourge, A. Smith, L. W. Stevenson, J. G. Bauman, and J. S. Yadav, "Champion Trial Rationale and Design: The Long-Term Safety and Clinical Efficacy of a Wireless Pulmonary artery Pressure Monitoring System," Journal of Cardiac Failure, Vol. 17, No. 1, 2011, pp. 3–10.
44. E. Y. Chow, A. L. Chlebowski, S. Chakraborty, W. J. Chappell, and P. P. Irazoqui, "Fully Wireless Implantable Cardiovascular Pressure Monitor Integrated with a Medical Stent," IEEE Transactions on Biomedical Engineering, Vol. 57, No. 6, Jun 2010, pp. 1487–1496.
45. P. Bingger, M. Zens, and P. Woias, "Highly Flexible Capacitive Strain Gauge for Continuous Long-Term Blood Pressure Monitoring," Biomedical Microdevices, Vol. 14, 2012, pp. 573–581.

46. Z. Yang, W. T. Liu, and E. Basham, "Inductor Modeling in Wireless Links for Implantable Electronics," IEEE Transactions on Magnetics, Vol. 43, No. 10, 2007, pp. 3851–3860.
47. A. K. RamRakhyani, S. Mirabbasi, and M. Chiao, "Design and Optimization of Resonance-Based Efficient Wireless Power Delivery Systems for Biomedical Implants," IEEE Transactions on Biomedical Circuits and Systems, Vol. 5, No. 1, Feb 2011, pp. 48–63.
48. A. Kurs, A. Karalis, R. Moffatt, J. D. Joannopoulos, P. Fisher, and M. Soljačić, "Wireless Power Transfer Via Strongly Coupled Magnetic Resonances," Science, Vol. 317, No. 5834, July 6, 2007 2007, pp. 83–86.
49. J. Gemio, J. Parron, and J. Soler, "Human Body Effects on Implantable Antennas for Ism Bands Applications: Models Comparison and Propagation Losses Study," Progress in Electromagnetics Research, Vol. 110, 2010, pp. 437–452.
50. E. Y. Chow, Y. Ouyang, B. Beier, W. J. Chappell, and P. P. Irazoqui, "Evaluation of Cardiovascular Stents as Antennas for Implantable Wireless Applications," IEEE Transactions on Microwave Theory and Techniques, Vol. 57, No. 10, 2009, pp. 2523–2532.
51. A. S. Y. Poon, S. O'Driscoll, and T. H. Meng, "Optimal Frequency for Wireless Power Transmission into Dispersive Tissue," IEEE Transactions on Antennas and Propagation, Vol. 58, No. 5, May 2010, pp. 1739–1750.
52. C. Y. Chen, Y. K. Lin, C. W. Hsu, C. Y. Wang, Y. L. Chueh, L. J. Chen, S. C. Lo, and L. J. Chou, "Coaxial Metal-Silicide Ni2si/C54-Tisi2 Nanowires," Nano Letters, Vol. 12, No. 5, May 2012, pp. 2254–2259.
53. M. Ganzhorn, A. Vijayaraghavan, A. A. Green, S. Dehm, A. Voigt, M. Rapp, M. C. Hersam, and R. Krupke, "A Scalable, Cmos-Compatible Assembly of Ambipolar Semiconducting Single-Walled Carbon Nanotube Devices," Advanced Materials, Vol. 23, No. 15, Apr 2011, pp. 1734–1738.
54. Z. L. Wang, "Towards Self-Powered Nanosystems: From Nanogenerators to Nanopiezotronics," Advanced Functional Materials, Vol. 18, No. 22, Nov 2008, pp. 3553–3567.
55. S. Vaddiraju, I. Tomazos, D. J. Burgess, F. C. Jain, and F. Papadimitrakopoulos, "Emerging Synergy between Nanotechnology and Implantable Biosensors: A Review," Biosensors and Bioelectronics, Vol. 25, No. 7, 2010, pp. 1553–1565.
56. D. M. Whelan, W. J. van der Giessen, S. C. Krabbendam, E. A. van Vliet, P. D. Verdouw, P. W. Serruys, and H. M. M. van Beusekom, "Biocompatibility of Phosphorylcholine Coated Stents in Normal Porcine Coronary Arteries," Heart, Vol. 83, No. 3, Mar 2000, pp. 338–345.
57. K. Nakano, K. Egashira, S. Masuda, K. Funakoshi, G. Zhao, S. Kimura, T. Matoba, K. Sueishi, Y. Endo, Y. Kawashima, K. Hara, H. Tsujimoto, R. Tominaga, and K. Sunagawa, "Formulation of Nanoparticle-Eluting Stents by a Cationic Electrodeposition Coating Technology: Efficient Nano-Drug Delivery Via Bioabsorbable Polymeric Nanoparticle-Eluting Stents in Porcine Coronary Arteries," JACC: Cardiovascular Interventions, Vol. 2, No. 4, 2009, pp. 277–283.
58. M. C. Loya, K. S. Brammer, C. Choi, L. H. Chen, and S. Jin, "Plasma-Induced Nanopillars on Bare Metal Coronary Stent Surface for Enhanced Endothelialization," Acta Biomaterialia, Vol. 6, No. 12, 2010, pp. 4589–4595.
59. A. W. Martinez and E. L. Chaikof, "Microfabrication and Nanotechnology in Stent Design," Wiley Interdisciplinary Reviews-Nanomedicine and, Nanobiotechnology, 3(3), May-Jun 2011, pp. 256–268.

Chapter 23
Integration of Various Health Record Systems

Ankur Agarwal, Borko Furht and Vivek Tyagi

This chapter discusses the integration between the Health Record Systems and Patient Record System. The chapter also highlights the importance of a Patient Centric Health Record system. Such systems can empower patients to participate in improving health care quality. It would also provide an economically viable solution to the need for better healthcare without escalating costs by avoiding duplication. The proposed system is cloud based system so patients and healthcare providers can access it from any location. The use of cloud computing architecture will allow consumers to address the challenge of sharing medical data that is overly complex and highly expensive to address with traditional technologies.

Introduction

Generally health information is scattered across many different providers and facilities. A visit to a new doctor or any member of a CDO often results in lengthy process of filling all the information in a new system from where which such information is not ported to any other system. A new hospital encounter often results in repeated tests and all previous conversations are ignored due to the absence of any central repository of all data. This naturally results in higher cost to the patients, health insurance companies and government. Most of the times this health information is stored in chapter files, which are difficult to organize and share with others. Moreover,

A. Agarwal (✉) · B. Furht · V. Tyagi
Department of Computer and Electrical Engineering and Computer Science, Florida Atlantic University, Boca Raton, FL 33431, USA
e-mail: Ankur@cse.fau.edu

B. Furht
e-mail: bfurht@fau.edu

V. Tyagi
e-mail: vtyagi@my.fau.edu

B. Furht and A. Agarwal (eds.), *Handbook of Medical and Healthcare Technologies*,
DOI: 10.1007/978-1-4614-8495-0_23, © Springer Science+Business Media New York 2013

the information is not stored in standardized formats. Allowing patients to access their own medical records will encourage patients to be involved in their own healthcare and that will further strengthen the patient–provider relationship. Such an effort will enhance and increase the effectiveness of healthcare management. Healthcare institutions around the world are encouraged to develop the Electronic Health Record (EHR) systems. Personal Health Record (PHR) Systems that would track all such EHRs from various encounters with a variety of health professionals over years can be seen as one of the means that can empower patients in their own healthcare. It is noted that consumers that are well informed about their illnesses tend to understand and follow instructions and ask more insightful questions [2, 10]. We can define the PHR as an electronic application through which individuals can access, manage and share their health information in a secure and confidential environment [3]. It allows people to access and coordinate their lifelong health information and make appropriate parts of it available to those who need it. Thus, it differs from the EHR [15], which is "an electronic version of the patient medical record" kept by physicians and hospitals. The data in the EHR are controlled by and intended for use by medical providers. EMR is the basic building block, the source of information that feeds the EHR. The EHR is the longitudinal record made possible by RHIO's (Regional Health Information organizations) and interoperability across care delivery organizations; and the PHR is the record owned, accessed, and managed by the consumer. The interdependencies are clear. Without linkages to the EMR, the PHR depends on the consumer to manually input vital data, like laboratory results. Without an EHR, the PHR cannot accept information from multiple providers.

EMR is the basic building block, the source of information that feeds the EHR. The EHR is the longitudinal record made possible by RHIO's (Regional Health Information organizations) and interoperability across care delivery organizations; and the PHR is the record owned, accessed, and managed by the consumer. The interdependencies are clear. Without linkages to the EMR, the PHR depends on the consumer to manually input vital data, like laboratory results. Without an EHR, the PHR cannot accept information from multiple providers [28].

This chapter discusses an emerging concept of a cloud computing based Patient Centric Medical Information System framework that will allow various authorized users to securely access patient records from various Care Delivery Organizations (CDOs) such as hospitals, urgent care centers, doctors, laboratories, imaging centers among others, from any location. Such a system must seamlessly integrate all patient records including images such as CT- SCANS and MRI'S which can easily be accessed from any location and reviewed by any authorized user. In such a scenario the storage and transmission of medical records will have be conducted in a totally secure and safe environment with a very high standard of data integrity, protecting patient privacy and complying with all Health Insurance Portability and Accountability Act (HIPAA) regulations. Such as system would allow us to overcome the challenges by allowing patients to collect and manage their health information such as medical history, past surgeries, medications, and allergies), to request self-referrals, and to store a record of their consultations among others.

Further, the sharing of medical records, specifically radiology imaging databases with CDOs will have potential to drastically reduce medical redundancies, exposure to radiations, costs to patients. In addition such system can empower the patients with the automated ownership of their secure personal medical information. It is essential to use the cloud computing in this application since it would allow the CDOs to address the challenge of sharing medical data that is overly complex and highly expensive to address with traditional technologies. In addition to providing community of care, proposed system can also serve as a valuable tool in clinical research, medical decision-making, epidemiology, evidence-based medicine, and in formulating public health policy. Figure 23.1 shows a high level simplified overview of the designed system.

The system is conceptualized to shift from institute centered hospital information system towards a regional/global medical information system by developing standards based Service-Oriented-Architecture (SOA) for interfacing heterogeneous medical information systems such that it would allow real-time access to all medical records from one medical information system to another. The system integrates a Lossless Presentation layer for viewing the radiology imaging. This chapter discuss a brief architecture of "Lossless Accelerated Presentation Layer" that will allow one to view all radiology images (Digital Imaging and Communication in Medicine (DICOM) objects) that reside in a cloud based distributed database. We further will demonstrate the web-based interface that will provide a holistic view of all medical records to every patient. Figure 23.2 shows the layered view of the proposed system.

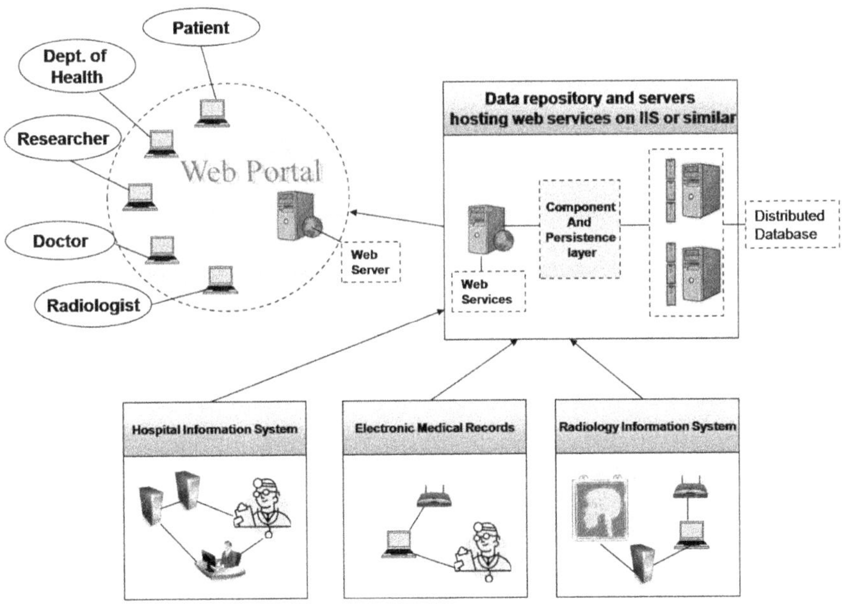

Fig. 23.1 Overview of global medical information system model

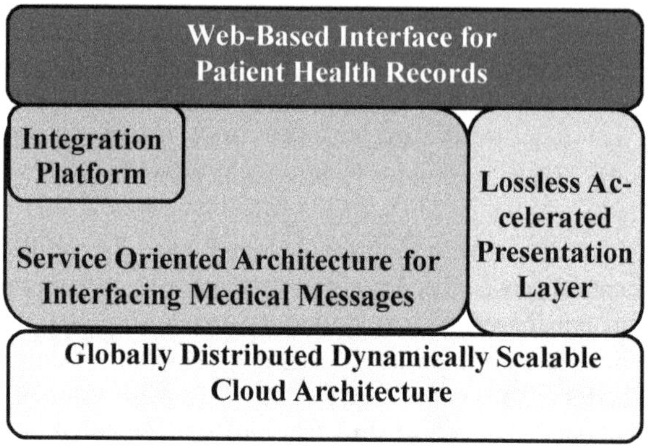

Fig. 23.2 Layered architecture for the proposed medical information system

Potential Impact of Proposed Medical Informatics System

This project focuses on the development of an architecture for integrating heterogeneous medical information systems such as (Hospital Information System, Radiology Information System, and Electronic Medical Records among others). These systems in their current form do not transfer information from one system into another outside a network. The proposed approach for a global medical informatics system would allow all medical records to be completely portable. In the current system a significant amount of delay is involved in transmitting medical records from one CDO to another, leading to repetitive medical testing and increased cost of healthcare to the patient, insurance companies and federal government. The development of a cloud based service oriented architecture that will provide all patients with an interactive view of all their medical records. Such a system would provide all patients with the ownership of their medical records, thereby eliminating the need to repetitive procedures.

The proposed system architecture drastically reduces the Medicare spending for imaging services. The sharing of medical records, specifically radiology imaging databases, will drastically reduce medical redundancies, and exposure to radiations. Total national healthcare spending is in excess of \$2.6 Trillion or about 17 % of our Gross Domestic Product. The proposed architecture would significantly contribute the reduction in national healthcare spending by eliminating the repetition of procedure due to unavailability of medical records. In year 2006 itself various medical imaging services accounted for 58 % of Medicare's physician office spending. In order to control this spending on medical imaging, the "Deficit Reduction Act" (DRA) was created in year 2005 to reduce medical imaging spending by \$2.8 Billion by 2011. This project will allow various CDOs to share the medical records and imaging thereby, eliminating the need to repeat the procedures during a defined time period thereby, serving the objectives of Deficit Reduction Act. Please note with the current technology radiology imaging can be shared within a CDO, however not among various CDOs. The development of a lossless accelerated presentation layer would allow to access all radiology images residing on a cloud based distributed database in a lossless manner through a web-based DICOM viewer. This layer would provide a seamless access to all radiology imaging from any location in real-time thereby increasing the efficiency of overall medical record systems.

Centralizing medical records can also create new and more intelligent perspectives in medicine. Such database with medical information will be extremely valuable for advanced data mining in clinical research. This will have potential to analytically evaluate and innovate new disease information and test methods that will improve the health care delivery and lead the exploration of new preventive treatment. In addition, the proposed project also serves the criteria of national Health Information Technology agenda.

Background and Related Work

The focus of healthcare has recently been shifted from healthcare providers' paternalistic approach to the consumer oriented approach. There are several efforts in such direction. Microsoft and Google's open source health initiatives are just two examples of big corporation's future interest in this domain. The Personal health record is a concept that has been developing over several years. The early form of PHR used to be paper-based records. Problems caused due to the lack of availability of chapter based medical records and the lack of data transferability has been well described. Moving these records into an electronic format that is used universally has been proposed as a way to solve some of these problems. As a result, the focus on electronic PHRs has steadily increased over the past several years, with more than 200 systems available in 2006 [12, 13, 19, 29]. Moreover, the effective use of information technology is a key focal point for improving healthcare in terms of patient safety, quality outcomes, and economic efficiency. The electronic PHR systems have many forms. In addition to Web-based systems, information in electronic PHRs may be stored on portable computer drives (such as USB "flash drives"), "smart cards," or other electronic storage devices. Functionally, PHRs are diverse. Some contain tools for managing care, such as delivering electronic test results, providing support for remote monitoring (e.g. weight, blood pressure, blood glucose), and providing secure communication services between patient/family and health care professional or access to health-related content. Some PHRs have the ability to transfer information using standardized data formats or to transfer data to a patient-controlled health data record or repository. System Integration has been always the most critical issue for the development of information systems in healthcare industry. Medical Information Systems (MIS) are heterogeneous in nature and therefore pose a severe challenge in their interoperability [16, 22, 23, 31]. A large number of healthcare applications are isolated and do not communicate with each other. Therefore, the integration of existing information systems represents one of the most urgent priorities of healthcare information systems [25]. Many efforts have been made on integrating the heterogeneous systems in hospitals. Healthcare industry has developed several standards through which relevant data can be transferred among different information systems. These standards are Health Language Seven (HL7), Electronic Data Interchange (EDI) X12 Version 4010, Health Insurance Portability And Accountability (HIPAA), Digital Image Communication in Medicine (DICOM), Integrating Healthcare Enterprise (IHE) among others [21]. All these standards are currently being widely used in healthcare industry. According to Open Source Clinical Research Group HL7 is the most widely used messaging standard in health, not only in North America, but also around the world. Further, a 1998 survey found the HL7 standard in use in more than 95 % of hospitals with more than 400 beds. Overall, more than 80 % of the respondents in that study reported using HL7 in their information system departments with another 13.5 % planning to do so. The proposed solution will be able to integrate all medical information systems that are in compliance with HL7 standard.

Standardized interfaces are available to many healthcare "Object Oriented Sevices" such as CORBAmed (Common Object Request Broker Architecture in Medicine), which realizes the share of common functionalities like access control among different systems. Others, like DICOM, HL7 (Health Level Seven) and the initiative of IHE (Integrating the Healthcare Enterprise) [7], specify the guidelines or standards for exchanging messages among different systems, which make the different systems work in harmony and implement the workflow integration [22] [30]. Broker, an embedded device facilitated the communication between HIS, RIS and Picture Archiving and Communication System (PACS) by integrating HL7 with DICOM. Broker accepted HL7 messages from RIS, translated and mapped the data to produce DICOM messages for transmission to PACS. However, the Broker system posed a challenge since it allowed RIS information to flow only in one direction resulting in the duplication of databases. IHE initiative, jointly established by Hospital Information Management Systems Society (HIMSS) and the Radiological Society of North America (RSNA), later addressed the issue by allowing the integration of clinical information within a healthcare delivery network. Later a consolidated solution with RIS/PACS/HIS integration was offered by healthcare companies. This was a major step towards the successful integration of patient records within a network [4]. Assurance of consumer control of privacy is essential to the acceptance and adoption of PHR's. With appropriate access controls, patients can allow portions of the PHR to be made available to family members, various care providers, and others.

Various researches have been conducted on personal health record systems such as Evaluation of Functionality and Utility [20], improvement of quality and usability of existing systems and analysis of security protection of personal health record systems. Mostly the current PHR research is focused on areas of PHR function that allow patients to manage their own health data and data/information exchange with others. However studies suggest that in these areas PHR has potential to improve the patient–provider relationship and enhance patient and shared decision making [18].

There have been some efforts to share the patient information within a limited group of in order to facilitate the teamwork and effective healthcare management. The Medical Informatics Network Tool (MTNL). The software included an intelligent engine that was used for treating only Schizophrenia, a chronic brain disorder [32]. The software allowed collecting useful information about the patient and facilitating the communication among all the team members in addition to other providing other useful information related to Schizophrenia. This system was very helpful in taking meaningful decisions quickly and therefore had a positive impact on the patient healthcare. Similarly, the proposed solution would provide all information regarding a patient in a centralized location. Aggregation of such information will have profound impact on the overall patient healthcare and would reduce the probability of making wrong decisions such as prescribing conflicting prescriptions. In 2006 Al-Busaidi et al. researched on introducing a personalized patient information that was extracted from a single patient database [5]. This research was more focused on web mining and intelligent information retrieval from web that can provide a simplified and meaningful description to the problem that a patient might be experiencing. Project was more focused towards analyzing the information based on conceptual integration of ontology. However in this project our focus is to integrate several patient record systems (Radiology Information System (RIS), Electronic Medical Records (EMR), Hospital Information System (HIS), Patient Health Record (PHR) and Clinical Information System (CIS) among others) and provide a cloud computing based patient centric interface for all patient records.

Recently service oriented architecture type IT platforms are emerging as solutions for clinical enterprises [26]. Web Services (WS) provide an open and standardized way to achieve interoperation between different software applications, running on a variety of platforms and/or frameworks. Therefore, they constitute an important technological tool toward the incremental delivery of advanced inter-enterprise services. Significant advantages of using WS on top of any existing middleware solution is location transparency, language and platform independence, together with their embracement by big vendors and the acceptance they enjoy between the users. WS, with their extensible markup language (XML) roots, open the door for the next generation, loosely coupled, coarse-grained, document-oriented architectures. The term "loosely coupled" is used to characterize services where the assumptions made by the communicating parties about each other's implementation, internal structure, and the communication itself are kept to a minimum. In [30] researchers have proposed the use of a SOA for combining few workflows for integrating various health information systems. Although the workflows are not complete however it is an important contribution towards integrating various informatics systems.

Harvard Medical School CIO John Halamka quoted, "Putting servers and exchanges into doctors' offices is not going to work". He suggested a better model is using regional health-care information technology centers that use cloud computing systems to work with doctors [11]. Computing done at cloud scale allows users to access virtual supercomputer-level [14]. Cloud computing's aim is to deliver tens of trillions of computations per second to problems such as delivering medical information in a way that users can tap through the Web. When implemented correctly, cloud computing allows the development and deployment of applications that can easily grow capacity, deliver needed performance, and have a high-degree of fault tolerance, all without any concern as to the nature and location of the underlying infrastructure

[6]. IBM announced that American Occupational Network and HyGen Pharmaceuticals are improving patient care by digitizing health records and streamlining their business operations using cloud-based software. GoogleHealth and Microsoft Vault health solutions are commercial steps in the direction of aggregating patient records in a unified environment. However, the major issue with their solution is the inability of CDOs to upload patient health records in a central data repository. In both systems patients must upload all the records, which require patients to first gain access to their medical history. It is important to note that EMR is the basic building block, the source of information that feeds the Electronic Health Record (EHR). The EHR is the longitudinal record made possible by Regional Health Information organizations (RHIOs). While he Patient Health Record (PHR) is the record owned, accessed, and managed by the consumer. The interdependencies among them are very clear. Without linking (interfacing) a EMR with a PHR, the consumer will have to manually input vital data, like laboratory results. Without an EHR, the PHR cannot accept information from multiple providers. This is the case in both solutions offered by Microsoft and Google. Often it takes several weeks before one can gain access to their medical records from a hospital thereby, limiting its usage. In addition, both Google and Microsoft health solutions do not provide a lossless solution to the imaging services, which are important component of the overall patient centric system. In this chapter, we discuss a framework that will allow us to interface all medical records systems those are HL7 compliant and store the data in a multi-cloud based distributed database system.

Brief Discussion of Medical Standards

Healthcare industry currently has several standards through which relevant data is transferred between different information systems, these standards are HL7, EDI X12 Version 4010 (EDI X12), HIPAA, DICOM, IHE among others. A brief discussion of these standards is discussed below:

Health Language 7: aims at enabling communication between applications provided by different vendors, using different platforms, operating systems, application environments (e.g. programming languages, tools). In principle, HL7 enables communication between any systems regardless of their architectural basis and their history. Therefore, HL7 supports communication between real-world systems, newly developed or legacy. This is achieved through syntactically and semantically standardized messages. HL7 interfaces realize the request/service procedure by sending and receiving these standardized messages. HL7 functional areas include typical health-care (clinical) domains as Admission Discharge and Transfers (ADT), Patient Registration, Orders, Results, Financial and Master files. More recent versions of HL7 also include Non-ASCII character sets, Query language support, Medical documents, Clinical trials, Immunization reporting, Ad6erse drug, Reactions, Scheduling, Referrals, and Problems and goals. An example of an HL7 transaction set is shown below:


```
MSH|^~\&|GHH LAB|ELAB-3|GHH OE|BLDG4|200202150930||ORU^R01|CNTRL-3456|P|2.4<cr>
PID|||555-44-4444||EVERYWOMAN^EVE^E^^^^L|JONES|19620320|F|||153 FERNWOOD DR.^
^STATESVILLE^OH^35292||(206)3345232|(206)752-121||||AC555444444||67-A4335^OH^20030520<cr>
OBR|1|845439^GHH OE|1045813^GHH LAB|15545^GLUCOSE|||200202150730|||||||||
555-55-5555^PRIMARY^PATRICIA P^^^^MD^^|||||||||F||||||444-44-4444^HIPPOCRATES^HOWARD H^^^^MD<cr>
OBX|1|SN|1554-5^GLUCOSE^POST 12H CFST:MCNC:PT:SER/PLAS:QN||^182|mg/dl|70_105|H|||F<cr>
```


Electronic Data Interchange: is a data format based on ASC (Accredited Standards Committee) X12 standards. It is used to exchange specific data between two or more trading partners. Term 'trading partner' may represent organization, group of organizations or some other entity. EDI X12 is governed by standards released by ASC X12. Each release contains set of message types like invoice, purchase order, healthcare claim, etc. Each message type has specific number assigned to it instead of name. For example: an invoice is 810, purchase order is 850 and healthcare claim is 837. Some key EDI transactions are:

- 837: Medical claims with subtypes for professional, institutional, and dental varieties
- 820: Payroll deducted and other group premium payment for insurance products
- 834: Benefits enrollment and maintenance
- 835: Electronic remittances
- 270/271: Eligibility inquiry and response
- 276/277: Claim status inquiry and response
- 278: Health services review request and reply

Health Insurance Portability and Accountability: regulation impacts those in healthcare that exchange patient information electronically. HIPAA regulations were established to protect the integrity and security of health information, including protecting against unauthorized use or disclosure of the information. HIPAA states that a security management process must exist in order to protect against "attempted or successful unauthorized access, use, disclosure, modification, or interference with system operations". In allows monitoring, reporting and sounding alert on attempted or successful access to systems and applications that contain sensitive patient information. Current version of HIPAA is X12 4010 and recently a new guideline X12 5010 was released and mandated by the Department of Health to be complied with and implemented by all care givers before January 2013.

Digital Imaging and Communication in Medicine: is the industry standard for storing and transferring all radiology images. The standard ensures the interoperability of system and can be use to produce, display, send, query, store, process, retrieve, and print DICOM objects. Patterned after the Open System Interconnection of the International Standards Organization, DICOM enables digital communication between diagnostic and therapeutic equipment and systems from various manufacturers. The DICOM 3.0 standard, developed by the American College of Radiology

(ACR) and National Electrical Manufacturers Association (NEMA), evolved from versions 1.0 and 2.0 which evolved in 1985 and 1988 respectively.

In addition to these standards it is must that the designed medical informatics system is in compliance with the following requirements.

Patient Safety: One of the most important requirements of any medical informatics system is the availability of consistent and correct information. At no point should the system show inaccurate, incomplete and unintended information that may jeopardize the safety of a patient.

Disaster Recovery: Since the proposed system is cloud computing based (hosted on Internet) there must be provision for backing up the entire system data incase of a system failure. A method must be included that would prevent the data from being corrupted or lost. If not done so this may lead to major crisis in terms of patient safety.

Accuracy, Availability and Accessibility: It is must that health informatics system must achieve the availability target of above 99 % since the system stores critical information. The data stored must be accurate, available and always accessible from any location.

Integration: As discussed above, for the system to serve as a global medical record that will include all patient records, all medical standards must be correctly and carefully integrated into the system. Several of these standards have already been discussed above.

Ease of use and Customer Satisfaction: It is expected that the system will be widely used by all patients, doctors, nurses and other entities involved in healthcare. Therefore, the system must provide a simple user interface for all entities (users) involved. Inability to achieve this may prohibit users in using the system thereby reducing the potential impact of the proposed informatics system.

Government Compliance: The most important system requirement is security and the HIPAA compliance. The system must support both. Each workflow must be carefully designed such that it meets the HIPAA standard.

Architecture Description and System Design

Currently clinical data, in standardized format, is distributed among Care Delivery Organizations (CDO) such as hospitals, pharmacies, insurance companies among others. We proposed an approach which would create and authorize and allow secured sharing of this data repository on cloud(s) based distributed database. In this section we provide an architecture description of each layer of our proposed medical information system as shown in Fig. 23.2.

A Service Oriented Architecture for Interfacing Medical Messages

This section discusses the approach that has been adopted for interfacing several medical systems in order to centralize all patient records. The proposed solution does not focus on the developing yet another standard which would try and enforce other organizations to comply with. Rather the federated approach was selected, based on a set of already existing healthcare industry standards through which medical messages are transferred between different information systems. Currently medical messaging standards enable data transfer between systems in a request—service manner, where in the data is sent from one system to another directly or via a modulator like an EDI VAN service provider. Such data transfer is occurs only upon the request and is not based on the occurrence of an event such as admission of patient.

Through a service oriented architecture various medical information systems can be integrated by collecting standardized data on a cloud based distributed database repository. In this architecture Web-services will be hosted securely on a cloud while the Web service clients serving as agents will be running on various health-information-systems. In order to facilitate a seamless integration of various medical information databases the schemas of the distributed database residing on cloud(s) will imitate the existing schema of healthcare standards like HL7, EDI and DICOM. During initial setup of the web-service clients, the schema of the existing HIS or EMR systems will be mapped to the proposed cloud based distributed database schema. This would allow the agent to periodically query the client databases through established connections which will facilitate the transfer of data to the cloud(s) over secure HTTP connection. Figure 23.3 shows the proposed approach as discussed above.

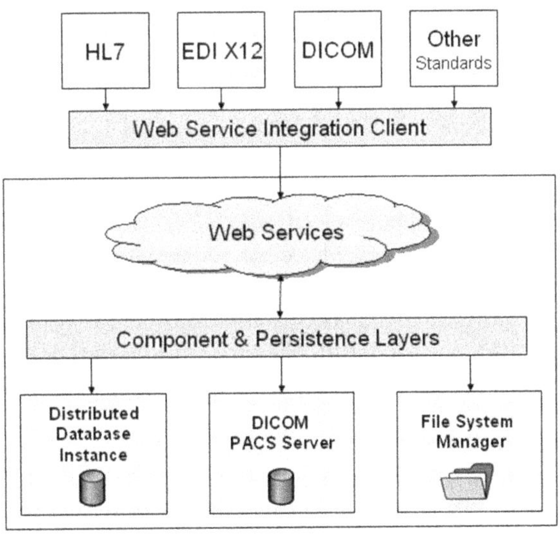

Fig. 23.3 Layered view of the proposed service oriented architecture for interfacing medical messages

Web-Services (WS) is major, service-oriented, connection technologies which is specification based and mostly open. In addition to its open source development potential in a technology neutral environment, major vendors are embracing World Wide Web Consortium (W3C) and the Internet Engineering Task Force (IETF) efforts. Significant advantages of using WS on top of any existing middleware solution are location transparency, language and platform independence, in addition to their adoption by big vendors and wide acceptance. WS, with their XML roots, open the door for the next generation, loosely coupled, coarse-grained, document-oriented architectures. Security should not be considered an afterthought but it should be built into the communication platform itself. WS were originally considered as an easy way to do business across the Internet since it allows tunneling through the hypertext transfer protocol that usually bypasses corporate firewalls. The use of transport layer security may not be enough to provide the desired levels of authentication, authorization, and trust. The use of technologies like XML-Signature, XML-Encryption, and WS-Security should be mandatory in order to achieve the necessary quality of protection for message integrity and confidentiality. Additional efforts such as WS-Trust, WS-Policy, and WS-Secure Conversation must be consideration as well. Currently, the most common technological tool to cover various security aspects is the Public Key Infrastructure (PKI). PKI is used to describe the processes, policies, and standards that govern the issuance, maintenance, and revocation of the certificates, public, and private keys that the encryption and signing operations require. PKI incorporates the necessary techniques to enable two entities that do not know each other to securely exchange information using an insecure network such as the Internet.

Lossless Accelerated Presentation Layer for Viewing DICOM Objects on Cloud

A key requirement for DICOM viewers is lossless image coding; users accessing DICOM images should receive lossless image to rule out any compression artifacts. Figure 23.4 shows the proposed architecture for the imaging sub-system. When users open a DICOM image, a DICOM viewer is executed in the cloud. The views rendered by the DICOM viewer have to be communicated to the users remotely accessing the image. Commercial remote access tools such as Citrix use lossy compression for remote viewing and hence are not suitable for medical imaging application. A few hospitals have used such solution for making the DICOM objects available outside the hospital network. However, such use of lossy compression may not be an acceptable solution under several medical conditions. For instance, such a lossy compression may provide wrong information about the size of a cancer cells that may be growing in any part of a body. Since the stage of a cancer is determined by the volume of the cancer cells; a lossy image may show a reduced volume by removing some pixels.

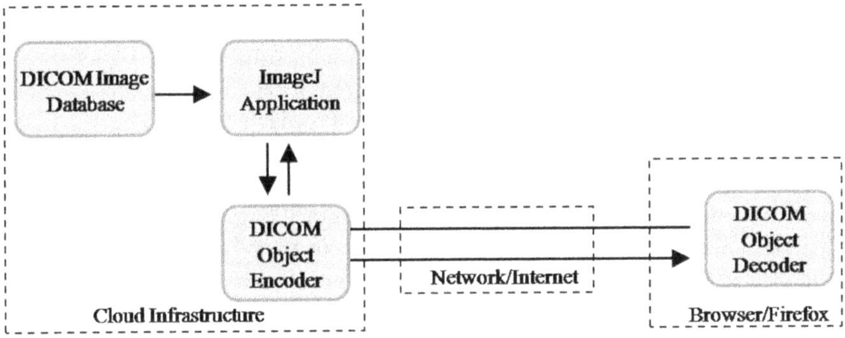

Fig. 23.4 The proposed architecture for the imaging sub-system

Our proposed solution is to use the open source remote control software TightVNC as a basis and modify the image coding engine to support lossless images. The complexity of encoding and the compression achieved varies with algorithms. One can easily evaluate and measure the compression performance for lossless JPEG-2000 and JPEG. High performing compression algorithms can then be selected to get maximum performance of the imaging sub-system.

Web Based Interface for Patient Health Records

Patient health records stored in a centralized data repository over the distributed cloud(s) can be instantly viewed by any authorized user connected to this system through a web-based interface designed as part of the proposed system. The data can be accessed by existing health information systems with the help of remote calls to cloud hosted web services as shown in Fig. 23.5. The proposed SOA would allow various medical information systems to interface with these web-services through

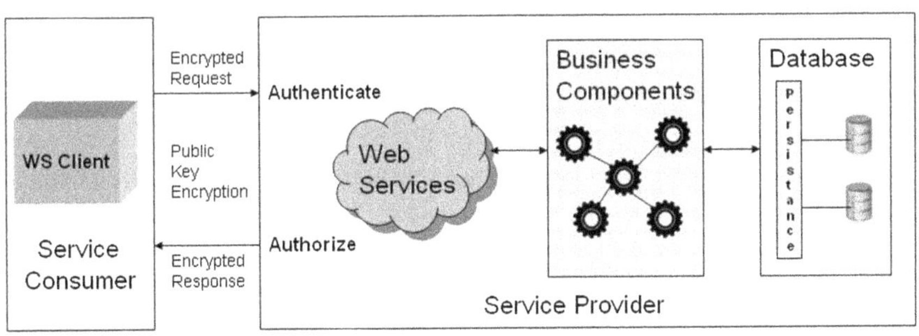

Fig. 23.5 Service oriented architecture for presentation layer

their interfacing clients. All clients will go through a standard layer of authentication and authorization through public key encryptions standards.

Since the data is stored in the standardized format (HL7 or EDI) on the cloud based GHIS database, we must present the data in a readable format. The web portal can provide all users with the ability to search for a patient's identity given a set of demographic criteria and retrieval of all the related health and medical information pertaining to the patient under consideration. Additional filtering of patient data will be possible if the consumer of the service is only restricted to view some parts of the patient's medical records. This will be accomplished by the use of user roles and access grants. Secured logins to access patient records for authorized users such as physicians, radiologists, laboratory technicians among others can be created using the existing methods like one-time passwords (OTP). OTP methods can be facilitated through the use of a standard medical hardware device such as a "Token" that would generate a time synchronized one time password to allow the access to patient database.

A web-based ImageJ interface can be easily made available through this web-portal system for viewing DICOM objects. ImageJ is a public domain Java image processing program inspired by NIH ImageJ for the Macintosh. It was designed with an open architecture that provides extensibility via Java plugins. ImageJ will be integrated with a PACS server on the cloud to read DICOM objects residing on the distributed database. The user interface of ImageJ viewer application would depend upon the role of the accessing user. For instance, a radiologist will have the permission to alter the DICOM object that will be stored as a new version in form of a separate image layer. A web-browser presents the remote 'desktop' from which an authorized user may launch ImageJ to open DICOM objects. Users interact with ImageJ directly using the controls provided by ImageJ. As the views of ImageJ change, a view encoder based on the TightVNC server compresses the 'desktop' and transmits this to the user. TightVNC uses the standard Remote Frame Buffering (RFB) protocol for desktop sharing and control. Since lossless compression will be used in the View Encoder, the users will see images that are identical to the images rendered by ImageJ.

A Globally Distributed Dynamically Scalable Cloud Based Application Architecture

The proposed medical information system concept is for patients, doctors and other care providers to have immediate access to medical records, images and other digital resources. Once connected to information system, the services available to a consumer will be filtered depending upon the consumer's role, type or responsibility. Figure 23.6 shows high level layered architecture for a proposed globally distributed dynamically scalable cloud that will be used for storing all medical data. Every tier in

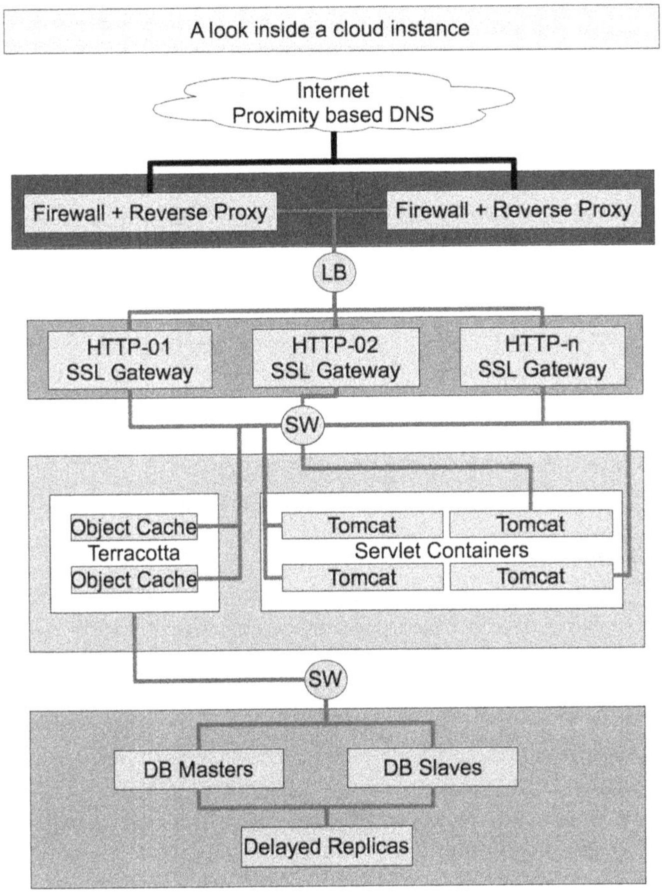

Fig. 23.6 Layered architecture for a globally distributed dynamically scalable cloud

the Fig. 23.6 includes multiple instances in the local and geographically distributed clouds.

Tier 1 (Security Tier) of each application partition would include firewall with VPN, traffic filtering, statistical reporting and balancing functionalities and capabilities. In order increase efficiency of the tier, one would explore combining few of these services together on the same host or device, though cross-cloud Virtual Private Network (VPN) services will reside on isolated hosts. Additionally, due to the sensitive nature of the Internet Protocol Security (IPSEC) hosts and to ensure data security, this separation is considered necessary.

Tier 2 (Presentation Tier) represents a web server for serving of http clients. Ultimately each instance on this tier should be able to detect a failed node on its tier and take over the load in order to provide fault tolerance in our overall proposed system. This can be accomplished by using the "Linux-Ha" clustering software in an active/active configuration (http://www.linux-ha.org/GettingStarted/TwoApaches). Secure Socket Layer (SSL)/Transport Layer Security (TLS) and http proxy services are somewhat compute intensive therefore their impact on overall performance is close to linear. Thus, resources on this layer can be estimated based on number of connections.

Tier 3 (Application Tier) is the actual application/business logic tier. The primary platforms in this tier are Apache Tomcat and Sun Java. Since the load balancing will be done mostly on the outer perimeter and http tier, high availability becomes the primary concern at this level. It being a healthcare domain, one of our prime objectives is to ensure the application availability all the time. Being data critical, healthcare applications cannot afford to lose the connection even during the major hardware outage of $x - 1$ nodes (where x is the number of nodes serving the application via Apache Tomcat), the layer would ensure the constant availability of all applications.

The final Tier, Tier 4 (Database Tier) of the server systems is the database systems. We discuss a brief architecture of our proposed system.

Distributed Data Consistency Across Clouds

One can easily carry out a detailed performance evaluation and benchmarking of various database storage methodologies such as traditional relational database management systems (RDBMS) Object Oriented Database Systems and Distributed Key-Value Persistence. The performing database architecture could then be implemented on a single-cloud in a standard master-slave topology with distributed reads and master-only writes.

A special replication server can be configured to replicate the data from the master database after every 20–60 min. Such configuration would allow us to preserve a consistent data state which is lagged by 20–60 min. In case of a system failure the data from this state can be recovered. All data-backups can be scheduled to run from the special replication server such as to avoid affecting read or write performance. The existence of multiple databases scattered over multiple clouds will pose a data consistence issue [17, 24]. Cross-cloud architecture can be developed to handle this issue safely and efficiently. Figure 23.7 shows the proposed method for distributed master database synchronization technique.

The proposed solution is to perform offline synchronization on a schedule. On the system being replicated to, we can develop an agent to stop and reroute new connections, pause all automated maintenance agents flush all the caches on each node of each system and then perform cross replication from a replica of the online system to its own master.

The agents responsible for this will also communicate amongst each other to ensure that it would be performed in a rolling pattern, where no more than 1/3 to 1/2 of the individual global cloud instances are unavailable at any given time. This will eliminate perceived service interruption. Since this data is ultra sensitive and must be protected at all costs, an industry standard IPSEC VPN must be implemented to facilitate this cross-cloud replication or synchronization (Fig. 23.8).

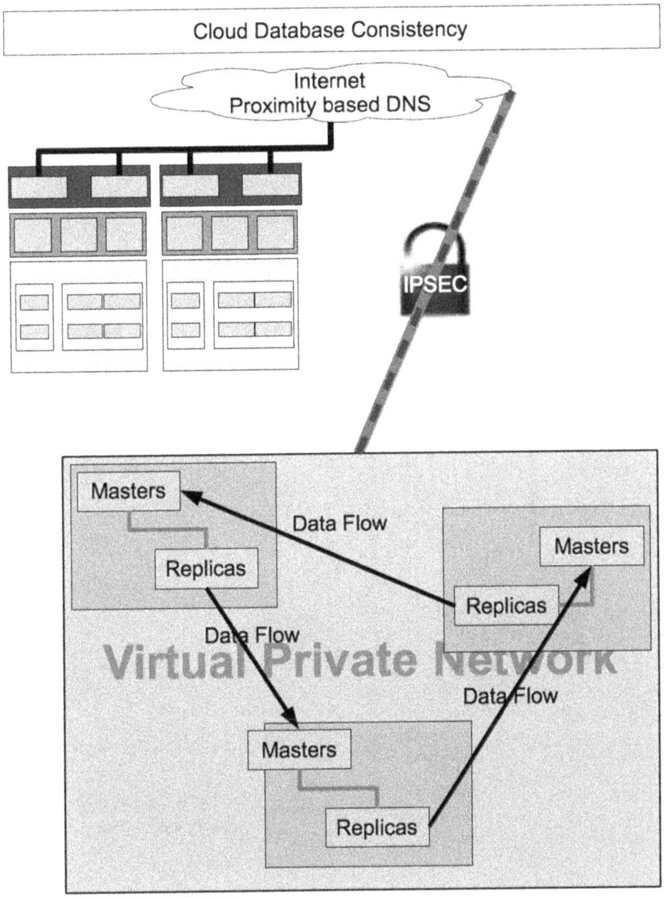

Fig. 23.7 Proposed method for distributed master database synchronization

Higher Availability and Application Scalability

We propose the architecture of a global medical information system that may have millions of users accessing the system for accessing personal health records. Therefore the system must ensure high scalability in order to serve increasing number of users on the system. Further, it will be imperative to ensure the persistence and integrity of the information store while maintaining high performance.

Once can easily explore and benchmark the methods for distributed HTTP serving [33]. One method distributed HTTP serving, referred to as Geographic Load Balancing, is controversial as to its effectiveness yet being quite heavily used among large web presences like Google, Inc. or Amazon.com. The premise of Geographic Load Balancing method is that any host with a public IP address can be cross referenced with the IP address block assignments on a per country basis [8].

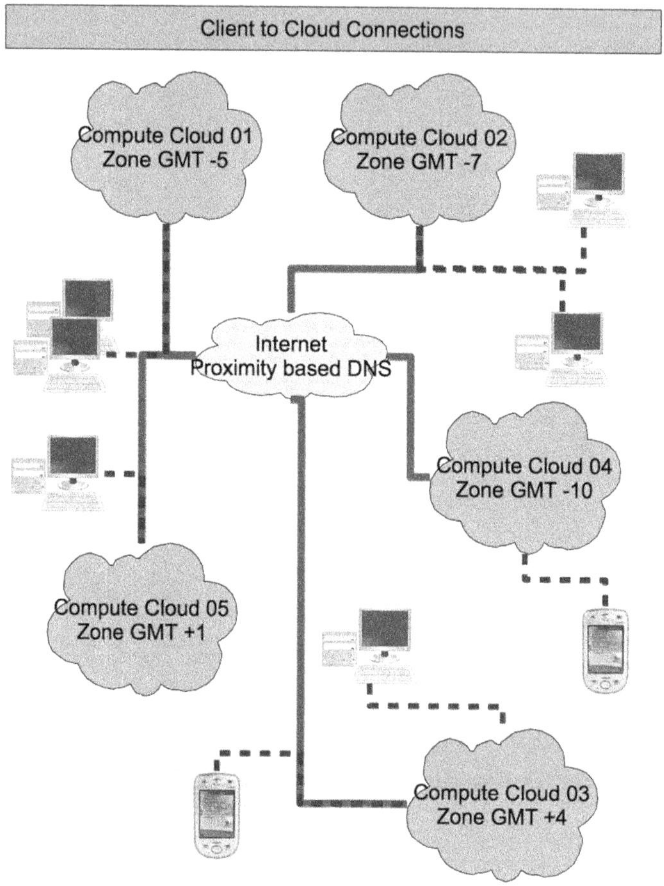

Fig. 23.8 Geographic proximity cloud selection

For the application tier, we propose to implement load balancing using the JK connector from the http layer in a weighted round robin load balancing scheme. The application cluster software stack will include Apache Tomcat on Sun Java™ and a JVM heap clustering suite, Terracotta (see Fig. 23.9) [9, 27].

On cloud computing clusters one can spawn new computing resources, virtual machines, dynamically. We propose to that one should develop a method that would allow us to effectively allocate/deallocate a new application instance in a timely manner. Such a method would further interface with the JK connector(s) in order to dynamically alter connection weights and notify the HTTP layer of a new resource against which it can balance [1]. The proposed system would include four application partitions: Core System Services, Hospital Information Web Services, PACS System and Accelerated DICOM Presentation Services. The agent will know which of these

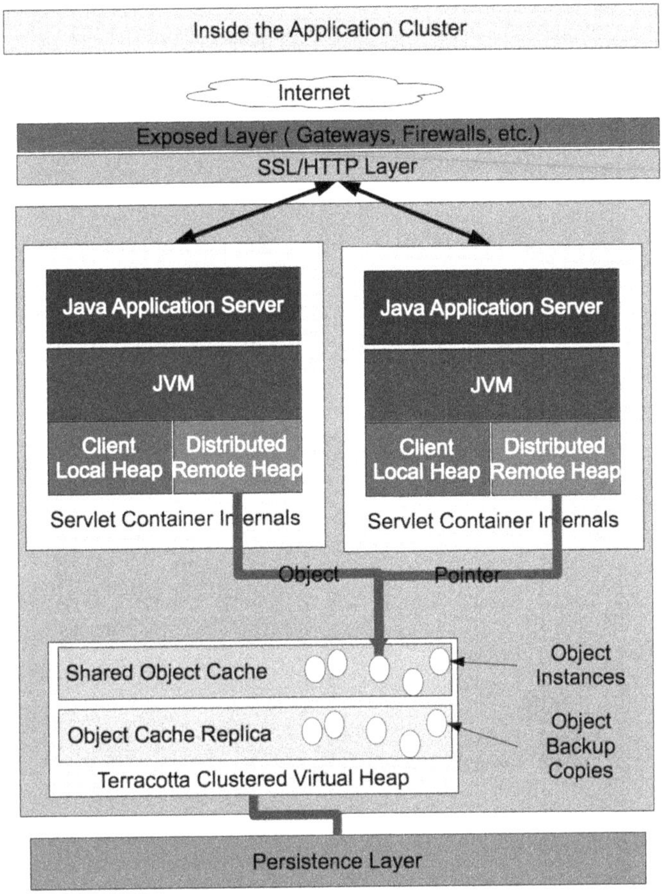

Fig. 23.9 Application cluster

services needs more resources. We will develop an algorithm to detect rate of load increase based on the special needs of each subsystem.

Concerning Low Level Security

Although user authentication and authorization will reside in the application and integration services, the GMIS Infrastructure must be developed in such a way so as to ensure trustworthy use of the cloud systems and networks. GMIS security components and layers will be enforced on any internet capable platform. The existing security methods such as use of firewalls with a minimum necessary access policy and Public key infrastructure will be deployed in order to ensure secured access to the healthcare cloud. Further, one must aim at certifying all clients by GMIS Root

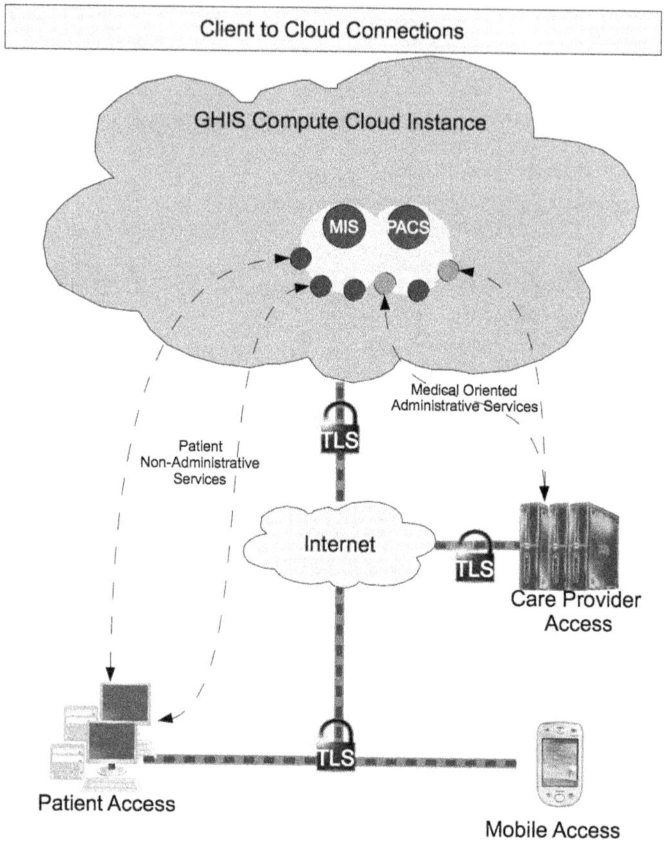

Fig. 23.10 Trusted client connection to the healthcare cloud

Certificate Authority which in-turn may be certified by a third party. Figure 23.10 shows a simplified view of trusted client connection to the healthcare cloud.

The public key infrastructure should be used for accessing the services and applications using Transport Layer Security (TLS) and require the servers to provide their credentials to the client. Additionally, by requiring the client also to present their security credentials (or certificate) we can easily establish a low level trust and assume that both parties are very likely to be who they claim. One must further configure the SSL/TLS processing servers with an HTTP based reverse proxy and Intrusion Detection suite.

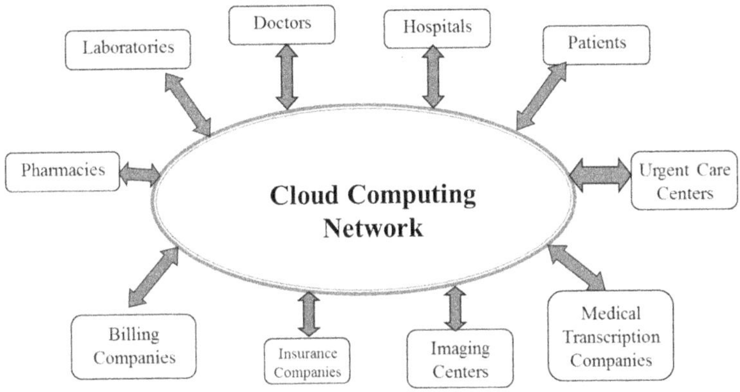

Fig. 23.11 Interaction of various CDO's and patient with the cloud computing network

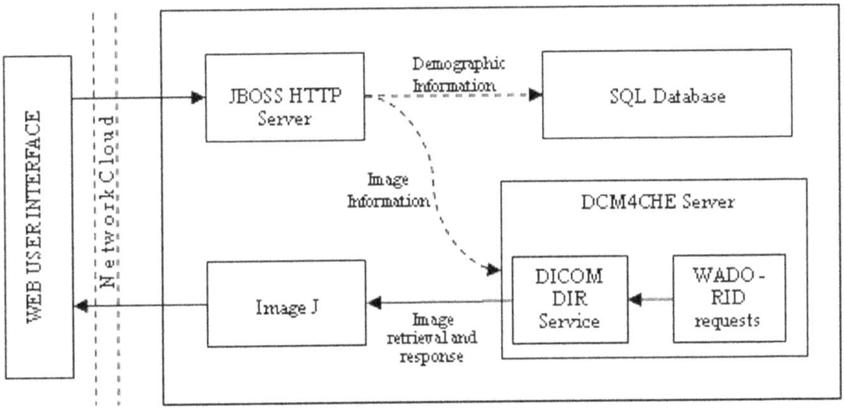

Fig. 23.12 Proposed personal health record system architecture

Implementation Example

The proposed cloud computing based PHR System can allow various authorized users to securely access patient records from various CDO from any location. The system will seamlessly integrate all patient records including images such as CTSCANS and MRI'S which can easily be accessed from any location and reviewed by any authorized user. Figure 23.11 shows the overall view of such a PHR.

The architecture of the proposed system is shown in Fig. 23.12. It is a web application that runs on J2EE platform and could be deployed on cloud computing network such as Amazon EC2 and uses Microsoft SQL Server 2005. The J2EE platform is chosen for its platform independent features and availability of rich web application framework library.

The user interface layer for PHRS is based on J2EE, a platform for web applications hosted by the JBOSS Application server. The user interface is divided into role-specific pages (system administrator, patient, CDO, researchers and insurance providers) and common pages (messaging and account maintenance).

The database layer of the system consists of two components: the First component is DCM4CHE server [16], which is a collection of open source applications and utilities for the healthcare enterprise. These applications have been developed in the Java programming language for performance and portability, supporting deployment on JDK 1.4 and up. Also contained within the dcm4che project is dcm4chee. Dcm4chee is an Image Manager/Image Archive (according to IHE). The application contains the DICOM, HL7 services and interfaces that are required to provide storage, retrieval, and workflow to a healthcare environment. DCM4CHEE is pre-packaged and deployed within the JBoss application server. The basic work of the DCM4CHE server is to handle the implementation of the DICOM standard images uploaded by the patient.

The second component, which is a SQL server, is needed to store the general demographic information of the patient along with other patient health related data, such as, Insurance provider details, frequent CDO visit logs and prescription, lab reports etc.

The Web viewer interface used is open source Image J [17] which is a Java based image processing program. Image J is chosen because it can work as an online application and can read a variety of image formats including TIFF, GIF, JPEG, BMP and DICOM. The scalable and modular personal health record system is capable of importing/Exporting information with various computer based medical record system such as Electronic Medical record (EMR), Electronic Health Record (EHR). The users can also share the information including medical imaging (DICOM images) with the various care providers.

To ensure the security of the data we plan to implement password protected access to the system and only registered patients, CDO's and specialists can log in to the system. Patients are restricted to viewing and modifying and sharing only their own records and CDO's and other care units can only access those records, which are shared with them. Patients can edit the access privileges on their records at the granularity of the categories.

Use Case for Personal Health Record System

One approach to establishing a foundation for evaluating information design in PHRS is "use cases" that categorize and describe discrete functional scenarios and how computer interactions are carried out. The use cases are intended to serve as a framework demonstrating and establishing the relationship between high-level clinical functions and related standards in information design and usability. Figures 23.13, 23.14 and 23.15 outline the use of the proposed PHRS.

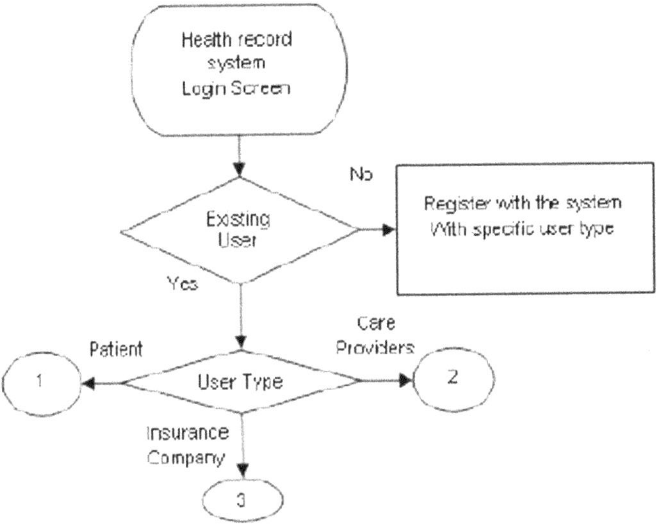

Fig. 23.13 Login flow usecase for the proposed system

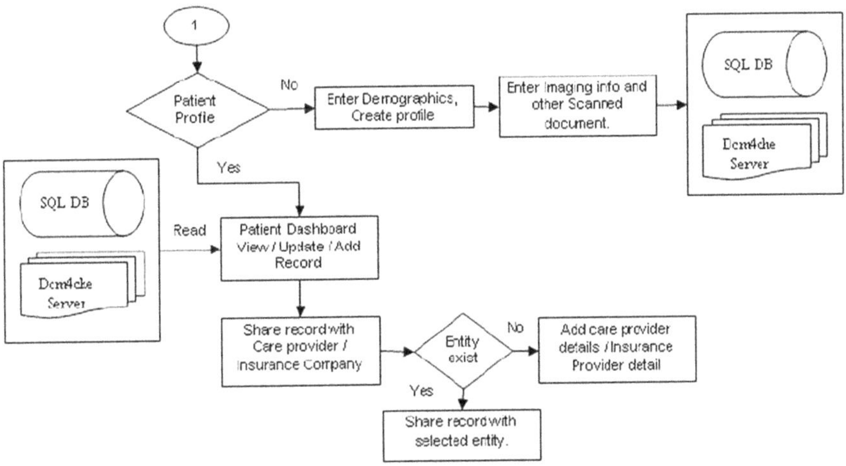

Fig. 23.14 Patient centric usecase flow for proposed PHRS system

The user first logs into the web based personal health record system (see Fig. 23.13). If the user is a first time customer then he/she will have to create a user account in system before storing/accessing the medical information. Once the account is created, user can select the desired user type and can login into the system.

As soon as users logs into the system with user type as Patient, they will be first asked to first create their profile. The data in the profile comprises of demographic information of the patient and the past laboratory results including images, MRI,

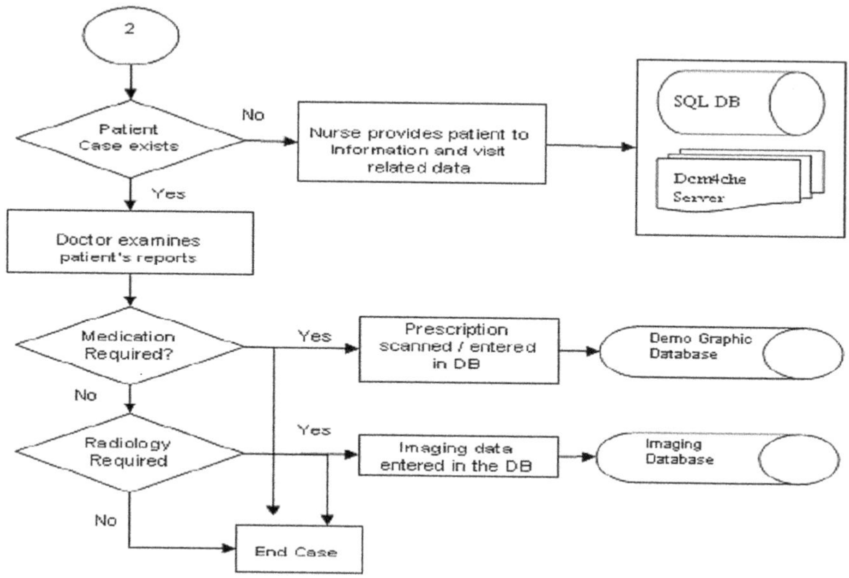

Fig. 23.15 CDO usecase for proposed PHRS system

X-rays and other scanned documents. All the demographic information entered by the patient will be stored in the SQL database and all the imaging data will be processed and stored by the Dcm4che server.

Patients can View/Update or Add new information in the exiting profile. The patients can also share the medical records and their laboratory test results (including imaging information) with various CDO's and insurance providers by giving access to them. The patients can control the data sharing mechanism and can either share the complete profile or only the selected information with the care provider or insurance provider companies.

When user shares any information to any of the registered CDO it will be displayed on that particular CDO's dashboard. Any information to the CDO can be shared either in read only mode or with the read/write mode. The patients control the access levels. Once any patient case is displayed in the dashboard, they can then examine the patient data and can suggests if any medication or radiology is required. Later the details can be stored into the database.

References

1. Emmanuel Arzuaga, David R. Kaeli, "Quantifying Load Imbalance on Virtualized Enterprise Servers", ACM Proceedings joint WOSP/SIPEW international conference on Performance, engineering, pp. 235–242, 2010.

2. Ankur Agarwal, Nathan Henehan, Vivek Somashakharappa, A. S., Pandya, Hari Kalva, Borko Furht, "Cloud Computing Based Patient Centric Medical Information System", Handbook of Cloud Computing, Springer, pp. 553–574, 2010.
3. Marion J. Ball, Jonathan Gold, "Banking on Health: Personal Records and Information Exchange", Journal of Healthcare Information Management, Vol. 20, No. 2.
4. Stephen S. Boochever, "HIS/RIS/PACS Integration: Getting to the Gold Standard", Radiology Management, Vol. 26, No. 3, pp. 16–24, 2004.
5. Asma Al-Busaidi, Alex Gray, Nick Fiddian "Personalizing Web Information for Patients: Linking Patient Medical Data with the Web via a Patient Personal Knowledge Base", Health Informatics Journal, Vol. 12, No. 17, pp. 27–39, 2006.
6. Rajkumar Buyya, Chee Shin Yeo, Srikumar Venugopal, James Broberg, Ivona Brandic, "Cloud Computing and Emerging IT Platforms: Vision, Hype, and Reality for Delivering Computing as the 5th Utility", Elsevier Future Generation Computer Systems, Vol. 25, pp. 599–616, 2009.
7. Christopher D. Carr, Stephen M. Moore, "IHE: a model for driving adoption of standards", Journal of Computerized Medical Imaging and Graphics, Vol. 27, pp. 137–147, 2003.
8. Michele Colajanni, Philip S. Yu, "Adaptive TTL Schemes for Load Balancing of Distributed Web Servers", ACM SIGMETRICS Performance Evaluation Review, Vol. 25, Issue 2, pp. 36–42, 1997.
9. Lieven Eeckhout, Andy Georges, Koen De Bosschere "How Java Programs Interact with Virtual Machines at the Microarchitectural Level", ACM Conference on Object Oriented Programming Systems Languages and Applications, pp. 169–186, 2003.
10. Eysenbach G, "Consumer health informatics: Recent advances", Br. Med. J, 320:1713–1716, 2000.
11. James Gallagher, "Harvard med dean sees long road to electronic records" Triangle Business Journal, April 23, 2009, http://triangle.bizjournals.com/triangle/stories/2009/04/20/daily53.html
12. Wilhelm Hasselbring, "Information system integration ", Communications of the ACM, Vol. 43, Issue 6, pp. 32–38, 2000.
13. Reinhold Haux, "Health Information Systems - Past, Present, Future", International Journal of Medical Informatics, Vol 75, pp. 268–281, 2006.
14. Brian Hayes, "Cloud Computing", Communications of the ACM, Vol. 51, Issue 7, pp. 9–11, 2008.
15. Thomas Handler, Rick Holtmeier, Jane Metzger, Marc Overhage, Sheryl Taylor, Charlene Underwood, "HIMSS Electronic Health Record Definitional Model Version 1.0", 2003.
16. William R. Hersh, "Medical Informatics Improving Health Care through Information", Journal of American Medical Association, Vol. 288 No. 16, pp. 1955–1958, 2002.
17. Edward P. Holden, Jai W. Kang, Dianne P. Bills, Mukhtar Ilyassov, Edward P. Holden, Jai W. Kang, Dianne P. Bills, Mukhtar Ilyassov, "Databases in the Cloud: A Work in Progress" ACM Conference on Information Technology, Education, pp. 138–143, 2009.
18. David C. Kaelber, MD, Phd, Ashish K. Jha, MD, MPH, Douglas Johnston, MTS, Blackford Middleton, MD, MPH, MSC, David W. Bates, MD, MSC, "A Research Agenda for Personal Health Records (PHRs)", Journal of the American Medical Informatics Association Volume 15 Number 6, 2008.
19. Dimitrios G. Katehakis, Stelios G. Sfakianakis, Georgios Kavlentakis, Dimitrios N. Anthoulakis, Manolis Tsiknakis, "Delivering a Lifelong Integrated Electronic Health Record Based on a Service Oriented Architecture", IEEE Transactions on Information Technology in Biomedicine, Vol. 11, No. 6, pp. 639–650, 2007.
20. Matthew I. Kim, Kevin B. Johnson, "Personal Health Records: Evaluation of Functionality and Utility", Journal of the American Medical Informatics Association, Volume 9 Number 2, 2002.
21. Richard Lenz, Mario Beyer, Klaus A Kuhn, "Semantic integration in healthcare networks, International Journal of Medical Informatics, Vol. 7 6, pp. 201–207, 2007.
22. Xudong Lu, Huilong Duan, Haomin Li, Chenhui Zhao and Jiye An, "The Architecture of Enterprise Hospital Information System", 27th Annual Conference Proceedings of IEEE Engineering in Medicine and Biology, Vol. 7, pp. 6957–6960, 2005.

23. Clement J. McDonald, "The Barriers to Electronic Medical Record Systems and How to Overcome Them", Journal of the American Medical Informatics Association, Volume 4 Number 3, pp. 213–221, 1997.
24. Yasushi Saito, Marc Shapiro, "Optimistic Replication", Journal of ACM Computing Surveys, Vol. 37, Issue 1, pp. 42–81, 2005.
25. S.S. Spyrou, P. Bamidis, I. Chouvarda, G. gogou, S. M. Tryfon, N. Maglaveras, "Healthcare Information Standards: Comparison of the Approaches", Health Informatics Journal, Vol. 8, pp. 14–19, 2002.
26. M. Strähle, M. Ehlbeck, V. Prapavat, K. Kück, F. Franz, J.-U. Meyer, "Towards a Service-Oriented Architecture for Interconnecting Medical Devices and Applications", IEEE Workshop on High Confidence Medical Devices, Software, and Systems and Medical Device Plug-and-Play Interoperability, pp. 153–155, 2007.
27. Guillermo L. Taboada, Juan Touriño, Ramón Doallo, "Java for High Performance Computing: Assessment of Current Research and Practice", ACM Proceedings of the 7th International Conference on Principles and Practice of Programming in, Java, pp. 30–39, 2009.
28. Vishesh Ved, Vivek Tyagi, Ankur Agarwal, A. S. Pandya, "Personal Health Record System and Integration Techniques with Various Electronic Medical Record Systems", IEEE High Assurance System, Engineering, 2011.
29. Tang PC, Ash JS, Bates DW, Overhage JM, Sands DZ, "Personal health records: definitions, benefits and strategies for overcoming barriers to adoption", J Am Med Inform Assoc. 2006; 13 (2):121–126.
30. Weiping Wang, Mingming Wang, Shijun Zhu, "Healthcare Information System Integration: A Service Oriented Approach", IEEE International Conference on Services Systems and Services Management, Vol. 2, pp. 1475–1480 2005.
31. Jens H. Weber-Jahnke, Morgan Price, "Engineering Medical Information Systems: Architecture, Data and Usability & Security", IEEE International Conference on Software Engineering, pp. 188–189, 2007.
32. Alexander S. Young, Jim Mintz, Amy N. Cohen, Matthew J. Chiman, "Network-Based System to Improve Care for Schizophrenia: The Medical Informatics Network Tool (MINT)", Journal of American Medical Informatics, Vol. 11, No. 5, pp. 358–367, 2004.
33. Ellen W. Zegura, Mostafa, H. Ammar, Zongming Fei, Samrat Bhattacharjee, "Application-Layer Anycasting: A Server Selection Architecture and Use in a Replicated Web Service", IEEE/ACM Transactions on Networking, Vol. 8, Issue 4, pp. 455–466, 2000.

About the Editors

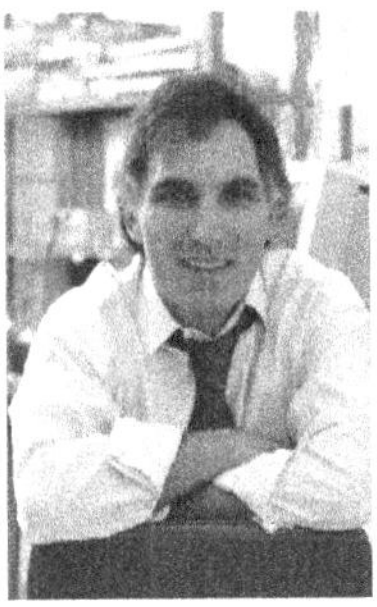

Borko Furht is a professor and chairman of the Department of Electrical and Computer Engineering and Computer Science at Florida Atlantic University (FAU) in Boca Raton, Florida. He is also Director of the NSF-sponsored Industry/University Cooperative Research Center on Advanced Knowledge Enablement. Before joining FAU, he was a vice president of research and a senior director of development at Modcomp (Ft. Lauderdale), a computer company of Daimler Benz, Germany, a professor at University of Miami in Coral Gables, Florida, and a senior researcher in the Institute Boris Kidric-Vinca, Yugoslavia. Professor Furht received Ph.D. degree in electrical and computer engineering from the University of Belgrade. His current research is in multimedia systems, video coding and compression, 3D video and image systems, wireless multimedia, and Internet and cloud computing. He is presently Principal Investigator and Co-PI of several multiyear, multimillion dollar projects including NSF PIRE project and NSF High-Performance Computing Center. He is the author of numerous books and articles in the areas of multimedia, computer architecture, real-time computing, and operating systems. He is a founder and editor-in-chief of *the Journal of Multimedia Tools and Applications* (Springer). He has received several technical and publishing awards, and has consulted for many high-tech companies including IBM, Hewlett-Packard, Xerox, General Electric, JPL, NASA, Honeywell, and RCA. He has also served as a consultant to various colleges and universities. He has given many invited talks, keynote lectures, seminars, and tutorials. He served on the Board of Directors of several high-tech companies.

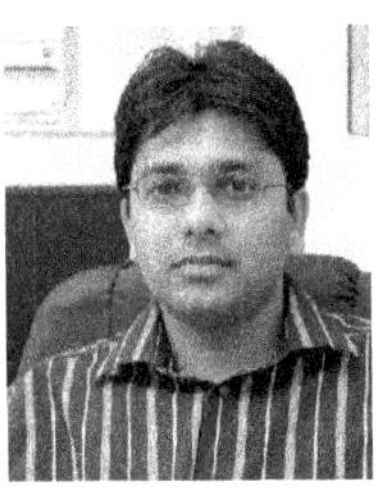

Ankur Agarwal has earned his doctorate in Computer Engineering from Florida Atlantic University, Boca Raton, FL. He also holds post graduate diplomas in VLSI design and Embedded Systems Design. He is an associate professor in Computer and Electrical Engineering and Computer Science at Florida Atlantic University. Ankur Agarwal has been widely funded in the area of healthcare technologies and innovative application design and development. His research interests include, Healthcare Informatics, System Design and Engineering, Multicore Architectures, Embedded Systems and Innovative Application Development. Professor Agarwal has served as the vice president of IEEE Palm Beach Chapter, and the chair of IEEE Computer Society at Palm Beach. He also serves as the Assistant Director of the college wide Center of Systems Integration at Florida Atlantic University and Assistant Director of Mobile Technology Consortium in South Florida. He serves as a reviewer

B. Furht and A. Agarwal (eds.), *Handbook of Medical and Healthcare Technologies*, DOI: 10.1007/978-1-4614-8495-0, © Springer Science+Business Media New York 2013 and an editor for ACM Computing Journal, International Journal of Computer Science and Engineering, International Journal of Electronics, Circuits and Systems, International Journal of Computer System Science and Engineering and Scientific International Journal of Engineering, Computing and Architectures. Ankur Agarwal has published more than 55 papers on low power processor designs, Network-on-Chips architecture, and medical information systems among other research areas. He has also been very active in corporate world. He has worked with a number of companies as their advisors and technology liaison. Currently he serves as an Advisor on the board of five companies.

Index

B. Furht and A. Agarwal (eds.), *Handbook of Medical and Healthcare Technologies*, DOI: 10.1007/978-1-4614-8495-0,

www.ingramcontent.com/pod-product-compliance
Lightning Source LLC
Chambersburg PA
CBHW060748150926
51501CB00003B/127
9781461484943